CORONARY DISEASE IN WOMEN

CONTEMPORARY CARDIOLOGY

CHRISTOPHER P. CANNON, MD
SERIES EDITOR

CORONARY DISEASE
IN WOMEN

Evidence-Based Diagnosis and Treatment

Edited by

LESLEE J. SHAW, PhD

Outcomes Research, American Cardiovascular Research Institute, Atlanta, GA

RITA F. REDBERG, MD, FACC

Division of Cardiology, University of California School of Medicine, San Francisco, CA

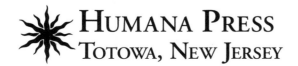

HUMANA PRESS
TOTOWA, NEW JERSEY

© 2004 Humana Press Inc.
999 Riverview Drive, Suite 208
Totowa, New Jersey 07512

www.humanapress.com

Production Editor: Robin B. Weisberg.
Cover design by Patricia F. Cleary.

For additional copies, pricing for bulk purchases, and/or information about other Humana titles, contact Humana at the above address or at any of the following numbers: Tel.: 973-256-1699; Fax: 973-256-8341, E-mail: humana@humanapr.com; or visit our Website: www.humanapress.com

This publication is printed on acid-free paper. ∞
ANSI Z39.48-1984 (American National Standards Institute) Permanence of Paper for Printed Library Materials.

Printed in the United States of America. 10 9 8 7 6 5 4 3 2 1

1-59259-645-2 (e-ISBN)

Library of Congress Cataloging-in-Publication Data

Coronary disease in women : evidence-based diagnosis and treatment / edited by Leslee J. Shaw and Rita F. Redberg.
      p. ; cm. -- (Contemporary cardiology)
   Includes bibliographical references and index.
   ISBN 0-89603-958-7 (alk. paper).
      1. Heart diseases in women. 2. Coronary heart disease. 3. Evidence-based medicine. I. Shaw, Leslee J., 1957–
II. Redberg, Rita F. (Rita Fran), 1956– III. Contemporary cardiology (Totowa, N.J. : unnumbered)
      [DNLM: 1. Coronary Disease--diagnosis. 2. Coronary Disease--therapy. 3. Evidence-Based Medicine. 4. Sex Factors. 5. Women's Health. WG 300 C82173 2004]
   RC685.C6C635 2004
   616.1'2'0082--dc21
                                                                                      2003049990

PREFACE

Coronary Disease in Women: Evidence-Based Diagnosis and Treatment provides a clinical management approach to the care of women with known or suspected coronary artery disease. Whereas previous books on the subject have focused on gender-based differences in the epidemiology of coronary disease as well as in gender bias in treatment, this text focuses on the daily clinical management of women using an evidence-based approach.

Because women's health is also a critical issue to health care administrators, an increasingly important decision maker in health care, additional chapters address managing women's health issues in our current era of managed care and organizing a women's health center. Topical issues on the effectiveness of using a gynecologist to diagnose or manage coronary disease, as well as the cost effectiveness of diagnosis and treatment are also included.

In the current health care era, there is an increased use of guidelines or pathways of care that are developed within managed care organizations to deal with coronary artery disease. *Coronary Disease in Women* includes special management issues with women in developing clinical pathways, including those of primary and secondary prevention of coronary heart disease. Primary care physicians, including cardiologists, family practitioners, and general internists should find this text both informative and timely.

ACKNOWLEDGMENT

We would like to thank Lesley Wood, MA, for her editorial assistance with this book.

Leslee J. Shaw, PhD
Rita F. Redberg, MD, FACC

CONTENTS

CONTRIBUTORS

ADAM ATHERLY, PhD, *Department of Health Policy and Management, Rollins School of Public Health, Emory University, Atlanta, GA*

MICHAEL S. BAILEY, MD, *Division of Cardiovascular Medicine, University of Florida, Gainesville, FL*

SHEELA BARHAN, MD, *Department of Obstetrics and Gynecology, Wright State University School of Medicine, Dayton, OH*

ANDRA L. BLOMKALNS, MD, *Department of Emergency Medicine, University of Cincinnati Medical Center, Cincinnati, OH*

PAUL R. CASPERSON, PhD, *Division of Cardiology, University of Texas Health Science Center at San Antonio, TX*

JONATHAN CHAN, MBBS, *Department of Medicine, University of Queensland, Brisbane, Australia*

ELISA YUEN MAN CHIU, RN, MS, *Department of Physiological Nursing, School of Nursing, UCSF, San Francisco, CA*

STEVEN D. CULLER, PhD, *Department of Health Policy and Management, Rollins School of Public Health, Emory University, Atlanta, GA*

ANNE B. CURTIS, MD, *Division of Cardiovascular Medicine, University of Florida College of Medicine, Gainesville, FL*

CHRISTI DEATON, PhD, RN, FAHA, *School of Nursing, Emory University, Atlanta, GA*

ERIKA SIVARAJAN FROELICHER, RN, PhD, FAAN, *Department of Epidemiology and Biostatistics, School of Medicine, UCSF, San Francisco, CA*

W. BRIAN GIBLER, MD, *Department of Emergency Medicine, University of Cincinnati Medical Center, Cincinnati, OH*

DARCY GREEN CONAWAY, MD, *Department of Cardiology, University of Missouri-Kansas City School of Medicine, Kansas City, MO*

WILLIAM W. HURD, MD, *Department of Obstetrics and Gynecology, Wright State University School of Medicine, Dayton, OH*

SHAWNA JACKSON, MS, *Aequitas Consulting Group, San Diego, CA*

ALICE K. JACOBS, MD, *Evans Department of Medicine, Boston Medical Center, Boston, MA*

MARIELL JESSUP, MD, FACC, FAHA, *Department of Medicine, University of Pennsylvania School of Medicine, Philadelphia, PA*

B. DELIA JOHNSON, PhD, *Epidemiology Data Center, Graduate School of Public Health, University of Pittsburgh, Pittsburgh, PA*

SHERYL F. KELSEY, PhD, *Epidemiology Data Center, Graduate School of Public Health, University of Pittsburgh, Pittsburgh, PA*

SUSAN KENDIG, RNC, MSN, WHCNP, *Barnes College of Nursing and Health Studies, University of Missouri-St. Louis, St. Louis, MO*

MARVIN A. KONSTAM, MD, *Division of Cardiology, Department of Medicine, Tufts-New England Medical Center, Boston, MA*

CHERIE L. KUNIK, MSN, RN, CS, *Shepherd Spinal Center, Atlanta, GA*

MICHAEL S. LAUER, MD, FACC, *Department of Cardiology, Cleveland Clinic Foundation, Cleveland, OH*

JANE A. LEOPOLD, MD, *Evans Department of Medicine, Boston Medical Center, Boston, MA*

THOMAS H. MARWICK, MD, PhD, FRACP, FACC, *Department of Medicine, University of Queensland, Brisbane, Australia*

MICHAEL E. MENDELSOHN, MD, *Molecular Cardiology Research Institute, Tufts-New England Medical Center, Boston, MA*

C. NOEL BAIREY MERZ, MD, *Preventive and Rehabilitative Cardiac Center, Cedars Sinai Medical Center, Los Angeles, CA*

JENNIFER H. MIERES, MD, *Division of Nuclear Medicine, North Shore University Hospital, Manhasset, NY*

D. DOUGLAS MILLER, MD, CM, MBA, FACC, FRCP(C), *Department of Internal Medicine, Saint Louis University School of Medicine, St. Louis, MO*

DANIEL P. MORIN, MD, MPH, *Division of Cardiology, Department of Medicine, Tufts-New England Medical Center, Boston, MA*

ANTHONY P. MORISE, MD, *Section of Cardiology, Department of Medicine, West Virginia University School of Medicine, Morgantown, WV*

LORI MOSCA, MD, MPH, PhD, *Division of Cardiology and Division of Preventive Medicine and Nutrition, New York-Presbyterian Hospital, Columbia and Cornell Universities, New York, NY*

SHARON MULVAGH, MD, *Division of Cardiovascular Diseases, Mayo Clinic, Rochester, MN*

L. KRISTIN NEWBY, MD, *Duke Clinical Research Institute, Duke University, Durham, NC*

ELIZABETH OFILI, MD, *Division of Cardiology, Morehouse School of Medicine, Atlanta, GA*

ROBERT A. O'ROURKE, MD, *Division of Cardiology, University of Texas Health Science Center at San Antonio, TX*

FRANK J. PAPATHEOFANIS, MD, MPH, PhD, *Aequitas Consulting Group and Advanced Medical Technology Assessment and Policy Program, University of California, San Diego, CA*

ERIC PETERSON, MD, FACC, *Duke Clinical Research Institute, Duke University, Durham, NC*

KIMBERLY J. RASK, MD, PhD, *Division of General Internal Medicine, Emory University School of Medicine, and Department of Health Policy and Management, Rollins School of Public Health, Emory University, Atlanta, GA*

RITA F. REDBERG, MD, FACC, *Department of Medicine, University of California School of Medicine, San Francisco, CA*

MARIA VIVINA T. REGIS, RN, MS, *Department of Physiological Nursing, School of Nursing, University of California, San Francisco, CA*

VÉRONIQUE L. ROGER, MD, MPH, *Division of Cardiovascular Diseases and Internal Medicine, Mayo Clinic and Foundation, Rochester, MN*

ROBERT E. ROGERS, MD, *Department of Obstetrics and Gynecology, Indiana University School of Medicine, Indianapolis, IN*

JOHN A. RUMBERGER, PhD, MD, FACC, *Division of Cardiology, Department of Medicine, The Ohio State University, Columbus, OH*

LAURA SAMPIETRO-COLOM, MD, MPH, *Catalan Agency for Health Technology Assessment, Barcelona, Spain*

LESLEE J. SHAW, PhD, *Outcomes Research, American Cardiovascular Research Institute, Atlanta, GA*

CLAIRE E. POTHIER SNADER, MA, *Department of Cardiology, Cleveland Clinic Foundation, Cleveland, OH*

JOHN SPERTUS, MD, MPH, FACC, *Department of Internal Medicine, University of Missouri-Kansas City School of Medicine, Kansas City, MO*

JAMES E. UDELSON, MD, *Division of Cardiology, Department of Medicine, Tufts-New England Medical Center, Boston, MA*

MARY NORINE WALSH, MD, *Department of Cardiology, The Care Group, Indianapolis, IN*

NANETTE K. WENGER, MD, *Division of Cardiology, Emory University School of Medicine, Atlanta, GA*

ERIN WILLIAMS, BSN, RN, *Aequitas Consulting Group, San Diego, CA*

BRANDI J. WITT, MD, *Division of Cardiovascular Diseases and Internal Medicine, Mayo Clinic and Foundation, Rochester, MN*

I INTRODUCTION

1

The Institute of Medicine Report, Women's Cardiovascular Health, and Evidence-Based Medicine

Nanette K. Wenger, MD

CONTENTS

THE INSTITUTE OF MEDICINE REPORT

The recently released Institute of Medicine (IOM) report *(1) Exploring the Biological Contributions to Human Health: Does Sex Matter?* advocated the study of sex differences "from womb to tomb" to improve the quality and appropriateness of health care services for women. This landmark IOM report reviews the pervasive gender bias in medical research, highlighting that a better understanding of the differences in human disease between the sexes is required, with the translation of these differences into clinical practice.

In the study of human subjects, the report recommends that the term *sex* should be used as a classification, generally as male or female, according to the reproductive organs and functions that derive from the chromosomal components. The term *gender* should be used to refer to a person's self-representation as a male or female or how that person is responded to by social institutions on the basis of the individual's gender presentation. Sex is biologic; gender is the term used to characterize people of different sexes in sociological, psychological, or behaviorial terms.

In the past decade, human biology discoveries have demonstrated that both normal physiological and pathological functions are directly influenced by sex-based biology differences. This underlies the need to consider sex in the design and analysis of all aspects and at all levels of biomedical and health-related research. The study of sex differences is evolving into a mature science, emphasizing that sex governs human physi-

From: *Contemporary Cardiology: Coronary Disease in Women: Evidence-Based Diagnosis and Treatment*
Edited by: L. J. Shaw and R. F. Redberg © Humana Press Inc., Totowa, NJ

ology and health far beyond the realm of reproduction, sex hormones and sex chromosomes.

Sex is a basic human variable that influences health and illness across the lifespan. There are differences between the sexes in the prevalence and severity of a wide range of diseases and medical conditions. Men and women have different patterns of illness, lifespans, metabolism, and they respond differently to therapies. There are sex differences in the susceptibility to diseases and responses to environmental stresses and drug treatments. Researchers must pay increased attention to the different ways in which women and men are affected by both diseases and disease treatments. The unique health profiles of minority populations, and in particular, cultural and racial effects on health, also require attention.

Both sex differences and similarities must be monitored in human diseases; this will be enabled by making sex-specific data more readily available. Since 1990, the National Institutes of Health (NIH) has required the inclusion of women in all NIH-sponsored research; since 1994, analysis of outcomes by sex has been required. The analysis and presentation of sex-based differences in clinical research results are requisite to ascertain and understand sex-specific components of disease pathogenesis, diagnostic modalities, preventive approaches, and therapeutic interventions, as well as to develop new approaches to disease prevention, diagnosis, and management. Scientific journal editors should encourage researchers to report the results of sex analyses. For example, why do females have a greater risk of developing life-threatening ventricular arrhythmias with a variety of potassium-channel blocking drugs? Why do females recover language ability more rapidly after a left hemisphere stroke?

Previously, men were viewed as the norm or standard, and sex differences tended to be underreported rather than highlighted. Other than differences in reproductive systems, the historical assumption was that men and women reacted comparably to diseases and drugs. There must be a change in this traditional male-oriented approach to fact finding. Basic genetic and physiological differences as well as environmental factors cause behavioral and cognitive differences between the sexes. Sex differences can affect behavior, perception, and overall health and wellness. What must be considered are the relative roles of biology and the environment.

It is imperative to include women in every aspect of health research, testing, and trials. Medical researchers must devote attention to differences between males and females even at the cellular level. Important sex differences that extend to the cellular and molecular levels involve all cells, not just the reproductive system. "Every cell has a sex." Many of the basic biochemical differences of cells derive from genetic, rather than hormonal differences; underlying mechanisms must be studied and explained. For example, the Y chromosome and an apparently inactive X chromosome likely plays a role in cell life. Little research has been done regarding sex differences at the cellular level, and there is rarely any delineation when cells or tissues are used in experiments as to whether they derive from men or from women. Do sex differences at the cellular level explain why diseases affect men and women differently? Previously, only epidemiological differences in whole organisms were examined for sex differences; basic biologic research is needed. In the materials and methods section, researchers should disclose the sex of origin of biological research material (i.e., whether cells or tissue cultures derive from male or female patients or animals). There must be a paradigm shift to address the pervasiveness of cellular genetic differences based on sex.

Until recently, medical researchers did little to ensure that women received the same representation as men in clinical studies and that studies were designed to allow analyses of data by sex. Often the trials were underpowered for statistical power, owing to inadequate numbers of women recruited. Particularly in phase I data, women remain underrepresented. Women's health requires the inclusion of women by researchers, with systematic analyses of the differences between the sexes. Once clinical trials show differences in how the sexes react to diseases and drugs, health care practitioners must consider these differences in their preventive, diagnostic, and therapeutic practices. Although sex differences in physiology extend far beyond the realm of reproduction, the effects of menstrual cycle phases, of menopause, and of menopausal hormone therapy on diseases and drugs must be ascertained in clinical studies. Sex differences must be explored in drug pharmacokinetics, pharmacodynamics, safety, and side effects.

OVERALL RECOMMENDATIONS: THE IOM REPORT

The IOM advises the federal government on health issues. The IOM report provides 14 recommendations for scientists:

Recommendations for research

- Promote research on sex at the cellular level
- Study sex differences from womb to tomb
- Mine cross-species information
- Investigate natural variations
- Expand research in sex differences in brain organization and function
- Monitor sex differences and similarities for all human diseases that affect both sexes

Recommendations for addressing barriers to progress

- Clarify the use of sex and gender terms
- Support and conduct additional research on sex differences
- Make sex-specific data more readily available
- Determine and disclose the sex of origin of biological research materials
- Conduct longitudinal studies and construct them so that their results can be analyzed by sex
- Identify the endocrine status of research subjects (an important variable that should be considered, when possible, in analyses)
- Encourage and support interdisciplinary research on sex differences
- Reduce the potential for discrimination based on identified sex differences

THE IOM REPORT AND CORONARY HEART DISEASE

The IOM report highlighted pervasive sex differences in the prevalence and severity of a wide range of diseases, disorders, and medical conditions. This report emphasized the need to examine sex differences in the incidence and severity of heart disease as well as the incidence and severity of pain and pain syndromes.

Specific to coronary heart disease (CHD) and highly relevant to this volume is the spectrum of sex differences. Cardiovascular disease (CVD) is the leading cause of death for American women; whereas men are experiencing a decline in deaths as a result of CVD, the number of CVD deaths in women is increasing. Age-adjusted incident CHD is greater in African-American women age 20–54 years than in white women, but lower in African-American men than in white men.

Men incur myocardial infarction (MI) approx 10–15 years earlier than women, yet men have a better 1-year postinfarction survival rate than women. However, men die at an earlier age. Heart attack symptoms show distinct sex differences, with men experiencing acute, crushing chest pain and many women experiencing shortness of breath and fatigue, in addition to classical chest pain.

Regarding coronary risk factors, hypertension and hypercholesterolemia are more prominent in men than women until their late 40s and early 50s; after that, the prevalence is higher in women. High triglyceride levels present a greater risk to women than to men; low high-density lipoprotein (HDL) cholesterol levels may be a better predictor than high low-density lipoprotein (LDL) for coronary risk in women. Mortality from CHD is two to four times greater in diabetic than nondiabetic men, but three to seven times greater in diabetic than nondiabetic women. It must be considered unlikely that menopausal hormone therapy has a cardioprotective effect. As a response, health care organizations, including the American Heart Association, have undertaken gender-specific coronary risk reduction programs. Yet, in a survey conducted by the Society for Women's Health Research, most women were unaware of gender-based medical differences *(2)*.

Women with CHD are more likely to have comorbidities, including heart failure, hypertension, and diabetes. Diabetic women are particularly vulnerable to complications of MI. Women hospitalized for acute MI are likely to be older than men and have more "silent" MIs. Women younger than 65 years of age are more than twice as likely to die from MI as men of the same age, possibly because diabetes, heart failure, and stroke are more prevalent in younger women; arterial narrowing is less and reactive platelet levels are higher in younger women; and plaque erosions are more common in premenopausal women who die.

Women are less likely to be given effective interventions, which include aspirin, beta blockers, and thrombolytic agents. Women are also less likely than men to undergo diagnostic and therapeutic tests and procedures. Possible reasons include discrepancies in physician perception of the severity of coronary disease in men vs women and physician perception of the risks and efficacies of diagnostic and therapeutic procedures; higher rates of admission for women with ischemic symptoms in the absence of documented CHD; patient perceptions and preferences (i.e., women may be more willing to adhere to lifestyle changes and medications than to choose surgery); and bias in health care delivery.

As data from large ongoing clinical trials become available, gender-specific cardiology is likely to expand.

THE GENERAL ACCOUNTING OFFICE (GAO) REPORT: RELEVANCE TO THE IOM REPORT

The 2001 GAO report *(3)* cited that the US Food and Drug Administration (FDA) allowed industry to ignore 1998 regulations for reporting sex difference data. More than one-third of drugs approved by the FDA between 1998 and 2000 did not provide information on gender-related responses in New Drug Application (NDAs). Twenty-two percent of reports failed to provide separate efficacy data for men and women, and

17% omitted sex-based safety data. The GAO suggested that the information was available, but was not reported. Thus, there remains a compelling need for the FDA to monitor the inclusion of women in all stages of drug research and to improve oversight of the analyses and presentation of data related to sex differences in clinical trials. Although later stage clinical trials currently include sufficient numbers of women for safety and efficacy determinations, in the initial small-scale safety trials, only 22% of participants are women.

In 1993, the FDA provided guidance to industry to include enough women in clinical drug trials to detect clinically significant differences in drug efficacy and safety, with the analysis of sex differences to be presented in NDAs. From 1992 to 2000, female participation in phase III trials increased from 44 to 56%; however, this includes trials for clinical issues involving only women.

The 1998 FDA regulations for NDAs required separate presentation of safety and efficacy data for women and men and tabulation of study participants by sex. However, one-third of current NDAs did not meet this requirement. A weakness of these regulations is the lack of specific criteria for the number of women needed and the lack of specific requirements regarding data analysis. Furthermore, there is currently no FDA system to track women in clinical trials, no procedures regarding requirements for NDA presentation of sex differences or drug side effects, and no information mandated about dose adjustment based on sex reflecting body weight, body fat distribution, differential drug absorption, metabolism or excretion, and resultant drug concentrations. Also unaddressed in the inclusion of women in drug clinical trials is, when appropriate, the identification of the menstrual cycle stages regarding hormonal variability or notation of menopausal status. Sex-based differences in drug response must be more broadly explored. Of the 10 prescription drugs withdrawn from the market since 1997, 8 caused more adverse events in women than men. In response to the GAO report, the FDA is currently implementing management systems to improve the review of sex-specific data. As well, the FDA Office of Women's Health is creating a clinical trials demographic database.

SUMMARY

The IOM report should be a wake-up call to clinical trial investigators and research scientists at the molecular, genetic, a cellular levels to encourage more detailed sex-based research to advance knowledge about sex differences and stimulate the understanding of gender differences in health, illness, and health care. This report should also provide guidance to the NIH, FDA, private foundations, and to industry.

REFERENCES

1. Wizemann TM, Pardue M-L (eds.). Exploring the Biological Contributions to Human Health. Does Sex Matter? Committee on Understanding the Biology of Sex and Gender Differences. Board on Health Sciences Policy, Institute of Medicine. National Academy Press, Washington, DC: 2001.
2. http://www.womens-health.org (Society for Women's Health Research survey): Accessed March 2003.
3. http://www.gao.gov/new.items/d01754.pdf (2001 GAO Report): Accessed March 2003.

2

Evidence-Based Medicine in the Assessment of Women at Risk for Cardiovascular Disease

Leslee J. Shaw, PhD

The diagnosis and treatment of cardiovascular disease (CVD) in women is perhaps one of the greatest clinical dilemmas in medicine. Coronary heart disease (CHD), including congestive heart failure (CHF), hypertensive disease, and other forms of atherosclerotic diseases, is an all-encompassing challenge that is a major cause of death and disability for women in most Westernized countries. The lifetime risk of coronary disease is substantial with approximately one in four women being at risk (1). Although CVD is manifested earlier for men, nearly 250,000 women die from ischemic heart disease every year. As a result of greater longevity, further growth in the number of deaths is anticipated (2).

Only in the last several decades has research focused on the CVD risk in women. A number of challenges and contradictions exist within the evaluation of the disease and in the risk estimation of women that currently hinder effective care for females. Despite the burden of the disease, dramatic improvements in therapeutic and surgical interventions have led to substantive declines in cardiovascular mortality. Since peaking in the 1960s, recent trends in mortality have revealed a 35–50% decline in CVD mortality (Fig. 1; 3). Declines in mortality have been less for lower socioeconomic, racial, ethnic, and female subsets of the population.

These data should be considered within our current era of evidence-based medicine, where optimal medical management is structured based on a substantial body of clinical effectiveness research on the diagnosis and treatment of at-risk women. Evidence-based medicine is divergent from prior clinical reasoning, where decision making was based on an accumulation of varied clinical experiences. Evidence-based medicine stands in contrast to the decision-making processes of the past in that patient outcomes data (in this case, derived from female populations) from published, peer-reviewed literature would be used to develop high-quality clinical guidelines for various clinical scenarios. Thus, for women, high-quality health care would require a threshold level of evidence such that effective guidelines of care could be established, including a sufficient (statistically powered sample) representation of women in large multicenter, observational series and randomized clinical trials in order to make definitive state-

From: *Contemporary Cardiology: Coronary Disease in Women: Evidence-Based Diagnosis and Treatment*
Edited by: L. J. Shaw and R. F. Redberg © Humana Press Inc., Totowa, NJ

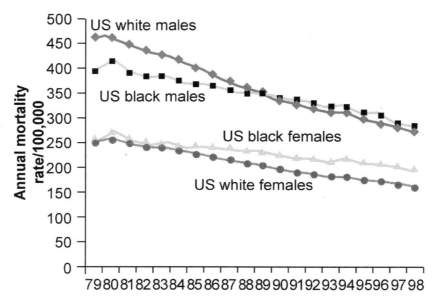

Fig. 1. CHD mortality trends by race and gender in United States 1979–1998. (From ref. *3.)*

ments about the diagnosis and treatment of women in both the primary and secondary prevention setting. This volume provides a present-day understanding of the epidemio-logical evidence of the disease, asymptomatic screening and diagnosis of symptomatic women, primary and secondary prevention strategies, as well as health care policy evaluations, including developing cost-effective care for women.

Within the area of women's health, evidence has grown dramatically over the last decade. In many cases, developments in the field have substantially outpaced educa-tional efforts for patients, consumers, and clinicians. This chapter serves to orient the reader as to the depth of knowledge on women's cardiovascular health as well as a the-oretical framework for current and future standards required for evidence in order to effectively guide care for women. Historically, women have been underrepresented in clinical trials and observational studies *(4,5),* despite the mandate from the US Food and Drug Administration (FDA) in 1990 to assure equivalent inclusion of women *(6).* Furthermore, in 1990, the National Institutes of Health (NIH) began requiring docu-mentation of recruitment strategies for women and minority subsets of the population. The lack of available evidence is one factor that has hindered wide-scale reductions in morbidity and mortality for women.

To further compound the challenge of diagnosing at-risk women, current data sug-gest that women more often present atypically with a greater frequency of nonexer-tional chest pain (or an equivalent, e.g., dyspnea) *(7–10).* The women who present atypically have often been considered to be at a decidedly lower risk when compared to their male counterparts *(7).* In the primary prevention setting, there are marked differ-ences in the incidence, prevalence, and outcome of women with traditional risk factors, including hypertension, hyperlipidemia, family history of premature coronary disease, and diabetes *(11–18).* Accumulating risk using a global risk score often classifies a disproportionate frequency of women as low risk (Fig. 2; *16).* Furthermore, women

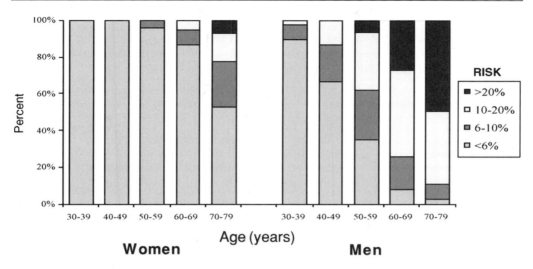

Fig. 2. Estimated 10-year hard CHD risk Framingham offspring and cohort. (From ref. *16.*)

generally have a lower prevalence of ischemia and obstructive coronary disease (i.e., approx 40–60% rate of normal coronaries), contributing to less intensive management patterns for women *(19–23)*. Gender differences in risk factor profiles, symptom presentation, and reports on reduced noninvasive test accuracy for women may contribute to greater case female fatality rates and challenge appropriate selection of at-risk women *(24–28)*.

New evidence reveals that there is a more complex interaction of risk factors and reproductive hormones that affect both vascular function and metabolism *(2)*. This includes new evidence on the role of conditional risk markers, such as high sensitivity C-reactive protein (CRP), an indicator of inflammation that both mediate and mark vascular disease abnormalities *(29,30)*. Additional challenges in the diagnosis and risk assessment of women is further challenged by the smaller artery size and evidence that microvascular abnormalities or subclinical disease may be more of a risk factor for CHD in women than in men *(31,32)*.

Evidence suggests that there may be gender-based differences in pain perception that may be acting on differential clinical presentation and evaluation of symptomatic women *(33)*. The perception of pain is further compounded by differences in societal roles and expectations for women that may constrain early and optimal health care-seeking behavior. Despite this, in the evaluation of a patient with new onset of chest pain symptoms, women report more anginal symptoms. Approximately 4 million women were evaluated for chest pain symptoms in 2000 in comparison to 2.4 million men. Women are also more often hospitalized for chest pain. However, at diagnostic cardiac catheterization, women have lower rates of obstructive coronary disease *(34)*. A large majority of women without a significant lesion in one of their epicardial coronary arteries have persistent symptoms and continue to consume large amounts of health care resources. Thus, for this large subset of women, few diagnostic strategies have been elucidated, but preliminary evidence suggests that a proportion of this group may have evidence of subendocardial flow heterogeneity or shifts in anaerobic metabolism that is suggestive of myocardial ischemia *(35–38)*. Additionally, very recent evidence suggests that when large subsets of women with chest pain symptoms are evaluated, cardiac imaging using stress echocardiographic or nuclear perfusion-based techniques may risk stratify women with normal and abnormal test results *(39–41)*.

For women with obstructive coronary disease, an abundance of evidence suggests a worsening short- and/or long-term prognosis, including acute coronary syndromes or myocardial infarction, poststent or coronary bypass surgery, and, in some cases, CHF *(42–52)*. Although women have less extensive disease and more often have normal left ventricular function, greater in-hospital and 30-day outcomes have been reported *(42–52)*. The acuity of presentation and greater comorbidity promotes differences in early outcome, especially for women with diabetes mellitus. For surgical interventions, such as percutaneous coronary interventions or bypass surgery, smaller body and artery size contributes to variations in procedural success and outcome differences, including a greater need for recurrent intervention and less symptom relief *(42)*, although overall procedural success rates are equally high for both men and women (i.e., >90–95%). Additionally, symptomatic women (especially diabetics) with evidence of provocative ischemia on conventional stress testing have a substantially worse event-free survival when compared to men with ischemia *(39)*.

For years, the reason for the worsening outcomes has been related to the older age of clinical presentation for women. However, recent evidence suggests younger women may be those at greatest risk *(48)*. This increase in risk may be the result of delays from chest pain onset to treatment-seeking, underrecognition of the disease in young women, a greater acuity of female presentation, a greater degree of comorbidity, and a less aggressive treatment pattern for women. Recent evidence suggests that greater mortality risk in women may be most likely driven by a greater degree of risk factor burden and comorbidity than to sex-related differences per se *(49)*.

Women with CHD also have worse functional capacity, a greater degree of physical disability, greater symptom burden, and an overall lower quality of life when compared to men *(2)*. As such, for female subsets of the population, there is a greater amount of health care resources consumed throughout the course of the disease process *(2)*. The reasons for the higher costs of care are most likely multifactorial and related to less intensive prevention management, resulting in greater use of higher cost hospitalization *(2)*, as well as less gender-tailored therapies and a lower evidence-base of female-oriented guidelines of care. As such, there is a need for considerations of strategies aimed at cost efficiency and cost-effectiveness analysis. The development of cost-effective diagnosis and treatment patterns for women is hampered by a lack of knowledge in the pathophysiology of the disease, the role of reproductive hormones, and the transition state into menopause, as well as influential factors that contribute to varying atherogenic processes in women.

Despite rapid advances in the field of gender-based evaluations in CVD, the pathophysiology of myocardial ischemia and CHD in women remains poorly understood and underdeveloped *(2)*. There is still a need to develop more wide-ranging strategies for research, diagnosis, management, and education oriented toward female patients. In particular, there is a growing body of evidence that the atherosclerotic disease process may vary by gender and may be mediated by sex hormones, an area of research that is vastly underdeveloped. For example, pathological evidence suggests that positive remodeling may occur more often in women *(53,54)*. From the Armed Forces Institute of Pathology registry, plaque erosion is a more common presentation for sudden cardiac death in women in comparison to plaque rupture in men *(53,54)*. This latter point is mediated by age, where older women present more typically with plaque rupture *(53,54)*. Additionally, there are NIH-sponsored studies, such as the Women's Ischemia Syndrome Evaluation (WISE), that may provide a theoretical model for the interplay between traditional risk factors, conditional risk markers, vascular function and abnormalities, as well as signs and symptoms suggestive of myocardial ischemia in a relatively large cohort of women.

Despite our research gap, there are also misunderstandings on the part of patients and clinicians alike. Although most women are at risk of developing CHD, most women still consider coronary disease only a remote health risk. In fact, many patients do not realize that mortality for men and women is higher than from all cancers combined (CVD deaths in 2002: women = 512,904, men = 445,871; cancer-related deaths: women = 264,006, men = 445,871). For women, awareness of higher morbidity and mortality in females dictates the need for early detection strategies and more aggressive therapeutic interventions. Thus, a paradigm shift in screening and diagnostic testing should be promoted. Currently, the evaluation of new or worsening coronary disease is prompted by an evaluation of symptoms. Typical symptoms, occurring less often in women, provide the mainstay for aggressive care of at-risk patients. If we allow symptoms to drive the testing and treatment of women, then we will be less accurate in risk detection. Thus, a broadened definition of symptoms or more female-specific symptom evaluation tools will need to be developed to foster efficient care for women. Chapter 17 provides a state-of-the-heart evidence primer for the work-up of women with stable chest pain symptoms and is based on strategies currently utilized in the Clinical Outcomes Using Revascularization and Aggressive Drug Evaluation (COURAGE) randomized trial. Strategies developed and aimed at improving outcomes in women provide a cornerstone for reducing the heavy clinical and economic burden of the disease in most Westernized societies. Furthermore, the development of female-oriented strategies offers a huge opportunity for improving the quality of care for women, as well as enhanced community goodwill, which translates into improved health care for women and their families, as women are often the gatekeepers for their family's health, making approximately two-thirds of all health care decisions. There are also economic benefits to targeting high-risk women that could result in increased early detection of the disease and aversion of costly downstream care that will impact improved societal productivity and the economic load of the disease.

In this era of evidence-based medicine, our current aim for the evaluation of at-risk women is to provide a solid base of research to guide both the diagnosis and management of this large subset of the population. For diagnostic decision making, this would include the fact that results from a noninvasive or laboratory test may be reliably used to determine the necessity for cardiac catheterization and determine the underlying disease burden. Chapters 12 and 13 discuss current evidence for the evaluation of asymptomatic and symptomatic women, including the detection of subclinical disease and tests for myocardial ischemia. For therapeutic decision making, clinical decision making would then be aimed at risk reduction using an array of medical and surgical interventions that have shown to be efficacious and effective in adequately studied female samples from rigorously controlled clinical trials.

REFERENCES

1. Lloyd-Jones DM, Larson MG, Beiser A, Levy D. Lifetime risk of developing coronary heart disease. Lancet 1999;353:89–92.
2. Bairey-Merz CN, Bonow R, Sopko G, et al. National Heart Lung Blood Insitute WISE workshop. Circulation 2003, in press.
3. Benjamin EJ, Smith SC Jr, Cooper RS, et al. Task force #1—magnitude of the prevention problem: opportunities and challenges. 33rd Bethesda Conference. J Am Coll Cardiol 2002;40:588–603.
4. Conrad DA, Maynard C, Cheadle A, et al. Primary care physician compensation method in medical groups: does it influence the use and cost of health services for enrollees in managed care organizations? JAMA 1998;279:853–858.
5. Shaw LJ, Peterson ED, Johnson LL. Non-invasive testing techniques: prognosis and diagnosis in coronary artery disease in women: What all Physicians Need to Know. In: P. Charney, ed., American College of Physician's Women's Health Series, Philadelphia, PA, 1999, pp. 327–350.
6. http://www.fda.gov. whole body screening: access date: June 2002.
7. Diamond GA, Forrester JS. Analysis of probability as an aid in the clinical diagnosis of coronary-artery disease. N Engl J Med 1979;300:1350–1358.
8. Smith SC Jr, Blair SN, Bonow RO, et al. AHA/ACC Scientific Statement: AHA/ACC guidelines for preventing heart attack and death in patients wyth atherosclerotic cardiovascular disease: 2001 update: A statement for healthcare professionals from the American Heart Association and the American College of Cardiology. Circulation 2001;104:1577–1579.
9. Goraya TY, Leibson CL, Palumbo PJ, et al. Coronary atherosclerosis in diabetes milletus: a population-based autopsy study. J Am Coll Cardiol 2002;40:946–953.
10. Legato MJ. Dyslipidemia, gender, and the role of high-density lipoprotein cholesterol: implications for therapy. Am J Cardiol 2000;86:15L–18L.
11. Ledru F, Ducimetiere P, Battaglia S, et al. New diagnostic criteria for diabetes and coronary artery disease: insights from an angiographic study. J Am Coll Cardiol 2001;37:1543–1550.
12. Poehlman ET. Menopause, energy expenditure, and body composition. Acta Obstet Gynecol Scan 2002;81:603–611.
13. http://www.cdc.gov. Cardiovascular disease in women: access date: July 2002.
14. http://www.nhlbi.nih.gov. Framingham risk score: access date: July 2002.
15. Kanaya AM, Grady D, Barrett-Connor E. Explaining the sex difference in coronary heart disease mortality among patients with type 2 diabetes mellitus: a meta-analysis. Arch Intern Med 2002;162:1737–1745.
16. Pasternak RC, Abrams J, Greenland P, et al. Bethesda Conference #34: Identification of CHD and CHD risk: is there a detection gap? J Am Coll Cardiol 2003; 41:1863-1874.
17. Vaitkus PT. Gender differences in the utilization of cardiac catheterization for the diagnosis of chest pain. Am J Cardiol 1995;75:79–81.
18. Shaw LJ, Miller DD, Romeis JC, et al. Gender differences in the noninvasive evaluation and management of patients with suspected coronary artery disease. Ann Intern Med 1994;120:559–556.
19. Bowling A, Bond M, McKee D, et al. Equity in access to exercise tolerance testing, coronary angiography, and coronary artery bypass grafting by age, sex and clinical indications. Heart (British Cardiology Society) 2001;85:680–686.
20. Battleman DS, Callahan M. Gender differences in utilization of exercise treadmill testing: a claims-based analysis. J Health Qual 2001;23:38–41.
21. Mosca L, Grundy SM, Judelson D, et al. Guide to preventive cardiology for Women. AHA/ACC Scientific Statement: Consensus Panel Statement. Circulation 1999;99:2480–2484.
22. Stafford RS. Aspirin use is low among United States outpatients with coronary artery disease. Circulation 2000;101:1097–1101.
23. Rathore SS, Chen J, Wang Y, et al. Sex differences in cardiac catheterization: the role of physician gender. JAMA 2001;286:2849–2856.
24. http://www.nhlbi.nih.gov/guidelines/cholesterol/index.html. Framingham risk score: access date: July 2002.
25. Lerner DJ, Kannel WB. Patterns of coronary heart disease morbidity and mortality in the sexes: a 26-year follow-up of the Framingham population. Am Heart J 1986;111:383–390.
26. Milner KA, Funk M, Richards S, et al. Gender differences in symptom presentation associated with coronary artery disease. Am J Cardiol 1999;84:396–399.

27. Bairey-Merz CN, Olson M, McGorray S, et al. Physical activity and functional capacity measurement in women: a report from the NHLBI-sponsored WISE study. J Womens Health Gend Based Med 2000;9:769–777.

28. Sharaf BL, Pepine CJ, Kerensky RA, et al. The WISE Study Group. Detailed angiographic analysis of women with suspected ischemic chest pain (pilot phase data from the NHLBI-sponsored Women's Ischemia Syndrome Evaluation [WISE] Study Angiographic Core Laboratory). Am J Cardiol 2001;87:937–941.

29. Ridker PM, Rifai N, Rose L, et al. Comparison of C-reactive protein and low-density lipoprotein cholesterol levels in the prediction of first cardiovascular events. N Engl J Med 2002;347:1557–1565.

30. Ridker PM, Buring JE, Shih J, et al. Prospective study of C-reactive protein and the risk of future cardiovascular events among apparently healthy women. Circulation 1998;98:731–733.

31. Wong TY, Klein R, Sharrett AR, et al. Retinal arteriolar narrowing and risk of coronary heart disease in men and women. The Atherosclerosis Risk in Communities Study. JAMA 2002;287:1153–1159.

32. Shaw LJ, Raggi P, Berman DS, Callister TQ. Prognostic value of coronary calcium screening in diabetes. World Congress of Cardiology, Sydney, Australia, 2002.

33. Sheps DS, Kaufmann PG, Sheffield D, et al. Sex differences in chest pain in patients with documented coronary artery disease and exercise-induced ischemia: Results from the PIMI study. Am Heart J 2001;142:864–871.

34. Shaw LJ, Gibbons RJ, McCallister B, et al. Gender Differences in Extent and Severity of Coronary Disease in the ACC National Cardiovascular Disease Registry. J Am Coll Cardiol 2002;39:321A.

35. Buchthal SD, Den Hollander JA, Hee-Won K, et al. Metabolic evidence of myocardial ischemai by 31-P NMR spectroscopy in women with chest pain by no significant coronary stenoses: pilot phase results from The NHLBI WISE Study. N Engl J Med 2000;342:829–835.

36. Panting JR, Gatehouse PD, Yang GZ, et al. Abnormal subendocardial perfusion in cardiac syndrome X detected by cardiovascular magnetic resonance imaging. N Engl J Med 2002;346:1948–1953.

37. Reis SE, Holubkov R, Conrad Smith AJ, et al. The WISE Investigators. Coronary microvascular dysfunction is highly prevalent in women with chest pain in the absence of coronary artery disease: results from the NHLBI WISE study. Am Heart J 2001;141:735–741.

38. Reis SE, Holubkov R, Lee JS, et al. Coronary flow velocity response to adenosine characterizes coronary microvascular function in women with chest pain and no obstructive coronary disease. Results from the pilot phase of the Women's Ischemia Syndrome Evaluation (WISE) study. J Am Coll Cardiol 1999;33:1469–1475.

39. Giri S, Shaw LJ, Murthy DR, et al. Impact of diabetes on the risk stratification using stress single-photon emission computed tomography myocardial perfusion imaging in patients with symptoms suggestive of coronary artery disease. Circulation 2002;105:32–40.

40. Marwick TH, Shaw LJ, Lauer MS, et al. The noninvasive prediction of cardiac mortality in men and women with known or suspected coronary artery disease. Economics of Noninvasive Diagnosis (END) Study Group. Am J Med 1999;106:172–178.

41. Arruda-Olson AM, Juracan EM, Mahoney DW, et al. Prognostic value of exercise echocardiography in 5,798 patients: is there a gender difference? J Am Coll Cardiol 2002;39:625–631.

42. American Heart Association. Heart Disease and Stroke Statistics—2003 Update. American Heart Association, Dallas, TX, 2002.

43. Ahmed JM, Dangas G, Lansky AJ, et al. Influence of gender on early and one-year clinical outcomes after saphenous vein graft stenting. Am J Cardiol 2001;87:401–405.

44. Cho L, Marso SP, Bhatt DL, Topol EJ. Optimizing percutaneous coronary revascularization in diabetic women: analysis from the EPISTENT trial. J Womens Health Gend Based Med 2000;9:741–746.

45. Mehilli J, Kastrati A, Dirschinger J, et al. Differences in prognostic factors and outcomes between women and men undergoing coronary artery stenting. JAMA 2000;284:1799–1805.

46. Nohria A, Vaccarino V, Krumholz HM. Gender differences in mortality after myocardial infarction. Why women fare worse than men. Cardiol Clin 1998;16:45–57.

47. Vaccarino V, Chen YT, Wang Y, et al. Sex differences in the clinical care and outcomes of congestive heart failure in the elderly. Am Heart J 1999;138:835–842.

48. Vaccarino V, Parsons L, Every NR, et al. Sex-based differences in early mortality after myocardial infarction. National Registry of Myocardial Infarction 2 Participants. N Engl J Med 1999;341:217–225.

49. Kanaya AM, Grady D, Barrett-Connor E. Explaining the sex difference in coronary heart disease mortality among patients with type 2 diabetes mellitus: a meta-analysis. Arch Intern Med 2002;162:1737–1745.
50. Ghali WA, Faris PD, Galbraith PD, et al. Alberta Provincial Project for Outcome Assessment in Coronary Heart Disease (APPROACH) Investigators. Sex differences in access to coronary revascularization after cardiac catheterization: importance of detailed clinical data. Ann Intern Med 2002;136:723–732.
51. Vaccarino V, Abramson JL, Veledar E, Weintraub WS. Sex differences in hospital mortality after coronary artery bypass surgery: evidence for a higher mortality in younger women. Circulation 2002;105:1176–1181.
52. Woodwell DA. National Ambulatory Medical Care Survey: 1996 summary. Advance Data 1997;1–25.
53. Burke AP, Farb A, Malcom GT, et al. Effect of risk factors on the mechanism of acute thrombosis and sudden coronary death in women. Circulation 1998;97:2110–2116.
54. Virmani R, Kolodgie FD, Burke AP, et al. Lessons from sudden coronary death: a comprehensive morphological classification scheme for atherosclerotic lesions. Arteriosclerosis, Thrombosis Vascular Biol 2000;20:1262–1275.

II

SCREENING AND DIAGNOSIS
OF CORONARY DISEASE IN WOMEN

A. Cardiovascular Epidemiology in Women

3

Population-Based Sex Differences in Disease Incidence and Prevalence

Brandi J. Witt, MD
and Véronique L. Roger, MD, MPH

CONTENTS

INTRODUCTION

Heart disease remains the leading cause of death for women in the United States, causing more female deaths than all types of cancers combined *(1,2)*. Although age-adjusted mortality from coronary heart disease (CHD) declined in the last four decades in the United States, evidence shows that the decline may have been of a lesser magnitude in women (http://www.cdc.gov/nchs) *(3)*. The decline in CHD mortality could be the result of decreasing disease incidence, decreasing case fatality rates, or a combination of the two. This underscores the need to analyze disease trends separately in men and women in order to understand the sex-specific patterns of disease occurrence and outcome.

Furthermore, heart disease is a major cause of illness and disability for women and, as life expectancy increases, women, who have a greater life expectancy than men, will represent an increasingly larger proportion of the population with prevalent CHD *(4)*. These considerations underscore the magnitude of heart disease as a public health problem in women, which this chapter addresses and also outlines the sex differences in disease incidence and prevalence of CHD. Recognition of the magnitude of this public health problem is essential to its prevention, timely identification, and appropriate treatment.

From: *Contemporary Cardiology: Coronary Disease in Women: Evidence-Based Diagnosis and Treatment*
Edited by: L. J. Shaw and R. F. Redberg © Humana Press Inc., Totowa, NJ

Although attention has been directed toward heart disease in women, not all studies that focus on the subject include comparable groups of men so that comparisons could be made either informally or formally. The importance of avoiding "unisex" studies to appropriately address issues of sex differences and sex specificity has been underscored *(5)*. To this end, in the present chapter, we only report on studies that include both men and women to examine the sex differences in disease incidence and prevalence.

DEFINITIONS OF CHD AND CARDIOVASCULAR DISEASE

The classification of the American Heart Association (AHA) relies on disease categories based on the 9th and 10th revision of the International Classification of Disease (ICD) codes, categorized into total cardiovascular diseases (CVDs) (ICD9 390-459, 745–747 and ICD 10 100-199, Q20-Q28) and coronary heart disease (ICD 9 410-414, 429.2 and ICD10 I20-25). The National Center for Health Statistics (NCHS) tabulates the mortality of "Diseases of the Heart," which represents approx 75% of total cardiovascular mortality as defined by the AHA. Cohort and community surveillance studies rely on standardized criteria to validate diagnoses.

DATA SOURCES TO MEASURE INCIDENCE AND PREVALENCE

Several sources are available to measure the incidence and prevalence of heart disease and to gain insight into CHD trends in the population. The National Hospital Discharge Survey samples hospital discharges, which are event-based and not person-based, allowing multiple hospitalizations for the same individuals to be counted *(6)*. They do not differentiate between first and subsequent admissions for a given condition and, thus, cannot provide true incidence rates. Furthermore, the diagnoses are not validated using standardized criteria and documented shifts in hospital discharge diagnoses after the introduction of the diagnostic-related groups (DRG) payment system raises questions about the validity of these sources for epidemiology research. This phenomenon, whereby certain diagnoses can be spuriously represented on discharge summaries because of reimbursement considerations, has been referred to as "DRG Creep" *(7)*.

The National Health and Nutrition Examination Survey (NHANES III) is part of a national public health survey conducted by the NCHS and the Center for Disease Control (CDC). It was conducted from 1988 to 1994 and included a CVD component that assessed cardiovascular health and risk factors, including blood pressure measurements, electrocardiograms (ECGs), heart auscultation, blood lipid levels, and questionnaires related specifically to CVDs. The ascertainment of angina in NHANES relied on the Rose questionnaire, the validity of which has been questioned among women *(9,10)*.

Cohort studies reported sex-specific prevalence and incidence estimates. Depending on the size of the cohort, in some instances, these may have limited power to assess population trends. Because they rely on standardized definitions in a rigorously ascertained population, these have strong internal validity. However, cohort subjects may not be fully representative of the general US population because of the "healthy volunteer effect" *(11–13)*.

Several community surveillance programs examine sex-specific patterns in coronary disease prevalence and incidence in geographically defined populations. These pro-

Table 1
Sex-Specific Estimates of CVD/CHD Prevalence

Author	Men	Women	Data source	Ascertainment
Ford *(14)*	13.9 ± 0.9	10.1 ± 0.7	NHANES III	Rose questionnaire, self-report for MI, and ECG
Furberg *(45)*	35.7	23.4	Cardiovascular health study—community-dwelling persons ages 65–100	Major ECG abnormalities
Furberg *(45)*	55	52	Cardiovascular health study—community-dwelling persons ages 65–100	Self-report validated of a physician's diagnosis
2002 AHA *(16)*	18.6	16.1	NHANES III and CDC/NCHS among persons ≥ 75 years	Variable according to data source
Burke *(46)*	12.3	9.4	ARIC study ages 45–64	Rose questionnaire, self-report, MD diagnosis, or ECG. Includes peripheral and cerebrovascular diseases

ARIC, Atherosclerosis Risk in Communities; AHA, American Heart Association; NHANES, National Health and Nutrition Examination Survey; CDC Center for Disease Control; NCHS, National Center for Health Statistics; MI, myocardial infarction; ECG, echocardiogram.

grams include the surveillance component of the Atherosclerosis Risk in Communities (ARIC) study, Worcester Heart Attack Study (WHAS), Minnesota Heart Survey (MHS), Olmsted County Study, Corpus Christi study, and the World Health Organization monitoring trends and determinants in cardiovascular disease (MONICA) study. Community surveillance studies rely on standardized diagnoses using validation algorithms and thus have superior validity when compared to vital statistics. The ARIC and MSH studies have an upper age limit of 74 whereas MONICA excludes persons over age 65. This fact needs to be taken into consideration to interpret their results, particularly for sex-specific patterns of CHD because women develop clinical CHD later in life in comparison to men.

PREVALENCE

Sex Differences in Disease Prevalence

Selected studies reporting on sex-specific myocardial infarction (MI) prevalence are summarized in Table 1. Data from NHANES III provide insight into differences in the prevalence of CHD ascertained using angina as measured by the Rose questionnaire *(9),* self-report of MI, and ECG *(14).* Using these three measures combined, the prevalence of CHD is similar in men and in women. However, when each measure of CHD was analyzed separately, sex differences emerged with a higher frequency of self-reported MI in men and a higher prevalence of angina in women. It is important to note in this regard that the validity of the Rose questionnaire among women has been challenged *(9)*.

Other studies, which also reported on the prevalence of CHD, are summarized in Table 1. Several observations can be made from this review. First, the measures used to ascertain disease differ between studies, with some including peripheral and cerebrovascular disease, thereby encompassing all CVDs, whereas others included only CHD. Second, within each broad category, the methods of ascertainment differed, and the ages included varied. Thus, the results cannot be compared across studies. Altogether these studies underscore the lower prevalence of disease in women in comparison to men, but also the importance of age on the observed prevalence rates.

Age and the Prevalence of CVDs and CHD

Irrespective of the measure used, the prevalence of CVDs increases with age, such that although it is lower in women in comparison to men in younger age groups, the gender gap markedly narrows as age increases. Estimates from NHANES III show an increase in the prevalence of CVDs in women from 4.6% of the total population between ages 20 and 24 to 79% in women age 75 and older, whereas the prevalence in men increases from 5.5% of the total population between the ages of 20 and 24 to 70.7% in men over the age of 75 *(1)*. Similar patterns are observed for CHD, the prevalence of which also increases with age from 2.8% among women ages 25–44 to 16.1% among women ages 75 and older *(1)*. Among men, 2% of individuals ages 25–44 have prevalent CHD increasing to 18.6% of men age 75 and older *(1)*.

Autopsy data from Olmsted County indicate that although the prevalence of significant CHD at postmortem examination is high among both genders, it is higher overall among men. Age-specific prevalence estimates are consistent with a narrowing of the gender gap with increasing age of the decedents. Among persons ages 60 or older at death, the prevalence of CHD was 70% among men compared to 56% in women *(15)*.

Race and Ethnicity and the Prevalence of CVDs and CHD

For total CVDs, the age-adjusted prevalence estimates for non-Hispanic white men are 30% and 23.8% for non-Hispanic white women. The prevalence estimates for Mexican-Americans are nearly equivalent (28.8% for men; 26.6% for women). However, the prevalence increases in African Americans to 40.5% for men and 39.6% for women *(16)*. For CHD, the estimated prevalence in NHANES III among non-Hispanic white men is 6.9% and 5.4% for women. Mexican-Americans have somewhat higher prevalence estimates of 7.2% for men and 6.8% for women. Prevalence in African-American men is similar at 7.1%, whereas African-American women have the highest prevalence estimate at 9% *(16)*. Regarding American Indians, data from the Strong Heart Study indicate that the prevalence of definite CHD is higher among Native American men when compared to their female counterparts *(17)*. When less stringent ascertainment criteria were used and possible CHD was included, the higher prevalence of CHD in men remained apparent, but the sex difference was somewhat blunted, seemingly related in part to the inclusion of angina as measured by the Rose questionnaire in women.

Trends in Disease Prevalence

Trends in disease prevalence are difficult to evaluate because ascertainment methods differ across studies and time. Trends in CVDs are often reported using hospital discharge diagnoses. Using this approach, CVDs as the first listed diagnosis on hospital discharge increased 28% from 1979 to 1998 in the United States *(1)*. Trends in CHD between 1979 and 1998 are similar to those observed in CVDs, with increases in prevalence reflected in hospital discharge diagnoses. In 1979, 1,014,000 men and 724,000 women were dismissed from US hospitals with the diagnosis of CHD. In 1998, those numbers had risen to 1,317,000 for men and 945,000 for women *(1)*.

As these are event-based, not person-based, this allows multiple hospitalizations for the same individuals to be counted without distinguishing between first and subsequent admission. Therefore, this approach is not a reliable measure of disease prevalence. Furthermore, the diagnoses are not validated using standardized criteria and shifts in hospital discharge diagnoses preferences, after the introduction of the DRGs payment systems have been documented *(18,19)*.

Notwithstanding the limitations of these data sources to measure prevalence, it is important to underscore that these trends document the relentless health care burden of CVDs and CHD. Furthermore, notwithstanding the methodological challenges to measure changes in prevalence over time, based on an incidence–prevalence–mortality modeling study conducted in the Netherlands, the decline in CHD mortality can be expected to lead to increases in CHD prevalence given the relatively constant incidence of CHD. Given their greater life expectancy *(20)*, this is particularly relevant to women.

INCIDENCE

The incidence of CHD is a critical measure of the new onset of disease and trends that indicate increasing or decreasing rates of developing disease. Because MI can be ascertained using standardized criteria *(21)*, it is often used in epidemiology studies as an indicator of incident CHD. Selected studies reporting on sex-specific MI incidence are summarized in Table 2.

Data from the ARIC study indicate that the incidence of MI in women decreased slightly from 1987 to 1994 at a rate of 0.2% per year. However, race-specific trends differed in blacks when compared to whites, with the incidence of MI decreasing 2.5% per year in white women, but increasing 7.4% per year in black women *(22)*. For men, the incidence of MI increased slightly by 0.1% per year, contrasting with the trends in incidence noted in women *(22)*. However, the upper age limit of 74 in the ARIC study may not capture the full burden of disease among women.

The WHAS had no age limit and showed large declines between 1975 and 1988 in MI incidence among elderly individuals, but an increase in incidence among some but not all age groups in women *(23)*. Recent analyses from Worcester indicated qualitatively flat trends in overall MI incidence from the mid-1980s to the mid-1990s *(24)*.

The Olmsted County CHD surveillance study also included all ages and indicated that the secular trends in the MI incidence exhibited marked age and sex differences, with an 8% decline in men over time that contrasts with a 36% increase in women *(25)*. These results indicate large differences in an MI incidence as a function of age and sex, with less favorable trends in women and the elderly. Indeed, the large decrease over time in MI incidence noted among younger men contrasted with an increase in inci-

Table 2
Sex-Specific Estimates of CVD/CHD Incidence

Author	Men	Women	Data source	Ascertainment
Sytkowski (26)*	216/1000	144/1000	Framingham Heart Study	CVDs
Jousilahti (47)	786/100,000 person-years	256/100,000 person-years	Surveys of provinces in Finland	Finnish National Hospital discharge acute coronary event
Rosamond (22)*	4.1/1000	1.9/1000	ARIC Study	MI; standardized criteria
Roger (25)*	298/100,000	155/100,000	Olmsted County Study	MI; standardized criteria
Goff (27)	MA 367.4/ 100,000 NHW 342.2/ 100,000	MA 205.3/ 100,000 NHW150/ 100,000	Corpus Christi	MI; standardized criteria

* Denotes studies reporting on time trends. CVD, cardiovascular disease; ARIC, Atherosclerosis Risk in Communities; MI, myocardial infarction; MA, Mexican-Americans; NHW, non-Hispanic whites.

dence among older women of similar magnitude. This contrast indicates that the shift in CHD mortality toward women and the elderly observed in Olmsted County during that time period (3) is linked partly to age and sex shifts in MI incidence.

Data from the Framingham Heart Study between 1950 and 1989 were reported by Sytkowski et al. in 1996 (26). Three cohorts aged 50–59 years and free of CVD at baseline were identified in 1950, 1960, and 1970 and followed for 20 years. The incidence of CVDs in the 1970 cohort is shown in Table 2.

Among women, the incidence of CHD defined by MI and angina declined steadily from one cohort to the next over time with rates per 1000 persons of 218 in the 1950 cohort, 184 in the 1960 cohort, and 175 in the 1970 cohort. Among men, the incidence of CHD remained stable at approx 350 per 1000 in all three cohorts. These data were interpreted as reflective of concurrent improvement in risk factors. Regarding race and ethnicity, as shown in Table 2, the incidence of hospitalized MI is higher in Mexican-American men and women when compared to their non-Hispanic white counterparts. Among Mexican- Americans, the hospitalized MI incidence is higher among men than women (27).

The World Health Organization MONICA study indicated that coronary event rates, defined as definite nonfatal MI and coronary deaths, were higher in men in comparison to women (28). Over time, CHD mortality rates decreased in both men and women, whereas CHD events rates decreased more than case fatality rates, leading MONICA investigators to conclude that declines in CHD mortality were chiefly related to decreasing disease incidence.

Interpretation of the Trends in MI Incidence

The recently reported trends in MI incidence in the context of the decline in CHD mortality underscore the complexity of coronary disease trends. As discussed previously, the MONICA study ascribed the decline in coronary deaths to changes in incidence *(28)*. Conversely, the ARIC study described mostly stable trends in MI incidence despite declining mortality, suggesting that the decline is largely attributable to improved medical care *(22)*. However, a notable limitation to both ARIC and MONICA lies in their exclusion of elderly persons, such that they do not account for a growing segment of the population. This is particularly problematic for measuring trends in women, who present with CHD 10 years later than men and MI 20 years later *(29,30)*. The Olmsted County data, which include all ages, noted a decline over time in MI incidence among younger men, suggesting that primary prevention is effective among this group. These data also underscore the need to revisit primary prevention measures in women and the elderly, who did not experience commensurate declines in MI incidence. In light of the aging of the population, these unfavorable trends have major public health implications and call for continuous monitoring of CHD trends, which is essential to gain insight into the determinants of the trends and direct prevention and treatment. These results also underscore the dynamic nature of the trends observed, as they vary across age, ethnicity, as well as time. This, in turn, further emphasizes the importance of continued heart disease surveillance.

PERCEPTIONS AND ASCERTAINMENT CHALLENGES

A review of the prevalence and incidence of CHD as it relates to sex requires an understanding of how sex differences in the perception and ascertainment of CHD can impact the measured CHD trends. Indeed, a common misconception is that heart disease is a "man's disease," when, in fact, more women than men die of CVDs.

Mosca et al. examined knowledge and perception of heart disease risk among US women and indicated that more women perceive cancer (particularly breast cancer), not CVDs, to be a more significant health concern for women *(31)*. Although these data underscore the informational gap in women's perceptions of CVD risk and preventive strategies, they also highlight an even larger gap, which exists for older women and some minority groups. These findings are important for the understanding of CHD prevalence as misconception of the CVD/CHD risk can likely influence care-seeking behaviors, which, in turn, can conceptually lead to underascertainment of CHD. Given the difference in CHD incidence and prevalence as a function of age, race, and ethnicity, these findings are particularly alarming.

As these data document the need for a better understanding of CVD risk factors by US women, enhanced and innovative strategies to disseminate knowledge should be developed and tailored to adequately communicate to diverse age and race/ethnicity groups. Additionally, the clinical presentation of CHD differs by sex. Women have higher rates of noncardiac chest pain than men *(32,33)* and experience heart disease approx 10 years later than men *(29,30)*, which may, in turn, contribute to the clinical differences between men and women with CHD *(2)*. For example, women with CHD often have comorbid conditions, such as diabetes, hypertension, and heart failure *(2,33)*. Women tend to present more often with angina, whereas men more often present with MI as the inaugural manifestation of CHD *(29)*. When they experience MI, women have atypical symptoms more frequently, including rest pain, jaw, neck, and back pain, nausea and vomiting, dyspnea, dizziness, fatigue, and malaise *(2,33)*. These factors could all contribute to the underrecognition of CHD both by women and their physicians *(32)*, possibly leading to known differences in the evaluation and procedure rates for men and women.

Several studies have shown that the diagnostic performance of stress tests is lower among women, emphasizing the diagnostic challenges in ascertaining chronic CHD in women (34–42). These diagnostic challenges are associated with sex differences in the delivery of care. When the diagnosis of CHD is not established, women are less likely than men to undergo cardiac procedures, particularly invasive ones (43,44). Although these differences could represent overuse in women or underuse in men, less aggressive evaluation of chest pain in women can conceivably lead to underascertainment of CHD. It is possible that the aforementioned perception and ascertainment challenges lead to underascertainment of incident and prevalence of CHD in women. These considerations need to be kept in mind when interpreting data on the incidence and prevalence of CHD in men and women, because in order to be measured accurately, CHD must first be recognized.

CONCLUSIONS

Although the overall prevalence and incidence of CHD is lower in women, age-specific estimates unequivocally indicate that the sex gap narrows substantially among older individuals. Furthermore, the magnitude of sex differences in the prevalence and incidence of CHD varies widely across age, race/ethnicity, and time, depending on the definitions used to ascertain CHD.

Finally, increased life expectancy will lead to increased prevalence of CHD, particularly for women. Secular trends in the incidence of CHD trends suggest a displacement of the burden of death and clinical CHD toward women, which should direct prevention strategies.

REFERENCES

1. American Heart Association. 2001 Heart and Stroke Statistical Update. American Heart Association, Dallas, TX, 2000.
2. Heim LJ, Brunsell SC. Heart disease in women. Prim Care 2000;27:741–766.
3. Roger VL, Jacobsen SJ, Weston SA, et al. Trends in heart disease deaths in Olmsted County, Minnesota, 1979–1994. Mayo Clin Proc 1999;74:651–657.
4. Kitler ME. Coronary disease: are there gender differences? Eur Heart J 1994;15:409–417.
5. Barrett-Connor E. Sex difference in coronary heart disease. Why are women so superior? Circulation 1997;95:252–264.
6. Dennison C, Pokras R, ed. Design and Operation of the National Hospital Discharge Survey. 1988 Redesign. Vital and Health Statistics-Series 1: Programs and Collection Procedures 2000;39:1-42.
7. Simborg DW. DRG creep: a new hospital-acquired disease. N Engl J Med 1981;304:1602–1604.
8. Vargas CM, Burt VL, Gillum RF. Cardiovascular disease in the NHANES III. Ann Epidemiol 1997;7:523–525.
9. LaCroix AZ, Haynes SG, Savage DD, Havlik RJ. Rose Questionnaire angina among United States black, white, and Mexican-American women and men. Prevalence and correlates from The Second National and Hispanic Health and Nutrition Examination Surveys. Am J Epidemiol 1989;129:669–686.
10. Garber CE, Carleton RA, Heller GV. Comparison of "Rose Questionnaire Angina" to exercise thallium scintigraphy: different findings in males and females. J Clin Epidemiol 1992;45:715–720.
11. Wilhelmsen L, Ljungberg S, Wedel H, Werko L. A comparison between participants and non-participants in a primary preventive trial. J Chronic Dis 1976;29:331–339.
12. Smith P, Arnesen H. Mortality in non-consenters in a post-myocardial infarction trial. J Intern Med 1990;228:253–256.
13. Lindsted KD, Fraser Ge, Steinkohl M, Beeson WL. Healthy volunteer effect in a cohort study: Temporal resolution in the adventist health study. J Clin Epidemiol 1996;49:783–790.
14. Ford ES, Giles WH, Croft JB. Prevalence of nonfatal coronary heart disease among American adults. Am Heart J 2000;139:371–377.

15. Roger VL, Weston S, Killian J, et al. Time Trends in the Prevalence of Atherosclerosis: A Population-Based Autopsy Study. Am J Med 2001;110:267–273.
16. American Heart Association. 2002 Heart and Stroke Statistical Update. American Heart Association, Dallas, TX, 2002.
17. Howard BV, Lee ET, Cowan LD, et al. Coronary heart disease prevalence and its relation to risk factors in American Indians. The Strong Heart Study. Am J Epidemiol 1995;142:254–268.
18. Simborg DW. DRG creep: a new hospital-acquired disease. N Engl J Med 1981;304:1602–1604.
19. Jollis JG, Ancukiewicz M, DeLong ER, et al. Discordance of databases designed for claims payment versus clinical information systems. Implications for outcomes research. Ann Intern Med 1993;119:844–850.
20. Bonneux L, Barendregt JJ, van der Maas PJ. The new old epidemic of coronary heart disease. Am J Public Health 1999;89:379–382.
21. White AD, Folsom AR, Chambless LE, et al. Community surveillance of coronary heart disease in the Atherosclerosis Risk in Communities (ARIC) Study: methods and initial two years' experience. J Clin Epidemiol 1996;49:223–233.
22. Rosamond WD, Chambless LE, Folsom AR, et al. Trends in the incidence of myocardial infarction and in mortality due to coronary heart disease. N Engl J Med 1998;339:861–867.
23. Goldberg RJ, Gorak EJ, Yarzebski J, et al. A community wide perspective of sex differences and temporal trends in the incidence and survival rates after acute myocardial infarction and out-of-hospital deaths caused by coronary heart disease. Circulation 1993;87:1947–1953.
24. Goldberg RJ, Yarzebski J, Lessard D, Gore JM. A two-decades (1975 to 1995) long experience in the incidence, in-hospital and long-term case-fatality rates of acute myocardial infarction: a community-wide perspective. J Am Coll Cardiol 1999;33:1533–1539.
25. Roger VL, Jacobsen SJ, Weston SA, et al. Trends in myocardial infarction incidence and survival. Olmsted County, Minnesota—1979 to 1994. Ann Intern Med 2002;136:341-348.
26. Sytkowski PA, D'Agostino RB, Belanger A, Kannel WB. Sex and time trends in cardiovascular disease incidence and mortality: the Framingham Heart Study, 1950–1989. Am J Epidemiol 1996;143:338–350.
27. Goff DC, Nichaman MZ, Chan W, et al. Greater incidence of hospitalized myocardial infarction among Mexican Americans than non-Hispanic whites. The Corpus Christi Heart Project, 1988–1992. Circulation 1997;95:1433–1440.
28. Tunstall-Pedoe H, Kuulasmaa K, Mahonen M, et al. Contribution of trends in survival and coronary-event rates to changes in coronary heart disease mortality: 10-year results from 37 WHO MONICA project populations. Monitoring trends and determinants in cardiovascular diseases. Lancet 1999;353:1547–1557.
29. Wenger NK. The Natural History of Coronary Artery Disease in Women. In: Charney P, ed. Coronary Artery Disease in Women: American College of Physicians, 1999, pp. 3–35.
30. Charney P, Walsh JM, Nattinger AB. Update in women's health. Ann Intern Med 1998;129:551–558.
31. Mosca L, Jones WK, King KB, et al. Awareness, perception, and knowledge of heart disease risk and prevention among women in the United States. American Heart Association Women's Heart Disease and Stroke Campaign Task Force. Arch Family Med 2000;9:506–515.
32. Fields SK, Savard AM, Epstein KR. The Female Patient. In: S. DP, ed. Cardiovascular Health and Disease in Women. WB Saunders, Philadelphia, PA, 1993.
33. Douglas PS. Coronary Artery Disease in Women. In: Braunwald E, ed. Heart Disease: A Textbook of Cardiovascular Medicine, 6th ed. WB Saunders, Philadelphia, PA, 2001. pp. 2038–2048.
34. Roger VL, Jacobsen SJ, Pellikka PA, et al. Gender differences in the use of stress testing and Minnesota. J Am Coll Cardiol 1998;32:345–352.
35. Roger VL, Pellikka PA, Chow CWH, et al. Sex and test verification bias: Impact on the diagnostic value of exercise echocardiography. Circulation 1997;95:405–410.
36. Weiner DA, Ryan TJ, McCabe CH, et al. Exercise stress testing. Correlations among history of angina, ST-segment response and prevalence of coronary-artery disease in the coronary artery surgery study (CASS). N Engl J Med 1979;301:230–235.
37. Diamond GA, Forrester JS. Analysis of probability as an aid in the clinical diagnosis of coronary-artery disease. N Engl J Med 1979;300:1350–1358.
38. Sketch MH, Mohiuddin SM, Lynch JD, et al. Significant sex differences in the correlation of electro-cardiographic exercise testing and coronary arteriograms. Am J Cardiol 1975;36:169–173.
39. Barolsky SM, Gilbert CA, Faruqui A, et al. Differences in electrocardiographic response to exercise of women and men: A non-Bayesian factor. Circulation 1979;60:1021–1027.

40. Tavel ME. Specificity of electrocardiographic stress test in women versus men. Am J Cardiol 1992;70:545–547.
41. Higginbotham MB, Morris KG, Coleman RE, Cobb FR. Sex-related differences in the normal cardiac response to upright exercise. Circulation 1984;70:357–366.
42. Hanley PC, Zinsmeister AR, Clements IP, et al. Gender-related differences in cardiac response to supine exercise assessed by radionuclide angiography. J Am Coll Cardiol 1989;13:624–629.
43. Schulman KA, Berlin JA, Harless W, et al. The effect of race and sex on physicians' recommendations for cardiac catheterization. N Engl J Med 1999;340:618–626.
44. Roger VL, Farkouh ME, Weston S, et al. Sex Differences in Evaluation and Outcome of Unstable Angina. JAMA 2000;283:646–652.
45. Furberg CD, Manolio TA, Psaty BM, et al. Major electrocardiographic abnormalities in persons aged 65 years and older (the Cardiovascular Health Study). Cardiovascular Health Study Collaborative Research Group. Am J Cardiol 1992;69:1329–1335.
46. Burke GL, Evans GW, Riley WA, et al. Arterial wall thickness is associated with prevalent cardiovascular disease in myocardial infarction middle-aged adults. The Atherosclerosis Risk in Communities (ARIC) Study. Stroke 1995;26:386–391.
47. Jousilahti P, Vartiainen E, Tuomilehto J, Puska P. Sex, age, cardiovascular risk factors, and coronary heart disease: a prospective follow-up study of 14 786 middle-aged men and women in Finland. Circulation 1999;99:1165–1172.

4   Risk Detection and Primary Prevention in Women

Lori Mosca, MD, MPH, PhD
and Leslee J. Shaw, PhD

CONTENTS

INTRODUCTION
EPIDEMIOLOGICAL PRINCIPLES INVOLVED IN PRIMARY PREVENTION
MAJOR RISK FACTORS
BARRIERS TO PREVENTION
CONCLUSION
REFERENCES

INTRODUCTION

Prevention of coronary heart disease (CHD) in asymptomatic individuals has traditionally been termed *primary prevention* because it aims to avert the clinical presentation of symptomatic disease along with major adverse cardiac events *(1)*. Our current management paradigm has been effective in reducing the burden of cardiovascular disease (CVD), with 35–50% declines in related mortality *(2)*. However, the CVD burden for most Westernized countries remains high. Prevention strategies are less often not instituted until after the clinical presentation of the atherosclerotic diseases. Primary CHD prevention offers the greatest opportunity to reduce the burden of disease in the United States *(3)*. This latter point becomes critical for the 40–60% of asymptomatic women whose initial presentation includes sudden cardiac death or acute myocardial infarction (AMI; *4*). There are a number of published guidelines from the American Heart Association (AHA), American College of Cardiology (ACC), and National Institutes of Health-National Heart, Lung, and Blood Institute (NIH-NHLBI, e.g., NCEP III-ATP) that detail management strategies for primary prevention risk-reducing methods for men and women *(3,5)*. Risk-reducing strategies, including control of major cardiac risk factors (e.g., weight, blood pressure, smoking, and regular exercise), can decrease a woman's risk for CHD by as much as 80% *(6,7)*. This chapter provides an introduction to primary prevention strategies and our current understanding of the traditional risk factors and emerging markers for CHD.

From: *Contemporary Cardiology: Coronary Disease in Women: Evidence-Based Diagnosis and Treatment*
Edited by: L. J. Shaw and R. F. Redberg © Humana Press Inc., Totowa, NJ

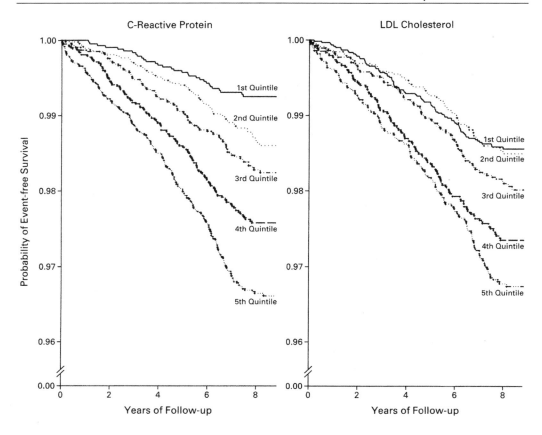

Fig. 1. Conditional risk factors: comparison of C-reactive protein (C-RP) (inflammatory marker) and low-density lipoprotein (LDL) cholesterol in prediction of first cardiovascular event. (From ref. 9. Copyright 2002, Massachusetts Medical Society.) Quintiles of C-RP are ≤0.49, 0.49–1.08, >1.08–2.09, >2.09–4.19, and >4.19 µg/L. Quintiles of LDL-cholesterol are ≤97.6, >97.6–115.4, >115.4–132.2, >132.2–153.9, and >153.9 µg/dL.

EPIDEMIOLOGICAL PRINCIPLES INVOLVED IN PRIMARY PREVENTION

Many risk factors have been shown to consistently increase an individual's risk of developing CHD *(8)*. By definition, a *risk factor* is a habit or trait that makes a person more likely to develop a disease. This chapter provides a synopsis of major cardiac risk factors that are associated with an increased risk of major adverse cardiovascular events. The basis for risk factor assessment is that the underlying risk of CHD varies for those individuals with and without the risk factor. For those with a documented risk factor, an individual's likelihood for CHD or cardiac events increases over time, which is commonly illustrated by the risk stratification principle (e.g., Kaplan-Meier or Cox survival curve). For example, in Fig. 1, 8-year event-free survival for 27,939 women *(9)* illustrates that a subset of this population had substantially higher risk than the compared group, and this risk variation yielded a statistical difference greater than that expected from chance alone. A person's absolute risk may be discerned from examining survival curves and plotting the time to cardiac events. Physicians often utilize absolute risk as a means of quantifying the expected event rate for a given patient or population series. Absolute risk considers the probability of a person with a certain characteristic or set of risk factors to develop CHD over a finite period of time (e.g., 10 years).

However, there are several other commonly employed measures of risk. *Relative risk* is the ratio of the likelihood of a cardiovascular event or disease in persons with and without a given risk factor. For example, diabetic women have an approximately threefold higher risk of dying than those without diabetes *(6)*. This multifold increase in risk is critical to understanding how significant the risk is in similar patients. However, relative risk is highly dependent on absolute risk, i.e., relative risk identifies the ratio of increased risk, but the baseline comparator's risk must also be understood. That is, recent evidence suggests that younger women have the highest mortality post myocardial infarction *(10)*. In fact, younger women have a 1.22-fold higher risk of dying postinfarction. This is an overall relative risk ratio but the underlying risk in a postinfarction population would vary substantially in comparison to the general population or from an outpatient series.

An additional consideration is that the relative risk is beneficial to determine causal relationships in CHD. As risk factors are highly correlated, relative risks (when considering their multifactorial relationship) often increase in additive or multiplicative manners. The multifactorial nature of cardiac risk factors can be discerned by examining multivariable regression equations, which examine the interactive relationship of risk and provides insight into how one risk factor (e.g., diabetes) may relate to other risk factors (e.g., hypertension or aging).

One final epidemiological measure to understand is *attributable risk,* where the CHD incidence rate is compared for those with and without risk factors. Any notable differences between population subsets provide an estimate of the potential disease amount that may be eradicated with appropriate control, management, or erasure of any risk factor *(8)*.

Currently, there are more than 200 identified risk factors that increase a woman's risk of heart attack or stroke. The core of traditional risk factors includes age, male gender, cigarette smoking, hypertension, dyslipidemia, diabetes, and a family history of premature CHD. Additional factors contributing to an increased CHD risk and compounding the frequency of other risk factors include obesity, sedentary lifestyle, and an atherogenic diet *(4,6)*. One of the challenges with both the identification and treatment of cardiac risk factors is that there are sex-based differences in the prevalence, age of onset, and treatment effectiveness for risk factor profiles that are discussed in this chapter.

MAJOR RISK FACTORS

Age

With increasing age, absolute CHD risk increases significantly as a result of the progressive accumulation of coronary atherosclerosis. For premenopausal women, endogenous estrogen may provide cardiac protection, and for women younger than 45 years of age, their likelihood for CHD is extremely low. Generally, a woman is considered postmenopausal after the age of 55 years; at this stage of a woman's life, absolute risk of CHD increases. For women, CHD development lags approx 10 years behind their male counterparts *(11)*. Differences exist in the age thresholds for men and women, where disease rates increase dramatically. The prevalence of the disease for men increases most significantly after the age of 45 years. Adding approx 10 years, the age threshold is more than 55 years of age for women. Women may further suffer an AMI as much as 20 years later than men *(11)*. On average, the majority of new-onset CHD occurs in women after the age of 65 years *(12)*. In particular, for women approaching menopause (average age = 51 years), the risk of heart disease and stroke begins to rise and continues to rise as age increases.

Advancing age is one of the strongest prognosticators for coronary artery disease (CAD) but can be confounded by the presence of other traditional and conditional risk factors and comorbid conditions. For example, in AMI presentation, women are at higher risk of complications and worsening survival. Despite this evidence, recent data from the National Registry of Myocardial Infarction 2 (NRMI-2) database reveal that younger women, because of differences in comorbidity, infarct severity, and management differences, may be at the highest risk *(10,13)*.

Tobacco Use

Tobacco use is the leading preventable cause of CHD in women, especially in those 50 years of age and younger *(14,15)*. Aggressive public health campaigns put forth over the last few decades have resulted in declining smoking rates for both women and men. However, the declining rate has been lower for women. Whereas 33.9% of women and 51.9% of men were smokers in 1965, 22% of women and 26.4% of men were smokers in 1998 *(14,15)*. Smoking prevalence is also affected by education level and ethnicity. For women with less than a high school education, the prevalence of smoking is threefold higher than for those with at least a college education *(14,15)*. The prevalence of female smokers in the Native American population is alarmingly high at 40.8%, nearly double that of non-Hispanic white and black women.

There appears to be a dose-dependent relationship between total tar consumption per day and risk of myocardial infarction (MI; *16*). As few as one to four cigarettes per day increases a patient's risk of fatal or nonfatal MI by as much as two- to threefold *(17)*. Several reports show an increased risk of first MI in female smokers when compared with male smokers *(18)*. There is also a well-established synergistic relative risk for women who smoke and also use oral contraceptives, including an elevated risk of thrombosis and CVD complications *(19)*. Clinicians should counsel female smokers to quit as smoking cessation decreases CVD morbidity and mortality *(17–21)*. One year after cessation, risk of MI decreases by 50% *(22)*, and in 10 years, the CVD rate approaches that of nonsmokers *(17,20)*.

Estrogen Loss and Hormone Therapy (HT)

As CHD prevalence increases for women in their postmenopausal years, the role of estrogen supplementation has been the focus of most research aimed at both primary and secondary prevention of CVD risk. In a woman's premenopausal years, estrogen levels are approx 10 times higher than that of an older-aged woman, which is accounted for primarily by the ovarian production of estrogen. Endogenous estrogen may serve to protect a woman's risk of CHD through higher levels of high-density lipoprotein (HDL) cholesterol, improved arterial compliance and coronary flow reserve, as well as improvements in global myocardial function responses to stress *(5,6,23,24)*.

During menopausal years, the gradual loss of ovarian estrogen production may make women more vulnerable to CHD. Although estrogen supplementation in post-menopausal years has been found to have favorable effects on lipid, glucose, and insulin levels *(24,25)*, it has also been found to increase levels of high sensitivity C-reactive protein (CRP), an inflammatory marker that is believed to be an independent predictor of CHD *(26)*. A more detailed discussion of HT is provided in Chapter 21. Currently, the AHA has cautioned against the use of HT for the purpose of primary and secondary prevention of CHD *(27)*. A key message from both the Heart and Estro-gen/Progestin Replacement Study (HERS) and Women's Health Initiative (WHI) studies is that the use of HT for CVD protection is ineffective, and for healthy lifestyles, physicians should focus on lifestyle changes (e.g., smoking cessation, dietary modifications, exercise) and interventional (i.e., therapeutic) risk reductions for the primary and secondary prevention of CVD.

For women currently taking HT, an individualized decision regarding continuation should include a discussion of the risks and benefits of treatment, but may also include the consideration of HT continuation if they are doing well and possibly for those women without other traditional risk factors and a low-risk high-sensitivity (Hs)-CRP *(27)*. The results from both studies are clear that postmenopausal women not taking any treatment should not start HT for the sole purpose of preventing CHD events *(28)*. Although data on cardiovascular effects in symptomatic women are limited, HT is still an accepted strategy for women with vasomotor symptoms.

Hypertension

Hypertension is considered to be a systolic blood pressure greater than 140 mm Hg and/or a diastolic number greater than 90 mm Hg *(29)*. Hypertension is a major risk factor for CHD, affecting one in four adult Americans *(30–36)*. For women, hypertension leading to diastolic dysfunction is a major cause of congestive heart failure, noted as the primary cause in 60% of cases of heart failure in women *(8)*. Generally, hypertension is more common in men than women, but the overall prevalence increases, being higher for women over the age of 55 years. There is gradual loss of arterial compliance with aging, such that blood pressure increases with age. For comparison, approximately one in two women are hypertensive prior to 45 years of age, whereas three of every four elderly women are hypertensive *(23,24)*.

Elevations in blood pressure increase a patient's risk of stroke as well as CHD. Recent evidence suggests that the relative risk for CHD death is increased twofold for white women with blood pressure measures that exceed 120/80 mm Hg when compared with white men *(33)*.

Although genetics do play a strong role in developing hypertension, modifiable and environmental factors can aid in blood pressure control. Initial steps to control hypertension include weight control and dietary changes. Particularly, dietary modifications as part of a primary prevention program should include the lowering of sodium intake and reduction in alcohol consumption as effective steps to lower blood pressure. For example, diets high in fruits and vegetables have been reported to lower blood pressure measures. Following initial care for weight control and dietary changes, some hypertensives may require drug therapy (e.g., beta blockers, diuretics, angiotensin-converting enzyme [ACE] inhibitors) to provide adequate blood pressure control.

Dyslipidemia

An estimated 100 million adult Americans have a total cholesterol value greater than or equal to 200 mg/dL, with approx 40% of this cohort having high-risk cholesterol measures of more than 240 mg/dL. Cholesterol values should be the average of at least two measurements from lipoprotein analysis *(37)*. Generally, men have higher average cholesterol values until the fifth decade of life, whereas after that, higher values are noted in women *(2,38–39)*. Recent statistics reveal that approx 40% of women over the age of 55 years have elevated total cholesterol values *(2)*. Women with total cholesterol levels of greater than or equal to 265 mg/dL have a two- to threefold increased CHD risk when compared to women with normal total cholesterol values.

For premenopausal women, endogenous estrogen is associated with higher HDL cholesterol values (e.g., >55 mg/dL). HDL cholesterol is significantly and inversely correlated with CHD. As women enter menopause, HDL cholesterol values decrease, and it is this loss of cardioprotection that is the rationale for the increasing disease prevalence in women after 55 years of age. Because of the higher rates of HDL cholesterol, some researchers have noted that a value of less than 50 mg/dL may be a differential high-risk threshold for women *(3)*. One of the best predictors for CHD risk in women is the ratio of total HDL cholesterol. A ratio of total cholesterol that is approximately four or more times that of HDL cholesterol is associated with an increase in CHD risk of fivefold when compared to those with normal cholesterol measures.

Elevated triglyceride levels appear to be a stronger risk factor for CHD in women than in men. Framingham study data reveal that individuals with triglyceride levels exceeding 150 mg/dL have an increased CHD risk greater than 1.5 *(39)*. Triglyceride values that exceed 350 mg/dL are associated with a twofold increased CHD risk. Although the exact role and mechanism that triglycerides play in the development of CAD is not yet completely understood, for women with elevated levels, it is important to reduce fat intake and restrict the intake of simple carbohydrates, as both can reduce triglyceride levels *(8)*.

Current cholesterol management has recently been published in the Third Report of the National Cholesterol Education Program (NCEP) Expert Panel on the detection, evaluation, and treatment of high blood cholesterol in adults *(3)*. Based on this recent guideline, the primary target of therapy is the lowering of low-density lipoprotein (LDL) cholesterol values. For primary prevention, optimal LDL cholesterol is less than 100 mg/dL. Despite this level being optimal, a woman's LDL treatment goal depends on her absolute risk of CHD (e.g., 10-year risk of death or MI). The higher the risk, the lower the LDL goal (e.g., LDL goals are <100, <130, and <160 md/dL for patients with diabetes or CHD, have two or more risk factors, or risk factor of one or less).

Certainly, initial clinical approaches to the management of women with elevated LDL cholesterol values include: reduced intake of saturated fat (<7% of total calories) and cholesterol (<200 mg/day), increased physical activity (or balance energy intake with expenditure), and weight control. Additionally, total fat intake should be restricted to 25–35% of total calories. Despite efforts at therapeutic lifestyle changes, there remain a number of patients whose cholesterol remains elevated. There are a number of over-the-counter drugs that exhibit cholesterol-lowering effects. The most commonly prescribed class of LDL-lowering drugs includes statins. The overall effects of this drug class includes 18–55% reduction in LDL cholesterol, 5–15% increase in HDL cholesterol, and 7–30% reduction in triglyceride levels. More modest effects have been noted for fibric acids, nicotinic acid, and bile acid sequesterants.

Statins are commonly prescribed for hyperlipidemia and have been extensively studied *(40)*. In the primary prevention setting, LDL-lowering drugs have been shown to reduce a woman's risk for major adverse cardiac events, including death from all causes and cardiovascular deaths *(40)*. Regarding statin use, LaRosa et al. found that the mean reduction (weighted by sample size) in total cholesterol, LDL cholesterol, and triglyceride levels was –20%, –28%, and –13%, respectively, and HDL cholesterol was increased by an average of 5% *(40)*. For women, a synthesis of this evidence reveals that the use of statins is associated with a significant reduction in cardiac events and, in many cases, reductions in all-cause mortality (Fig. 2). This evidence supports the effectiveness of cholesterol-lowering therapy with the use of statins to reduce CHD risk *(41–45)*.

Despite the effectiveness of this class of drugs for reducing a woman's risk for CHD events, a large percentage of women remain undertreated and/or do not meet the current NCEP III goals for optimal risk reduction *(46)*. However, it is clear that aggressive lipid-lowering should be integrated within a well-rounded primary prevention program to further reduce CHD risk *(47)*.

The Metabolic Syndrome

The metabolic syndrome represents a constellation that results from insulin resistance (with or without glucose intolerance), dyslipidemia (elevated triglycerides, small LDL particles, low HDL cholesterol), hypertension, and abdominal obesity that place an individual's CHD risk as intermediate between normal glucose homeostasis and diabetes *(48,49)*. The NCEP Adult Treatment Panel (ATP)-III has defined the metabolic syndrome in women by the presence of three or more of the following factors: (1) waist circumference larger than 88 cm, (2) fasting triglycerides of 150 mg/dL or above, (3) HDL cholesterol less than 50 mg/dL, (4) hypertension (systolic blood pressure ≥ 130 mm Hg, diastolic blood pressure ≥ 85 mm Hg or use of antihypertensive drug therapy), and (5) fasting glucose of ≥ 110 mg/dL or more. Patient management with the metabolic syndrome includes directed care at the underlying causes, including (at least initially) weight reduction and increased physical activity (ATP), to be followed by lipid control *(3)*.

Diabetes

Diabetes mellitus defined as fasting plasma glucose value of 126 md/dL or more is a major risk factor for CHD for both men and women *(50–54)*. Recent data form a Center for Disease Control (CDC) cross-sectional telephone survey showed a significant increase in the prevalence of diabetes in the US population from 4.9% in 1990 *(51)* to 7.3% in 2000 and 7.9% in 2001 *(55)*. In fact, some have noted that diabetes has become an epidemic in the United States as a result of marked increases in the majority of adults being overweight.

Because of an increased risk of death and prevalence for CHD, diabetes is now considered a coronary disease risk equivalent, based on the most recent NCEP III guidelines *(3)*. Diabetes is associated with an increased risk of fatal and nonfatal CVD events *(56)*. Nearly two out of three diabetics die of some type of CVD *(2,12,57)*. Often, type

Major Coronary Events by Sex

Trial	No. of Participants	No. of Major Coronary Events Placebo	Statin
Women			
4S,[1] 1994	827	91	60
CARE,[4,5] 1996	576	39	23
AFCAPS/TexCaps,[7] 1998	997	13	7
LIPID,[8] 1998	1516	104	90
Overall	**3916**	**247**	**180**
Men			
4S	3617	531	371
WOSCOPS,[3] 1995	6595	248	174
CARE	3583	235	189
AFCAPS/TexCaps	5608	170	109
LIPID	7498	611	467
Overall	**26901**	**1795**	**1310**

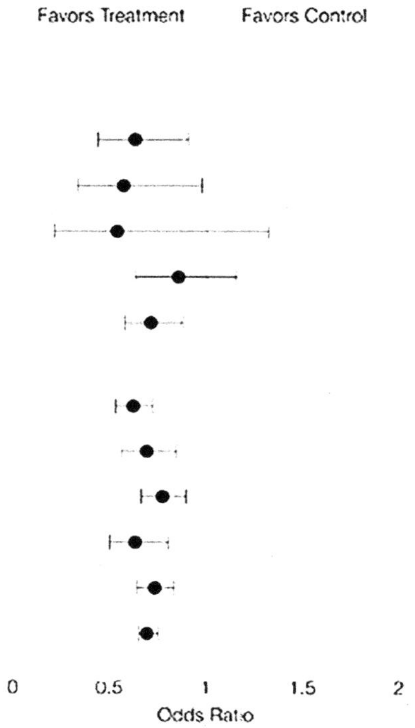

Favors Treatment
Favors Control
0
0.5
1
1.5
2
Odds Ratio

Fig. 2. Synthesis of this evidence reveals that the use of statins for women is associated with a significant reduction in cardiac events and often all-cause mortality.

Change in Total Body Fat (%)
2
1
0
-1
-2
-3
-4
-5
Control
Low
Intermediately
High

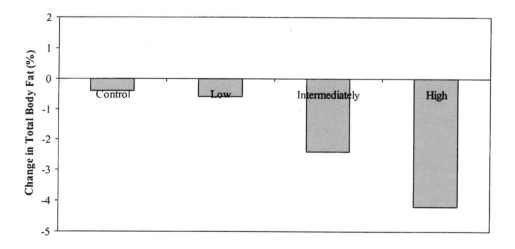

Fig. 3. Percent change in total body fat at 12 months by duration and change in fitness level. For this figure, low, intermediately, and highly active women are defined as ≤135, 136–195, and >195 minutes per week (p<0.05). (From ref. *60*.)

II diabetics have additional risk factors for CHD, including hypertension, hyperlipidemia, and obesity.

In numerous population-based studies, diabetic women have a three- to sevenfold increase in CHD death when compared to a two- to threefold increase in death for diabetic men *(2,38,58,59)*. Obesity is more often associated with mild glucose intolerance and higher CHD risk in women (AHA). In addition to CVD death, patients with diabetes often have subclinical disease, including atheromatous plaque in the carotid and femoral arteries, as well as measurable amounts of coronary calcium.

A key to effective blood glucose control is the maintenance of a diet low in saturated fats and cholesterol along with optimal weight control. Patients are also recommended to adopt a regular (monitored) aerobic exercise regimen as the risk of diabetes increases with increased weight and body mass index (BMI). For women, a BMI greater than 30 is associated with an increased risk for diabetes, hypertension, heart failure, as well as other major adverse cardiac events *(54)*. For diabetics, current guidelines (using secondary prevention goals) require aggressive risk factor reductions for blood glucose, cholesterol, and high blood pressure *(3)*. Optimal risk reduction strategies can be effective at reducing the risk of heart disease and its associated adverse sequelae.

A recent meta-analysis pooled all of the population-based studies to examine sex-related differences in CHD mortality between male and female diabetics *(59)*. These results were interesting in that unadjusted and age-adjusted summary odds ratios for death showed trends or significant differences by sex, whereas risk-adjusted results (i.e., controls for age, hypertension, total cholesterol, and smoking) revealed no gender difference in CHD mortality. For diabetic women, optimal control of comorbidity and other traditional risk factors can lead to effective risk reduction. As such, it is more often suboptimal control of other risk factors in women that may lead to higher CHD death rates, rather than any sex-related differences per se.

Obesity

There is a rising epidemic of obesity among US women, especially among minority populations. Approximately one in four women are classified as obese based on a BMI of 30 or more *(50,54)*. There is a linear relationship between BMI and mortality risk *(1)*. The relative risk for death is increased approx 30–50% for patients with a BMI equal to or greater than 30. Central obesity (i.e., >35 in.) is a risk factor for diabetes, hypertension, CHD, and worsening outcome. In order to maintain optimal body weight, patients have to achieve a balance between energy expenditures and food intake.

Obesity is closely linked with poor diet and the lack of physical activity. Consequently, overweight patients should be encouraged to engage in regular aerobic physical exercise and eat a well-balanced diet. In a recent randomized controlled trial of 173 sedentary, overweight, postmenopausal women (ages 50–75 years), moderate intensity aerobic exercise (45 minutes x 5 days per week for 12 months) resulted in reduced body weight and body fat. As measured by computed tomography, subcutaneous abdominal fat decreased by 29 g/cm^2. Furthermore, there was a significant dose response for greater body fat loss with increasing duration of exercise (see Fig. 3; *60*).

Table 1
Estimate of 10-Year Risk for Women (Framingham Risk Scores)

Age	Points
20–34	−7
35–39	−3
40–44	0
45–49	3
50–54	6
55–59	8
60–64	10
65–69	12
70–74	14
75–79	16

	Age				
	20–39	40–49	50–59	60–69	70–79
Total cholesterol					
<160	0	0	0	0	0
160–199	4	3	2	1	1
200–239	8	6	4	2	1
240–279	11	8	5	3	2
≥280	13	10	7	4	2

	Age				
	20–39	40–49	50–59	60–69	70–79
Nonsmoker	0	0	0	0	0
Smoker	9	7	4	2	1

HDL (mg/dL)	Points
≥60	−1
50–59	0
40–49	1
<40	2

Systolic BP (mm Hg)	If untreated	If treated
<120	0	0
120–129	1	3
130–139	2	4
140–159	3	5
≥160	4	6

(continues)

Table 1
(Continued)

Point total	10-Year risk %
<9	<1
9–12	1
13–14	2
15	3
16	4
17	5
18	6
19	8
20	11
21	14
22	17
23	22
24	27
≥25	≥30

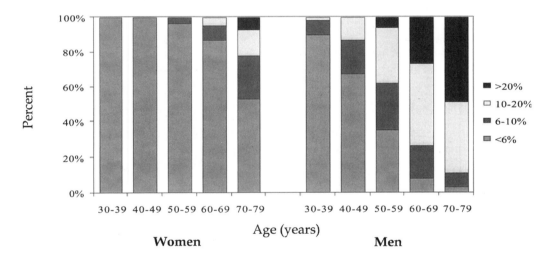

Fig. 4. Estimated 10-year hard CHD risk Framingham offspring and cohort men and women.

Global Risk Scores

There is a complex interplay between sex and traditional risk factors (as noted previously) with the frequency of risk factors resulting in a differential synergistic increase in CHD risk. As such, accounting for the global risk for major CHD events has become a central method to estimating a patient's likelihood for major adverse cardiac events (Table 1; 3). A commonly applied global risk score was developed based on the Framingham study participants and their offspring. Figure 4 details a recent analysis of the percent of low (<6% 10-year risk of cardiac death or MI) to high (>20% 10-year risk of cardiac death or MI) risk subsets of this study cohort in women and men across the age spectrum (1). A patient whose risk exceeds 20% is considered to be the equivalent of a

CHD patient (i.e., 2%/year risk of cardiac death or MI) with subsequent initiation of secondary prevention treatment strategies. Generally, across the ages, women are at lower risk than men. However, a woman's risk does increase by her 50s; such that, approx 5, 15, and 50% of women in their 50s, 60s, and 70s, accordingly, have an elevated risk of CHD events.

One challenge with using global risk scores (like using Framingham risk score) is that they explain less of the variance in outcome for women when compared to men *(1)*. In one recent example, coronary calcium, a measure of subclinical disease, was noted in 47% of women classified as low risk by the recent NCEP III guidelines *(61)*, which has led many investigators and clinicians to search for additional laboratory markers or imaging measures that may further delineate risk in women.

Emerging Risk Markers (Fig. 1)

Emerging risk markers include lipoprotein-a, homocysteine, prothrombotic factors, proinflammatory factors (i.e., hs-CRP), impaired fasting glucose, and subclinical atherosclerosis measures. hs-CRP is an acute-phase reactant marker for inflammation. CRP levels are elevated in patients with hypertension, smokers, impaired glucose tolerance patients, and obese patients *(62–64)*. Its ease, consistency, and measurement cost make it a very attractive marker for increased CVD risk. hs-CRP levels are generally higher in African-Americans and women. Interestingly, higher CRP levels are noted for women after the age of 12 or 13 years. As well, hs-CRP levels generally increase with age.

In the Women's Health Study, a prospective cohort of 30,000 middle-aged, predominantly postmenopausal American women CVD-free at study entry, the relative risk of future vascular events increased as the level of CRP went from low-normal to high-normal *(9,65)*, which was true for all cardiovascular events, as well as for the specific combined endpoint of MI or stroke. Figure 1 illustrates the 8-year event-free survival for hs-CRP and LDL values *(9)*. Despite the ability of hs-CRP to predict future events, it remains unclear whether it is a risk marker or a risk factor, and routine screening of all adults remains controversial *(66)*. Although there are several drugs that have been known to reduce hs-CRP, including aspirin *(67)* and statins *(68)*, it is not known if therapy should be altered as a result of the CRP level.

Measures of Subclinical Disease

Imaging markers of subclinical disease have examined the abnormalities of microvascular disease and function, including most commonly carotid-intima media thickness (C-IMT) or electron beam tomographic (EBT) measures of coronary calcium *(69,70)*. A number of reports have noted abnormal internal or common carotid thickness as a marker for increased CHD risk. Recent evidence from the Cardiovascular Health Study of elderly men and women revealed that internal carotid thickness and a carotid stenosis greater than 25% as a marker for diabetes *(71)*.

Another commonly applied procedure, electron beam computed tomography, measures coronary calcium. In the United States, approx 300,000 EBT procedures are performed annually in 79 centers *(72)*. Coronary calcium is common and increases with age; a high risk score (>400) ranges from 10% of a middle-aged women to approx 50% of elderly women *(73,74)*. Coronary calcium does not occur in a normal vessel wall, being a part of atherosclerosis development and occurs in advanced plaques. Coronary calcium is considered a marker for plaque burden, where scores range from 0 to greater than 1000. Age and gender percentile scores have been established *(75,76)*. Recent evidence suggests that because of smaller body surface area and arterial size, the relative risk associated with dying may be greater for every extent of coronary calcium in women when compared with men *(70)*. That is, a coronary calcium score of 100 in a woman has similar mortality risk to that of a man with a score of 400. These results suggest that lower thresholds for risk-reducing therapies may have to be implemented for women with measurable calcium amounts, although precise treatment strategies have yet to be elucidated.

BARRIERS TO PREVENTION

Primary prevention strategies have been shown to be highly effective to reduce both the incidence and recurrence of cardiac events in women. However, in a recent report using the National Ambulatory Care Survey conducted by the CDC, women were found to be less often counseled about diet, exercise, smoking cessation, and weight reduction *(77,78)*. Suboptimal treatment for women also includes lower rates of using beta blockers, aspirin, statins, antiarrhythmic therapies, as well as an underuse of cardiac catheterization, percutaneous coronary interventions, and coronary bypass surgery *(79–83)*.

The issue of optimal primary prevention is complex and includes a variety of matters, e.g., patient compliance, physician factors like physician gender, access, and organizational barriers, along with ethnic and societal barriers that may affect women in particular. The knowledge gap for women and their understanding of CHD and its associated risk factors (especially modifiable risk factors) is of primary importance. Interestingly, women perceive and rate barriers to making healthy lifestyle changes quite differently than men *(84)*. Women should be encouraged to participate in further clinical research that provides a better understanding of any sex-related differences and provides a venue for improved diagnostic and treatment strategies for CHD, because historically, women have constituted only a very small portion of CVD clinical trials.

CONCLUSION

A large number of differences in risk-factor prevalence and outcome, as well as in the global risk scores, exist between men and women. Generally, women have a greater degree of comorbidity, an older age of presentation, and a risk-factor burden, which play important roles in clinical outcomes (especially for younger women). A compilation of evidence suggests that there is sex-related variation in the interplay of risk factors; hormonal factors, and disease burden that further impact on outcome.

Much of our current health care system is based on a reactive approach to care. Optimal risk reduction requires a more proactive and preventive approach to care. For optimal prevention, the aim of a healthy lifestyle is to prevent the future evolution of cardiac risk factors, including an annual examination for men and women at or following their age of increasing disease prevalence (i.e., >55 years of age). The examination should check blood pressure, blood glucose, and cholesterol levels, etc. Women should know their own risk factors and develop a rapport with their doctor for optimal interchanges about hurdles in lifestyle changes. Generally, this examination should have some measure of global risk, where higher risk women are targeted for more aggressive management, resulting in long-term proportional risk reduction.

Using this tenet, resources and programs can then be allocated to higher risk patients, which leads to a greater degree of risk reduction. Low-risk patients should be encouraged to maintain healthy lifestyles that can prevent them from becoming high risk. A large body of evidence suggests the rate-limiting step for prevention is the implementation of risk-factor modification and the utilization of laboratory and other diagnostic tests that identify a high-risk female population. Optimal utilization of risk scores, identification and management of risk factors, provides the platform for reducing a large percentage of the population attributable risk for CHD in women.

REFERENCES

1. Pasternak RC, Abrams J, Greenland P, et al. Identification of CHD and CHD Risk: Is there a detection gap? J Am Coll Cardiol 2003; 41:1863–1874.
2. American Heart Association. 2003 Heart and Stroke Update. American Heart Association, Dallas, TX, 2002.
3. http:/www.nhlbi.nih.gov/guidelines/cholesterol/atp3xsum.pdf. Framingham risk score: access date: July 2002.
4. Women and Cardiovascular Disease: AHA Biostatistical Fact Sheet.
5. Mosca L, Grundy SM, Judelson D, et al. Guide to preventive cardiology for women. AHA/ACC Scientific Statement Consensus panel statement. Circulation 1999;99:2480–2484.
6. Mosca L, Manson JE, Sutherland SE, et al. Cardiovascular disease in women: a statement for healthcare professionals from the American Heart Association. Writing Group. Circulation 1997;96:2468–2482.
7. Mosca L, Jones WK, King KB, et al. Awareness, perception, and knowledge of heart disease risk and prevention among women in the United States. American Heart Association Women's Heart Disease and Stroke Campaign Task Force. Arch Fam Med 2000;9:506–515.
8. Mosca L. Epidemiology and prevention of coronary artery disease. In: Humes D, ed. Kelley's Textbook of Internal Medicine, 4th Edition. Lippincot, Williams and Wilkins Philadelphia, PA, 2000, pp. 182–191.
9. Ridker PM, Rifai N, Rose L, et al. Comparison of C-reactive protein and low-density lipoprotein cholesterol levels in the prediction of first cardiovascular events. N Engl J Med 2002;347:1557–1565.
10. Vaccarino V, Parsons L, Every NR, et al. Sex-based differences in early mortality after myocardial infarction. National Registry of Myocardial Infarction 2 Participants. N Engl J Med 1999;341:217–225.
11. Lerner DJ, Kannel WB. Patterns of coronary heart disease morbidity and mortality in the sexes: a 26-year follow-up of the Framingham population. Am Heart J 1986;111:383–390.
12. Grundy SM, Balady GJ, Criqui MH, et al. Primary prevention of coronary heart disease: guidance from Framingham: a statement for healthcare professionals from the AHA Task Force on Risk Reduction. American Heart Association. Circulation 1998;97:1876–1887.
13. Ayanian JZ. Increased mortality among middle-aged women after myocardial infarction: searching for mechanisms and solutions. Ann Int Med 2001;134:239–241.
14. Women and smoking: a report of the surgeon general. Executive summary. MMRW 2002;51:1–30.
15. Tobacco use-United States, 1900–1999. MMWR 1999;48:986–993.
16. Sauer WH, Berlin JA, Strom BL, et al. Cigarette yield and the risk of myocardial infarction in smokers. Arch Intern Med 2002;162:300–306.
17. Willett WC, Green A, Stampfer MJ, et al. Relative and absolute excess risks of coronary heart disease among women who smoke cigarettes. N Engl J Med 1987;317:1303–1309.
18. Nyboe J, Jensen G, Appleyard M, Schnohr P. Smoking and risk of first acute myocardial infarction. Am Heart J 1991;122:438–447.
19. Castelli WP. Cardiovascular disease: pathogenesis, epidemiology, and risk among users of oral contraceptives who smoke. Am J Ob Gyn 1999;180:S349–S356.
20. LaCroix AZ, Lang J, Scherr P, et al. Smoking and mortality among older men and women in three communities. N Engl J Med 1991;324:1619–1625.

21. Kawachi I, Colditz GA, Stampfer MJ, et al. Smoking cessation in relation to total mortality rates in women. A prospective cohort study. Ann Intern Med 1993;119:992–1000.
22. Rich-Edwards JW, Manson JE, Hennekens CH, et al. The primary prevention of coronary heart disease in women. N Engl J Med 1995;332:1758–1766.
23. Mosca L, Grundy SM, Judelson D, et al. AHA/ACC scientific statement: consensus panel statement. Guide to preventive cardiology for women. American Heart Association/American College of Cardiology. J Am Coll Cardiol 1999;33:1751–1755.
24. Mosca L. The role of hormone replacement therapy in the prevention of postmenopausal heart disease. Arch Int Med 2000;160:2263–2272.
25. Mendelsohn ME, Karas RH. The protective effects of estrogen on the cardiovascular system. N Engl J Med 1999;340:1801–1811.
26. Cushman M, Legault C, Barrett-Connor E, et al. Effect of postmenopausal hormones on inflammation-sensitive proteins: the Postmenopausal Estrogen/Progestin Interventions (PEPI) Study. Circulation 1999;100:717–722.
27. Mosca L, Collins P, Herrington DM, et al. American Heart Association. Hormone replacement therapy and cardiovascular disease: a statement for healthcare professionals from the American Heart Association. Circulation 2001;104:499–503.
28. Writing Group for the Women's Health Initiative Investigators. Risks and benefits of estrogen plus progestin in healthy postmenopausal women: principal results From the Women's Health Initiative randomized controlled trial. JAMA 2002;288:321–333.
29. Wilansky S. Pathophysiology, clinical recognition, therapy, and prevention of hypertension. In: Wilansky S, Willerson JT, eds. Heart Disease in Women. Churchill Livingstone, New York, NY, 2000, pp. 339–341.
30. Stokes J III, Kannel WB, Wolf PA, et al. The relative importance of selected risk factors for various manifestations of cardiovascular disease wmong men and women from 35 to 64 years old: 30 years of follow-up in the Framingham Study. Circulation 1987;75:V-64–V-73.
31. Stokes J III, Kannel WB, Wolf PA, et al. Blood pressure as a risk factor for cardiovascular disease: the Framingham Study-30 years of follow-up. Hypertension 1989;13:I-13–I-18.
32. Kannel WB. Blood pressure as a cardiovascular risk factor: prevention and treatment. JAMA 1996;275:1571–1576.
33. Stamler J. Blood pressure and high blood pressure: aspects of risk. Hypertension 1991;18:I-95–I-107.
34. Burt VL, Whelton P, Roccella EJ, et al. Prevalence of hypertension in the US adult population. Results from the Third National Health and Nutrition Examination Survey, 1988–1991. Hypertension 1995;25:305–313.
35. Hayes SN, Taler SJ. Hypertension in women: current understanding of gender differences. Mayo Clin Proceedings 1998;73:157–165.
36. Stamler J, Stamler R, Neaton JD. Blood pressure, systolic and diastolic, and cardiovascular risks. US population data. Arch Int Med 1993;153:598–615.
37. hin.nhlbi.nih.gov/atpiii/calculator.asp?usertype=prof. Framingham risk score: access date: July 2002.
38. Kannel WB. Metabolic risk factors for coronary heart disease in women: perspective from the Framingham Study. Am Heart J 1987;114:413–419.
39. Castelli WP. Cholesterol and lipids in the risk of coronary artery disease—the Framingham Heart Study. Can J Cardiol 1988; (4 Suppl) A:5A-10A.
40. LaRosa JC, He J, Vupputuri S. Effect of statins on risk of coronary disease: a meta-analysis of randomized controlled trials. JAMA 1999;282:2340–2346.
41. Sacks FM, Pfeffer MA, Moye LA, et al. The effect of pravastatin on coronary events after myocardial infarction in patients with average cholesterol levels. Cholesterol and Recurrent Events Trial Investigators. N Engl J Med 1996;35:1001–1009.
42. Lipid Study Group. Prevention of cardiovascular events and a broad range of initial cholesterol levels. The Long-Term Intervention with Pravastatin in Ischemic Disease (LIPID) Study Group. N Engl J Med 1998;339:1349–1357.
43. Scandinavian Simvastatin Survival Study. Randomized trial of cholesterol lowering in 4444 patients with coronary heart disease: the Scandinavian Simvastatin Survival Study. Lancet 1994;344:1383.
44. Shepherd J, Cobbe SM, Ford I, et al. Prevention of coronary heart disease with pravastatin in men with hypercholesterolemia. West of Scotland Coronary Prevention Study Group. N Engl J Med 1995;333:1301–1307.

45. Downs JR, Clearfield M, Weis S, et al. Primary prevention of acute coronary events with lovastatin in men and women with average cholesterol levels: Results of AFCAPS/TexCAPS. Air Force/Texas Coronary Atherosclerosis Prevention Study. JAMA 1998;279:1615–1622.

46. Schrott HG, Bittner V, Vittinghoff E, et al. Adherence to National Cholesterol Education Program Treatment goals in postmenopausal women with heart disease. The Heart and Estrogen/Progestin Replacement Study (HERS). The HERS Research Group. JAMA 1997;277:1281–1286.

47. LaRosa JC. The role of diet and exercise in the statin era. Prog Cardiovasc Dis 1998;41:137–150.

48. Lakka H-M, Laaksonen DE, Lakka TA, et al. The Metabolic Syndrome and Total and Cardiovascular Mortality in middle aged men. JAMA 2002;288:2709–2716.

49. Isomaa B, Almgren P, Tuomi T, et al. Cardiovascular morbidity and mortality associated with the metabolic syndrome. Diabetes Care 2001;24:683–689.

50. Winkleby MA, Pudaric S. Cardiovascular disease risk factors among older black, Mexican-American, and white women and men: an analysis of NHANES III, 939 women1988–1994. Third National Health and Nutrition Examination Survey. J Am Ger Soc 2001;49:109–116.

51. Anonymous. Preventive Cardiology: How can we do Better? Proceedings of the 33rd Bethesda Conference. December 18, 2001, Bethesda, MD. J Am Coll Cardiol 2002;40;580–651.

52. Goraya TY. Leibson CL. Palumbo PJ. Coronary atherosclerosis in diabetes mellitus: a population-based autopsy study. J Am Coll Cardiol 2002;40:946–953.

53. Ledru F, Ducimetiere P, Battaglia S, et al. New diagnostic criteria for diabetes and coronary artery disease: insights from an angiographic study. J Am Coll Cardiol 2001;37:1543–1550.

54. Poehlman ET. Menopause, energy expenditure, and body composition. Acta Obst Gynecol Scand 2002;81:603–611.

55. Mokdad AH, Ford ES, Bowman BA, et al. Prevalence of obesity, diabetes, and obesity-related health risk factors, 2001. JAMA 2003;289:76–79.

56. Orlander PR. Diabetes mellitus. In: Wilansky S, Willerson JT, eds. Heart Disease in Women. Churchill Livingstone, New York, NY, 2000, pp. 102–119.

57. Bakris GL. Williams M. Dworkin L, et al. Preserving renal function in adults with hypertension and diabetes: a consensus approach. National Kidney Foundation Hypertension and Diabetes Executive Committees Working Group. Am J Kid Dis 2000;36:646–661.

58. Orchard TJ, Forrest KY, Ellis D, Becker DJ. Cumulative glycemic exposure and microvascular complications in insulin-dependent diabetes mellitus. The glycemic threshold revisited. Arch Int Med 1997;157:1851–1856.

59. Kanaya AM, Grady D, Barrett-Connor E. Explaining the sex difference in coronary heart disease mortality among patients with type 2 diabetes mellitus: a meta-analysis. Arch Int Med 2002;162:1737–1745.

60. Irwin ML, Yasui Y, Ulrich CM, Bowan D, et al. Effect of exercise on total and intra-abdominal body fat in post-menopausal women. JAMA 2003;289:323–330.

61. Hecht HS, Superko HR. Electron beam tomography and National Cholesterol. Education Program guidelines in asymptomatic women. J Am Coll Cardiol 2001;37:1506–1511.

62. Festa A, D'Agostino R Jr., Howard G, et al. Chronic subclinical inflammation as part of the insulin resistance syndrome: the Insulin Resistance Atherosclerosis Study (IRAS). Circulation 2000;102:42–47.

63. Tracy RP, Psaty BM, Macy E, et al. Lifetime smoking exposure affects the association of C-reactive protein with cardiovascular disease risk factors and subclinical disease in healthy elderly subjects. Art Thromb Vasc Biol 1997;17:2167–2176.

64. Redberg RF, Rifai N, Gee L, Ridker PM. Lack of association of C-reactive protein and coronary calcium by electron beam computed tomography in postmenopausal women: implications for coronary artery disease screening. J Am Coll Cardiol 2000;36:39–43.

65. Ridker PM, Buring JE, Shih J, et al. Prospective study of C-reactive protein and the risk of future cardiovascular events among apparently healthy women. Circulation 1998;98:731–733.

66. Mosca L. C-reactive protein—to screen or not to screen? N Engl J Med 2002;347:1615–1617.

67. Ridker PM, Cushman M, Stampfer MJ, et al. Inflammation, aspirin, and the risk of cardiovascular disease in apparently healthy men. N Engl J Med 1997;336:973–979.

68. Ridker PM, Rifai N, Pfeffer MA, et al. Inflammation, pravastatin, and the risk of coronary events after myocardial infarction in patients with average cholesterol levels. Cholesterol and Recurrent Events (CARE) Investigators. Circulation 1998;98:839–844.

69. Wong TY, Klein R, Sharrett AR, et al. Retinal arteriolar narrowing and risk of coronary heart disease in men and women. The Atherosclerosis Risk in Communities Study. JAMA 2002;287:1153–1159.

70. Shaw LJ, Raggi P, Berman DS, Callister TQ. Gender differences in the prognostic value of coronary calcium. World Congress of Cardiology 2002, Sydney, Australia.

71. Barzilay JI, Spiekerman CF, Kuller LH, et al. The Cardiovascular Health Study. Prevalence of clinical and isolated subclinical cardiovascular disease in older adults with glucose disorders: the Cardiovascular Health Study. Diabetes Care 2001;24:1233–1239.

72. Mark DB, Shaw LJ, Lauer MS, et al. Bethesda Conference #34 – Task Force 5: Is Atherosclerosis Imaging Cost Effective? J Am Coll Cardiol 2003; 41:1906–1917.

73. Newman AB, Naydeck BL, Sutton-Tyrrell K, et al. Coronary artery calcification in older adults to age 99: prevalence and risk factors. Circulation 2001;104:2679–2684.

74. Shaw LJ, Raggi P, Schisterman E, et al. Prognostic value of cardiac risk factors and coronary artery calcium screening for all cause mortality. Radiol, in press.

75. Wong ND, Budoff MJ, Pio J, Detrano RC. Coronary calcium and cardiovascular event risk: evaluation by age- and sex-specific quartiles. Am Heart J 2002;143:456–459.

76. Hoff JA, Chomka EV, Krainik AJ, et al. Age and gender distributions of coronary artery calcium detected by electron beam tomography in 35,246 adults. Am J Cardiol 2001;87:1335–1339.

77. Health United States, 1998 with Socioeconomic Status and Health Chartbook. www.cdc.gov/nchs. National Center for Health Statistics, Hyattsville, MD, 1998.

78. Missed Opportunities in preventative counseling for cardiovascular disease: United States 1995. MMWR Morb Mortal Wkly Rep 1998;47:91–95.

79. Stafford RS. Aspirin use is low among United States outpatients with coronary artery disease. Circulation 2000;101:1097–1101.

80. Shaw LJ, Miller DD, Romeis JC, et al. Gender differences in the noninvasive evaluation and management of patients with suspected coronary artery disease. Ann Int Med 1994;120:559–566.

81. Bowling A, Bond M, McKee D, et al. Equity in access to exercise tolerance testing, coronary angiography, and coronary artery bypass grafting by age, sex, and clinical indications. Heart 2001;85:860–866.

82. Battleman DS. Callahan M. Gender differences in utilization of exercise treadmill testing: a claims-based analysis. J Healthcare Qual 2001;23:38–41.

83. Rathore SS, Chen J, Wang Y, et al. Sex differences in cardiac catheterization: the role of physician gender. JAMA 2001;286:2849–2856.

84. Mosca L, McGillen C, Rubenfire M. Gender differences in barriers to lifestyle change for cardiovascular disease prevention. J Wom Health 1998;7:711–715.

5

Early Detection of Coronary Artery Disease in Women

Role of Coronary Artery Calcium Scanning With EBT

John A. Rumberger, PhD, MD, FACC

CONTENTS

INTRODUCTION

The total number of men who develop clinically manifested heart disease during their lifetime is greater than that number diagnosed in women, but currently more women die as a result of coronary artery disease (CAD) than men. It has been estimated that 63% of these deaths occur in women who had no antemortem CAD diagnosis.

The following general facts have been established: (1) women develop CAD symptoms later than men (average of 10 years); (2) chest pain is generally a poor predictor of epicardial coronary disease in women; and (3) women often have more extensive disease than their male counterparts when they do develop symptoms, thus their overall prognosis at presentation is worse than men.

The incidence of coronary disease in women increases dramatically after menopause, and this is *not* necessarily established in the traditional Framingham risk assessment, which places chronologic age as the most powerful risk factor, but considers female sex (regardless of age) as a separate and "negative" risk factor. Elevated total serum cholesterol is another important cardiovascular risk, but a high-density lipoprotein (HDL) cholesterol of more than 60 mg/dL is considered a "negative" (i.e.,

From: *Contemporary Cardiology: Coronary Disease in Women: Evidence-Based Diagnosis and Treatment*
Edited by: L. J. Shaw and R. F. Redberg © Humana Press Inc., Totowa, NJ

beneficial) for the whole population. However, there is emerging evidence that suggests this may not always be true for women *(1)*.

Many cardiologists therefore suggest that clinicians consider testing women on an individual basis for signs of subclinical atherosclerosis, rather than relying on traditional broad-based population National Cholesterol Education Program (NCEP) or Framingham "risk equations" to identify those at greatest risk. Current and emerging measures for clinicians to predict coronary plaque burden generally involve direct imaging of the vascular system, including direct coronary angiography, ultrasonography (carotid, peripheral, and intravascular), and quantification of coronary artery calcium by electron beam tomography (EBT).

Coronary artery calcium is intimately associated with mural atheromatous plaque *(2–6)*. A direct relationship has been established between coronary artery calcium as measured by EBT and both histologic *(7,8)* and in vivo intravascular ultrasound *(9,10)* measures of atherosclerotic plaque on a heart-by-heart, vessel-by-vessel, and segment-by-segment basis. Additionally, there is increasing evidence that the common clinical measure of coronary calcium by EBT, the "calcium score" *(11)*, has a significant predictive value for subsequent cardiac events in both symptomatic and asymptomatic patients *(12–16)*, having predictive value over and above the traditional risk factors *(15)*. The following discussion examines the role of EBT in the diagnosis of CAD in women.

CORONARY ARTERY CALCIUM

General Pathology of Coronary Calcium

Atherosclerosis is the only disease known to be associated with coronary calcification *(2,3,6)*. Recent studies have shown that calcium can be seen in all degrees of atherosclerotic involvement and is an active process *(17–20)*.

Coronary calcification is common in patients with known CAD *(21–25)*, being strongly related to age and increasing dramatically after age 50 *(23–25)*. McCarthy *(21)* studied 65 consecutive autopsy-derived hearts (death not necessarily of cardiac causes) and found 63% to have some coronary artery calcification, nearly always associated with a degree of luminal CAD. Of the coronary arteries studied from patients older than 60 years, 94% demonstrated some degree of calcification. In a series of 360 (living) patients undergoing cardiac catheterization and coronary fluoroscopy, Bartel *(26)* found a 43% prevalence of calcification, and roughly 60% of patients studied over age 60 had some calcification as noted by fluoroscopic examination. In a separate study of individuals from the general population not known to have coronary disease, the calcification prevalence by fluoroscopy has been reported to be roughly 20% *(24)*. Because Faber *(27)* noted in 1912 that Mönckeberg's calcific medial sclerosis does not occur in the coronary arteries, atherosclerosis is the only vascular disease known to be associated with coronary calcification.

Many reports relate the amount of coronary calcification to the severity of stenoses. For example, in the autopsy series mentioned previously *(21)*, significant stenosis and/or occlusion was virtually certain if calcification was present in segments longer than 1 cm. This link has been borne out by other studies as well *(2,3,28)*. Hamby *(29)* found that 81% of patients with angiographic two- or three-vessel disease had coronary artery calcification. Mintz et al. *(30)* studied 110 men and women undergoing coronary angioplasty for symptomatic CAD. The presence of target lesion calcification was identified in 75% of these individuals using intravascular ultrasound.

Coronary remodeling associated with the development and progression of athero-sclerotic disease is a recently described phenomena, whereby the luminal cross-sectional area and/or external vessel dimensions enlarge in compensation for increasing areas of mural plaque *(31)*. Coronary artery calcium is an intimate component of some plaques. In a histopathology investigation, Clarkson *(32)* has shown that plaques with microscopic evidence of mineralization were much larger and were associated with much larger coronary arteries than those sections without microscopic evidence of calcification; this was true in humans and in nonhuman primates. The compensatory enlargement of atherosclerotic coronary segments may explain why coronary angiography frequently underestimates the severity of coronary disease when compared with histopathological studies. Studies that attempt to correlate the site and amount of coronary calcium with percent luminal narrowing at the same anatomic site have shown a positive but nonlinear relationship with large confidence limits *(7)*. However, coronary plaque and its associated coronary calcification may have only a poor correlation with the extent of histopathological stenosis *(32,33)*, which, in turn, is largely accounted for because of individual variations in coronary artery remodeling. On the other hand, *in situ* coronary calcium is associated with plaque size *(33)*.

A study by Rumberger et al. *(8)* emphasized that the total area of coronary artery calcification is correlated in a linear fashion with the total area of coronary artery plaque on a segmental, individual, and whole coronary artery system basis. However, the areas of coronary calcification were on the order of one fifth that of the associated coronary plaque. Additionally, there were clear plaque areas without associated coronary calcium as detected with EBT. These data suggest that there may be a coronary plaque size most commonly associated with coronary calcium but, in the smaller plaques, the calcium is either not present or is undetectable. However, coronary plaque disease is a diffuse process; although calcium may not be seen in one particular area, if the overall plaque burden is sufficient, coronary artery calcium will be identified.

Molecular Biology of Coronary Calcium

Calcium phosphate (in the hydroxyapatite form) and cholesterol accumulate in atherosclerotic lesions. Circulating proteins that are normally associated with bone remodeling play an important role in coronary calcification. Although the true role of calcium in the atherosclerotic process is unknown, within the past several years, new insights into the pathophysiology of coronary calcification have developed. Fitzpatrick et al. *(34)* used *in situ* hybridization to identify mRNA of matrix proteins that are associated with mineralization in coronary artery specimens. Specifically, they identified a cell attachment protein (osteopontin) from autopsy coronary artery specimens, which is a protein associated with calcium (osteonectin) and a gamma carboxylated protein that regulates mineralization (osteocalcin). Similar studies have shown that osteopontin can be seen in tissue that demonstrates atherosclerotic involvement and appears to be present only in sites of concomitant coronary atherosclerotic disease. Hirota et al. *(19)* demonstrated by Northern blotting that osteopontin mRNA expression is related to the severity of atherosclerosis. Additionally, osteonectin mRNA expression decreased with atherosclerosis development. Shanahan *(20)* and Ideda *(18)* have independently demonstrated that the predominant cell types in these areas are macrophage-derived foam cells, although some smooth muscle cells were also identified. Finally, Bostrom et al. *(17)* recently identified bone morphogenetic protein-2a, a potent factor for osteoblastic differentiation in calcified human atherosclerotic plaque. Cultured cells from the vascular wall formed calcified nodules similar to those found in bone cell cultures. The predominant cells in these nodules had immunocytochemical features characteristic of microvascular pericytes, which are capable of osteoblastic differentiation. These findings suggest that arterial calcium in atherosclerosis is a regulated process similar to bone formation, rather than a passive precipitation of calcium phosphate crystals.

In summary, recent studies have confirmed that arterial calcium development is intimately associated with vascular injury and atherosclerotic plaque evolution, being largely controlled by common cellular and subcellular mechanisms. Calcium can be seen in all degrees of atherosclerotic involvement and is an active process; thus, the long-held notion of so-called *degenerative* calcification of the coronary arteries with aging is incorrect. Although there is an increasing incidence of coronary calcification in patients, as one grows older, this simply parallels the increased incidence of coronary atherosclerosis with advancing age.

OVERVIEW OF ELECTRON BEAM COMPUTED TOMOGRAPHY

Although it has been clinically available for nearly 20 years, EBT (also referred to as Ultrafast-CT, Imatron Inc., South San Francisco, CA) employs unique technology that enables ultrafast scan acquisition times of 50–100 ms per slice. EBT is distinguished by the use of a scanning electron beam, rather than a traditional X-ray tube and mechanical rotation device used in current spiral scanners. The electron beam (cathode) is steered by an electromagnetic deflection system that sweeps the beam across the distant anode, a series of fixed tungsten target rings. Thus, as opposed to physically moving the X-ray tube in a circle about the patient, as is done by the so-called "subsecond" mechanical computed tomography (CT) scanners, only the electron beam is moved in EBT. Current mechanical CT systems take images with scanning 3–10 times slower than EBT and may or may not also use retrospective gating of images and postprocessing to attempt to mathematically or visually reduce cardiac motion artifacts. There are very few studies published with the use of these mechanical scanners, and their information is generally considered by experts in cardiac CT to be limited regarding the reliable quantification of coronary artery calcium scores. The following discussions apply only to the EBT imaging system.

Standardized methods for the imaging, identification, and quantification of coronary artery calcium using EBT have been established *(6)*. The scanner is operated in the high-resolution, single-slice mode with continuous nonoverlapping slices of 3-mm thickness and an acquisition time of 100 ms per tomogram. Patients are positioned supine and, after localization of the main pulmonary artery, a sufficient number of tomographic slices are obtained to cover the complete heart through the left ventricular apex (usually 36–40 slices). Electrocardiographic triggering is done at the end-diastole at the prespecified phase of the relative risk (RR) interval, determined from the continuous electrocardiogram (ECG) recording. The presence of coronary calcium is sequentially evaluated in all levels. Coronary calcium is defined as a hyperattenuating lesion above a threshold of 130 "Hounsfield Units," with an area of three or more adjacent pixels (at least 1 mm². CT Hounsfield Unit densities range from −1000 [air],

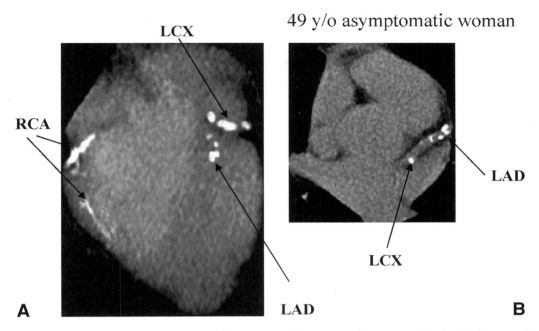

Fig. 1. Noncontrast EBT of a 49-year-old asymptomatic woman with an extensive family history of premature coronary disease. (**A**) A single tomogram at the heart base showing prominent calcification in the left anterior descending (LAD) and left circumflex (LCX) arteries. (**B**) A three-dimensional volume rendering that shows the extent of calcification in both the LAD and LCX. Additionally, there is prominent calcification of the proximal, mid, and distal (lower arrow) right coronary arteries (RCA) evident when the entire scan set was reviewed.

through 0 [water], and up to +1000 [dense cortical bone]). Figure 1 shows a representative EBT tomogram at the base of the heart, demonstrating ossification of mural arterial segments in the left anterior descending coronary artery, left circumflex, and right coronary arteries of 49-year-old women with normal lipids, but family history or premature CAD. To the right of the figure is also a three-dimensional rendering that shows the coronary calcium extent in several vascular beds. The *calcium score (6,11)* is a product of the area of calcification per coronary segment and a factor rated 1–4 dictated by the maximum calcium CT density within that segment. A calcium score is reported for a given coronary artery and for the entire coronary system; however, most research studies have reported data related to the sum or total score for the entire epicardial coronary system.

CORONARY ARTERY CALCIUM BY EBT AND CORONARY DISEASE

Coronary Calcium, EBT, and Estimates of Atherosclerotic Plaque Burden

A fundamental requirement for the use of EBT coronary calcium quantification to define coronary artery plaque is to establish how these two measures relate to each other. Additionally, the potential for fundamental differences in plaque determination by EBT between men and women must be established before broad clinical application.

My colleagues and I initially examined random autopsy hearts and compared coronary calcium measures using EBT when compared with direct histologic plaque areas and percent luminal stenosis (8,35,36). This study determined that the total area of coronary artery calcification quantified by EBT is linearly correlated ($r = 0.90$), with the total area of histologic coronary artery plaque. Here, although the total atherosclerotic plaque burden was tracked by the total calcium burden, not all plaque was found to be calcified, and the total calcium area was approx 20% of the total atherosclerotic plaque area. An article by Baumgart et al. (9) compared direct intracoronary ultrasound measures during angiography with EBT scanning and confirmed a direct association of coronary calcium score with the localization and extent of atherosclerotic plaques in vivo.

Our original autopsy study evaluating EBT consisted of 13 hearts (5 women and 8 men). In this study, the three major epicardial arteries were dissected, each artery straightened and scanned using EBT in contiguous 3-mm thick cross-sections. After imaging, histologic sections were prepared at corresponding intervals, and luminal area obstruction was determined by planimetry. A total of 522 (182 female and 340 male) histologic specimens were examined and paired with corresponding EBT scans. Receiver-operating characteristic (ROC) analysis was used to define site specificity of calcium area for luminal area narrowing by atherosclerosis (36). ROC curve areas for segmental EBT calcium and prediction of mild (maximum lumen stenosis <50% diameter narrowing), moderate (maximum stenosis at least 50% diameter narrowing), and severe (maximum stenosis at least 75% diameter narrowing) were 0.712, 0.843, and 0.857 for women and 0.732 ($p = $ NS), 0.793 ($p = $ NS), and 0.841 ($p = $ NS) for men, respectively. Curves relating false-positive rate sclerotic narrowing vs EBT-quantified coronary calcium area were curvilinear. Examples of those data for women are shown in Fig. 2. Figure 2A is the ROC curve for women based on calcium area and the presence in the same histologic region of varying luminal stenoses. Figure 2B represents the linear measure of the calcium area in a given histologic section and the false-positive rate (defined as 1-specificity). In both men and women, an EBT measured coronary calcium area of 1 mm^2 in any histologic specimen gave a false-positive rate of 0%. For both men and women, a segmental calcium area of 2.0–2.5 mm^2 by EBT showed no false-positives for the presence of moderate coronary stenoses, whereas a segmental EBT calcium area of 3.0–3.5 mm^2 was positively associated with the presence of severe luminal disease at the same anatomic site.

Angiographic Correlates

The direct pathological study noted previously thus suggested that coronary artery calcium defined by EBT had similar predictive values for similar extents of coronary disease, regardless of sex. The next step was then to assess the effect of patient sex on EBT studies done in patients undergoing direct coronary angiography.

We studied 50 women and 89 men who had EBT scans done 1 day after cardiac catheterization. The women were roughly a decade older than the men, but were matched for clinical indications for angiography and luminal disease extent as confirmed by angiography. Sixteen women (32%) had normal coronary arteriograms; 6 women (12%) had trivial stenoses (maximum <20%); 10 women (20%) had moderate stenoses (>20% but <50%); and 18 women (36%) had significant stenoses (>50%) ($p = $ NS for all in comparison to men). Sensitivity, specificity, and positive and negative pre-

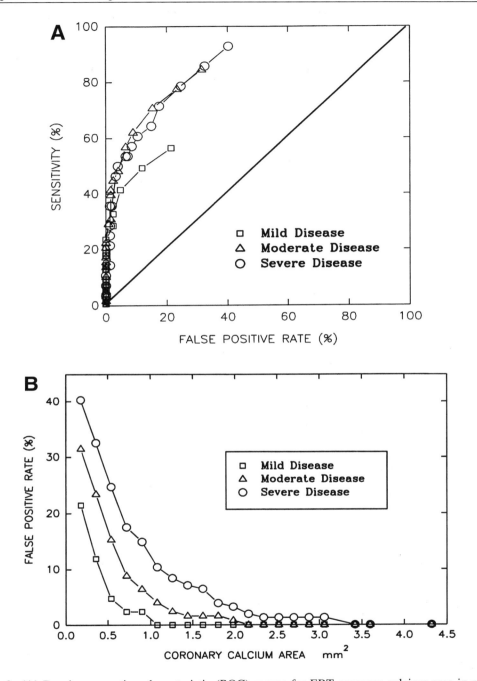

Fig. 2. (A) Receiver-operating characteristic (ROC) curves for EBT coronary calcium area in predicting mild, moderate, and severe luminal atherosclerotic disease in coronary artery pathologic specimens from women. (Adapted from ref. *36, see* text for details.) False-positive rate is defined as the quantity (1-specificity). Each of these ROC curve areas indicates the positive association between EBT calcium area and coronary disease. **(B)** False-positive rate vs coronary artery calcium area from pathological specimens in women, relating to the prediction of mild, moderate, and severe luminal atherosclerotic disease. (Adapted from ref. *36, see* text for details.) A false-positive rate of 0.5 corresponds to a 50% specificity, whereas a false-positive rate of 0 corresponds to 100% specificity.

Table 1
Sensitivity, Specificity, Predictive Values, and Standard Errors for EBT Detection of Coronary
Calcium and Angiographic Disease Severity

EBT and coronary calcium	Any arteriographic disease		Significant arteriographic disease	
	Women	Men	Women	Men
Sensitivity	97 ± 3%	94 ± 3%	100 ± 0%	98 ± 2%
Specificity	38 ± 12%	35 ± 10%	66 ± 8%	57 ± 8%
Positive predictive value	85 ± 6%	89 ± 4%	46 ± 8%	66 ± 6%
Negative predictive value	91 ± 9%	79 ± 9%	100 ± 0%	95 ± 5%

Any angiographic disease—presence of at least minimal luminal irregularities. Significant angiographic disease—presence of any luminal stenosis representing greater than or equal to 50% diameter narrowing. (Based on data in ref. *37.)*

dictive values for coronary calcium were nearly identical for men and women, regardless of the degree of angiographic stenoses (*see* Table 1). Overall, negative predictive values were 91% in women for any angiographic disease and 100% in women for significant angiographic disease. ROC curve areas in women for angiographic disease prediction using EBT was 0.92 ± 0.02; for prediction of significant angiographic disease in women using EBT, the ROC curve area was 0.83 ± 0.06 (p = NS for both when compared to men).

Based on this study, we concluded that in this middle-aged population, noninvasive definition of coronary calcium by EBT had similar predictive value for angiographic coronary artery stenoses in men and women.

CLINICAL EPIDEMIOLOGY, RELATIONSHIPS TO RISK FACTORS, AND PREDICTION OF RISK IN FUTURE CARDIAC EVENTS

Epidemiology of Coronary Artery Calcium by EBT

A prospective study of more than 14,000 men and women found that CAD risk increases with age, and this increase is more dramatic in women. Most risk factors were more favorable in women, but the gender affect on risk factors diminishes with increasing age *(38)*. Another study found that CAD incidence is lower in premenopausal women when compared with men. However, following menopause, the mortality risk from CAD increases in women.

The incidence of coronary artery calcium by EBT as a function of age has been shown to mimic the incidence of cardiovascular atherosclerotic disease in men and women. Figure 3 shows coronary calcification incidence by EBT in an unselected patient population of men and women between the ages of 20 and 80 *(39)*. These data show the following: (1) the incidence of coronary artery calcium increases from only a few percent in the second decade of life to nearly 100% by the eighth decade in men and women; (2) the general incidence of coronary artery calcium in women is similar to that in men a decade younger; and (3) this separation in incidence with age is eliminated by approximately ages 65–70, when coronary calcium incidence is similar to men of the same age.

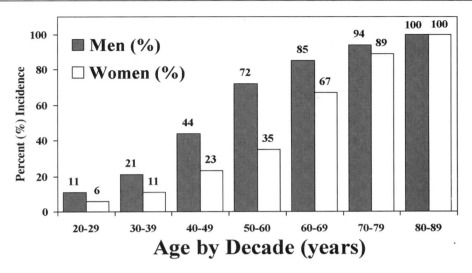

Fig. 3. Incidence of coronary artery calcium by EBT as a function of age and gender. (Adapted from ref. *39*.)

Table 2
Calcium Scores of 9728 Adults

Age/Men							
Percentile rank	*35–39*	*40–44*	*45–49*	*50–54*	*55–59*	*60–64*	*65–69*
25th	0	0	0	0	3	14	28
50th	0	0	3	16	41	118	151
75th	2	11	44	101	187	434	569
90th	21	64	176	320	502	804	1178
Age/Women							
Percentile rank	*35–39*	*40–44*	*45–49*	*50–54*	*55–59*	*60–64*	*65–69*
25th	0	0	0	0	0	0	0
50th	0	0	0	0	0	4	24
75th	0	0	0	10	33	87	133
90th	4	9	23	66	140	310	362

Age, chronologic age in years. (Adapted from ref. *40.*)

As a measure of the extent of coronary disease, coronary artery calcium score also increases with age, but the magnitude of the estimated atherosclerotic plaque burden by EBT is quite different in men vs women. Table 2 shows calcium scores in a large group (9728) of unselected consecutive male and female adults seen at one EBT scanning center *(40).* Data are given as a function of age, sex, and percentile rank of EBT calcium scores. The median coronary calcium score is zero for women until their mid- to late 50s. In men of similar ages, already moderate EBT calcium scores are noted—

again consistent with an overall low prevalence of advanced coronary atherosclerotic disease in men and, in particular, women until their fifth decade of life.

EBT Coronary Calcium and Risk Factors in Women

Kuller and colleagues recently examined coronary and aortic calcification by EBT in a group of postmenopausal women relating to premenopausal risk factors (41). From the Healthy Women Study, Dr. Kuller measured conventional risk factors in 169 women at age 48, then followed up with an EBT scan at age 59. Thirty-seven percent of these healthy women (with no known heart or vascular disease) had positive EBT coronary scans; the 75th percentile score was 13, the 90th percentile score was 138, and the 95th percentile score was 332. These calcium scores are consistent with the data obtained in a separate asymptomatic female population between the ages of 50 and 59, as given in Table 2.

Coronary and aortic calcification (an indicator of extracardiac atherosclerosis) was positively associated with each other. There were very strong associations between low-density lipoprotein (LDL) cholesterol and coronary calcification. Among women with premenopausal LDL cholesterol less than 100 mg/dL, only 9% had a calcium score above 100 when compared with 30% of women with an LDL cholesterol greater than 160 mg/dL. Approximately 5% of women with an HDL cholesterol greater than 60 mg/dL had coronary calcium, and the level of HDL cholesterol had an especially strong inverse relationship with coronary calcium scores. Other premenopausal risks associated with postmenopausal coronary calcium (coronary plaque) were cigarette smoking, higher systolic blood pressure, serum triglycerides levels, and 2-hour postprandial serum glucose. These data strongly indicated that premenopausal risk factors were powerful predictors of postmenopausal coronary and aortic calcification by EBT. However, despite the general linear association, risk factor values on an individual basis were only moderate predictors of the extent of coronary plaque.

EBT Coronary Calcium and Risk of Future Cardiac Events

Because EBT calcium scores do relate to conventional risk, yet also provide an assessment that cannot be obtained by a blood test (that is, the actual site and severity of atherosclerotic plaque disease), it is important to explore how EBT might be an independent predictor of risk.

EBT coronary calcium scores have been shown to be predictive of cardiac and coronary vascular events in several studies. The data discussed are consistent with the area or score for coronary calcification quantified by EBT being viewed as a surrogate for the overall atherosclerotic plaque burden. Although calcification may be a histological feature of stable as well as unstable plaques, it is reasonable to assume that a greater overall plaque burden increases the likelihood of greater proportions of both plaque subtypes. Indeed, the extent of coronary atheromatous disease remains the most powerful predictor of subsequent or recurrent cardiac events (42). The prognostication implications using coronary calcium quantification by EBT should not be predicated solely on the site and severity of the calcified plaque per se or even the probable severity of luminal narrowing, but that the extent of atherosclerotic disease and the presence of plaques of variable morphologic characteristics increase in direct proportion to the amount of detectable calcified plaques.

There have been several recent studies regarding cardiac prognosis and EBT calcium score. Arad and colleagues *(13)* initially reported a follow-up study of 1173 initially asymptomatic patients (average age 53 ± 11 years) with no known coronary disease for a mean of 19 months after a screening EBT coronary calcium scan. The magnitude of the coronary calcium score at the time of the index EBT scan was highly predictive of subsequently developing symptomatic cardiovascular disease during follow-up. Odds ratios ranged from 20:1 for a calcium score of 100 to 35:1 for a calcium score of 160. This study has now been carried out for a total of 3.6-year follow-up *(16)*. Complete follow-up was available in 99.6% of the original 1177 patients. There were 39 total subjects with coronary events (only one event/patient was considered, even if some had multiple events), including 3 coronary deaths, 15 nonfatal myocardial infarctions (MIs) and 21 coronary artery revascularization procedures. For the prediction of "hard" events only (nonfatal MI or coronary death), areas under the ROC curve were 0.86, and a coronary calcium score above 160 was associated with an odds ratio of 22.2. The odds ratios for all cardiac events remained high (14.3–20.2) after adjustment for self-reported cardiovascular risk factors. However, the study by Arad did not specifically evaluate female risk and, in fact, 71% of the participants were men.

Wong et al. have reported on a group of 926 initially asymptomatic men ($n = 735$) and women ($n = 191$) for cardiovascular event follow-up a mean of 3.3 years after a baseline EBT scan *(12)*. Although there were 41 total new cardiovascular events reported by the patients, only 28 could be verified by careful review of medical records and included 6 MIs, 2 strokes, and 20 coronary revascularization procedures. Cox proportional-hazards regression showed coronary artery calcium by EBT to be associated with a greater risk for a cardiovascular event independent of age, sex, and other risk factors. Importantly, the relative risk for any cardiovascular event increased with the numerical value of the calcium score. In comparison to scores of 1–15, those with scores exceeding 271 (highest quartile of plaque burden) were 8.8 times higher. That these data were found independent of sex is at least consistent with the data suggesting that, at a given EBT calcium score, women have similar disease extents when compared to men and should thus be expected to have similar numbers of events based on estimates of total atherosclerotic plaque burden.

The magnitude of the risk to an individual with moderate or greater coronary artery calcium, viewed as a surrogate to measures of total coronary atherosclerotic burden, is underscored when one considers relative risks of developing symptomatic coronary disease using conventional risk analysis. Exercise thallium scintigraphy was recently shown to predict coronary death and nonfatal MI with an odds ratio of 4.4 at 6 years in an already high-risk cohort *(43)*. Bostom *(44)* reported a 15-year follow-up in 2191 middle-aged initially asymptomatic men (20–54 years old at entry) as part of the Framingham database. The relative risk of developing symptomatic CAD in this group was 1.9:1 (95% CI, 1.2–2.9) for an elevated Lp(a), 1.8:1 (95% CI, 1.2–2.6) for total cholesterol greater than 240 mg/dL, 1.8:1 (95% CI, 1.2–2.6) for an HDL less than 35 mg/dL, 3.6:1 (CI, 2.2–5.5) for cigarette smoking, and 1.2:1 (CI, 0.8–1.8) for systolic hypertension. Thus, based on these comparisons, EBT calcium score alone appears to be more predictive of cardiac events than traditional risk factors individually, and as the only noninvasive method to localize and quantitate the extent of the total coronary atherosclerotic plaque burden, it offers a measurable tool for improved risk stratification and prognosis.

CLINICAL APPLICATIONS

EBT is completely noninvasive, requires no injections, and scanning the entire heart is completed in a single breathhold. Coronary calcium scanning (CAS) using EBT is intended to assist clinical decision making and to consequently improve outcomes in patients with suspected coronary disease and in those at risk for its development. Based on the previous discussions, EBT has applications in women with and without cardiovascular symptoms.

Symptomatic Women

Women with a variety of symptoms (chest pain/pressure, unusual dyspnea with effort, and so forth) may have angina. The cardiac testing objective in most symptomatic individuals is to rule in or rule out the presence of obstructive CAD. The usual clinical scenario is to perform a provocative stress test to determine if there is inducible ischemia. If the test is abnormal, further testing, treatment, or intervention is indicated. If the test is normal or negative, the patient is reassured or sent for further testing to look for a noncardiac cause for their symptom(s). However, not all patients with symptoms are similar and conventional, and radionuclide stress testing in women is notoriously imprecise, mainly because of issues related to pre- and posttest likelihood of obstructive disease, as well as the referral bias issues that cloud the sensitivity and specificity related to conventional stress testing in men and women. Determining which investigations (if any) are needed beyond the initial history and physical examination requires the physician to first estimate the likelihood that the patient does or does not have angina.

Age, sex, contributing risks, and the nature or severity of symptoms are the usual clinical variables that provide useful clues to the need for additional testing. The commonly employed terms *atypical chest pain* vs *typical angina* imply a low to intermediate likelihood of ischemic disease vs a high likelihood of ischemic disease, respectively.

Using EBT as a probabilistic model for examining the likelihood of obstructive disease in women (and in men) was recently presented by Bielak and colleagues *(45)*. A total of 213 clinical patients were examined with clinically indicated coronary angiography, based on the symptoms or results of prior conventional stress examinations. Each of these individuals had an EBT scan 1 day after the angiogram. An additional 765 research patients were examined with EBT alone to assist in refining issues of referral (or verification) bias. Referral bias is a common problem with conventional stress testing; sensitivity for obstructive disease in comparison with angiography is falsely elevated, because mostly only "abnormal" stress results end up with requests for confirmatory angiograms. However, in general, the specificity of stress tests is actually falsely lowered, because "normal" patients do not usually get angiography referrals. To adjust for the bias potential, data on sex, age, and calcium scores from the research participants were incorporated into the overall sensitivity and specificity analysis.

In the angiography group, 53.6% had at least one obstructive lesion, and only 1 patient (0.9%) with obstructive CAD had a calcium score of zero. Conversely, 46.4% of the patients with obstructive CAD had a calcium score greater than 500, but few (3 of 101; 3%) without obstructive CAD had a calcium score greater than 500. Among

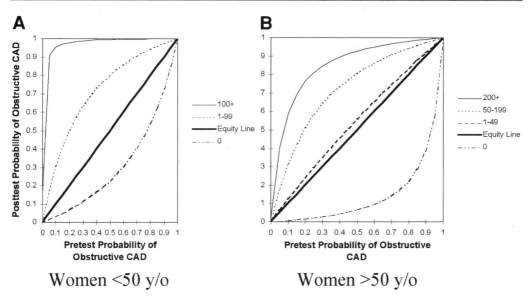

Fig. 4. (A) Pre- and **(B)** posttest likelihood of obstructive CAD using EBT calcium score strata. (Adapted from ref. *45.*) Individuals with low-to-moderate pretest likelihood of obstructive disease are most likely to have the likelihood estimate significantly reduced or increased, depending on the corresponding EBT calcium score strata (*see* text for discussion).

patients older than 50 years, 39 women were in the angiography group and 196 women were in the nonangiography group. Among patients younger than 50 years, 12 women were in the angiography group, and 194 women were in the nonangiography group. After adjustments for verification bias, the overall EBT sensitivity for obstructive disease for men and women was 97%; the specificity was 73%. Four optimal strata were then identified for men and women based on age and EBT calcium score for the diagnosis of obstructive CAD.

The likelihood ratio reflects the odds that a given test result will occur in an individual with the disease as opposed to an individual without the disease, where values can range from zero to infinity. In women older than 50 years, a calcium score of zero gave a likelihood ratio close to zero (0.07), where calcium score greater than 200 gave a likelihood ratio of 12.85. In women over 50, a calcium score equal to zero again had a likelihood ratio of 0.29, where the same age group had a calcium score above 100, optimal with a likelihood ratio of 189.69.

Figure 4 shows the probabilistic curves for women based on the previous information; LRs were constructed for each of the strata. For a specific pretest probability, the vertical distance between a point on the line that shows the posttest probability and the equity line indicates the size of the difference between the pretest and posttest probabilities, as well as the direction of the revision. As noted, when the obstructive disease pretest probability (based on clinical information, e.g., history, physical, and laboratory work) is close to zero or 1 (i.e., 100%), the gain in information from the EBT examination is small, as is the case with any specific test that fits into a probabilistic model and Bayesian statistics. However, the most incremental value is in the patient with an intermediate pretest likelihood of obstructive disease, where (specifically for women above and below age 50) the use of the EBT scan result helps to determine if further testing may be necessary.

Two recent studies using EBT have confirmed that its use in patients with an intermediate pretest probability as a clinical test is highly cost-effective (46,47). Furthermore, recent studies have confirmed that a zero calcium score is associated with a 95–98% event-free survival at a median follow-up of 3.5 years (16).

A positive coronary calcium scan indicates unequivocally that there is coronary atherosclerotic plaque disease present. Although one cannot use the magnitude of the calcium score to define percent luminal stenosis on a one-to-one basis, the calcium score can be used to define the likely severity of associated coronary luminal disease (48). In a symptomatic patient with an abnormal EBT scan, further cardiac testing is indicated. Low to moderate scores (10–400) increase the likelihood of disease from low/intermediate to intermediate/high, and provocative stress testing would be the reasonable next step. A high coronary calcium score (>400) in a patient with chest pain, however, increases the likelihood of obstructive disease significantly, and, in some cases, direct coronary angiography may be the most prudent next step in the work-up.

Asymptomatic Women

Traditional cardiac risk factors predict coronary disease in only 50% of cases. Although a traditional determination of risk is clinically useful, the most powerful predictor of coronary events is a measure of current disease severity. EBT can determine the calcium score, which measures the overall atherosclerotic plaque burden (8).

CAD is a complex process, resulting from a combination of environmental, hereditary, habitual, and perhaps infectious influences that affect its occurrence and severity in an imprecise manner. Yet, heart disease is not inevitable. There are effective means to reduce the chances of developing manifest heart disease, but truly determining the magnitude of the risk in any given patient has been traditionally difficult. Deciding whether or not to use expensive drug therapy in very high- vs very low-risk patients is relatively straightforward in clinical practice. However, these decisions in individuals at intermediate risk are clinically difficult. Overtreatment of truly low-risk patients with drugs, such as statins, is not cost-effective and subjects them to a low, but real, long-term risk of harmful side effects. Undertreatment of true high-risk patients with such drugs may limit the potentially life-saving benefits verified in multiple treatment trials.

EBT and coronary artery calcium scanning can determine the severity of atherosclerotic plaque disease. Based on the magnitude of the calcium score, clinical treatment and/or additional work-up guidelines have arisen (49,50). Recommendation details based on absolute and relative calcium scores (based on age and sex) are given in Fig. 5. More recently, Grundy (51) took an alternative approach to incorporate EBT calcium score into the traditional Framingham analysis. Because chronological age has the most dominant effect on the actual risk calculation, Grundy suggested using coronary calcium percentile ranking as a more precise measure for atherosclerotic plaque burden. In this way, the intermediate-risk patient might benefit from a refinement in risk stratification to determine if they are indeed at median risk or fall at a calcium score that suggests they more properly belong in the low or alternatively high cardiac risk subclasses.

EBT has also the potential to follow the progression and/or regression of atherosclerotic plaque disease (52,53). Thus, when recommended, repeat scanning may provide

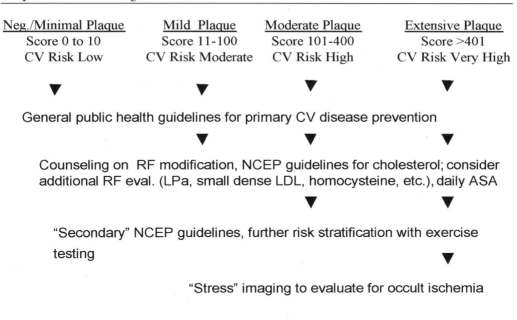

Neg./Minimal Plaque	Mild Plaque	Moderate Plaque	Extensive Plaque
Score 0 to 10	Score 11-100	Score 101-400	Score >401
CV Risk Low	CV Risk Moderate	CV Risk High	CV Risk Very High

▼   ▼   ▼   ▼

General public health guidelines for primary CV disease prevention

▼   ▼   ▼

Counseling on RF modification, NCEP guidelines for cholesterol; consider additional RF eval. (LPa, small dense LDL, homocysteine, etc.), daily ASA

▼   ▼

"Secondary" NCEP guidelines, further risk stratification with exercise testing

▼

"Stress" imaging to evaluate for occult ischemia

Caveat: If calcium score >75th percentile for age or gender - *move to next level*

Fig. 5. Overview of suggested interpretation of EBT calcium scoring in women and men based on the total or absolute calcium score, as well as the percentile rank, which is dependent on both age and gender.

information for the clinician and patient that indicates if the disease process is under control. Such information can also provide motivation for the patient to follow a healthy lifestyle or continue to take prescribed medications. Unfortunately, statistics show that up to four out of five patients without known heart disease starting on lipid-lowering medications will stop them within the first 1 to 2 years.

Women with negative EBT scans can be reasonably reassured that there is no detectable disease and no further testing is presently indicated. Furthermore, in such patients with borderline cholesterol elevation diet and exercise is the most prudent and cost-effective therapy, reserving pharmacological therapy for those with abnormal scans. This has important implications in the overall costs for preventive therapies. A negative EBT scan may allow deferring statin therapy initiation based on the absence of detectable disease. Utilization of repeat scanning at a later date may allow this issue to be readdressed with indications for drug therapy reserved for those who have developed measurable disease since the last scan.

Women between the ages of 45 and 70 with no known heart disease and atleast one significant conventional risk factor are potential candidates for EBT scanning. Advice on scanning younger patients would depend on mitigating factors (e.g., history of very early heart disease in a first- or second-degree relative, familial hypercholesterolemia, juvenile-onset diabetes).

CONCLUSIONS

EBT can be used to estimate the overall coronary atherosclerotic plaque burden in women. It can also be used to diagnose its presence and determine its extent; furthermore, information from the calcium score can be used to assess the likelihood of advanced obstructive disease and to provide prognostic information, and as discussed, these findings appear to be gender-independent. Finally, EBT has the potential to determine the consequences of therapeutic interventions regarding progression, stabilization, or regression of coronary atherosclerotic disease.

EBT application is seen in both symptomatic and asymptomatic women, but the clinical questions vary between these individuals. In the symptomatic woman, the clinical question is "Does this patient have obstructive coronary disease?" In older and younger women, it can function as a convenient and low-cost alternative to conventional stress testing in those with a low to intermediate pretest likelihood of ischemic heart disease. Additional considerations for EBT in lieu of conventional stress testing could also be in women with preexisting resting echocardiogram abnormalities, women unable to adequately exercise, women with a question of noncardiac chest pain, and in women with equivocal prior stress test results. If negative for coronary calcium, no further cardiac testing is recommended. If positive, then the magnitude of the total score can be used as a guide for further testing. Regardless, even if further testing does not confirm the presence of advanced obstructive coronary disease, the presence of subthreshold coronary plaque can be used to address the need for intervention relating to risk factor modification.

In the asymptomatic woman, EBT is most useful in the intermediate-risk patient in whom there is often a clinical conundrum as to the need or level of aggression for risk factor intervention. Traditional estimates of risk for women, such as lipids and even the use of age-adjusted Framingham estimates, cannot provide a measure of current plaque disease severity as EBT can. Currently, there are published guidelines for the use of EBT in men and women.

REFERENCES

1. Bittner V, Simon JA, Fong J, et al. Correlates of high HDL cholesterol among women with coronary heart disease. Am Heart J 2000;139:288–296.
2. Blankenhorn DH, Stern D. Calcification of the coronary arteries. Am J Roentgen 1959;81:772–777.
3. Frink RJ, Achor RWP, Brown AL, et al. Significance of calcification of the coronary arteries. Am J Cardiol 1970;26:241–247.
4. McCarthy JH, Palmer FJ. Incidence and significance of coronary artery calcification. Brit Heart J 1974;36:499–506.
5. Rifkin RD, Parisi AF, Folland E. Coronary calcification in the diagnosis of coronary artery disease. Am J Cardiol 1979;44:141–147.
6. Wexler L, Brundage B, Crouse J, et al. Coronary artery calcification: pathophysiology, epidemiology, image methods and clinical implications. A scientific statement from the American Heart Association. Circulation 1996;94:1175–1192.
7. Mautner SL, Mautner GC, Froehlich J, et al. Coronary artery disease: Prediction with in vitro electron beam CT. Radiology 1994;192:625–630.
8. Rumberger JA, Simons DB, Fitzpatrick LA, et al. Coronary artery calcium areas by electron beam computed tomography and coronary atherosclerotic plaque area: A histopathologic correlative study. Circulation 1995;92:2157–2162.
9. Baumgart D, Schmermund A, Goerge G, et al. Comparison of electron beam computed tomography with intracoronary ultrasound and coronary angiography for detection of coronary atherosclerosis. J Am Coll Cardiol 1997;30:57–64.

10. Schmermund A, Baumgart D, Adamzik M, et al. Comparison of electron-beam computed tomography and intracoronary ultrasound in detecting calcified and noncalcified plaque in patients with acute coronary syndromes and no or minimal to moderate angiographic coronary artery disease. Am J Cardiol 1998;81:141–146.
11. Agatston AS, Janowitz WR, Hildner FJ, et al. Quantification of coronary artery calcium using ultrafast computed tomography. J Am Coll Cardiol 1990:15:827–832.
12. Detrano R, Tzung H, Wang S, et al. Prognostic value of coronary calcification and angiographic stenoses in patients undergoing coronary angiography. J Am Coll Cardiol 1996;27:285–290.
13. Arad Y, Spadaro LA, Goodman K, et al. Predictive value of electron beam computed tomography of the coronary arteries: 19-month follow-up of 1173 asymptomatic subjects. Circulation 1996;93:1951–1953.
14. Secci A, Wong N, Tang W, et al. Electron Beam Computed tomographic coronary calcium as a predictor of coronary events: comparison of two protocols. Cir 1997;96:1122–1129.
15. Wong ND, Hsu JC, Detrano RC, et al. Coronary artery calcium evaluation by electron beam computed tomography and its relation to new cardiovascular events. Am J Cardiol 2000;86:495–498.
16. Arad Y, Spadaro LA, Goodman K, et al. Prediction of coronary events with electron beam computed tomography. J Am Coll Cardiol 2000;36:1253–1260.
17. Bostrom K, Watson KE, Horn S, et al. Bone morphogenetic protein expression in human atherosclerotic lesions. J Clin Invest 1993;91:1800–1809.
18. Ideda T, Shirasawa T, Esaki Y, et al. Osteopontin mRNA is expressed by smooth muscle-derived foam cells in human atherosclerotic lesions of the aorta. J Clin Invest 1993;92:2814–2820.
19. Hirota S, Imakita M, Kohri K, et al. Expression of osteopontin messenger RNA by macrophages in atherosclerotic plaques. A possible association with calcification. Am J Pathol 1993;143:1003–1008.
20. Shanahan CM, Cary NR, Metcalfe JC, Weissberg PL. High expression of genes for calcification-regulating proteins in human atherosclerotic plaque. J Clin Invest 1994;93:2393–2402.
21. McCarthy JH, Palmer FJ. Incidence and significance of coronary artery calcification. Brit Heart J 1974;36:499–506.
22. Tampas JP, Soule AB. Coronary artery calcification: Its incidence and significance in patients over forty years of age. Am J Roentgenol Radium Ther Nucl Med 1966;97:369–376.
23. Lieber A, Jorgens J. Cinefluorography of coronary artery calcification. Am J Radiol 1961; 86:1063–1067.
24. McGuire J, Schneider HJ, Chou T. Clinical significance of coronary artery calcification seen fluoroscopically with the image intensifier. Circulation 1968;37:82–87.
25. Uretsky B, Rifkin R, Sharma S, Reddy P. Value of fluoroscopy in the detection of coronary stenosis: influence of age, sex, and number of vessels calcified on diagnostic efficacy. Am Heart J 1988 Feb;115:323–333.
26. Bartel AG, Chen JT, Peter RH, et al. The significance of coronary calcification detected by fluoroscopy. Circulation 1974;49:1247–1253.
27. Faber A. Die Arteriosklerose, from Pathologische Anatomie, from Pathogenese Und Actiologie. G. Fischer (ed.), Verlag Spieler, Berlin, 1912.
28. Eggen DA, Strong JP, McGill HC Jr. Coronary calcification: Relationship to clinically significant coronary lesions and race, sex, and topographic distribution. Circulation 1965;32:948–955.
29. Hamby RI, Tabrah F, Wisoff BG, Hartstein ML. Coronary artery calcification: clinical implications and angiographic correlates. Am Heart J 1974;87:565–570.
30. Mintz GS, Douek P, Pichard AD, et al. Target lesion calcification in coronary artery disease: an intravascular ultrasound study. J Am Coll Cardiol 1992;20:1149–1155.
31. Glagov S, Elliot W, Zarins CK, et al. Compensatory enlargement of human atherosclerotic coronary arteries. N Engl J Med 1987;316:1371–1375.
32. Clarkson TB, Prichard RW, Morgan TM, et al. Remodeling of coronary arteries in human and nonhuman primates. JAMA 1994;271:289–294.
33. Sangiorgi G, Srivatsa SS, Rumberger JA, et al. Arterial calcification and not lumen stenosis is highly correlated with atherosclerotic plaque burden in humans: a histologic study of 723 coronary artery segments using nondecalcifying methodology. J Am Coll Cardiol 1998;31:126–133.
34. Fitzpatrick LA, Severson A, Edwards WD, Ingram RT. Diffuse calcification in human coronary arteries: Association of osteopontin with atherosclerosis. J Clin Invest 1994;94:1597–1604.
35. Simons DB, Schwartz RS, Edwards WD, et al. Non-invasive definition of anatomic coronary artery disease by ultrafast CT: A quantitative pathologic study. J Am Coll Cardiol 1992; 20:1118–1126.

36. Rumberger JA, Schwartz RS, Simons DB, et al. Relations of coronary calcium determined by electron beam computed tomography and lumen narrowing determined at autopsy. Am J Cardiol 1994;73:1169–1173.

37. Rumberger JA, Sheedy PF, Breen JR, Schwartz RS: Coronary calcium as determined by electron beam computed tomography, and coronary disease on arteriogram: Effect of patient's sex on diagnosis. Circulation 1995;91:1363–1367.

38. Jousilahti P, Vartiainen E, Tuomilehto J, Puska P. Sex, age, cardiovascular risk factors, and coronary heart disease: a prospective follow up study of 14,786 middle aged men and women in finland. Circulation 1999;99:1165–1172.

39. Janowitz WR, Agatston AS, Kaplan G, Viamonte M. Differences in prevalence and extent of coronary artery calcium detected by ultrafast computed tomography in asymptomatic men and women. Am J Cardiol 1993;72:247–254.

40. Raggi P, Callister TQ, Booil B, et al. Identification of patients at increased risk of first unheralded acute myocardial infarction by electron beam computed tomography. Circulation 2000;101:850–855.

41. Kuller LH, Matthews KA, Sutton-Tyrrell K, et al. Coronary and Aortic calcification among women 8 years after menopause and their premenopausal risk factors: the healthy women study. Arterioscler Thromb Vasc Biol 1999;19:2189–2198.

42. Hasdai D, Bell MR, Grill DE, et al. Outcome greater or equal to 10 years after successful percutaneous transluminal coronary angioplasty. Am J Cardiol 1997;79:1005–1011.

43. Blumenthal RS, Becker DM, Moy TF, et al. Exercise thallium tomography predicts future clinically manifest coronary heart disease in a high risk asymptomatic population. Circulation 1996;93:915–923.

44. Bostom AG, Cupples LA, Jenner JL, et al. Elevated plasma lipoprotein (a) and coronary heart disease in men aged 55 years and younger. JAMA 1996;276:544–548.

45. Bielak LF, Rumberger JA, Sheedy PF, et al. A probabilistic model for prediction of angiographically defined obstructive coronary artery disease using electron beam computed tomography calcium score strata. Circulation 2000;102:380–385.

46. Rumberger JA, Behrenbeck T, Breen JF, Sheedy PF. Coronary calcification by electron beam computed tomography and obstructive coronary artery disease: a model for costs and effectiveness of diagnosis as compared with conventional cardiac testing methods. J Am Coll Cardiol 1999;33:453–462.

47. Raggi P, Callister TQ, Cooil B, et al. Evaluation of chest pain in patients at low to intermediate pretest probability of coronary artery disease by electron beam computed tomography. Am J Cardiol 2000;85:283–288.

48. Rumberger JA, Sheedy PF, Breen JF, Schwartz RS. Electron beam CT coronary calcium score cutpoints and severity of associated angiographic luminal stenosis. J Am Coll Cardiol 1997;29:1542–1548.

49. Rumberger JA, Brundage BH, Rader DJ, Kondos G. Electron beam CT coronary calcium scanning: a review and guidelines for use in asymptomatic individuals. Mayo Clinic Proc 1999;74:243–252.

50. Hecht HS, for the Society of Atherosclerosis Imaging. Practice guidelines for electron beam tomography: a report of the Society of Atherosclerosis Imaging. Am J Cardiol 2000;86:705–706.

51. Grundy SM. Cholesterol management in the era of managed care. Am J cardiol 2000;85:3A-9A.

52. Callister TQ, Raggi P, Cooil B, et al. Effect of HMG-CoA reductase inhibitors on coronary artery disease as assessed by electron beam computed tomography. N Engl J Med 1998;339:1972–1978.

53. Budoff MJ, Lane KL, Bakhsheshi H, et al. Rates of progression of coronary calcium by electron beam tomography. Am J Cardiol 2000;86:8–11.

6   Heart Failure in Women

Epidemiology, Gender Differences in Pathophysiology, and Implications for Therapy

Daniel P. Morin, MD, MPH,
Marvin A. Konstam, MD,
Michael E. Mendelsohn, MD,
and James E. Udelson, MD

CONTENTS

INTRODUCTION

In terms of morbidity, mortality, and economic expense, heart failure (HF) is a syndrome of great importance in contemporary society. Despite recent advances in the treatment of other types of heart disease, the impact of HF continues to increase. HF is now the most common reason for hospital admission in the Medicare population *(1)*. Given the aging of the adult population *(2)*, along with the increasing incidence and prevalence of HF with age *(3)*, the clinical and economic burden of HF is likely to continue to rise (Fig. 1; *3a*).

Nearly every large study of HF etiology and treatment has predominantly involved men as subjects, and results largely have been secondarily generalized to women. However, recent investigations have revealed that men and women with HF differ significantly regarding epidemiology, etiology, diagnosis, prognosis, and possibly even treatment effects *(4)*.

From: *Contemporary Cardiology: Coronary Disease in Women: Evidence-Based Diagnosis and Treatment*
Edited by: L. J. Shaw and R. F. Redberg © Humana Press Inc., Totowa, NJ

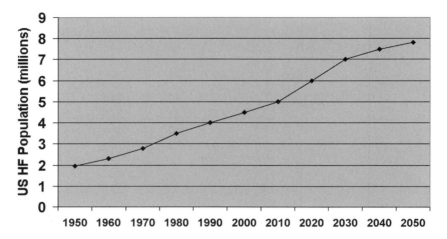

Fig. 1. Effect of the aging US population on the prevalence of heart failure (HF) (actual and predicted). (Adapted from ref. *3a.*)

EPIDEMIOLOGY

Incidence and Prevalence

Many physicians primarily regard HF as a male disease. This is likely the result of the fact that risk factors for coronary artery disease (CAD) are common in men and because most large HF trials have enrolled mostly men as subjects *(5)*. Although the age-adjusted incidence of HF in women is one-third lower (relative risk [RR] = 0.6) than that in men (Fig. 2; *6)* population studies have shown that overall HF prevalence is approximately equal in men and women. For example, during the 20-year follow-up of an initially normal population, the Framingham Heart Study identified the development of HF in 3.7 per 1000 men and 2.4 per 1000 women *(7)*. Despite the similarity in total numbers of HF cases, important differences exist in gender-related HF demographics.

As depicted in Fig. 3, differences between women and men in the prevalence of HF are age-related. Studies have shown a doubling in the prevalence with each decade over 50 years *(3,8)*. On average, men are diagnosed at a younger age, whereas HF is more common among women older than 75 years *(9)*. It is women's longer HF survival (see below) and their population predominance among older age groups that consequently boosts the overall prevalence to be approximately equal to that of men. Because of these factors, the number of women with HF is expected to increase dramatically as the population ages. This trend will cause the diagnosis and treatment of this disorder to be of substantial importance in future patient care.

Differences in Etiology

As a population, women present with a different profile of HF risk factors than do men. Women with HF more often present with hypertension, diabetes, obesity, and smoking—and less CAD and left ventricular (LV) systolic dysfunction. Additionally, pregnant women are at risk for peripartum cardiomyopathy. This section discusses these distinctions and their implications.

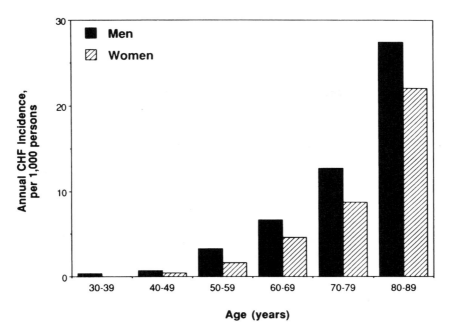

Fig. 2. Incidence rates of congestive heart failure by gender and age, showing that the incidence of heart failure is slightly lower in women than in men at all age groups. (Reprinted from ref. *6,* Copyright 1993, with permission from American College of Cardiology Foundation.) CHF, congestive heart failure.

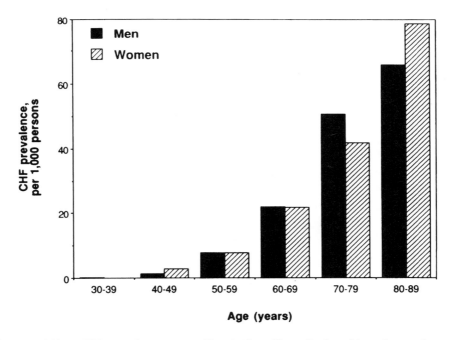

Fig. 3. Heart failure (HF) prevalence among Framingham Heart Study subjects by gender and age, illustrating that HF prevalence approximately doubles with each decade of age past 50 years, and prevalence in women was particularly high at older ages. (Reprinted from ref. *6,* Copyright 1993, with permission from American College of Cardiology Foundation.) CHF, congestive heart failure.

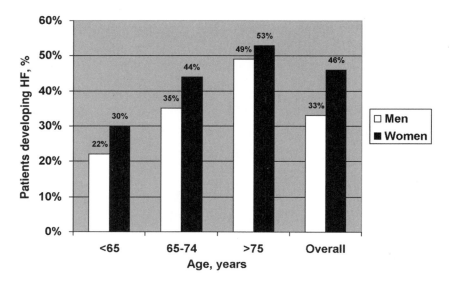

Fig. 4. Age-specific incidence rates of heart failure (HF) in the Worcester Heart Attack Study, showing that at all ages examined women had higher myocardial infarction-associated incidence rates of HF than did men. (Adapted from ref. *11.*)

In large population studies, hypertension is the most commonly identified etiology of HF in both genders. However, among patients with hypertension, women appear to have a higher risk than men of developing HF *(10)*. Analysis of the Studies of Left Ventricular Dysfunction (SOLVD) database, for example, found a similar prevalence of hypertension among both genders of HF patients, but a higher population attributable risk for women than for men (55% vs 39%; *10*).

CAD and its resultant effects on myocardial tissue—ischemia and infarction—are also important risk factors for HF. CAD is less often identified in women with HF than in men with HF *(22)*. Although more men than women have CAD (and, thereby, myocardial infarction [MI]), women may be more likely to develop HF in the post-MI period. As an example, in the 1980s, Kimmelstiel and Goldberg examined data from the Worcester Heart Attack Study (WHAS) database of patients with acute MI and/or out-of-hospital cardiac arrest and noted a significantly higher risk of MI-associated HF for women than for men (Fig. 4; *11*). This finding was preserved even after controlling for potentially confounding factors (e.g., CAD, diabetes, and MI location), indicating that the female sex was independently related to the development of infarct-associated HF. This increased risk of post-MI HF development in women has also been reported by others *(12,13)*.

Diabetics are at risk for HF because of the common association of diabetes with CAD, hypertension, and obesity. Additionally, a cardiomyopathy more directly related to the perturbed metabolism of diabetes mellitus (DM) patients has been identified *(3,5)*. Large clinical trials have found that more female than male patients with HF have concomitant diabetes *(12)*. As an example, in the SOLVD trial, Schindler et al. reported that women made up 33% of the diabetic HF population, but only 26% of the entire HF population *(12)*. Additionally, the Framingham Heart Study showed a higher prevalence of DM in women with HF when compared with similarly affected men (26% vs 14%; *13*). Furthermore, the HF risk among diabetics is higher than that for nondiabetics, and the risk among female diabetics is more than double that of diabetic men even after the adjustment for comorbidities, such as age, hypertension, and CAD *(13)*.

Obesity has also been shown to be an independent predictor of HF risk *(3,14)*. Data from the Framingham study suggest that the risk of HF from being overweight may be even more important in women than in men (men RR = 1.3, women RR = 1.7, $p < 0.05$; *3*). Recent continued analysis by Kenchaiah et al., however, showed a graded increase in the risk of HF across categories of body mass index (BMI; normal vs overweight vs obese), with similar intercategory hazard ratios for both genders (1.46 for women, 1.37 for men) *(14)*. In this study, 11% of HF cases among men and 14% of cases among women were attributable to obesity alone.

Analysis of Framingham data also has shown cigarette smoking to increase HF incidence among women (RR = 1.3), but not among men *(15)*. Although smoking has been more prevalent among men than among women in the past (42% of men, 24% of women; *16*), recent trends show an increase in smoking among women *(17)*, which may contribute to an increasing HF incidence among women in the future.

Peripartum cardiomyopathy results in HF in previously healthy women during the peripartum period. It is severe, with a reported mortality rate of 18–56%, but mercifully rare (1/3000–4000 live births; *18*). By definition, this form of HF develops within the last month of pregnancy or within 5 months after delivery. Risk factors include multiparity, advanced maternal age, multifetal pregnancy, gestational hypertension/preeclampsia, and African-American race. The etiology of peripartum cardiomyopathy is unclear, but several possible causes have been suggested (e.g., myocarditis, autoimmunity, maladaptive response to pregnancy's physical stress, and cytokine cascades; *18*). This cardiomyopathy resolves over roughly 6 weeks in approximately half of cases, but patients with prolonged cardiac dysfunction can have dire outcomes. In one series, for example, 7 of 14 patients had a complete recovery within 6 weeks, and 6 of the remaining 7 patients died *(19)*. The recurrence risk in subsequent pregnancies remains controversial, but expert consensus suggests that any gestation that follows an episode of resolved peripartum cardiomyopathy should be managed in a high-risk perinatal center *(18)*.

As in most syndromes, there are some HF patients for whom no etiology is identified. Among these idiopathic cases, there is a male predominance that ranges from 61% to 92% *(23)*. The reason for excess male representation among this subpopulation of HF patients is not clear. One hypothesis is that perhaps men are more likely to have covert alcoholism (which predisposes to HF) and/or asymptomatic CAD *(4)*.

There are gender-specific differences in the profile of LV dysfunction that results in HF. Population-based studies have shown that although men more often have systolic dysfunction (with ventricular dilatation) as the underlying pathophysiology driving their symptoms, women more often have a preserved ejection fraction (EF) with a nondilated ventricle and thus presumed diastolic dysfunction. For example, in their review of echocardiograms from a cohort of 73 patients with HF in the Framingham Heart Study, Vasan et al. showed that HF with a normal EF is more common in women than in men (Fig. 5), a finding also reported by others *(20,21)*.

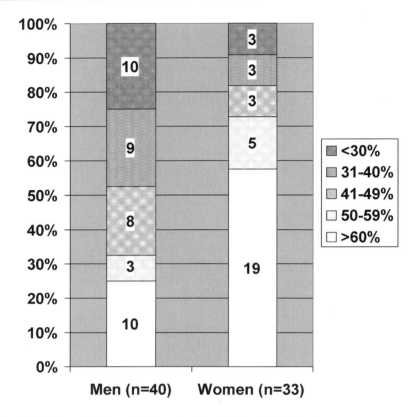

Fig. 5. The distribution of left ventricular ejection fraction (LVEF) values among men and women with heart failure, showing higher EF among women than men. Of men, 67.5% (27/40) had a reduced EF, compared to only 27% (9/33) of women. (Adapted from ref. *20,* Copyright 1999, with permission from American College of Cardiology Foundation.)

Morbidity and Mortality

Women with HF tend to have a poorer quality of life and also tend to experience more symptoms than their male counterparts. The SOLVD investigators found that women report more exertional shortness of breath than men, and experience a higher New York Heart Association (NYHA) class of symptoms *(22).* These women also tended to have edema more frequently than men with HF (22% in women, 15% in men), and those with idiopathic dilated cardiomyopathy have been shown to have lower exercise tolerance than men *(23).*

Patterns in HF hospitalization rates parallel the trends in prevalence previously specified. Whereas some (but not all) studies report a higher admission rate for HF for men *per patient,* there is a higher absolute number of hospitalizations among women than among men *(4,24,25).* Most of the difference in absolute hospitalization numbers likely is a result of the fact that there are more older women than men in most parts of the developed world, and HF prevalence increases with age.

Although women with HF tend to be more symptomatic than male HF patients, longitudinal studies of the natural history of HF have revealed longer survival for

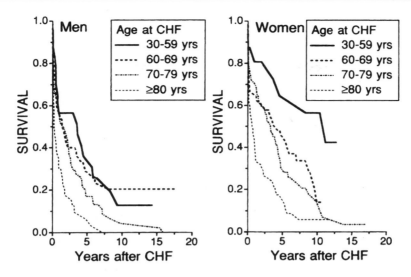

Fig. 6. Survival after heart failure diagnosis for men and women by age, showing a survival advantage for women. CHF, congestive heart failure. (Adapted from ref. *26.)*

women than men (Fig. 6; *26*). In the Framingham Heart Study, median survival after diagnosis of HF was 1.7 years among men and 3.2 years among women. Further observation revealed consistently higher survival among women at 1, 2, 5, and 10 years after diagnosis *(26)*. Later, the NHANES trial corroborated the Framingham finding of prolonged survival in women, estimating a 10-year mortality of clinical HF at 54% in men and 24% in women (at 15 years, mortality rates were 79% and 51%, respectively; *27*). In an analysis of the population with severe HF from the Flolan International Randomized Survival Trial (FIRST; a randomized trial of epoprostenol as a novel treatment for HF), Adams et al. reported that female gender is an independent predictor of survival by calculating for men an adjusted RR of 2.18 for death from advanced HF (Fig. 7; *28*). Subgroup analysis further suggested that women's mortality advantage is strongest among patients with a nonischemic cause of HF (RR = 3.08, $p = 0.001$). A similar survival advantage among women with HF was seen in the Cardiac Insufficiency Bisoprolol Study (CIBIS II; *28a*). In that study, there was a 36% reduction in all-cause mortality in women when compared to men (hazard ratio 0.64, 95% CI 0.47–0.86, $p = 0.003$), as well as significant cardiovascular reductions and pump failure deaths.

In addition to the previous evidence regarding the survival advantage for women with HF from therapeutic clinical trials (which consist of selected populations), a recent large community database has demonstrated similar findings. In a population-based study of 38,702 consecutive patients with first-time admissions for HF in Ontario, Canada, women were found to have a more favorable 1-year survival (odds ratio [OR] = 0.84, 95% confidence interval [CI] 0.80–0.88, $p < 0.001$), independent of many other factors in a multivariate model. Interactions existed with other factors, in that this survival advantage diminished with increasing age and number of comorbidities.

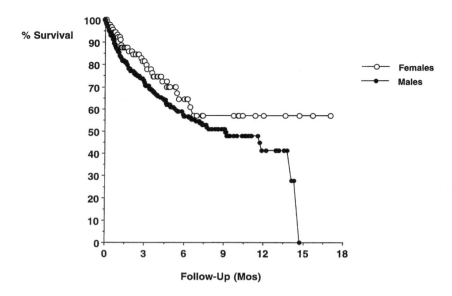

Fig. 7. Unadjusted survival curves for male vs female heart failure patients, revealing a strong trend toward a survival advantage for women vs men ($p = 0.074$) among 430 study patients. (Adapted from ref. *28.*)

This study repeatedly demonstrated survival advantage among women is even more impressive upon recognition that women are, on average, significantly older at the time of HF diagnosis (72 vs 68 years; *26*).

CARDIOVASCULAR PHYSIOLOGICAL DIFFERENCES BETWEEN GENDERS

The understanding of gender-specific differences in HF epidemiology parallels the understanding of the physiological basis of HF. Gender disparities in physical size, hormonal balance, blood pressure response to loading and exercise, ventricular remodeling trends, and electrophysiology may each have an effect on the natural history of HF.

Physical Size

One difference between men and women is their dissimilarity in average physical size; the discrepancy in heart size is even larger. Adult women have smaller hearts than men, even when corrected for total body mass *(29)*. The difference in heart size is much smaller (~6%) before puberty than in postpubescent subjects (25–38%; *30*). These observations are consistent with the testosterone-induced cardiac weight increase that has been seen in animal models *(31)*. Women also have smaller coronary arteries than men, even after correction for heart size *(32)*.

Although young adult women have smaller hearts than age-matched men, the aging process has a more detrimental effect on men's hearts. With aging, women's hearts tend to have preserved myocardial structure and mass. In contrast, men lose nearly 1 g of myocardium per year, and the remaining cells tend to hypertrophy. In their morphome-

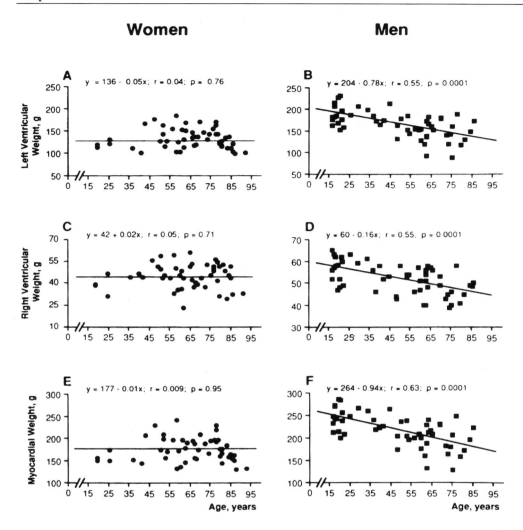

Fig. 8. The effect of aging on myocardial weight by gender. Myocardial weight is preserved with age in women, whereas men suffer a loss of nearly 1 g of myocardium per year. (Used with permission from ref. *33,* Copyright 1995, with permission from American College of Cardiology Foundation.)

tric analysis of the number and size of myocytes in the hearts of 53 women and 53 men, Olivetti et al. showed that myocardial mass decreased by an average of 0.94 g/year in men (Fig. 8), whereas LV myocyte cell diameter increased by an average of 78 nm/year (Fig. 9; *33*). In contrast, with aging in women, there was preserved ventricular mass and myocyte morphology, which suggest that gender accounts (at least in part) for differences in the spectrum of cardiac diseases suffered by men and women, as well as for the clinical expression of disease.

Response to Exercise

The heart is able to achieve dramatic changes in output in response to exercise. However, men and women accomplish this dynamic adjustment through distinct physi-

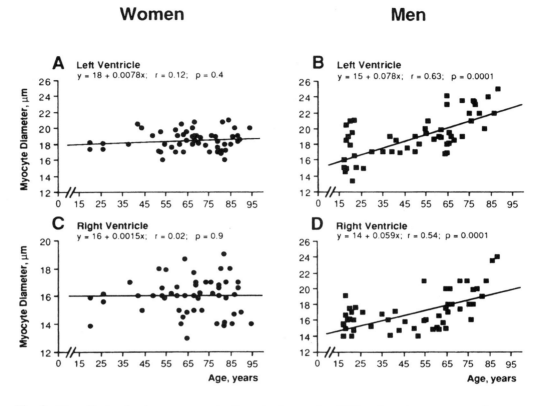

Fig. 9. The effects of aging on myocyte diameter by gender. With aging, the myocytes of women remain approximately the same diameter, whereas men's myocytes tend to hypertrophy. (Used with permission from ref. *33,* Copyright 1995, with permission from American College of Cardiology Foundation.)

ological responses. As depicted in Figs. 10 and 11, Higginbotham et al. reported that when stressed by exercise, men increase stroke volume and cardiac output predominantly by decreasing end-systolic volume. In contrast, healthy women in that study increased stroke volume by increasing their end-diastolic LV volume with little change in end-systolic volume (i.e., by using preload reserve; *34*). This difference may help to explain possible differential pharmacological responses between genders (*see* Pharmacological Response section).

Hormonal Milieu

Sex steroid hormones have been linked to differences in myocardial architecture along with biochemical and mechanical function (*35,36*). Both estrogen and testosterone, for example, have each been shown in a variety of experiments to augment cardiac size and performance in both animals and humans (*8,37,38*). There also is substantial evidence to support the existence of estrogens' (and estrogen receptor [ER] regulated genes') impact on each of the key pathophysiological processes that influence HF progression. Although the effects of estrogen on the myocardium in MI and HF are not completely understood, myocardial expression of the functional ERs,

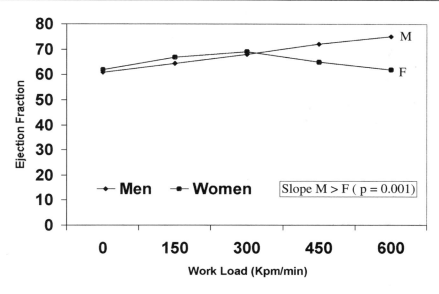

Fig. 10. Ejection fraction (EF) response during exercise in which the workload was increased every 3 minutes, showing a steady increase in EF for men with a flat response (i.e., little change) in women. (Adapted from ref. *34.*)

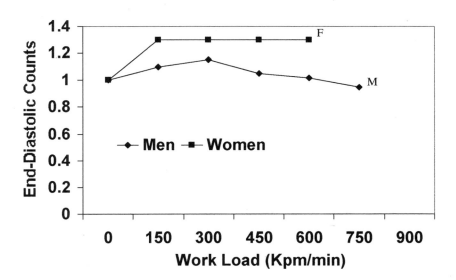

Fig. 11. End-diastolic volume (EDV) responses to progressive exercise (as in Fig. 10) by gender, showing an increase in end-diastolic counts ($EDV_{exercise}/EDV_{rest}$) with exercise in women but not in men. (Adapted from ref. *34.*)

ER-α and ER-β, implies a role for direct estrogen effects on the heart. One such effect is estrogen-induced inhibition of cardiac myocyte apoptosis seen in the in vitro rat myocyte model of Pelzer et al. *(39,40)*. Additional evidence is outlined in the following section.

Neurohormonal Activation and Vascular Loading

Neurohormonal activation and altered autonomic reflexes are important components of HF pathophysiology. Reduced ventricular function is associated with the chronic activation of adrenergic nervous and renin-angiotensin (RA) systems, as well as increased secretion of vasopressin, natriuretic factors, cytokines, and endothelin *(41)*. In addition to their influence on systemic hemodynamics and the handling of sodium and water, activation of these systems on a local tissue level mediates myocardial and vascular responses to HF.

There are several mechanisms by which stimulation of ERs may moderate the unfavorable effects of angiotensin II on the myocardium and vasculature. Animal data show that estrogen leads to the downregulation of angiotensin II receptor expression in ovarectomized rats *(42)*. In humans, estrogen replacement therapy results in diminished renin and angiotensin-converting enzyme (ACE) activity *(43,44)*. These effects may then be associated with a reduction in the RA system's hypertensive effect, as well as the attenuation of angiotensin's direct drive toward myocyte apoptosis *(45)*.

Gender differences in autonomic tone may be regulated in part by ERs and their target genes. Studies have used muscle sympathetic nerve activity (MSNA) analysis and heart rate variability (HRV) to demonstrate that women have significantly lower MSNA *(46)* and greater parasympathetic modulation of heart rate when compared to men *(47)*. Further trials revealed that hormone replacement therapy (HRT) favorably increases HRV in postmenopausal women *(48)*. These clinical observations suggest that estrogen has an important influence on autonomic reflexes.

Estrogen has vasodilator properties in vivo *(49)*. It has been shown to diminish the release of the potent endogenous vasoconstrictor endothelin, and to increase production of the vasodilator nitric oxide *(50,51)*. Indeed, such changes have been seen in postmenopausal women following the initiation of HRT *(52)*. As an example, Best et al. found that following treatment with 17β-estradiol for 6 months and a 10-day course of methoxyprogesterone every 3 months, the mean nitric oxide level increased from 27.5 to 34.7 nmol/mL ($p = 0.04$), whereas endothelin-1 levels decreased from 16.4 to 12.5 pg/mL *(52)*. Such effects are expected to result in enhanced endothelial relaxation. Improved levels of these important vasoactive substances also are expected to have a favorable effect on LV dysfunction through afterload reduction and diminution of the mechanical and neurohormonal drives to remodel. Direct cardioprotective effects may also result from the reduction of endothelin's untoward effects on collagen regulation *(53)*, perhaps accounting for the decreased myocardial fibrosis in females with HF (*see* following section).

Ventricular Remodeling

The myocardial response to a sustained pressure load (via systemic hypertension or aortic stenosis) includes LV hypertrophy (LVH) and remodeling. Distinct differences in this response have been observed between genders. For example, among elderly patients with aortic stenosis, men were found to have considerably greater increases in

LV wall mass, cavity dilatation, and reduced systolic function, whereas women manifested greater increases in wall thickness, leading to concentric LVH with less EF reduction *(54)*. In an analogous rat model using aortic banding, Douglas et al. reported that gender influenced the early response to pressure overload *(55)*. Although LV remodeling, LVH extent, and LV function were similar in male and female rats at 6 weeks postbanding, more male rats showed an early transition to HF, accompanied by greater cavity dilation, more eccentric remodeling, and greater wall stress elevation with more diastolic dysfunction. In a subsequent report from the same investigative group, Weinberg et al. *(56)* reported that at 6 weeks post-aortic banding, female rats had more preservation of contractile reserve and a more favorable molecular remodeling profile, including preservation of the sarcoplasmic reticulum Ca^{2+}-ATPase mRNA levels in female rats. ER transcript was detected in cardiac myocytes and LV tissue in both genders. The investigators concluded that estrogen signaling may contribute to the gender differences observed in the pressure overload response.

Animal models have improved our understanding of possible gender-based hormonal effects on myocardial histology in hypertensive pressure overload. The average diameter of myocytes in spontaneously hypertensive rats (SHRs) is significantly smaller in females than in males, and significantly less myocardial fibrosis is observed in female SHRs than in males *(55)*. In a cardiac remodeling model using volume-overloaded rats, Gardner et al. found that there was less overt HF in female rats when compared to male rats, survival was improved, and cardiac volume and compliance increased more prominently *(58)*.

Remodeling is a major pathophysiological mechanism of long-term morbidity and mortality following MI *(59)*. Post-MI remodeling includes increased cardiac myocyte length, myocardial fibroblast proliferation, and collagen deposition *(60)*. Macroscopically, often there is progressive LV dilatation, loss of normal chamber eccentricity, and increased myocardial mass. These changes are associated with progressive reduction in systolic EF, and this process continues to progress long after the original injury. Interestingly, recent studies have shown that these post-MI changes occur to different degrees between genders.

Several investigations suggest that gender (and thus perhaps ER-mediated phenomena) influences the course of LV remodeling following MI *(61)*. For example, data suggest that men tend to have a greater degree of remodeling than women late after MI (Fig. 12; *62*). For example, in an analysis of a subpopulation of the SOLVD trial, there was an interaction between gender and the rate of end-diastolic volume (EDV) change over time. Men increased EDV more than women, and thus the enalapril effect on attenuation of remodeling was predominantly seen in men *(62)*. This difference may partly explain the potential differential gender-specific benefit of ACE inhibition post-MI (*see* the Pharmacological Response section).

Arrhythmia

There are gender-specific differences in cardiac electrophysiology—both with and without HF. For example, women tend to have a longer rate-corrected QT interval (QTc) more than men, caused by in large part to differences in repolarizing potassium current densities *(63,64)*. The higher prevalence of abnormal ventricular repolarization places women at greater risk for torsade de pointes following treatment with the antiarrhythmic agents quinidine and sotalol, certain antibiotics, and antihistamines.

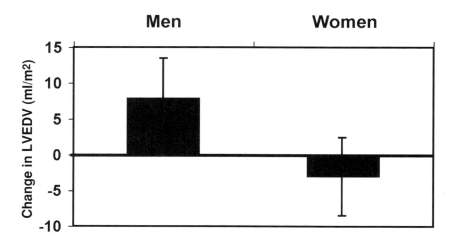

Fig. 12. Influence of gender on change in left ventricular end-diastolic volume (LVEDV) index (mL/m^2) in placebo-treated patients with LV systolic dysfunction (EF ≤ 35%) in the SOLVD trial. There was a significant difference in the rate of change in LVEDV index over 1 year ($\dot{p} < 0.05$), with men demonstrating an increase in LVEDV index when compared to a trend toward a slight decrease in women. (Adapted from data used in ref. *62.*)

The long QTc syndrome is also associated with increased mortality in post-MI patients *(65,66)*.

Certain arrhythmias tend to affect HF patients differently than others. In the general population, atrial fibrillation (AF) incidence is significantly higher in men than in women (RR = 1.5), but in the HF population, this difference is much less pronounced (calculated RR = 1.1; *67*). The morbidity and mortality associated with AF—in stroke, serious symptomatology, and decreased exercise tolerance—tends to be worse for women than for men *(65)*. This difference may have implications in the presence of HF, because these patients rely heavily on atrial contraction to support stroke volume.

GENDER-RELATED DIFFERENCES IN HF MANAGEMENT

Differences in Treatment Patterns

In recent years, some large trials have shown that women with HF tend to receive less appropriate medical therapy than do similarly affected men. One of the most concerning aspects of these data is that in some analyses, women received ACE inhibitors less often than men. In one analysis, for instance, women with HF were treated with ACE inhibitors 50% of the time, whereas the rate of such treatment in men was 56% (Table 1; *69*). In this study, treatment with ACE inhibitors showed a better risk reduction (RR ≅ 0.5) than any other medical therapy studied, suggesting that the lower utilization of ACE inhibitors in women may have been directly associated with more unfavorable outcomes (Fig. 13). However, it should be noted that not all such analyses support a gender-based bias in therapy. As an example, a study by Vaccarino et al. of 2445 elderly patients showed no gender-based difference in medical treatment of HF patients admitted to Connecticut hospitals *(70)*.

Table 1
Percentage of Patients with CHF Treated with Various Medications

Medication	Men	Women
Diuretics	83%	82%
ACE inhibitors[a]	56	50
Nitrates[a]	51	47
Digoxin	47	44
ASA[a]	39	32
Calcium-channel blockers	20	21
Warfarin	19	16
Beta-blockers	15	14

N: male = 2381, female = 2225.
[a] $p < 0.01$. (Adapted from ref. 69.)

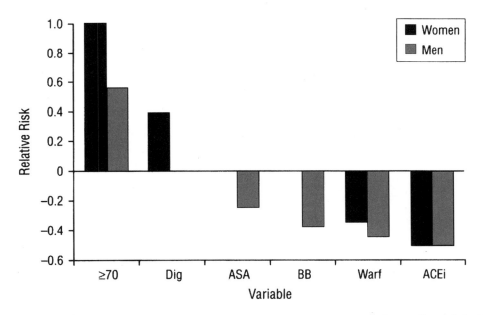

Fig. 13. Analysis of demographic and clinical variables relative to in-hospital mortality risk in 2381 men and 2225 women with heart failure from eight hospitals during 1992–1993. ≥70 = age greater than 70 years; Dig, digoxin; ASA, aspirin; BB, beta-blocker; Warf, warfarin; ACEi, ACE inhibitor. (Adapted from ref. 69.)

The reason for the possible underuse of ACE inhibition in women is unclear; perhaps physicians recognize women to be at greater risk for adverse side effects, although this would seem to be an extreme avoidance of proven therapy. More investigation is needed in order to determine the causes of sex differences in prescription patterns.

Evaluation and Referral Patterns

It has been suggested that women are referred for intensive and/or invasive evaluation of heart disease less often than men are (17,71). This concerning trend includes a

Table 2
Care Processes for 45,894 Patients With Congestive Heart Failure, Stratified by Gender

Care process	Women (n = 25,915)	Men (n = 19,979)
Cardiac specialist care	18.3%	23.1%
Cardiac catheterization	3.5%	4.8%
Revascularization (any)	0.3%	0.4%
Heart transplantation	0.02%	0.09%
Any cardiac surgery	0.4.%	0.5%
Electrophysiology testing	0.2%	0.4%
Permanent pacemarker placement	1.0%	1.3%

$p < 0.05$ for all comparisons between men and women. (Adapted from ref. *72*, Copyright 1998, with permission from American College of Cardiology Foundation.)

tendency against women's evaluation and referral for HF. For example, studies have shown that women are more likely to be treated in the community by their general practitioners rather than to be referred for hospital evaluation *(4,72)*. Even when women are admitted to hospitals for evaluation, they may be managed less frequently by cardiology specialists than men are (18.3% vs 23.1%) and may undergo invasive procedures less often *(72)*. For example, in one review of 45,894 HF patients, women underwent significantly less coronary revascularizations, cardiac surgery, electrophysiology testing, and pacemaker implantations (Table 2; *72*). However, Vaccarino et al. analyzed a similar (although smaller) population and showed no significant difference in gender-based utilization patterns for cardiac catheterization or revascularization *(70)*. It is unclear whether these possible differences in procedure utilization reflect true biological differences, physician bias, or patient preference. It is also unclear whether differential practice patterns have significant effects on morbidity and mortality.

Utilization of Heart Transplant and Associated Outcomes

When pharmacological HF treatment options fail, heart transplantation is sometimes a viable option. However, as with other parameters of HF diagnosis and treatment, there is a gender-based discrepancy of transplant rates: only 20% of patients undergoing transplantation are female *(4,73)*. This can be partly explained by the fact that men tend to present with HF earlier in life and may have more rapid disease progression. Furthermore, as noted previously, physicians seem to act less aggressively in the evaluation and HF treatment in women. But in 1994, Aaronson et al. investigated the reasons for the divergence in transplant rates and showed that female transplant candidates were more likely than men to refuse transplant as a treatment option (29% vs 9%, $p < 0.001$; *73*). The reasons for refusal are unclear, but Aaronson et al. speculate that societally enforced sex roles have a strong influence. Additionally women may be more accepting of reduced exercise tolerance, less tolerant of the transplant risks, or more likely to accept "fate."

Another factor leading to lower rates of transplantation in women may be differential outcome posttransplant. Women suffer more episodes of allograft rejection *(74)*. In addition, the Society of Heart and Lung Transplantation has reported that women who receive heart transplants have a 17% higher 1-year mortality than transplanted men (RR = 1.17, $p = 0.026$; *75*).

DIFFERENTIAL PHARMACOLOGICAL RESPONSE

Therapy for HF is detailed comprehensively elsewhere *(5).* As a result of the many gender-specific differences in cardiovascular physiology detailed previously, the response to pharmacological treatment may differ between men and women *(76).* Furthermore, there are differences in drug metabolism and side-effect profiles.

Pharmacological Differences

Currently, no gender-based difference in HF treatment is recommended by professional society guidelines based on evidence from clinical trials *(5).* However, as HF treatment regimens continue to evolve, so does the understanding of potential gender-specific differences in response to such treatment. Clinicians presently tailor therapy based on comorbid conditions, as well as the severity and/or type (systolic, diastolic, or mixed) of LV dysfunction; in the near future, studies may show that outcomes are favorably affected by customizing treatment based on gender and/or pharmacogenomic parameters.

ACE INHIBITORS/ANGIOTENSIN-RECEPTOR BLOCKERS (ARBs)

Blockade of the RA-aldosterone axis by ACE inhibitors has been shown to reduce HF morbidity and mortality *(77).* HF treatment patients with ACE inhibitors results in modulation of the effects of the RA-aldosterone system, which may cause slowing or reversal of LV dilatation and remodeling *(78).*

Although ACE inhibitors are now a mainstay in HF treatment for both genders, several studies have suggested smaller benefit in women than in men. In a subgroup analysis of the Cooperative North Scandinavian Enalapril Survival Study (CONSENSUS) trial, for example, there was a trend toward mortality benefit for men only (RR = 0.49 for men, 0.94 for women) *(4,11,79).* Similarly, examination of the Survival and Ventricular Enlargement (SAVE) trial of the use of captopril in post-MI patients with LV dysfunction showed a smaller morbidity and mortality reduction in women than in men *(80),* as was also seen in the SOLVD trial *(81).* As is the case for most cardiovascular trials, the subject populations in these studies consisted mostly of men, which reduces the power of data analyses pertaining to the isolated female population within the individual trials.

However, once the trials of ACE inhibitor use in HF were pooled via meta-analysis, a similar degree of benefit was found for both women and men. In their examination of pooled data, Garg and Yusuf showed that ACE inhibition yielded an odds ratio for mortality of 0.76 (0.65–0.88) for the 5399 men represented in the studies and 0.79 (0.59–1.06) among the 1587 women *(77).* It seems likely that ACE inhibition is useful in both genders.

Beneficial effects of ACE inhibition are likely mediated through modulation of factors other than angiotensin suppression *(5).* For this reason, ARBs are second-line agents usually reserved for those patients intolerant of ACE inhibition. The Evaluation of Losartan in the Elderly (ELITE) trial compared treatment with the ARB, losartan, to the ACE inhibitor, captopril, and showed a statistically significant mortality reduction that favors losartan, even though mortality was not a prespecified primary endpoint *(82).* However, further evaluation in the ELITE II trial revealed that losartan was not, in fact, superior to captopril regarding mortality *(83).* In this study, the reported hazard

Table 3
Percentage of Females in Large Mortality
Trials of Beta-Blockers in HF

Trial	% Women
MDC, 1993	27.5%
MERIT-HF, 1999	22.0%
CIBIS I, 1994	27.0%
CIBIS II, 1999	20.0%
US Carvedilol, 1996	23.4%
COPERNICUS, 2001	20.5%
BEST, 2001	22.0%

Adpated from ref. 85.

ratio for captopril in comparison to losartan was similar for both genders (women 1.12, men RR = 1.14, p = NS for both).

BETA-ADRENERGIC BLOCKERS

As noted previously, sustained activation of the sympathetic nervous system in HF results in the down-regulation of cardiac β_1 receptors, chronic blunting of the cardiac response to exercise and other forms of adrenergic demand, and an increase in morbidity and mortality related to the degree of activation of adrenergic activity (84,85). Beta-blockers are now a key therapy for HF in both genders because these drugs improve both morbidity and mortality among a wide range of functional classes (85).

To date, all major trials examining beta-blockers have involved predominantly men as subjects, leading to low power in regard to reaching gender-specific conclusions (Table 3). Although it is now well-established that adrenergic blockade improves outcome for HF patients with varying degrees of symptoms and LV dysfunction, several large studies' subgroup analyses have failed to show a statistically significant mortality benefit for women (86–88). In the MERIT-HF trial, for example, beta blockade in women showed no clear mortality benefit, whereas most other major groups did benefit significantly (87). However, a recent pooled analysis of the three major mortality trials of beta blockade in HF (Cardiac Insufficiency Bisoprolol Study II [CIBIS II], MERIT-HF, and COPERNICUS) showed that combining these data revealed a very similar survival benefit for men and women (Fig. 14; 89). This suggests that the underpowering of gender-specific outcome analysis remains important, even in relatively large HF trials.

DIURETICS

Gender-based differential response to diuretic therapy has not been reported. Because of the longer average QTc in women, however, one could hypothesize that diuretic-induced hypokalemia leads to more arrhythmias in women than in men (76). Potassium levels should therefore be monitored closely. The addition of potassium-sparing diuretics (e.g., spironolactone) may be of particular benefit in this regard.

ANTICOAGULATION

One adverse HF consequence is its associated increased risk for thromboembolic events, which stems primarily from HF patients' sluggish flow in poorly contracting

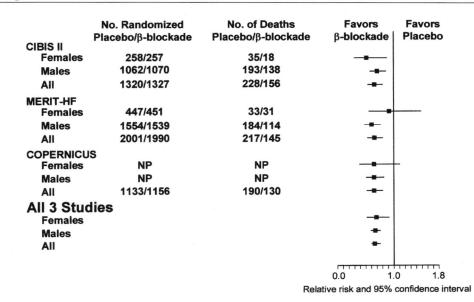

	No. Randomized Placebo/β-blockade	No. of Deaths Placebo/β-blockade	Favors β-blockade	Favors Placebo
CIBIS II				
Females	258/257	35/18		
Males	1062/1070	193/138		
All	1320/1327	228/156		
MERIT-HF				
Females	447/451	33/31		
Males	1554/1539	184/114		
All	2001/1990	217/145		
COPERNICUS				
Females	NP	NP		
Males	NP	NP		
All	1133/1156	190/130		
All 3 Studies				
Females				
Males				
All				

0.0   1.0   1.8
Relative risk and 95% confidence interval

Fig. 14. Point estimates for hazard ratios and 95% confidence intervals for total mortality by gender in major heart failure/beta-blocker trials. Note that although the individual studies were sometimes unable to show statistically significant benefit for females, analysis of pooled data revealed a significant benefit that was approximately equal to that for men. (From ref. *89.*)

ventricles. The resultant hypodynamic state results in deep venous thrombi, pulmonary embolism, and arterial embolic phenomena, including stroke *(90,91).* HF patients' limited physical activity also predisposes to peripheral thrombi formation. Often seen in HF patients, AF is an independent risk factor for thrombotic events that compounds these patients' risk. Additionally, some HF patients manifest a hypercoagulable state, further predisposing to thrombus formation *(92).*

The annual incidence of thromboembolic events in HF patients has been estimated by large studies at 0.9–5.5% *(90).* Dries et al. analyzed the SOLVD registry and showed that women with HF were at even higher risk for thrombotic events than were similarly afflicted men (2.4% vs 1.8%; *90).* Interestingly, in this study, an EF decline was associated with higher risk in women but not in men (Table 4). Most of this increased risk was the result of a higher incidence of pulmonary embolism (PE) in women (rather than stroke or peripheral embolism), but even when PE was excluded from the analysis, the association between females' reduced EF and increased risk for thromboembolic events persisted *(90).* The cause of this difference is unknown, but these data suggest that there may be physiological gender differences in thromboembolism formation in patients with LV systolic dysfunction. Based on women's possible increased risk of thromboembolic events, the use of antithrombotic therapy should be carefully considered.

Some available evidence supports the use of warfarin as routine prophylaxis of thrombosis in patients with HF *(91).* Analysis of the SOLVD registry of 6797 patients with LV systolic dysfunction, for example, showed a significant reduction in mortality (HR = 0.76) that was independent of potentially confounding factors like gender *(93).* It is unknown whether this benefit would be observed in patients with preserved EF but with diastolic dysfunction.

Table 4
Incidence and Crude Relative Risk (RR) of Thromboembolic Events According
to Gender and Ejection Fraction (EF)

EF	Men (n = 5457)		Women (n = 921)	
	Incidence	RR (95% CI)	Incidence	RR (95% CI)
≥30%	1.70	1.00	1.78	1.00
21–30%	1.83	1.08 (0.83–1.41)	2.41	1.35 (0.74–2.47)
11–20%	2.01	1.21 (0.86–1.70)	3.80	2.17 (1.10–4.30)
≤10%	1.96	1.21 (0.30–4.92)	4.20	2.43 (0.32–18.26)

CI, confidence interval. (Adapted from ref. 90, Copyright 1997, with permission from American College of Cardiology Foundation.)

HORMONE THERAPY

There is mixed evidence regarding HRT's effects on HF prognosis. One retrospective analysis has shown a benefit from estrogen replacement therapy on patients with HF, but results of other trials of HRT's effects on cardiovascular survival have been equivocal—some show a benefit, but others do not (94,95). As shown in Fig. 15, in a retrospective cohort analysis of a randomized trial of vesnarinone by Reis et al., women with symptomatic HF using unopposed estrogen had a significant survival benefit when compared to hormone nonusers (RR = 0.68, CI 0.48–0.96, $p = 0.03$; 49). It should be noted that in this analysis, those patients who were treated with both estrogen and progesterone had survival that was intermediate between users of unopposed estrogen and hormone nonusers. In this study, the estrogen-induced mortality benefit persisted on subgroup analysis by HF etiology: patients with both ischemic and nonischemic cardiomyopathy had lower mortality if treated with estrogen (18.6% vs 29.7% and 12.8% vs 24.5%, respectively). These results suggest that in older women with HF, estrogen use may be associated with lower mortality.

Other data do not support a favorable effect of HRT on morbidity in more general populations of women with cardiovascular disease. As an example, reports of continued surveillance of 2321 members of the Heart and Estrogen/Progestin Replacement Study (HERS) cohort concluded that hormone therapy did not reduce hospitalization for congestive heart failure (RR = 1.06, $p = 0.79$; 96), and in this study, HRT showed an unfavorable effect on the incidences of venous thromboembolism (RR = 2.08, $p = 0.003$), biliary disease (RR = 1.48, $p = 0.005$) and other noncardiovascular disease (97). HRT's potential adverse effect on cancer risk, the extent of which remains a topic of intense research, must also be taken into account when deciding whether to prescribe estrogen and/or progestin replacement.

As of mid-2003, ongoing research was examining ways in which manipulation of estrogen's effects on the development and progression of HF could be used to improve outcomes. Because of HRT's possibly unfavorable effects on morbidity from cardiovascular and noncardiovascular disease listed previously, clinical trials are examining the effects of selective estrogen receptor modulators (SERMs) on various cardiovascular outcomes. Members of this pharmaceutical class take advantage of polymorphisms among various tissues' ERs, and are thus estrogenic in some tissues and antiestrogenic in others. Research is currently investigating the impact of ER modulation on ventricu-

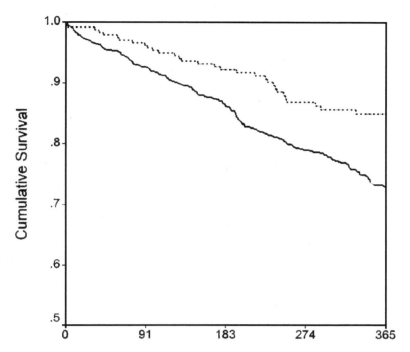

Fig. 15. Kaplan-Meier curves for all-cause mortality according to estrogen use, showing a mortality benefit among estrogen users; $p = 0.004$. Dotted line: estrogen users; Solid line: non-estrogen users. (Reprinted from ref. *49*, Copyright 2000, with permission from American College of Cardiology Foundation.)

lar remodeling and endothelial function. Given the presence of functionally relevant ERs on myocytes, cardiac fibroblasts and vascular tissue as well as the potential neuro-hormonal effects already noted, it may be hypothesized that *selective* ER modulation may have favorable effects on the remodeling process, on ameliorating endothelial dys-function and on neorohormonal activation. If so, this suggests a potentially favorable effect on the HF course in women and perhaps even in men. Laboratory benchwork is examining the effects of SERMs on myocytes, myocardial fibroblasts, and the vascular wall. As examples of ongoing clinical research, further subset analysis of the Multiple Outcomes of Raloxifene Evaluation (MORE; *98*) Registry may provide some insight, and the Raloxifene Use for the Heart (RUTH) trial is an ongoing investigation designed to determine the cardiovascular effects of ER modulation in women at risk for cardio-vascular disease *(99)*. One or more SERMs may be shown in these trials to cause estro-gen's beneficial effects on cardiovascular prevention and/or treatment, while avoiding the potentially harmful side effects of conventional HRT.

Drug Metabolism

Gender-based differences in drug efficacy may in part (and perhaps in large part) result from differences in pharmacokinetics and pharmacodynamics. These differences arise from the gender disparities in physical size, percentage of adipose tissue, and bio-chemical makeup. As in all drug therapies, gender-based differences in cardiovascular pharmakokinetics lie in the absorption, metabolism, and excretion of drugs. Not all of these factors' effects on cardiovascular therapy has been investigated completely, but several studies have provided insight *(100)*.

For example, aspirin absorption in women slows near the middle of the menstrual cycle *(100)*. Gender-related differences in hepatic cytochromes have been shown to be responsible for decreased clearance of digoxin and flecainide (and for increased clearance of other medications), whereas gender-specific differences in renal clearance have been described for other drugs, including quinidine *(100)*. In the Beta Blocker Heart Attack Trial (BHAT), which examined use of beta-blockers following MI, steady-state propranolol concentration was 80% higher in women than in men—again thought to be a result of sex hormones' effects on subsets of the cytochrome P450 system *(100,101)*. Future evaluations are required to define these differences more definitively and to suggest therapeutic situations in which gender-specific alteration in treatment should be considered.

Differences in Side-Effect Profiles

Published data on the side-effect profiles of HF medications are not generally reported in a format that allows any conclusions regarding gender-specificity, but some interesting differences have been reported. For example, it has been suggested that women's smaller volume of distribution is associated with a higher rate of side effects *(100)*. With this in mind, some have advised that the dose of loop diuretics does be adjusted for patient size, because the ototoxicity risk of these drugs is related to serum concentration *(102)*. It also has been noted that thiazide-induced hypokalemia is more common among women than men *(102)*.

Other differences in untoward reactions are independent of concentration. For instance, ACE inhibitors have been shown to induce cough nearly twice as frequently in women as in men *(100)*. Kubota et al. used prescription-event monitoring to examine side effects experienced by patients and found that women treated with ACE inhibitors complained of cough 1.1–1.8 times as much as similarly treated men *(103)*. These authors also noted an excess (RR = 1.2–1.8) of reported adverse drug events (ADEs) in women for a variety of cardiovascular and noncardiovascular drugs and for a variety of ADEs (e.g., back pain, dizziness, headache, and nausea). In contrast, investigators in the Randomized Aldactone Evaluation Study reported side effects of the potassium-sparing diuretic spironolactone (e.g., gynecomastia or breast pain) in 10 times as many men as women *(104)*. As clinical trials are now required to include more significant numbers of women, our understanding of gender-based side-effect profiles likely will continue to expand.

CONCLUSION

As detailed in this chapter, HF in women differs significantly from that in men. In women, HF is more often caused by hypertension, diabetes, obesity, and/or smoking, while CAD and systolic dysfunction seem less prevalent than in men. Differences in anatomy and physiology, including physical size, exercise response, and cardiac remodeling in response to physical and neurohormonal burdens, are likely important determinants of dissimilar course of disease between women and men. Although women with HF are more symptomatic than men, a survival advantage for women has been demonstrated consistently.

Some aspects of HF therapy are similar between the genders, but others are not. Women may undergo intensive evaluation for HF less frequently than men, and women may receive optimal medical treatment less often. Despite the differences in epidemiology, physiology, and outcomes previously summarized, currently there is a lack of definitive evidence that shows an obvious outcome difference in response to major medical HF therapies (e.g., ACE inhibitors and beta-blockers). One major surgical therapy—heart transplant—may be underutilized among women with HF, perhaps most importantly because of patients' refusal to accept transplant as a therapeutic option. Finally, there are likely gender-based differences in side-effect profiles and possible differences in the rate of HF complications, including thromboembolic events.

HF is a very common condition with an increasingly major impact on patients and society as a whole. Our understanding of HF has increased dramatically in recent years, and this syndrome remains a major topic of research. As more is learned about HF, and as gender-specific data accumulate regarding its causes and treatments, hopefully we, will be able to offer our future patients better evidence-based treatments, a better quality of life, and lower mortality.

REFERENCES

1. Health Care Financing Review. Statistical Supplement. US Department of Health and Human Services, Baltimore, MD, 1995, p. 56.
2. Foot DK, Lewis RP, Pearson TA, Beller GA. Demographics and cardiology, 1950–2050. J Am Coll Cardiol 2000;35:1067–1081.
3. Kannel WB, Belanger AJ. Epidemiology of heart failure. Am Heart J 1991;121:951–957.
3a. Bristow MR. Management of heart failure. In Braunwald E, Zipes DP, Libby P (eds.). Heart Disease: A Textbook of Cardiovascular Medicine, 6th ed. W.B. Saunders, Philadelphia, PA: 2001, pp. 635–658.
4. Petrie MC, Dawson NF, Murdoch DR, et al. Failure of women's hearts. Circulation 1999;99:2334–2341.
5. Hunt SA, Baker DW, Chin MH, et al. ACC/AHA guidelines for the evaluation and management of chronic heart failure in the adult: a report of the American College of Cardiology/American Heart Association Task Force on Practice Guidelines (Committee to Revise the 1995 Guidelines for the Evaluation and Management of Heart Failure). American College of Cardiology website, 2001. Available at: http://www.acc.org/clinical/guidelines/failure/hf_index.htm
6. Ho KKL, Pinsky JL, Kannel WB, Levy D. The epidemiology of heart failure: the Framingham study. J Am Coll Cardiol 1993;22(Suppl A):6A–13A.
7. McKee PA, Castelli WP, McNamera PM, Kannel WB. The natural history of congestive heart failure in Framingham Heart Study subjects. Circulation 1993;88:107–115.
8. Kimmelstiel CD, Konstam MA. Heart failure in women. Cardiology 1995;86:304–309.
9. Kannel WB, Plehn JF, Cupples LA. Cardiac failure and sudden death in the Framingham study. Am Heart J 1988;115:869–875.
10. Levy D, Larson MG, Vasan RS, et al. The progression from hypertension to heart failure. JAMA. 1996;275:1557–1562.
11. Kimmelstiel C, Goldberg RJ. Congestive heart failure in women: focus on heart failure due to coronary artery disease and diabetes. Cardiology 1990;77(Suppl 2):71–79.
12. Shindler DM, Kostis JB, Tusuf S, et al. Diabetes mellitus: a predictor of morbidity and mortality in the Studies of Left Ventricular Dysfunction (SOLVD) Trials and Registry. Am J Cardiol. 1996;77:1017–1020.
13. Kannel WB, Hjortland M, Castelli WP. Role of diabetes in congestive heart failure: the Framingham Heart study. Am J Cardiol 1974;34:29–34.
14. Kenchaiah S, Evans JC, Levy D, et al. Obesity and the risk of heart failure. N Engl J Med 2002;347:305–308.
15. Kannel WB. Epidemiological aspects of heart failure. Cardiol Clin 1989;7:1–9.
16. Ho KKL, Pinsky JL, Kannel WB, Levy D. The epidemiology of heart failure: The Framingham Study. J Am Coll Cardiol 1993;22(Suppl A):6A–13A.

17. Wenger NK, Speroff L, Packared B. Cardiovascular health and disease in women. N Engl J Med 1993;329:247–256.
18. Pearson GD, Veille J-C, Rahimtoola S, et al. Peripartum cardiomyopathy: National Heart, Lung, and Blood Institute and Office of Rare Diseases (National Institutes of Health) Workshop recommendations and review. JAMA 2000;283:1183–1188.
19. O'Connell JB, Costanzo-Nordin MR, Subramanian R, et al. Peripartum cardiomyopathy: clinical, hemodynamic, histologic, and prognostic characteristics. J Am Coll Cardiol 1986;8:52–56.
20. Vasan RS, Larson MG, Benjamin EJ et al. Congestive heart failure in subjects with normal versus reduced left ventricular ejection fraction: prevalence and mortality in a population-based cohort. J Am Coll Cardiol 1999;1948–1955.
21. Aronow WS, Ahn C, Kronzon I. Normal left ventricular ejection fraction in older persons with congestive heart failure. Chest 1998;113:867–869.
22. Johnstone D, Limacher M, Rousseau M, et al. Clinical characteristics of patients in the Studies of Left Ventricular Dysfunction. Am J Cardiol 1992;70:894–900.
23. De Maria R, Gavazzi A, Recalcati F, et al. Comparison of the clinical findings in idiopathic dilated cardiomyopathy in women versus men. Am J Cardiol 1993;72:580–585.
24. Ghali JK, Cooper R, Ford E. Trends in rates for heart failure in the United States 1973–1986: evidence for increasing population prevalence. Arch Intern Med 1990;150:769–773.
25. McMurray JJV, McDonagh TA, Morrison CE, Dargie HJ. Trends in hospitalisation for heart failure in Scotland. Eur Heart J 1993;14:1158–1162.
26. Ho KKL, Anderson KM, Kannel WB, et al. Survival after the onset of congestive heart failure in Framingham Study subjects. Circulation 1993;88:107–115.
27. Schocken DD, Arieta MI, Leaverton PE, Ross EA. Prevalence and mortality rate of congestive heart failure in the United States. J Am Coll Cardiol 1992;20:301–306.
28. Adams KF, Sueta MD, Gheorghiade M, et al. Gender differences in survival in advanced heart failure: insights from the FIRST Study. Circulation 1999;99:1816–1821.
28a. Simon T, Mary-Krause M, Funck-Brentano C, et al. Sex differences in the prognosis of congestive heart failure: Results from the Cardiac Insufficiency Bisoprolol Study (CIBIS II). Circulation 2001;103:375–380.
28b. Jong P, Vowinckel E, Liu PP, et al. Prognosis and determinanats of survival in patients newly hospitalized for heart failure. Arch Intern Med 2002;162:1689–1694.
29. Hinderliter AL, Light KC, Willis PW. Gender differences in left ventricular structure and function is young adults with normal or marginally elevated blood pressure. Am J Hypertens 1992;5:32–36.
30. De Simone G, Devereux RB, Daniels SR, Meyer RA. Gender differences in left ventricular growth. Hypertension 1995 Dec;26:979–983.
31. Schaer JA, Schaible TF, Capasso J. Effects of gonadectomy and hormonal replacement on rat hearts. Circ Res 1987;61:12–19.
32. Kucher N, Lipp E, Schwerzmann M, et al. Gender differences in coronary artery size per 100 g of left ventricular mass in a population without cardiac disease. Swiss Med Wkly 2001;131:610–615.
33. Olivetti G, Diordano G, Corradi D, et al. Gender differences and aging: effects on the human heart. J Am Coll Cardiol 1995;26:1068–1079.
34. Higginbotham MB, Morris KG, Coleman RE. Sex-related differences in the normal cardiac response to upright exercise. Circulation 1984;70:357–366.
35. McGill HC, Anselmo JC, Buchannan JM, Sheridan PH. The heart is a target organ for androgen. Science Wash DC 1980;2107:775–777.
36. McGill HC, Sheridan PH. Nuclear uptake of sex steroid hormones in the cardiovascular system of the baboon. Circ Res 1981;48:238–244.
37. Rosano GM, Panina G. Cardiovascular pharmacology of hormone replacement therapy. Drugs Aging 1999;15:219–234.
38. Giraud GD, Morton MJ, Davis LE, et al. Estrogen-induced left ventricular chamber enlargement in ewes. Am J Physiol 1993;264:E490–E496.
39. Pelzer T, Schumann M, Neumann M, et al. 17β-Estradiol prevents programmed cell death in cardiac myocytes. Biochem Biophys Res Commun 2000;268:192–200.
40. Pelzer T, Neumann M, de Jager T, et al. Estrogen effects in the myocardium: inhibition of NF-kappaB DNA binding by estrogen receptor-alpha and – beta. Biochem Biophys Res Commun 2001;286:1153–1157.

41. Francis GS, Benedict C, Johnstone DE, et al. Comparison of neuroendocrine activation in patients with left ventricular dysfunction with and without congestive heart failure. A substudy of the Studies of Left Ventricular Dysfuncton (SOLVD). Circulation 1990;82:1724–1729.
42. Nickenig G, Baumer AT, Hrohe C, et al. Estrogen modulates AT1 receptor gene expression in vitro and in vivo. Circulation 1998;97:2197–2201.
43. Schunkert H, Danser AHJ, Hense HW, et al. Effects of estrogen replacement therapy on the renin-angiotensin system in postmenopausal women. Circulation 1997;95:39–45.
44. Proudler AJ, Hasib AI, Crook D, et al. Hormone replacement therapy and serum angiotensin converting enzyme activity in postmenopausal women. Lancet 1995;346:89–90.
45. Kajstura J, Cigola E, Malhotra A, et al. Angiotensin II induces apoptosis of adult ventricular myocytes in vitro. J Cell Cardiol 1997;29:859–870.
46. Ng AV, Callister R, Johnson DG, Seals DR. Age and gender influence muscle sympathetic nerve activity at rest in healthy humans. Hypertension 1993;21:498–503.
47. Liao D, Barnes R, Chambless LE, et al. Age, race, and sex difference in autonomic cardiac function measured by spectral analysis of heart rate variability—The ARIC Study. Am J Cardiol 1995;76:906–912.
48. Huikuri H, Pikkujamsa S, Airaksinen KEJ, et al. Sex-related differences in autonomic modulation of heart rate in middle aged subjects. Circulation 1996;94:122–125.
49. Reis SE, Holubkov R, Young JB, et al. Estrogen is associated with improved survival in aging women with congestive heart failure: Analysis of the vesnarinone Studies. J Am Coll Cardiol 2000;36:529–533.
50. Weiner CP, Lizasoain I, Baylis SA, et al. Induction of calcium-dependent nitric oxide synthesis by sex hormones. Proc Natl Acad Sci USA 1994;91:5212–5216.
51. Zhu Y, Bian Z, Lu P, et al. Abnormal vascular function and hypertension in mice deficient in estrogen receptor beta. Science 2002;295:505–508.
52. Best PJM, Berger PB, Miller VM, Lerman A. The effects of estrogen replacement therapy on plasma nitric oxide and endothelin-1. Ann Intern Med 1998;128:285–288.
53. Guarda E, Katwa LC, Myers PR, et al. Effects of endothelins on collagen turnover in cardiac fibroblasts. Cardiovascular Res 1993;27:2130–2134.
54. Carroll JD, Carroll EP, Feldman T, et al. Sex-associated differences in left ventricular function in aortic stenosis of the elderly. Circulation 1992;86:1099–1107.
55. Douglas PS, Katz SE, Weinberg EO, et al. Hypertrophic remodeling: Gender digfferences in the early response to left ventricular pressure overload. J Am Coll Cardiol 1998;32:1118–1125
56. Wienberg EO, Thienelt CD, Katz SE, et al. Gender differences in molecular remodeling in pressure overload hypertrophy. J Am Coll Cardiol 1999;34:264–273.
57. Pfeffer JM, Pfeffer MA, Fletcher P, et al. Favorable effects of therapy on cardiac performance in spontaneously hypertensive rats. Am J Physiol 1982;242:H776–H784.
58. Gardner JD, Brower GL, Janicki JS. Gender differences in cardiac remodeling secondary to chronic volume overload. J Cardiac Failure 2002;8:101–107.
59. McKay RG, Pfeffer MA, Pasternak RC, et al. Left ventricular remodeling after myocardial infarction: a corollary to infarct expansion. Ciculation 1986;74:693–702.
60. Weber KT, Sun Y, Katwa LC. Wound healing following myocardial infarction. Clin Cardiol 1996;19:447–455.
61. Mendelsohn ME, Karas RH. Mechanisms of disease: the vascular protective effects of estrogen. N Engl J Med 1999;340:1801–1811.
62. Udelson JE, Kronenberg MW, Rousseau MF, et al. for the SOLVD Investigators. Determinants of progressive left ventricular dilatation in patients with left ventricular systolic dysfunction. Circulation 1992;86:I-251.
63. Ebert S, Liu X-K, Woosley R. Female gender as a risk factor for drug-induced cardiac arrhythmias: Evaluation of clinical and experimental evidence. J Women's Health 1998;7:547–557.
64. Lehmann MH, Hardy S, Archibald D, et al. Sex difference in risk of torsade de pointes with d,l-sotalol. Circulation 1996;94:2535–2541.
65. Schatzkin A, Cupple A, Heeren T, et al. Framingham heart study. Am J Epidemiol 1984;120:888–899.
66. Myerburg R. Epidemiology of ventricular tachycardia/fibrillation and sudden cardiac death. PACE 1986;9:1334–1338.

67. Benjamin EJ, Levy D, Vaziri SM, et al. Independent risk factors for atrial fibrillation in a population-based cohort. The Framingham Heart Study. JAMA 1994 Mar 16;271:840–844.
68. Wolbrette D, Naccarelli G, Curtis A, et al. Gender differences in arrhythmias. Clin Cardiol 2002;25:49–56.
69. Clinical Quality Improvement Network Investigators. Mortality risk and patterns of practice in 4606 acute care patients with congestive heart failure. The relative importance of age, sex, and medical therapy. Arch Int Med 1996;156:1669–1673.
70. Vaccarino V, Chen YT, Wang Y, et al. Sex differences in the clinical care and outcomes of congestive heart failure in the elderly. Am H J 1999;135:835–842.
71. Ayanian JZ, Epstein AM. Differences in the use of procedures between women and men hospitalized for coronary heart disease. N Engl J Med 1991;325:221–225.
72. Philbin EF, DiSalvo TG. Influence of race and gender on care process, resource use, and hospital-based outcomes in congestive heart failure. Am J Cardiol 1998;82:76–82.
73. Aaronson KD, Schwartz JS, Goin JE, Mancini DM. Sex differences in patient acceptance of cardiac transplant candidacy. Circ 1995;91:2753–2761.
74. Crandall BG, Renland DG, O'Connell JB, et al. Increased frequency of cardiac allograft rejection in female heart transplant recipients. J Heart Lung Transplant 1988;7:419–423.
75. Hosenpud JD, Novick RJ, Breen TJ, Daily OP. The Registry of the International Society for Heart and Lung Transplantation: Eleventh Official Report—1994. J Heart Lung Trans 1994;13:561–570.
76. Schwartz JB. Congestive heart failure medications: Is there a rationale for sex-specific therapy? J Gender-Specific Med 2000;3:17–22.
77. Garg R, Yusuf S. Overview of randomized trials of angiotensin-converting enzyme inhibitors on mortality and morbidity in patients with heart failure. Collaborative Group on ACE Inhibitor Trials. JAMA 1995;273:1450–1456.
78. Konstam MA, Kronenberg MW, Rousseau MF, et al. Effects of the angiotensin converting enzyme inhibitor enalapril on the long-term progression of left ventricular dilatation in patients with asymptomatic systolic dysfunction. Circulation 1993;88:2277–2283.
79. The CONSENSUS Trial Study Group. Effects of enalapril on mortality in severe congestive heart failure: Results of the Cooperative North Scandinavian Enalapril Survival Study (CONSENSUS). N Engl J Med 1987;316:1429–1435.
80. Pfeffer MA, Braunwald E, Moye LA, et al. Effect of captopril on mortality and morbidity in patients with left ventricular dysfunction after myocardial infarction. Results of the survival and ventricular enlargement trial. The SAVE Investigators. N Engl J Med 1992;327:669–677.
81. The SOLVD Investigators. Effect of enalapril on survival in patients with reduced left ventricular ejection fractions and congestive heart failure. N Engl J Med 1991;325:293–302.
82. Pitt B, Segal R, Martinez FA, et al. Randomised trial of losartan versus captopril in patients over 65 with heart failure (Evaluation of Losartan in the Elderly Study, ELITE). Lancet 1997;349:747–752.
83. Effect of losartan compared with captopril on mortality in patients with symptomatic heart failure: randomised trial – the losartan heart failure survival study ELITE II. Lancet 2000;355:1582–1587.
84. Goldstein S. Benefits of β-blocker therapy for heart failure. Arch Int Med 2002;162:641–648.
85. Foody JM, Farrell MH, Krumholz HM. β-blocker therapy in heart failure. Scientific Review. JAMA 2002;287:883–889.
86. The Beta-Blocker Evaluation of Survival Trial Investigators. A trial of the beta-blocker bucindolol in patients with advanced chronic heart failure. N Eng J Med 2001;344:1659–1667.
87. Hjalmarson A, Goldstein S, Fagerberg B, et al. Effects of controlled-release metoprolol on total mortality, hospitalizations, and well-being in patients with heart failure. The Metoprolol CR/XL Randomized Intervention Trial in Congestive Heart Failure (MERIT-HF). JAMA 2000;283:1295–1302.
88. Packer M, Coats AJS, Fowler MB, et al. Effect of carvedilol on survival in severe chronic heart failure. N Engl J Med 2001;344:1651–1658.
89. Ghali JK, Pina IL, Gotleib SS, Deedwania PC, Wikstrand JC; on behalf of the MERIT-HF Study Group. Metoprolol CR/XL in female patients with heart failure: analysis of the experience in metoprolol extended-release randomized intervention trial in heart failure (MERIT-HF). Circulation 2002;105:1585–1591.
90. Dries DL, Rosenberg YD, Waclawiw MA, Domanski MJ. Ejection fraction and risk of thromboembolic events in patients with systolic dysfunction and sinus rhythm: evidence for gender differences in the Studies of Left Ventricular Dysfunction trials. J Am Coll Cardiol 1997;29:1074–1080.

91. Koniaris LK, Goldhaber SZ. Anticoagulation in dilated cardiomyopathy. J Am Coll Cardiol 1998;31:745–748.
92. Yamamoto K, Ikeda U, Furuhashi K, et al. The coagulation system is activated in idiopathic cardiomyopathy. J Am Coll Cardiol 1995;25:1634–1640.
93. al-Khadra AS, Salem DN, Rand WM, et al. Warfarin anticoagulation and survival: a cohort analysis from the Studies of Left Ventricular Dysfunction. J Am Coll Card 1998;31:749–753.
94. Grodstein F, Stampfer MJ, Manson JE, et al. Postmenopausal estrogen and progestin use and the risk of cardiovascular disease. N Engl J Med 1996;335:453–461.
95. Grady D, Rubin SM, Petitti DB, et al. Hormone therapy to prevent disease and prolong life in postmenopausal women. Ann Int Med 1992;117:1016–1037.
96. Grady D, Herrington D, Bittner V, et al. for the HERS Research Group. Cardiovascular disease outcomes during 6.8 years of hormone therapy: Heart and Estrogen/Progestin Replacement Study follow-up (HERS II). JAMA 2002;288:49–57.
97. Hulley S, Furberg C, Barrett-Connor E, et al. for the HERS Research Group. Noncardiovascular disease outcomes during 6.8 years of hormone therapy: Heart and Estrogen/Progestin Replacement Study Follow-up (HERS II). JAMA 2002;288:58–66.
98. Barrett-Connor E, Grady D, Sashegyi A, for the MORE Investigators (Multiple Outcomes of Raloxifene Evaluation). Raloxifene and cardiovascular events in osteoporotic postmenopausal women: four-year results from the MORE (Multiple Outcomes of Raloxifene Evaluation) randomized trial. JAMA 2002;287:847–857.
99. Mosca L, Barrett-Connor E, Wenger NK, et al. Design and methods of the Raloxifene Use for The Heart (RUTH) study. Am J Cardiol 2001;88:4 392–395
100. Thurmann PA, Hompesch BC. Influence of gender on the pharmacokinetics and pharmacodynamics of drugs. Int J Clin Pharma Therapeutics 1998;36:586–590.
101. Charney P, Meyer BR, Frishman WH, et al. Gender, race, and genetic issues in cardiovascular pharmacotherapeutics. In: Frishman WH, Sonnenblick EH, eds. Cardiovascular Pharmacotherapeutics. McGraw-Hill, New York, 1997, pp. 1347–1361.
102. Greenberg A. Diuretic complications. Am J Med Sci 2000;319:10–24.
103. Kubota K, Kubota N, Pearce GL, Inman WH. ACE-inhibitor-induced cough, an adverse drug reaction unrecognised for several years: studies in prescription-event monitoring. Eur J Clin Pharmacol 1996;49:431–437.
104. Pitt B, Zannad F, Remme WJ, et al. The effect of spironolactone on morbidity and mortality in patients with severe heart failure. N Engl J Med 1999;341:709–717.

7   Diastolic Dysfunction in Women

Mary Norine Walsh, MD
and Mariell Jessup, MD, FACC, FAHA

CONTENTS

INTRODUCTION

Not surprisingly, approximately half of the nearly 5 million people in the United States who have congestive heart failure (CHF) are women. Between 1985 and 1995, the number of hospitalizations for patients with heart failure increased from 1.7 to 2.6 million, and more than half of these patients were women. More than 500,000 new cases of CHF occur every year, and this disorder accounts for a major and ever-increasing number of hospitalizations. The aging population plays a significant role in this upswing. Improvements in survival, resulting from an array of new treatments, has resulted in more patients living longer with (often) more extensive disease. Thus, increasing the development of CHF in patients who previously would not have survived. Advances in the treatment of acute myocardial infarction, such as thrombolytic therapy and urgent angioplasty, have allowed more patients to survive what may have been a terminal event in the past. The aggressive use of hydroxymethylglutaryl coenzyme A (HMG-CoA) reductase inhibitors in patients with coronary artery disease (CAD) and the treatment of lethal arrythmias with implantable defibrillators have also contributed to the growing number of patients with symptomatic CHF and left ventricular (LV) dysfunction.

But not all patients with CHF have reduced LV systolic function. A significant number suffer from a similar symptom complex, but with evidence of normal or preserved systolic function. This condition has been termed *diastolic heart failure* or CHF with diastolic dysfunction (DD). Patients with DD constitute a substantial portion of those

From: *Contemporary Cardiology: Coronary Disease in Women: Evidence-Based Diagnosis and Treatment*
Edited by: L. J. Shaw and R. F. Redberg © Humana Press Inc., Totowa, NJ

requiring hospitalization and treatment for CHF. Moreover, the diagnosis of CHF with normal systolic function carries with it significant increases in both morbidity and mortality when compared to an aged-matched population without heart failure symptoms. Accordingly, this chapter reviews current understanding of the prevalence, prognosis, causes, and treatment of DD in women.

DEFINITION AND DIAGNOSIS

Standard cardiology textbooks define *heart failure* (HF) as "the pathophysiological state in which the heart is unable to pump blood at a rate commensurate with the requirements of the metabolizing tissues or can do so only from an elevated filling pressure" *(1)*. This definition emphasizes the clinical syndrome of CHF without specific reference to abnormalities of systolic or diastolic dysfunction. LV systolic function can be measured noninvasively with echocardiography, radionuclide techniques, or magnetic resonance imaging, being typically called the ejection fraction (EF). Contrast ventriculography can be performed invasively in the catheterization laboratory. Despite slight variations in LVEF assessment among the techniques used, a reduction in LV systolic function can be fairly easily identified and the definition can be agreed on.

On the other hand, a precise definition of DD is more problematic, which has prompted some authors to call for standardized diagnostic criteria *(2,3)*. Diastolic function abnormalities are most accurately evaluated with simultaneous measurements of LV pressure and volume via cardiac catheterization. (An abnormal result, suggesting diastolic HF, would be elevated end-diastolic pressure in the setting of a normal LV volume.) Because of the invasive nature of this type of assessment, noninvasive estimates of LV diastolic function have been used as a surrogate. In particular, Doppler echocardiography has been utilized to assess LV filling patterns and identify impairment of LV relaxation *(4–7)*. But for busy clinicians and the purposes of epidemiological studies, DD has been assumed to be the cause of HF in patients with CHF symptoms and normal or preserved LV systolic function as measured by a normal EF. Because the current data on DD in women have primarily derived from such epidemiological surveys, the following discussion assumes this latter definition (i.e., DD is present in patients who have signs and symptoms of CHF and with evidence of preserved LV systolic function).

EPIDEMIOLOGY

From the Framingham data, it is known that although the incidence of CHF is higher in men than in women in every age group, the prevalence of the disease is the same *(8)*. CHF is a disease of the elderly, with up to 10% of the population over 65 years being affected *(9)*. The annual incidence of CHF in men from Framingham increased from 3 cases per 1000 in men aged 50–59 years to 27 cases per 1000 in men aged 80–89. In women, the annual incidence increased from 2 cases per 1000 in those 50–59 years to 22 cases per 1000 in those in their eighth decade of life *(8)*.

Estimates of the number of patients with CHF as a result of DD vary widely. The percentage of patients with DD in any given study of CHF patients is influenced by several variables. In an elderly patient population, a higher incidence of normal systolic function is generally reported. Conversely, studies of patients presenting with acute, rather than chronic, CHF often report lower EFs. The criteria used for defining CHF also affect the reported prevalence of CHF because of DD *(10)*. Thus, it can be challenging, indeed, to accurately report the incidence and prevalence of DD in women from the studies published to date.

Vasan et al. *(11)* reported on a series of 31 small uncontrolled studies of CHF patients published from 1970 to 1995. In this series, the prevalence of normal LV function varied from 13 to 74%. The patient population studied clearly influenced the prevalence of DD. Studies restricted to middle-aged patients with chronic CHF had a prevalence of normal LV function of less than 15%, whereas elderly patients surveyed had a significantly higher prevalence of normal LV function (41–45%). Of the 12 studies in this series that reported information regarding the clinical predictors of normal systolic function in the presence of CHF, only 3 identified female gender as a predictor of preserved systolic function.

Of the 216 patients in Olmsted County, Minnesota, who received a primary diagnosis of CHF in 1991, 63% had an assessment of LV systolic function by echocardiography within 3 weeks of diagnosis. Of these patients, 43% had a LVEF equal to or greater than 50% *(12)*. Nearly half of the patients with preserved LV function were 80 years or older, and 69% were women. This is in comparison with 41% women in the CHF patient group with lower EF.

A CHF diagnosis in both the Framingham and Framingham offspring studies was made with a scoring system based on signs and symptoms of CHF *(13)*. Information regarding LV function was not included as part of the data set. Inferences about differences between patients in the Framingham population with CHF and preserved LV function, as well as those with reduced LV function are therefore impossible. However, a nested case-control study from Framingham involving 73 patients and 146 control subjects does provide insight into differences between patients with CHF and normal vs abnormal LV function *(14)*. Of these 73 patients, 40 were men and 33 were women, with a mean age of 73 years. Of the 33 women, 24 (73%) had normal systolic function, whereas only 13 of the 40 men (33.5%) had a preserved EF.

Another prospective study of elderly CHF patients used echocardiography to assess LV function *(15)*. In this elderly cohort, normal EF was found in 116 (47%) of 247 patients. However, in the patients with coronary disease, fewer (41%) had a normal EF. Unfortunately, baseline characteristics were provided only for those patients with CAD, not the entire cohort. The large majority of these elderly patients with CAD were women, 142 (86%) of 166 patients. Interestingly, although elderly age was a predictor of normal EF, female gender was not. The average age of the 68 patients with normal EF was 84 years vs 81 years for the 98 patients with abnormal EF. Of the patients with normal EF, 78% were women, and 64% of those with abnormal EF were women. Although a higher percentage of the group with normal EF was female, this did not reach statistical significance. Obviously, this study group included only patients with CAD and already had a large majority of female patients. Thus, conclusions about broader epidemiological principles regarding gender and DD are difficult.

Wong *(16)* studied a group of elderly patients presenting to a community hospital in a single year. In this group, there was a significant association of normal systolic function with increasing age. Additionally, 82% of the patients with normal systolic function were women, whereas women represented only 38% of those patients with decreased systolic function. Significantly fewer patients with preserved systolic function had CAD, and atrial fibrillation (AF) was more common in the patients with normal systolic function.

Two studies from the same authors *(17,18)* assessed the clinical characteristics associated with preserved systolic function (DD) and systolic dysfunction (low EF) in both a university hospital and a community hospital. In both studies, female gender predicted the presence of preserved systolic function in patients with CHF. In the first study, 75% of those with normal LV function were women; in the second, 71% were women. Of the entire patient population, 31% men and 39% women, respectively, had CHF and normal LV function.

Finally, data from both the Coronary Artery Surgery Study (CASS; *19*) and the Management to Improve Survival in Congestive Heart Failure Study (MISCHF; *20*) registries demonstrate the association of female gender and preserved LV function in patients with CHF. In the CASS registry, 284 of 13,355 patients with normal LV function had CHF, 80% of whom were women. The CHF patients were also older and had more comorbid conditions (e.g., diabetes, hypertension, and lung disease). In the MIS-CHF registry, 312 of 1291 (24%) patients with CHF had an EF greater than or equal to 50%, the large majority (70%) were women.

Thus, although recent reviews *(21,22)*, editorials *(23)*, and published guidelines *(24)* estimate the CHF incidence with preserved LV function to be present from 20% to 60% of patients with CHF, the patient population under study is obviously of great importance in making this estimate. The older the patient population, the higher the incidence of preserved LV function. Women constitute a significant majority of this elderly population. It is quite clear that if only female patients with CHF are considered, a large majority will be subsequently found to have normal LV function. CHF with DD affects women disproportionately to men.

CAUSES OF DD

Table 1 lists the conditions commonly associated with DD. Chronic ischemic heart disease and systemic hypertension commonly underlie DD, as can other conditions that result in significant LV hypertrophy (LVH; *25*). Studies have demonstrated that LV diastolic function declines as a function of normal aging *(26)*. Thus, elderly patients are at higher risk for DD development, particularly if other conditions that further impair diastolic function (e.g., hypertension or ischemia) are imposed on the normal aging process. AF is common in patients with DD *(15,16)*, and its development often results in a worsening of CHF symptoms *(27)*.

Whether or not women have a greater AF incidence in conjunction with DD is not clearly defined. However, there is a dramatic gender difference regarding hypertension. Data from Framingham have demonstrated that hypertension conferred the greatest population attributable risk for CHF development of all the risk factors considered. However, this risk was significantly greater for women than for men. A hypertensive woman's relative risk of developing CHF was 3.35 vs a relative risk of only 2.07 for a man with hypertension *(28)*. Although these data cannot be used to determine whether or not hypertension carried a higher risk of DD development specifically, the currently known prevalence of DD in women with CHF would argue that it does.

The role that gender plays in cardiac adaptation to the physiological stress of hypertension may explain the differential risks for CHF development in women and men

Table 1
Conditions Commonly Associated With DD

Coronary artery disease
Hypertension
Hypertrophic cardiomyopathy
Changes associated with aging
Diabetes mellitus
Aortic stenosis
Obesity
Atrial fibrillation
Pulmonary disease/sleep apnea

with hypertension. In an echocardiographic substudy from Framingham, 564 men and 797 women were evaluated *(29)*. Isolated systolic hypertension was associated with higher values of LV mass/height in both men and women. However, the prevalence of LVH was higher in women. Women with hypertension had a 57% prevalence of LVH when compared to a 17% prevalence seen in normotensive women.

The difference in prevalence for hypertensive vs normotensive men was 31 vs 12%. The relative odds of developing LVH associated with hypertension was 2.58 in men and 5.94 in women. Men with hypertension have been demonstrated to have a larger LV internal dimension without increased LV wall thickness. Women had greater wall thickness without increased LV size.

Other data support the hypothesis that women tend to develop increased LV wall thickness more vigorously than men. Hypertensive hypertrophic cardiomyopathy of the elderly, which is characterized by an increase in LV wall thickness and a small LV cavity, has been observed more often in women *(30)*. Also, women with calcific aortic stenosis have been demonstrated to have supernormal LVEF and smaller thick-walled left ventricles when compared to men *(31)*.

There is also a difference in gender regarding patients with normal LV function and CAD. In symptomatic patients with coronary disease, the prevalence of heart failure is found to be significantly higher in women; there was no gender difference in LVEF *(32)*. As previously noted, in the CASS registry *(19)*, women with preserved LV function were significantly more likely to present with symptoms of CHF than were men with matched EFs.

In a series of consecutive patients with CAD who underwent coronary angiography *(33)*, women had a higher prevalence of CHF (13% vs 10%), despite the fact that the frequency of three-vessel disease was lower in women in comparison to men. The women were older (63 vs 60 years), and more women had hypertension and diabetes when compared to men. Interestingly, the higher frequency of CHF symptoms in the women was associated with significantly higher EF in women vs men (61% vs 56%). Also, more women had normal EFs (79%) than did men (69%). Similarly, women had smaller LV volumes whether or not CHF was present. Clearly, the pathophysiology underlying DD demonstrates significant and important gender differences. Developing a better understanding of these differences will be crucial in any treatment approach.

PROGNOSIS

The Framingham study demonstrated that life expectancy after a clinical diagnosis of CHF was markedly reduced *(13)*. As noted previously, a CHF diagnosis in Framingham was made without the assessment of LV function. The criteria for a diagnosis of CHF were based on the physical exam, chest radiography, and response to diuretic therapy. From this population-based study, it is hard to extrapolate survival data for CHF patients and normal LV function. The natural history of CHF as a result of DD has yet to be well characterized.

Several studies have now examined mortality rates in patients with CHF and normal LV function, and the results are discordant. In the Vasodilator Heart Failure Trial *(34)*, the annual mortality rate was 8% in the group of CHF patients with normal EF when compared to 19% in the group with low EF. Similarly, in a study of 78 African-American patients with CHF admitted to Cook County Hospital during a 10-week period in 1984, many more patients with low EF died *(35)*. By the end of 4 years, 64% of the reduced EF group had died vs 36% in the preserved LV systolic function group (39% had normal LV function; 59% were women).

In the nested case-control study from Framingham *(14)*, Vasan reported a mortality rate of 46% for the normal LV function group and a 75% mortality rate for the patients with reduced function. In the elderly cohort described by Aronow *(15)*, patients with abnormal LVEF had significantly higher mortality rates than those with normal LV function. Unfortunately in this study, mortality statistics were only reported for patients with CAD.

Conversely, several other studies have shown no significant difference in mortality rates in CHF patients regardless of LV systolic function *(12,18,36,37)*. In a prospective study of more than 600 elderly patients admitted to a university hospital with CHF, 34% had normal LV function *(36)*. As has been seen in other data sets, significantly more women than men had preserved LV function (71% vs 29%). Although the patients with normal LV function had a better prognosis at 3 months, the mortality rate from 3 to 12 months was not different stratifying the data based on EF. Additionally, in a study of 52 patients referred to a nuclear cardiology laboratory with a diagnosis of CHF and LVEF greater than or equal to 45%, the mortality rate after 7 years was 56%, not substantially different from that reported for patients with reduced LV function *(37)*. McDermott *(18)* reported a survival rate of 65% at 27 months of follow-up for both patients with systolic dysfunction and those with preserved systolic function.

A recent review by Senni and Redfield *(21)* attempts to reconcile the differing outcomes in these studies. The authors consider that factors, such as age of the cohort studied, diagnostic criteria used to define CHF, and variations in the study populations, may play a significant role in accounting for the variable prognoses observed. They further point out that studies of patients with incident CHF may have different results than studies that include patients with both incident and recurrent CHF. In their view, racial and socioeconomic differences between studies may influence results, as might differences in therapeutic management of the patients studied.

The prognosis of women with CHF and preserved EF is not reported separately in any of these studies. Mortality rates for women with CHF in several epidemiological studies have been demonstrated to be significantly better than for men *(8,38,39)*. But these studies have not always been stratified according to degrees of LV dysfunction. Whether or not the high prevalence of DD in women with CHF plays a role in this apparent survival benefit is not clear. Further research on all patients with CHF and DD may shed light on this important question.

TREATMENT

If information about the true prevalence and prognosis of CHF with DD is in short supply, our knowledge of how to successfully treat it is even more limited. As yet, there is no proven treatment for DD. Multiple randomized, controlled trials have demonstrated the benefits of specific therapies for patients with CHF and reduced LV function, including angiotensin-converting enzyme (ACE) inhibitors, beta blockers, and spironolactone. In contrast, only small trials and meta-analyses are available to guide therapy for patients with DD.

ACE inhibitors *(40)*, angiotensin receptor blockers (ARBs) *(41)*, calcium blockers *(42)*, and beta blockers *(43)* have all been shown to benefit patients with CHF and DD in small trials. And, as did the larger group of patients with abnormal LV systolic function and CHF, patients with relatively well-preserved systolic function showed a reduction in hospitalization rates and worsening HF when they were treated with digoxin *(44)*. Of course, all of these trials were either too small or limited in scope to address the specific benefits of these therapies on women with DD.

The cornerstone of therapy for CHF with DD remains to be treatment of the underlying disease process. This is outlined in the recently revised American College of Cardiology (ACC)/American Heart Association (AHA) Guidelines for the Evaluation and Management of Chronic Heart Failure in the Adult *(24)*. Treatment of ischemia and adequate blood pressure control are paramount. The maintenance of fluid balance is stressed, as is the control of ventricular rate in patients with AF. There are several large randomized controlled trials that are investigating or will investigate the utility of some of these therapies in patients with DD. The role of ACE inhibitors, ARBs, and beta blockers in this patient population may soon become more clear.

FUTURE DIRECTIONS

No data regarding DD therapy will be of value unless a significant number of female patients are enrolled in upcoming and planned therapeutic trials. The preponderance of women with CHF and preserved LV function makes it imperative that women with this disease be investigated. Because the underlying pathophysiology of the disease may be gender-specific, therapies for DD in women will only prove to be therapeutic if they are investigated.

Although CHF is quite clearly a prevalent disease in females, relatively few women have been enrolled in previous CHF trials. In recently completed trials of medical therapy for CHF, only approx 20% of the subjects were women *(45)*. The absence of women in these studies may be a direct result of the tendency toward higher EF in women with CHF and their exclusion from the trials because of criteria that requires the presence of reduced systolic function. Only when women with DD are finally studied in clinical trials will we have a better understanding of "real-world" HF and its appropriate treatment.

REFERENCES

1. Braunwald E, Colucci WS. Pathophysiology of heart failure. In: Braunwald E, Zipes DP, Libby P, eds. Heart Disease. Saunders, Philadelphia, PA, 2001, p. 503.
2. Vasan RS, Levy D. Defining diastolic heart failure. A call for standardized diagnostic criteria. Circulation 2000;101:2118–2121.
3. The Task Force on Heart Failure of the European Society of Cardiology. Guidelines for the diagnosis of heart failure. Eur Heart J 1995;16:741–751.
4. Davie AP, Francis CM, Caruana L, et al. The prevalence of left ventricular diastolic filling abnormalities in patients with suspected heart failure. Eur Heart J 1997;18:981–984.
5. Presti CF, Walling AD, Montemayor I, et al. Influence of exercise-induced myocardial ischemia on the pattern of left ventricular filling: a doppler echocardiographic study. J Am Coll Cardiol 1991;18:75–82.
6. Nishimura RA, Tajik AJ. Evaluation of diastolic filling of left ventricle in health and disease: doppler echocardiography is the clinician's Rosetta Stone. J Am Coll Cardiol 1997;30:8–18.
7. Garcia MJ, Thomas JD, Klein AL. New doppler echocardiographic applications for the study of diastolic function. J Am Coll Cardiol 1998;32:865–875.
8. Ho KKL, Pinsky JL, Kannel WB, Levy D. The epidemiology of heart failure: the Framingham study. J Am Coll Cardiol 1993;22:6A–13A.
9. Kannel WB. Epidemiology and prevention of cardiac failure: Framingham Study insights. Eur Heart J 1987;8 Suppl F:23–26.
10. Marantz PR, Tobin JN, Wassertheil-Smoller S, et al. The relationship between left ventricular systolic function and congestive heart failure diagnosed by clinical criteria. Circulation 1988;77:607–612.
11. Vasan RS, Benjamin EJ, Levy D. Prevalence, clinical features and prognosis of diastolic heart failure: an epidemiologic perspective. J Am Coll Cardiol 1995;26:1565–1574.
12. Senni M, Tribouilloy CM, Rodeheffer RJ, et al. Congestive heart failure in the community: A study of all incident cases in Olmsted County, Minnesota, in 1991. Circulation 1998;98:2282–2289.
13. Ho KKL, Anderson KM, Kannel WB, et al. Survival after the onset of congestive heart failure in Framingham heart study subjects. Circulation 1993;88:107–115.
14. Vasan RS, Larson MG, Benjamin EJ, et al. Congestive heart failure in subjects with normal versus reduced left ventricular ejection fraction. J Am Coll Cardiol 1999;33:1948–1955.
15. Aronow WS, Ahn C, Kronzon I. Prognosis of congestive heart failure in elderly patients with normal versus abnormal left ventricular systolic function associated with coronary artery disease. Am J Cardiol 1990;66:1257–1259.
16. Wong WF, Gold S, Fukuyama O, Blanchette PL. Diastolic Dysfunction in elderly patients with congestive heart failure. Am J Cardiol 1989;63:1526–1528.
17. McDermott MM, Feinglass J, Sy J, Gheorghiade M. Hospitalized congestive heart failure patients with preserved versus abnormal left ventricular systolic function: clinical characteristics and drug therapy. Am J Med 1995;99:629–635.
18. McDermott MM, Feinglass J, Lee PI, et al. Systolic function, readmission rates, and survival among consecutively hospitalized patients with congestive heart failure. Am Heart J 1997;134:728–736.
19. Judge KW, Pawitan Y, Caldwell J, et al. Congestive heart failure symptoms in patients with preserved left ventricular systolic function: analysis of the CASS registry. J Am Coll Cardiol 1991;18:377–383.
20. Phillbin EF, Rocco TA, Lindenmuth NW, et al. Systolic versus diastolic heart failure in community practice: clinical features, outcomes, and the use of angiotensin-converting enzyme inhibitors. Am J Med 2000;109:605–613.
21. Senni M, Redfield MM. Heart failure with preserved systolic function. J Am Coll Cardiol 2001;38:1277–1282.
22. Vasan RS, Benjamin EJ, Levy D. Congestive heart failure with normal left ventricular systolic function: clinical approached to the diagnosis and treatment of diastolic heart failure. Arch Intern Med 1996;156:146–157.
23. Banerjee P, Banerjee T, Khand A, et al. Diastolic heart failure: neglected or misdiagnosed? J Am Coll Cardiol 2002;39:138–141.
24. ACC/AHA guidelines for the evaluation and management of chronic heart failure in the adult. A report of the American College of Cardiology/American Heart Association task force on practice guidelines (Committee to revise the 1995 guidelines for the evaluation and management of heart failure). J Am Coll Cardiol 2001;38:2101–2113.

25. Litwin SE, Grossman W. Diastolic dysfunction as a cause of heart failure. J Am Coll Cardiol 1993;22[Supplement A] :49A–55A.
26. Bonow RO, Udelson JE. Left ventricular diastolic dysfunction as a cause of congestive heart failure: mechanisms and management. Ann Intern Med 1992;117:502–510.
27 Robinson K, Frenneaux MP, Stockins B, et al. Atrial fibrillation in hypertrophic cardiomyopathy: a longitudinal study. J Am Coll Cardiol 1990;15:1279–1285.
28. Levy D, Larson MG, Ramachandran RS, et al. The progression from hypertension to congestive heart failure. JAMA 1996;275:1557–1562.
29. Krumholz HM, Larson M, Levy D. Sex differences in cardiac adaptation to isolated systolic hypertension. Am J Cardiol 1993;72:310–313.
30. Topol EJ, Traill TA, Fortuin NJ. Hypertensive hypertrophic cardiomyopathy of the elderly. N Engl J Med 1985;312:277–283.
31. Carroll JD, Carroll EP, Feldman T, et al. Sex-associated differences in left ventricular function in aortic stenosis of the elderly. Circulation 1992;86:1099–1107.
32. Tofler GH, Stone PH, Muller JE, et al. and the MILIS study group. Effects of gender and race on prognosi after myocardial infarction: adverse prognosi for women, particularly black women. J Am Coll Cardiol 1987;9:473–482.
33. Mendes LA, Davidoff R, Cupples A, et al. Congestive heart failure in patients with coronary artery disease: the gender paradox. Am Heart J 1997;134:207–212.
34. Cohn JN, Johnson G, and the Veterans Administration Cooperative Study Group. Heart failure with normal ejection fraction: the V-HeFT study. Circulation 1990;81(Suppl III):III-48–III-53.
35. Ghali JK, Kadakia S, Bhatt A, et al. Survival of heart failure patients with preserved versus impaired systolic function: the prognostic implication of blood pressure. Am Heart J 1992;123:993–997.
36. Pernenkil R, Vinson JM, Shah AS, et al. Course and prognosis in patients > or = 70 years of age with congestive heart failure and normal versus abnormal left ventricular ejection fraction. Am J Cardiol 1997;79:216–219.
37. Setaro JF, Soufer R, Remetz MS, et al. Long-term outcome in patients with congestive heart failure and intact systolic left ventricular performance. Am J Cardiol 1992;69:1212–1216.
38. Schocken DD, Arrieta MI, Leaverton PE, Ross EA. Prevalence and mortality rate of congestive heart failure in the United States. J Am Coll Cardiol 1992;20:301–306.
39. Adams KF, Dunlap SH, Sueta CA, et al. Relation between gender, etiology and survival in patients with symptomatic heart failure. J Am Coll Cardiol 1996;28:1781–1788.
40. Aronow WS, Kronzon I. Effects of enalapril on congestive heart failure treated with diuretics in elderly patients with prior myocardial infarction and normal left ventricular function. Am J Cardiol 1993;71:602–604.
41. Warner JG, Metzger C, Kitzman DW, et al. Losartan improves exercise tolerance in patients with diastolic dysfunction and a hypertensive response to exercise. J Am Coll Cardiol 1999;33:1567–1572.
42. Seatro J, Zaret BL, Schueman DS, et al. Usefulness of verapamil for congestive heart failure associated with abnormal left ventricular performance. Am J Cardiol 1990;66:981–986.
43. Aronow WS, Ahn C, Kronzon I. Effects of propranolol versus no propranolol on total mortality plus nonfatal myocardial infarction in older patients with prior myocardial infarction, congestive heart failure, and left ventricular ejection fraction > or = 40% treated with diuretics plus angiotensin-converting enzyme inhibitors. Am J Cardiol 1997;80:207–209.
44. The Digitalis Investigative Group. The effect of digoxin on mortality and morbidity in patients with heart failure. N Engl J Med 1997;336:525–533.
45. Lindenfeld J, Krausse-Steinrauf H, Salerno J. Where are all the women with heart failure? J Am Coll Cardiol 1997;30:1417–1419.

8 Functional Capacity and Activities of Daily Living in Women

Claire E. Pothier Snader, MA
and Michael S. Lauer, MD, FACC

CONTENTS

INTRODUCTION

An extensive literature search that involves diverse populations has convincingly and consistently shown a very powerful and inverse association between functional capacity and risk of death *(1–12)*. Although most studies have focused on men, more recent work has shown that a very similar pattern exists among women: those more physically active or who have a greater exercise capacity are substantially less likely to die or experience major cardiovascular events *(13–16)*. This chapter reviews the evidence relating functional capacity in women to cardiovascular outcome and also discusses the ongoing sedentary lifestyle epidemic among women of all ages.

DEFINITIONS AND MEASUREMENT OF FUNCTIONAL CAPACITY

Definitions

A physiological definition of *physical activity* is any body movement produced by a contraction of skeletal muscle, which results in a substantial increase over resting energy expenditure *(17)*. Muscle contraction has both mechanical and metabolic properties. Mechanical classifications are isometric (same length), isotonic (same tension), or dynamic exercise if there is limb movement. Metabolic classification includes aerobic (oxygen available) or anaerobic (oxygen unavailable) processes.

Physical fitness is the ability to carry out daily tasks with sufficient energy, enjoy leisure-time pursuits, and meet unforeseen physical and health emergencies *(18)*. Mea-

From: *Contemporary Cardiology: Coronary Disease in Women: Evidence-Based Diagnosis and Treatment*
Edited by: L. J. Shaw and R. F. Redberg © Humana Press Inc., Totowa, NJ

sures of physical fitness include cardiorespiratory endurance, skeletal muscular endurance, strength, power, speed, flexibility, agility, balance, reaction time, and body composition. Physical fitness has two distinct but related components: health and performance. Neither can be easily defined in terms of a single measurement *(19)*. The relative importance of any fitness attribute depends on the particular performance or health goal.

Health is defined as a human condition with physical, social, and psychological dimensions, each characterized on a continuum of positive and negative poles *(18)*. Positive health is associated with the capacity to enjoy life and withstand challenges, despite the presence of diseases or risk factors. Negative health is associated with morbidity (and at the extreme, premature mortality), an endpoint that has been extensively studied relating to physical inactivity and impaired functional capacity *(2–4,8,11,12)*.

Exercise is a form of planned physical activity with the goal of achieving or preserving physical fitness *(18)*. Endurance exercise involves dynamic, high-repetition movements against low resistance, also referred to as isotonic or aerobic exercise because muscle shortening develops without much tension. Examples of aerobic exercise include walking, jogging, swimming, cycling, and dancing. Resistance training involves exercise designed to increase muscle strength, which can be defined as the ability to exert force. The *training effect* is the ability to achieve a higher peak work rate and maximum oxygen uptake with lower heart rate responses to submaximal levels of exercise when compared with pretraining conditions.

Measurements

Physical activity, physical fitness, physical training, and exercise are related terms that are often used interchangeably, yet are based on multiple kinds of measures *(20)*. In children and adolescents, for example, physical fitness has been measured by time performing a 1-mile walk or run, the number of sit-ups performed in 1 minute, sports participation at school and in the community, self-administered surveys, and behavioral observations by teachers and parents. In adults, investigations have used estimated metabolic equivalents (METS; where 1 MET is the oxygen amount typically consumed at waking rest, namely 3.5 mL/kg/min), heart rates at submaximal levels of exercise *(6)*, and directly measured maximum oxygen consumption *(21)* with the use of treadmill or bicycle stress tests, as well as reports of leisure-time activities, job classifications, and structured questionnaires. In seniors, where stress testing can be prohibitive because of unsteady gait, fitness may be measured by activities of daily living (ADL) and leisure-time activities.

In practice, measures of functional capacity are most often divided into two major types: (1) exact or estimated measures of exercise capacity based on symptom-limited exercise testing, and (2) structured questionnaires. Exact measures of exercise capacity are typically based on expired gas analysis obtained during treadmill or bicycle exercise testing; these techniques are accurate and of prognostic value, but as a result of expense and logistical issues, they are typically limited to specific patient subsets, like those with severe heart failure *(22–25)*. In the vast majority of patients undergoing routine exercise testing, exercise capacity in METs is estimated based on the specific protocol used and time until exhaustion *(26)*. Functional capacity can then be classified as high, good, average, fair, or poor according to age and sex; one such scheme that has been prognostically validated *(3)* is shown in Table 1.

Table 1
Classification of Estimated Functional Capacity According to Age and Sex

Age	Estimated functional capacity (METs)				
	Poor	Fair	Average	Good	High
Women					
<29	<7.5	8–10	10–13	13–16	>16
29–30	<7	7–9	9–11	11–15	>15
40–49	<6	6–8	8–10	10–14	>14
50–59	<5	5–7	7–9	9–13	>13
60–69	<4.5	4.5–6	6–8	8–11.5	>11.5
70–79	<3.5	3.5–4.5	4.5–6.5	6.5–8	>8
≥80	<2.5	2.5–4	4–5.5	5.5–7	>7
Men					
< 29	<8	8–11	11–14	14–17	>17
29–30	<7.5	7.5–10	10–12.5	12.5–16	>16
40–49	<7	7–8.5	8.5–11.5	11.5–15	>15
50–59	<6	6–8	8–11	11–14	>14
≥60–69	<5.5	5.5–7	7–9.5	9.5–13	>13
70–79	<4.5	4.5–5.5	5.5–8	8–9.5	>9.5
≥80	<3.5	3.5–4.5	4.5–6.5	6.5–7.5	>7.5

(Adapted from ref. *3*.)

Questionnaires attempt to estimate the maximal functional capacity without the performance of a formal exercise study. One example is Goldman's *(27)*, the Specific Activity Scale (SAS) shown in Table 2, along with MET equivalents. Another validated questionnaire, the Duke Activity Scale Index (DASI), consists of 12 "Can you...?" questions regarding personal care, ambulation, household tasks, sexual function, and recreational activities *(28)*.

Heart Rate Recovery: A New Correlate of Functional Capacity

Although most studies of adults have focused on estimated or measured exercise capacity during treadmill testing or activity self-reports, recent work has suggested that another prognostically important correlate of physical fitness may be *heart rate recovery* or the decrease in heart rate during the first 1–2 minutes postexercise *(29)*. Heart rate recovery is considered to be a function of centrally mediated postexercise vagal reactivation *(29)*, whereas vagal tone is closely correlated with physical fitness *(30–32)*. In a recent report of 2428 men and women who underwent symptom-limited exercise nuclear testing, there was a close correlation between functional capacity and heart rate recovery in both sexes (Fig. 1; *33*).

PHYSICAL ACTIVITY AND CARDIOVASCULAR PROGNOSIS

Mortality

A number of groups have shown quite consistently that women who report lower levels of physical activity have as much as twice the mortality rate of women who

Table 2
Specific Activity Scale (SAS) of Goldman

Class and METs	Activity limits
Class I (≥ 7 METs)	A patient can perform any of the following:
	Carry 24 lbs up eight steps
	Carry an 80 lb object
	Shovel snow
	Ski
	Play basketball, touch football, squash, or handball
	Jog or walk at 5 mph
Class II (5–7 METs)	A patient does not meet Class I criteria, but can do any of the following:
	Carry anything up eight steps
	Have sexual intercourse
	Garden, rake, weed
	Walk 4 mph
Class III (2–5 METs)	A patient does not meet Class II criteria, but can do any of the following:
	Walk down eight steps
	Take a shower
	Change bed sheets
	Mop floors, clean windows
	Walk 2.5 mph
	Push a power lawn mower
	Bowl
	Dress without stopping
Class IV (≤ 2 METs)	None of the above

(Adapted from ref. 27.)

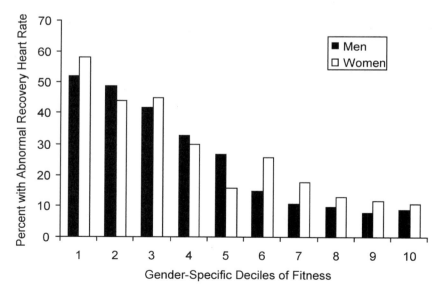

Fig. 1. Association of sex-specific deciles of physical fitness, as estimated by peak METs, with abnormal 1-minute recovery heart rate fall (≤12 beats), among 2428 adults referred for SPECT testing. Increasing physical fitness levels were strongly correlated with decreasing rates of abnormal 1-minute recovery heart rate fall (in men χ^2 for trend = 207, $p < 0.001$; in women χ^2 for trend = 97, $p < 0.001$). (Reproduced from ref. 33 with permission.)

exercise regularly *(13,34,35)*. Recently, a very large study reported the outcomes of 7080 women who underwent symptom-limited treadmill exercise testing as part of a preventive medicine program evaluation *(36)*. Low physical fitness was defined as a treadmill time in the lowest 20th percentile for each age–sex group, whereas moderate fitness was defined as a treadmill time in between the 20th and 40th percentiles for each age–sex group. During 52,982 person-years of follow-up, 89 women died. In a multivariable model there were only two independent predictors of death in women: smoking and low physical fitness (adjusted relative risk [RR] 2.10, 95% confidence interval [CI] 1.36–2.31). Low physical fitness was also independently predictive of cardiovascular death in women (adjusted RR 2.42, 95% CI 0.99–5.92). Stratified analyses demonstrated that low or moderate physical fitness was associated with increased mortality, irrespective of the number of standard cardiovascular risk factors present.

As previously discussed, heart rate recovery has recently been described as an easily obtainable and objective measure that is closely correlated with functional capacity *(33)*. Three studies that involved both men and women investigated the ability of an attenuated heart rate recovery to predict death. Among 2428 adults (including 905 women) who underwent symptom-limited nuclear testing, an abnormal heart rate recovery was defined as a heart rate decrease of 12 beats per minute or less during the first minute after exercise *(33)*. An abnormal heart rate recovery was noted in 252 women (28%) and 387 men (25%), being associated with a markedly increased 6-year mortality in both men (22% vs 6%, hazard ratio 3.9, 95% CI 2.8–5.3) and women (14% vs 4%, hazard ratio 4.4, 95% CI 2.6–7.5).

Another similar study focused on 9454 adults (including 2123 women) who underwent symptom-limited exercise electrocardiographic testing without concurrent imaging *(37)*. During the 5-year follow-up, 68 women (3%) died. As with men, an abnormal heart rate recovery was associated with an increased risk of death (8% vs 2%, hazard ratio 4.4, 95% 2.7–7.1). In a multivariable model, the only independent predictors of death were age, an abnormal heart rate recovery (adjusted hazard ratio 2.7, 95% CI 1.7–4.5), and the number of standard cardiovascular risk factors.

Finally, a third study followed the outcomes of 5234 healthy adults (including 2037 women) who underwent submaximal exercise testing as part of the Lipid Research Clinics Prevalence Study *(38)*. An abnormal heart rate recovery was defined as a heart rate decrease of 42 beats per minute or less during the first 2 minutes after exercise, which was noted in 613 women (30%). As with men, an abnormal heart rate recovery was associated with an increased risk of death during the 12-year follow-up (7% vs 4%, hazard ratio 2.1, 95% CI 1.4–3.1)

Coronary Events

The Nurses' Health Study is one of the largest epidemiological studies of cardiovascular disease in women *(39)* and has been a primary source of our understanding of the importance of lifestyle factors as correlates of risk for death and coronary heart disease events *(40)*. Recently, Manson and colleagues performed a systematic analysis of the association between self-reported physical activity and coronary risk among 72,488 female nurses between the ages of 40 and 65 years who were free of clinical coronary disease in 1986. The women were asked about the amount of time spent per week in eight activities: walking or hiking, jogging, running, bicycling, swimming, playing ten-

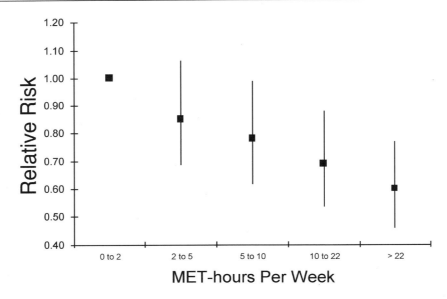

Fig. 2. Relative risk of major coronary events according to self-reported physical activity in the Nurses' Health Study. (Adapted from ref. *40.*)

nis or squash, and other types of formal aerobic exercise. Answers to these questions, as well as information about the number of stairs climbed per week, were used to calculate physical activity in MET hour units. The women were followed for 8 years, during which time 645 coronary events occurred.

There were important baseline differences between women who were and were not physically active. When compared to women in the highest quintile of activity (>21.7 MET hours/week), women in the lowest quintile (0–2.0 MET hours/week) were heavier (body mass index [BMI] 25.1 vs 23.5 kg/m^2), drank less alcohol (5.9 vs 7.0 g/day), were more likely to smoke (28% vs 18%) or have diabetes (4.2% vs 2.6%), and were less likely to use vitamin E supplements (12.8% vs 19.4%).

Even after adjusting for these and other differences, increasing physical activity levels were independently associated with substantially lower rates of coronary events (Fig. 2). Furthermore, stratified analyses found that this association was entirely independent of smoking status and BMI. Among women who did not engage in vigorous exercise (defined as an activity that required 6 or more METs per hour) a similar inverse association was noted. In comparison to women in the lowest quintile of weekly walking activity, there was a decrease in coronary event risk as the level of physical activity increased (multivariate adjusted relative risk for women in quintile 4 with exercise activity of 4–10 MET hours/week 0.70, 95% CI 0.51–0.95, and for women in quintile 5 with exercise activity, greater than or equal to 10 MET hours/week 0.65, 95% CI 0.47–0.91).

The authors also examined the association of walking pace with coronary risk among women who did not engage in any vigorous exercise. When compared to women who typically walked at a rate less than 2 miles per hour (mph), those who walked at a rate of 2–2.9 mph had a substantially lower risk of coronary events (multivariate adjusted RR 0.75), whereas those who walked briskly, defined as greater than or equal to 3 mph, were at even lower risk (multivariate adjusted RR 0.64).

Despite the increasing evidence that links regular physical activity and greater functional capacity to lower coronary risk, an interesting "paradox of exercise" has recently been described, whereby vigorous physical activity is actually associated with a higher acute risk of myocardial infarction (MI; *41*). Two now classic papers found that 4–7% of patients suffering from MI were engaged in heavy physical activity at the time or just before the onset of symptoms and that acute physical activity was associated with an increased acute infarction risk *(42,43)*. However, people who exercise regularly had a lower relative risk of infarction during vigorous physical activity. For example, in the study by Mittelman and colleagues *(42)*, sedentary adults had a relative risk of 107 (95% CI 67–171) for triggering an infarction, whereas those who exercised once a week had a much lower relative risk of 19 (95% CI 10–38), and those who exercised five or more times per week had a relative risk of only 2.4 (95% CI 1.5–3.7). Both studies found that there was no sex-based interaction. For both men and women, acute vigorous exercise was associated with increased risk of infarction, but this acute risk was much less among those who exercised regularly.

Stroke

Several studies have now reported an inverse association between physical activity and the risk of stroke in women. The Nord-Trondelag Health Survey studied 14,101 middle-aged and elderly women with specific attention to different levels of leisure-time activities and stroke mortality during the 10-year follow-up *(44)*. The relative risk of dying of stroke decreased with an increase in physical activity. When compared to sedentary women, the most active women by age groups 50–69, 70–79, and 80–101 had an adjusted relative risk of 0.42 (95% CI 0.24–0.75), 0.56 (95% CI 0.36–0.88), and 0.57 (95% CI 0.30–1.09). By multivariate analysis, the relative risk of death from stroke for all women 50 years or older by low, moderate, and high levels of physical activity were 1.0, 0.87, and 0.47, respectively.

The Nurses' Health Study also examined the association between physical activity and risk of total stroke in 72,488 women aged 40–65 years during the 8-year follow-up *(14)*. Increasing physical activity was strongly and inversely associated with the risk of total stroke. Relative risks from the lowest to highest MET quintiles were 1.00, 0.98, 0.82, 0.74, and 0.66. A brisk or stride walking pace was associated with a lower risk of stroke when compared to average or casual pace (0.36, 95% CI 0.27–0.48 vs 0.66, 95% CI 0.52–0.83). These data indicate that physical activity is associated with a substantial reduction in the risk of total stroke in a dose-response manner.

Other reports have also demonstrated that physically active women are at a markedly reduced stroke risk. These include the analyses of The Northern Manhattan Stroke Study *(16)*, National Health and Nutrition Examination Survey (NHANES I) database *(45)*, and the Copenhagen City Heart Study *(46)*.

POSSIBLE MECHANISMS LINKING FUNCTIONAL CAPACITY TO CARDIOVASCULAR RISK

Although the strong association between functional capacity and cardiovascular risk is now widely accepted, the precise mechanism(s) by which physical fitness protects

Table 3
Possible Biological Links Between Functional Capacity and Cardiovascular Outcome

Type of link	Links
Determinants of functional capacity	Greater regularity of exercise
	Greater intensity of exercise
	Genetics
	Lower body weight
	Healthy diet
	No cigarette smoking
	Increased total blood volume
	Decreased central arterial stiffness
	Medications (e.g., beta blockers)
Standard cardiovascular risk factors	Lower blood pressure
	Lower blood glucose
	Lower tryglyceride and LDL cholesterol
Biological markers of atherosclerosis	Quantitative coronary angiography
	Carotid intimal thickness by ultrasound
Physiological effects of exercise	Increased HDL cholesterol
	Improved autonomic balance
	Increased parasympathetic tone
	Decrease sympathetic tone
	Improved endothelial function
	Decreased oxidative stress
	Decreased heart rate

See text for details and references.

against major life-threatening cardiovascular events is not clearly known. Research in this area has focused on the determinants and cross-sectional correlates of functional capacity, association of functional capacity with changes in other biological markers, and physiological effects of exercise training (Table 3).

Not surprisingly, regular physical activity is a powerful determinant of measured functional capacity in both men and women (47,48), although the intensity of exercise, rather than the regularity, may be a stronger predictor of functional capacity (49). Nonetheless, both regularity and intensity are only modestly associated with measured physical fitness, arguing that other factors are likely to be related. For example, based on twin studies, it has been suggested that genetic factors account for 25–50% of the functional capacity variability (50,51). Other possible determinants of functional capacity include body weight and dietary factors (1,52,53), cigarette smoking (54,55), total blood volume (56), central arterial stiffness (57), and the use of medications (e.g., beta-blockers).

A number of groups have carefully analyzed the associations of physical activity and physical fitness with standard cardiovascular risk factors (58–63). In a very recent study, LaMonte and colleagues performed cross-sectional analyses of 2175 men and 980 women who were participants of the Latter Day Saints Hospital Fitness Institute in Salt Lake City, Utah (60). All subjects underwent symptom-limited exercise testing with exercise capacity estimated according to standard methods (64). Cardiorespiratory fitness was classified as low, moderate, or high based on age- and sex-specific criteria (65). The authors found that among both men and women, decreasing cardiorespiratory

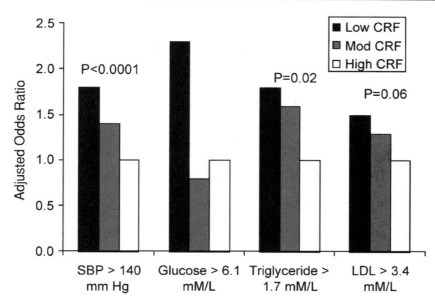

Fig. 3. Adjusted odds ratios for risk factors related to insulin-resistance metabolic syndrome according to cardiorespiratory fitness (CRF) in 980 women studied at the Latter Day Saints Fitness Institute. (From ref. *60* with permission.)

fitness was independently associated with higher rates of hypertension, elevated blood sugar, hypertriglyceridemia, and an elevated low-density lipoprotein (LDL) cholesterol (Fig. 3), even after adjusting for age, percent body fat, presence or absence of coronary heart disease, and family history of coronary heart disease. Of note, these risk factors have been linked to insulin-resistance metabolic syndrome.

Several recent studies have specifically examined the impact of functional capacity and physical exercise training on biological markers of atherosclerotic disease *(66)*, such as carotid intimal thickness and coronary artery stenoses as measured by quantitative angiography. For example, one recent study of a population-based sample of middle-aged men found that higher levels of functional capacity were predictive of slower rates of atherosclerotic disease progression as assessed by carotid ultrasound *(51)*; this study exclusively enrolled men. Similarly, other groups have found that an aggressive exercise regimen was associated with slowed coronary athetherosclerosis progression according to quantitative angiography measures *(67–69)*; these studies also specifically enrolled men. Analogous studies in women need to be performed.

Finally, other investigators have focused on the potentially beneficial biological effects of exercise training. For example, data collected as part of the National Runners' Health Study demonstrated substantial increases in high-density lipoprotein (HDL) cholesterol with vigorous exercise *(62)*. This study involved 1827 women (mean age 40) who were regular runners for an average of 6 years; the authors found an increase of HDL cholesterol by 0.133 mg/dL for each additional kilometer run per week. In another interventional study, it was again noted that women who participated in an exercise program had an increase of HDL cholesterol, but only after 2 years of regular exercise *(63)*. Other potentially beneficial effects of exercise programs include improved autonomic balance *(30–32)*, improved risk factor profiles

(70), improved endothelial function *(71,72),* decreased oxidative stress *(73),* and decreased heart rate *(74).*

THE SEDENTARY EPIDEMIC AMONG AMERICAN WOMEN

Despite the well-known association between physical activity and better health, as well as the extensive media coverage that has been dedicated to it, recent surveys have found no material change in leisure-time physical activities among American adults during the last 15 years *(75).* Furthermore, a number of surveys have found that throughout the life cycle, females tend to be less physically active than males.

Children and Adolescents

Lower levels of routine physical activity among girls begin during childhood. Crocker and colleagues found that among children and adolescents aged 9–15, boys were consistently more active than girls, and younger children were more active than adolescents *(76).* Katzamarzyk and colleagues surveyed 356 boys and 284 girls in three age groups and noted a marked decrease in activity among girls aged 13–15 that was (at least in part) correlated with increased time spent watching television *(19).*

Several large surveys have found disturbingly low levels of regular physical activity among adolescent girls. Gordon-Larsen and colleagues surveyed 13,157 students in grades 7–12 *(77).* Questionnaires were used to assess time spent in moderate-to-vigorous physical activity, defined as at least five bouts per week of 5–8 METs, and in inactivity, primarily defined as time spent watching television or videos. Girls were consistently less active than boys, with particularly high levels of inactivity observed among African-American and Asian girls. In 1995, the Youth Risk Behavior Survey *(78)* found that only 54% of high school girls participated in vigorous physical activity, at least 20 minutes three times a week in comparison to 72% of boys.

The observed low levels of physical activity among female children and adolescents might be partly related to inadequate physical education. Although formal physical education is required by 95% of school districts in the United States *(7,79),* only 26% of states require schools to offer a course at the high school level in lifetime physical activity, and only 15% of all physical education teachers require students to develop individualized fitness programs to prepare them to be physically active adults. Other important factors among girls and female adolescents may include sociocultural factors that pressure girls to curtail "masculine" activity and decreased self-esteem when girls enter junior and senior high school *(18,80–82).*

Adults

Data on frequency of physical activity in the American adult population have been derived from three major surveys *(18,75):* (1) the National Health Interview Survey (NHIS, sample size in 1991: 43,732), (2) the Behavioral Risk Factor Surveillance System (BRFSS, sample size in 1994: 106,040), and (3) the NHANES III (sample size 1988–1991: 9901). Overall, 22–30% of all adults reported no participation in leisure-time physical activity. In each survey and in all age groups, women were consistently more likely than men to be physically inactive, especially at older ages (18; *see* Fig. 4). Conversely, only 20–25% of adults reported participating in regular, sustained physical

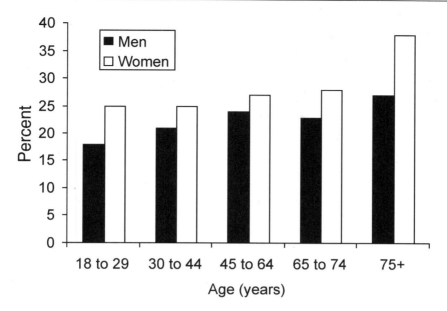

Fig. 4. Percentage of adults reporting no participation in leisure time physical activity according to sex and age as measured by the 1991 National Health Interview Survey (NHIS). (Reproduced from ref. *18.* US government publication.)

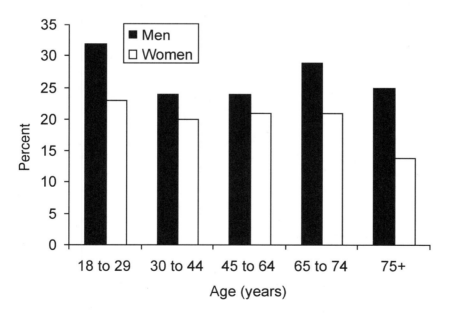

Fig. 5. Percentage of adults reporting participation in regular sustained physical activity, defined as five times per week for at least 30 minutes per session, according to sex and age as measured by the 1991 National Health Interview Survey (NHIS). (Reproduced from ref. *18.* US government publication.)

activity at least five times per week for at least 30 minutes per session. Again, for all age groups, women were less likely to be physically active than men (Fig. 5). Women were much less likely than men to have participated in strengthening exercises within 2 weeks of being surveyed (20% vs 9%), but were as likely as men to have participated in stretching exercises (25% vs 26%; *18*).

It is not entirely clear why women are less physically active than men, although a number of age-specific factors are likely important to consider. Among college-aged women, reasons cited for lower activity levels have included inadequate social support *(83)*, lack of awareness of available exercise facilities, and engaging in potentially harmful weight loss practices *(84)*, such as the use of diet pills or laxatives and self-induced vomiting. Among middle-aged adult women, possible barriers to physical activity include time constraints related to work and parenting responsibilities, cost, mood disturbances, and lack of self-discipline *(18)*. One questionnaire study involving 1336 women found that inactivity was associated with smoking, fatigue, frequent snacking, and obesity *(85)*. Seasonal and geographical factors have also been correlated with physical activity in women, with greater physical activity levels during the spring and summer and in the Western states *(18)*. Among older women, factors that contribute to physical inactivity include decreased skeletal muscle mass accompanied by increased body fat *(86,87)*, increased number of activity-limiting chronic diseases *(88–91)*, and concerns about falling *(92)*.

CONCLUSIONS

Evidence linking impaired functional capacity to increased risk for death and cardiovascular morbidity among both men and women is overwhelming. We recommend that an assessment of functional capacity, whether by formal exercise testing or by structured questionnaire, be an essential part of any comprehensive health assessment. Females who are physically active should be encouraged by physicians and other health care providers to maintain their levels of activity. Women who are physically inactive or who have a low functional measured capacity should be considered to be at increased risk. Physical inactivity is quite common among females, therefore, physicians, both as health care professionals and concerned citizens, should promote and encourage social and educational policies that will lead to higher levels of physical activity among females of all ages.

The US Surgeon General recently published physical activity recommendations that are similarly relevant to women and men *(18)*. Included among these recommendations is that *all people* age 2 years and older should engage in regular physical activity for at least 30 minutes *every day*. Inactive women over the age of 50 and any women with or at high risk for cardiovascular disease who wish to initiate an exercise program should consult with a physician first; a consultation might include a formal exercise test. Muscle strengthening exercises at least twice a week are also strongly recommended. Although these recommendations seem reasonable and strong biological links are present between regular exercise and improved cardiovascular profiles *(70)*, randomized trial data supporting physical activity as a means of preventing coronary events do not yet exist. Therefore, future research will be needed to determine how best to optimally improve overall and cardiovascular outcomes among physically inactive women.

REFERENCES

1. Blair SN, Jacobs DR, Jr., Powell KE. Relationships between exercise or physical activity and other health behaviors. Public Health Rep 1985;100:172–180.
2. Blair SN, Kohl HW, Paffenbarger RS, et al. Physical fitness and all-cause mortality. A prospective study of healthy men and women. JAMA 1989;262:2395–2401.
3. Snader CE, Marwick TH, Pashkow FJ, et al. Importance of estimated functional capacity as a predictor of all-cause mortality among patients referred for exercise thallium single-photon emission computed tomography: report of 3,400 patients from a single center. J Am Coll Cardiol 1997;30:641–648.
4. Wei M, Kampert JB, Barlow CE, et al. Relationship between low cardiorespiratory fitness and mortality in normal-weight, overweight, and obese men. JAMA 1999;282:1547–1553.
5. Weiner DA, Ryan TJ, Parsons L, et al. Long-term prognostic value of exercise testing in men and women from the Coronary Artery Surgery Study (CASS) registry. Am J Cardiol 1995;75:865–870.
6. Ekelund LG, Haskell WL, Johnson JL, et al. Physical fitness as a predictor of cardiovascular mortality in asymptomatic North American men. The Lipid Research Clinics Mortality Follow-up Study. N Engl J Med 1988;319:1379–1384.
7. Pate RR, Pratt M, Blair SN, et al. Physical activity and public health. A recommendation from the Centers for Disease Control and Prevention and the American College of Sports Medicine. JAMA 1995;273:402–407.
8. Paffenbarger RS, Hyde RT, Wing AL, Hsieh CC. Physical activity, all-cause mortality, and longevity of college alumni. N Engl J Med 1986;314:605–613.
9. Lakka TA, Venalainen JM, Rauramaa R, et al. Relation of leisure-time physical activity and cardiorespiratory fitness to the risk of acute myocardial infarction. N Engl J Med 1994;330:1549–1554.
10. Sandvik L, Erikssen J, Thaulow E, et al. Physical fitness as a predictor of mortality among healthy, middle-aged Norwegian men . N Engl J Med 1993;328:533–537.
11. Paffenbarger RS, Hyde RT, Wing AL, et al. The association of changes in physical-activity level and other lifestyle characteristics with mortality among men. N Engl J Med 1993;328:538–545.
12. Erikssen G, Liestol K, Bjornholt J, et al. Changes in physical fitness and changes in mortality. Lancet 1998;352:759–762.
13. Lissner L, Bengtsson C, Bjorkelund C, Wedel H. Physical activity levels and changes in relation to longevity. A prospective study of Swedish women. Am J Epidemiol 1996;143:54–62.
14. Hu FB, Stampfer MJ, Colditz GA, et al. Physical activity and risk of stroke in women. JAMA 2000;283:2961–2967.
15. Manson JE, Hu FB, Rich-Edwards JW, et al. A prospective study of walking as compared with vigorous exercise in the prevention of coronary heart disease in women. N Engl J Med 1999;341:650–658.
16. Sacco RL, Gan R, Boden-Albala B, et al. Leisure-time physical activity and ischemic stroke risk: the Northern Manhattan Stroke Study. Stroke 1998;29:380–387.
17. Garcia AW, Pender NJ, Antonakos CL, Ronis DL. Changes in physical activity beliefs and behaviors of boys and girls across the transition to junior high school. J Adolesc Health 1998;22:394–402.
18. US Department of Health and Human Services. Physical Activity and Health: A Report of the Surgeon General. Centers for Disease Control and Prevention, National Center for Chronic Disease Prevention and Health Promotion, US Department of Health and Human Services, Atlanta, GA, 1996.
19. Katzmarzyk PT, Malina RM, Song TMK, Bouchard C. Physical activity and health-related fitness in youth: a multivariate analysis. Med Sci Sports Exerc 1998;30:709–714.
20. LaPorte RE, Montoye HJ, Caspersen CJ. Assessment of physical activity in epidemiologic research: problems and prospects. Public Health Rep 1985;100:131–146.
21. Andersen LB. A maximal cycle exercise protocol to predict maximal oxygen uptake. Scand J Med Sci Sports 1995;5:143–146.
22. Kleber FX, Vietzke G, Wernecke KD, et al. Impairment of ventilatory efficiency in heart failure: prognostic impact. Circulation 2000;101:2803–2809.
23. Mancini D, LeJemtel T, Aaronson K. Peak VO(2): a simple yet enduring standard. Circulation 2000;101:1080–1082.
24. Myers J, Gullestad L, Vagelos R, et al. Clinical, hemodynamic, and cardiopulmonary exercise test determinants of survival in patients referred for evaluation of heart failure. Ann Intern Med 1998;129:286–293.
25. Robbins M, Francis G, Pashkow FJ, et al. Ventilatory and heart rate responses to exercise: better predictors of heart failure mortality than peak oxygen consumption. Circulation 1999;100:2411–2417.

26. Gibbons RJ, Balady GJ, Beasley JW, et al. ACC/AHA Guidelines for Exercise Testing. A report of the American College of Cardiology/American Heart Association Task Force on Practice Guidelines (Committee on Exercise Testing). J Am Coll Cardiol 1997;30:260–311.

27. Goldman L, Hashimoto B, Cook EF, Loscalzo A. Comparative reproducibility and validity of systems for assessing cardiovascular functional class: advantages of a new specific activity scale. Circulation 1981;64:1227–1234.

28. Hlatky MA, Boineau RE, Higginbotham MB, et al. A brief self-administered questionnaire to determine functional capacity (the Duke Activity Status Index). Am J Cardiol 1989;64:651–654.

29. Imai K, Sato H, Hori M, et al. Vagally mediated heart rate recovery after exercise is accelerated in athletes but blunted in patients with chronic heart failure. J Am Coll Cardiol 1994;24:1529–1535.

30. O'Sullivan SE, Bell C. The effects of exercise and training on human cardiovascular reflex control. J Auton Nerv Syst 2000;81:16–24.

31. Molgaard H, Hermansen K, Bjerregaard P. Spectral components of short-term RR interval variability in healthy subjects and effects of risk factors. Eur Heart J 1994;15:1174–1183.

32. Gallagher D, Terenzi T, de Meersman R. Heart rate variability in smokers, sedentary and aerobically fit individuals. Clin Auton Res 1992;2:383–387.

33. Cole CR, Blackstone EH, Pashkow FJ, et al. Heart-rate recovery immediately after exercise as a predictor of mortality. N Engl J Med 1999;341:1351–1357.

34. Kampert JB, Blair SN, Barlow CE, Kohl HW. Physical activity, physical fitness, and all-cause and cancer mortality: a prospective study of men and women. Ann Epidemiol 1996;6:452–457.

35. Stessman J, Maaravi Y, Hammerman-Rozenberg R, Cohen A. The effects of physical activity on mortality on mortality in the Jerusalem 70-year-olds longitudinal study. J Am Geriatr Soc 2000;48:499–504.

36. Blair SN, Kampert JB, Kohl HW, et al. Influences of cardiorespiratory fitness and other precursors on cardiovascular disease and all-cause mortality in men and women. JAMA 1996;276:205–210.

37. Nishime EO, Cole CR, Blackstone EH, et al. Heart rate recovery and treadmill exercise score as predictors of mortality in patients referred for exercise ECG. JAMA 2000;284:1392–1398.

38. Cole CR, Foody JM, Blackstone EH, Lauer MS. Heart rate recovery after submaximal exercise testing as a predictor of mortality in a cardiovascularly healthy cohort. Ann Intern Med 2000;132:552–555.

39. Colditz GA, Manson JE, Hankinson SE. The Nurses' Health Study: 20-year contribution to the understanding of health among women. J Womens Health 1997;6:49–62.

40. Stampfer MJ, Hu FB, Manson JE, et al. Primary prevention of coronary heart disease in women through diet and lifestyle. N Engl J Med 2000;343:16–22.

41. Maron BJ. The paradox of exercise. N Engl J Med 2000;343:1409–1411.

42. Mittleman MA, Maclure M, Tofler GH, et al. Triggering of acute myocardial infarction by heavy physical exertion. Protection against triggering by regular exertion. Determinants of Myocardial Infarction Onset Study Investigators. N Engl J Med 1993;329:1677–1683.

43. Willich SN, Lewis M, Lowel H, et al. Physical exertion as a trigger of acute myocardial infarction. Triggers and mechanisms of Myocardial Infarction Study Group. N Engl J Med 1993;329: 1684–1690.

44. Ellekjaer H, Holmen J, Ellekjaer E, Vatten L. Physical activity and stroke mortality in women. Ten-year follow-up of the Nord-Trondelag health survey, 1984–1986. Stroke 2000;31:14–18.

45. Gillum RF, Mussolino ME, Ingram DD. Physical activity and stroke incidence in women and men. The NHANES I Epidemiologic Follow-up Study. Am J Epidemiol 1996;143:860–869.

46. Lindenstrom E, Boysen G, Nyboe J. Lifestyle factors and risk of cerebrovascular disease in women. The Copenhagen City Heart Study. Stroke 1993;24:1468–1472.

47. Seals DR, Hurley BF, Schultz J, Hagberg JM. Endurance training in older men and women II. Blood lactate response to submaximal exercise. J Appl Physiol 1984;57:1030–1033.

48. Seals DR, Hagberg JM, Hurley BF, et al. Endurance training in older men and women. I. Cardiovascular responses to exercise. J Appl Physiol 1984;57:1024–1029.

49. Lakka TA, Salonen JT. The Physical Activity Questionnaire of the Kuopio Ischemic Heart Disease Study (KIHD). Med Sci Sports Exerc 1997;29:S46–S56.

50. Bouchard C, Malina RM, Perusse L. Genetics of Fitness and Physical Performance. Human Kinetics, Champaign, IL, 1997.

51. Lakka TA, Laukkanen JA, Rauramaa R, et al. Cardiorespiratory fitness and the progression of carotid atherosclerosis in middle-aged men. Ann Intern Med 2001;134:12–20.

52. Katzel LI, Bleecker ER, Colman EG, et al. Effects of weight loss vs aerobic exercise training on risk factors for coronary disease in healthy, obese, middle-aged and older men. A randomized controlled trial. JAMA 1995;274:1915–1921.

53. Allison DB, Fontaine KR, Manson JE, et al. Annual deaths attributable to obesity in the United States. JAMA 1999;282:1530–1538.

54. Hirsch GL, Sue DY, Wasserman K, et al. Immediate effects of cigarette smoking on cardiorespiratory responses to exercise. J Appl Physiol 1985;58:1975–1981.

55. Morton AR, Holmik EV. The effects of cigarette smoking on maximal oxygen consumption and selected physiological responses of elite team sportsmen. Eur J Appl Physiol 1985;53:348–352.

56. Jones PP, Davy KP, DeSouza CA, et al. Absence of age-related decline in total blood volume in physically active females. Am J Physiol 1997;272:H2534–2540.

57. Tanaka H, DeSouza CA, Seals DR. Absence of age-related increase in central arterial stiffness in physically active women. Arterioscler Thromb Vasc Biol 1998;18:127–132.

58. Manson JE, Colditz GA, Stampfer MJ, et al. A prospective study of obesity and risk of coronary heart disease in women.. N Engl J Med 1990;322:882–889.

59. Manson JE, Stampfer MJ, Hennekens CH, Willett WC. Body weight and longevity. A reassessment. JAMA 1987;257:353–358.

60. LaMonte MJ, Eisenman PA, Adams TD, et al. Cardiorespiratory fitness and coronary heart disease risk factors : the LDS hospital fitness institute cohort. Circulation 2000;102:1623–1628.

61. Haskell WL, Montoye HJ, Orenstein D. Physical activity and exercise to achieve health-related physical fitness components. Public Health Rep 1985;100:202–212.

62. Williams PT. High-density lipoprotein cholesterol and other risk factors for coronary heart disease in female runners. N Engl J Med 1996;334:1298–1303.

63. King AC, Haskell WL, Young DR, et al. Long-term effects of varying intensities and formats of physical activity on participation rates, fitness, and lipoproteins in men and women aged 50 to 65 years. Circulation 1995;91:2596–2604.

64. Bruce RA, Kusumi F, Hosmer D. Maximal oxygen intake and nomographic assessment of functional aerobic impairment in cardiovascular disease. Am Heart J 1973;85:546–562.

65. Pollock ML, Schmidt DH, Jackson AS. Measurement of cardiorespiratory fitness and body composition in the clinical setting. Compr Ther 1980;6:12–27.

66. Kramsch DM, Aspen AJ, Abramowitz BM, et al. Reduction of coronary atherosclerosis by moderate conditioning exercise in monkeys on an atherogenic diet. N Engl J Med 1981;305:1483–1489.

67. Niebauer J, Hambrecht R, Velich T, et al. Attenuated progression of coronary artery disease after 6 years of multifactorial risk intervention: role of physical exercise. Circulation 1997;96:2534–2541.

68. Schuler G, Hambrecht R, Schlierf G, et al. Regular physical exercise and low-fat diet. Effects on progression of coronary artery disease. Circulation 1992;86:1–11.

69. Hambrecht R, Niebauer J, Marburger C, et al. Various intensities of leisure time physical activity in patients with coronary artery disease: effects on cardiorespiratory fitness and progression of coronary atherosclerotic lesions. J Am Coll Cardiol 1993;22:468–477.

70. Shephard RJ, Balady GJ. Exercise as cardiovascular therapy. Circulation 1999;99:963–972.

71. Hambrecht R, Wolf A, Gielen S, et al. Effect of exercise on coronary endothelial function in patients with coronary artery disease. N Engl J Med 2000;342:454–460.

72. Niebauer J, Cooke JP. Cardiovascular effects of exercise: role of endothelial shear stress. J Am Coll Cardiol 1996;28:1652–1660.

73. Parthasarathy S, Santanam N, Ramachandran S, Meilhac O. Potential role of oxidized lipids and lipoproteins in antioxidant defense. Free Radic Res 2000;33:197–215.

74. Beere PA, Glagov S, Zarins CK. Retarding effect of lowered heart rate on coronary atherosclerosis. Science 1984;226:180–182.

75. Cooper R, Cutler J, Desvigne-Nickens P, et al. Trends and disparities in coronary heart disease, stroke, and other cardiovascular diseases in the united states: findings of the national conference on cardiovascular disease prevention. Circulation 2000;102:3137–3147.

76. Crocker PE, Bailey DA, Faulkner RA, et al. Measuring general levels of physical activity: preliminary evidence for the physical activity questionnaire for older children. Med Sci Sports Exerc 1997;29:1344–1349.

77. Gordon-Larsen P, McMurray RG, Popkin BM. Adolescent physical activity and inactivity vary by ethnicity: The National Longitudinal Study of Adolescent Health. J Pediatr 1999;135:301–306.

78. Centers for Disease Control and Prevention. Youth Risk Behavior Survey, 1993 data tape. US Department of Health and Human Services, Public Health Service, Centers for Disease Control and Prevention, National Center for Chronic Disease Prevention and Health Promotion. National Technical Information Service Order no. PB95-503363, Atlanta, GA, 1993.

79. Pate RR, Small ML, Ross JG, et al. School physical education. J School Health 1995;65:312–318.

80. Vijhjalmsson R, Thorlindsson T. Factors related to physical activity: a study of adolescents. Soc Sci Med 1998;47:665–675.

81. Pate RR, Trost SG, Felton GM, et al. Correlates of physical activity behavior in rural youth. Research Quarterly Exercise Sport 1997;68:241–248.

82. Boyd KR, Hrycaiko DW. The effect of a physical activity intervention package on the self-esteem of pre-adolescent and adolescent females. Adolescence 1997;32:693–708.

83. Leslie E, Owen N, Salmon J, et al. Insufficiently active Australian college students: perceived personal, social, and environmental influences. Prev Med 1999;28:20–27.

84. Lowry R, Galuska DA, Fulton JE, et al. Physical activity, food choice, and weight management goals and practices among US college students. Am J Prev Med 2000;18:18–27.

85. Hiraoka J, Ojima T, Nakamura Y, Yanagawa H. A comparative epidemiological study of the effects of regular exercise on health level. J Epidemiol 1998;8:15–23.

86. Evans WJ, Cyr-Campbell D. Nutrition, exercise, and healthy aging. J Am Diet Assoc 1997;97:632–638.

87. Evans JE. Exercise and nutritional needs of elderly people: effects on muscle and bone. Gerodontology 1998;15:15–24.

88. Fried LP, Bandeen-Roche K, Kasper JD, Guralnik JM. Association of comorbidity with disability in older women: the Women's Health and Aging Study. J Clin Epidemiol 1999;52:27–37.

89. Laukkanen P, Sakari-Rantala R, Kauppinen M, Heikkinen E. Morbidity and disability in 75-and 80-year-old men and women: a five-year follow-up. Scandinavian J Social Med 1997;53:79–106.

90. Laukkanen P, Leskinen E, Kauppinen M, et al. Health and functional capacity as predictors of community dwelling among elderly people. J Clin Epidemiol 2000;53:257–265.

91. Morrissey S. Resources and characteristics of elderly women who live alone. Health Care Women International 1998;19:411–421.

92. Satariano WA, Haight TJ, Tager IB. Reasons given by older people for limitation or avoidance of leisure time physical activity. J Am Geriatr Soc 2000;48:505–512.

9 Special Considerations for Minority Women

Jennifer H. Mieres, MD
and Elizabeth Ofili, MD

CONTENTS

THE MAGNITUDE OF THE PROBLEM

Heart disease is the leading cause of death in women in the United States. However, the burden of heart disease is not equally distributed among racial and ethnic groups. Recognizing major differences in health care in the minority populations of the United States, in February 1998 and at the direction of then President Bill Clinton, the US Department of Health and Human Services launched the Initiative to Eliminate Racial and Ethnic Disparities in Health. One of the major goals of the initiative was to eliminate disparities in heart disease by the year 2010 *(1)*.

Although heart disease is prevelant in society as a whole, several epidemiological studies have shown that African-American women experience higher rates of heart disease when compared to white and Hispanic women. In a landmark publication by Casper et al., African-American women were identified as being at much greater risk of dying from heart disease in comparison to women of other ethnic and racial groups *(1)*.

From: *Contemporary Cardiology: Coronary Disease in Women: Evidence-Based Diagnosis and Treatment*
Edited by: L. J. Shaw and R. F. Redberg © Humana Press Inc., Totowa, NJ

In 1995 in the United States, the death rate from heart disease in African-American women was 555 deaths per 100,000, followed by white women with 388 deaths per 100,000, Hispanic women of all races with 265 deaths per 100,000, and Native American and Alaskan native women with 259 deaths per 100,000 (1).

Although mortality from heart disease has been declining in the past few decades, the decline rate has varied by racial and ethnic groups. For African-American women, the rates of morbidity and mortality from coronary heart disease (CHD) have not improved to the same extent that they have in white women. In a 1997 publication of an analysis of the National Health and Nutrition Examination Survey (NHANES I) data, Gillium and colleagues demonstrated that the overall relative risk for African-American women between the ages of 25 and 54 was 1.76 for coronary artery disease (CAD) and 1.0 for acute myocardial infarction (MI), with a 2.25 relative risk for death from CAD (2).

This chapter discusses the recent advances in our knowledge of the occurrence and heart disease determinants in the community of African-American women in the United States because they are the minority group at greatest risk for mortality and morbidity from heart disease.

EPIDEMIOLOGY

Since 1950, it has been documented that African-American women, in comparison to white women, are at a higher risk for death from heart disease, as well as more prone to MI at an earlier age. Furthermore, when MI occurs in young African-American women, it is usually accompanied by major complications and worse outcomes when compared to white women (2–5).

In 1995, the death rate from heart disease was 65% higher in African-American women than in Caucasian women (American Heart Association [AHA] 1997). This startling fact is most likely the result of social, economic, and biological circumstances, which have a strong influence on important primary cardiovascular risk factors that are highly prevalent in African-American women: obesity, hypertension, diabetes mellitus (DM), and physical inactivity (6–8). Low socioeconomic status (SES) has also been strongly linked with CHD risk, which is especially relevant for African-American women because 30% live below the poverty level when compared to 10% of white women (9). Higher risk factor levels in African-American women may explain the excess risk of CAD. Differences in risk factors, health-seeking behavior, and access to health care may account for some of the gap in health status and clinical outcomes from heart disease in African-American women in the United States.

RISK FACTORS FOR CHD

There is a growing consensus that the disparity between African-American and white women in morbidity and mortality from CAD is related to the difference in the prevalence and impact of established risk factors for CAD, especially hypertension, DM, and obesity. In addition, other risk factors, such as smoking, insulin resistance, and stress, may contribute to the racial differences in morbidity and mortality from CAD.

Until recently, the risk factors for CHD in African-American women were not well studied. However, in an important publication, Rosenberg and colleagues investigated factors associated with CHD in data provided by the 64,530 participants of the Black

Women's Heart Study *(10)*. These data implied that conventional risk factors for CAD (hypertension, smoking, DM, hypercholesterolemia, and family heart disease history before age 50) were strongly correlated with CAD. Of note is that the odds ratio for CAD was increased for participants with lower education levels and lower SES. Thus, conventional risk factors for CHD are similar in both African-American and white women.

SPECIFIC RISK FACTORS IN AFRICAN-AMERICAN WOMEN

Hypertension

Epidemiologic studies demonstrate that elevated blood pressure is strongly and consistently linked to risk for CAD, as hypertension accelerates the atherosclerotic process *(11)*. The incidence of hypertension increases with age among all racial groups; however, the increase rate is much greater in African-American women. Among US women over 45 years of age, 60% of white women and 79% of African-American women have hypertension *(12)*. The prevalence of hypertension in African-Americans age 20 or older far exceeds that of the overall US population and has been estimated at 34.2% for African-American women vs 19.3% for white women *(13)*. The impact of hypertension is also much greater among African-American women than white women in the United States. In 1995, the death rate from hypertension was 352% higher for African-American women than for white women *(12)*.

Hypertension remains a key contributing factor to the development of atherosclerotic heart disease. Accordingly, with a significantly higher prevalence of hypertension, the African-American woman is at great risk for morbidity and mortality from CAD. A recent meta-analysis has demonstrated the impact of treatment of African-American women with primary hypertension on cardiovascular morbidity and mortality outcome based on data from 11 randomized controlled trials. In this meta-analysis, treatment of hypertension in African-American women reduced the risk of fatal and nonfatal coronary events by 33% *(14)*. Because hypertension plays such a pivotal role in CAD development, control of hypertension may be one of the most important aspects of CAD prevention in African-American women.

Obesity and Sedentary Lifestyle

Obesity and a sedentary lifestyle have reached epidemic proportions in the United States and are two important factors that contribute to an increased risk of heart disease. A high body mass index (BMI) and central obesity are important independent predictors of CHD in women *(15)*. Physical inactivity is a major contributing factor to obesity and is an independent risk factor for the development of CHD *(16)*.

Recent studies have demonstrated that 67% of African-American women are overweight (BMI >25 kg/m^2), and 68% have an inactive lifestyle *(17)*. The fact that there is a high prevalence of obesity and inactive lifestyle in African-Americans is directly correlated with the high incidence of CHD.

DIABETES MELLITUS

DM (more than 90% of which is type 2 diabetes with onset in adulthood) is an independent risk factor for CHD. Diabetes is associated with a three- to sevenfold increase in CHD risk in women *(18)*. Data from the NHANES III demonstrated that among women older than 20 years of age, 9.1% of African-American women when compared to 4.6% of white women, had DM (19). Because obesity is linked to type 2 diabetes, and with 67% of African-American women being obese, the high incidence of diabetes in this group is expected.

HYPERHOMOCYSTEINEMIA

Elevated plasma homocysteine concentration is an independent risk factor for CAD and subsequent mortality (20). In a recent study of 89 African-American women and 90 white women, Gerhard and colleagues demonstrated that the former had higher plasma total homocysteine levels and lower plasma folate levels (21). The higher plasma homocysteine levels and low folate levels were felt to be the result of lower folate and multivitamin intake in African-American women, who were included in this study. Thus, in addition to traditional risk factors, elevated homocysteine levels may be an additional potent risk factor for CAD in African-American women.

CHEST PAIN: THE PARADOX OF CAD IN AFRICAN-AMERICAN WOMEN

Angina as a presenting symptom of CHD has been found to be higher in African-American women in comparison to white women (22). Yet, despite this higher incidence of angina, there is a lower prevalence of angiographically significant disease. Angiographic prevalence of CAD was found to be 12% in African-American women in comparison to 20% in white women in the Coronary Artery Surgery Study (CASS) study (23). However, it appears that when CAD is present in the African-American woman, it is usually significant and has a poor prognosis. Thus, anginal chest pain in African-American women is a less specific marker and less predictive of CAD.

Possible causes of the high chest pain incidence in African-American women include resistance vessel disease in hypertensive women with left ventricular hypertrophy (LVH) and microvascular disease in the setting of diabetes and hypertension—two disease states that are present in large percentages in African-American women.

Despite the limited prognostic value of chest pain in African-American women, it remains the most common manifestation of CHD. Thus, chest pain and possible atypical symptoms of angina should be pursued in African-American women, given the appropriate clinical context and underlying probability of coronary disease.

IDENTIFICATION AND MANAGEMENT OF AFRICAN-AMERICAN WOMEN WITH CAD DIAGNOSIS

Noninvasive

The choice and interpretation of noninvasive tests pose unique challenges in women. Limited data exist on the use of the standard noninvasive test (e.g., exercise stress testing, stress echocardiography, and nuclear perfusion studies) in African-American women. One important factor that may have a significant influence on the diagnostic accuracy of noninvasive tests in African-American women is the high prevalence of LVH. Exercise electrocardiogram (ECG), for example, loses its diagnostic accuracy in the LVH setting.

The sensitivity and specificity of exercise treadmill testing can be greatly enhanced by adding imaging techniques, such as myocardial perfusion imaging and echocardiography. Myocardial perfusion imaging with the radioisotope technetium-99m Sestamibi with gated single photon emission tomography (SPECT) has been shown to have excellent sensitivity and specificity for detecting CAD in women (24) and has similar prognostic value in African-American and white subjects (25).

Stress echocardiography has been shown to be an accurate cost-effective approach to diagnosing CAD in women (26) and is a sensitive tool for the detection and quantification of LVH. Thus, with a high prevalence of hypertension and LVH in African-American women, stress echocardiography is a reliable, noninvasive diagnostic tool in detecting CAD in African-American women.

CARDIAC CATHETERIZATION AND CORONARY REVASCULARIZATION

Several studies have confirmed the existence of race-related disparities in the utilization of coronary procedures. African-Americans are less likely than whites to receive diagnostic and therapeutic cardiac procedures in the CAD setting (2,27,28). Several factors that may affect racial disparity in referral for cardiac procedures include financial barriers, differences in severity of disease, patient preferences, and the amount of patient contact with hospitals that offer invasive cardiac procedures (27,29). Peterson and colleagues demonstrated that patient choice is a contributing factor in the underutilization of coronary procedures in African Americans. Despite equivalent referral patterns to cardiac catheterization at Duke University, fewer African-American patients chose revascularization over medical therapy (27).

Physician referral bias is another important factor in the race-related disparity in referral for coronary procedures. In a recent publication, Schulman and colleagues demonstrated that the race and sex of a patient independently influence physicians'

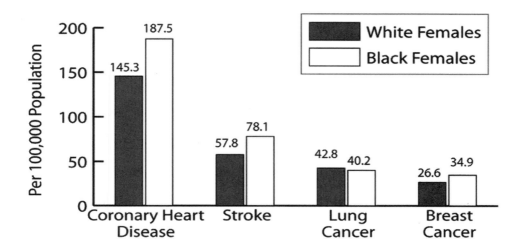

Fig. 1. Age-adjusted death rates for coronary heart disease, stroke, lung and breast cancer for white and black females. (From ref. 32.)

treatment strategies for chest pain. In this study, physicians were asked to outline a diagnostic and treatment plan based on a given history and videotapes of subjects of different races and sexes *(30)*. Given the same history, physician referral for cardiac catheterization was less frequent for women and African Americans. Thus, despite the increase in performance of coronary revascularization (coronary artery bypass graft surgery and percutaneous transluminal coronary angioplasty) in African Americans *(31)*, racial disparities still exist in the utilization of coronary procedures.

CONCLUSION

The fact that the African-American woman is vulnerable to CHD is undisputable, as it is the leading cause of death in African-American women. Despite the fact that heart disease mortality and morbidity have improved significantly over the past decade, African-American women continue to have worse life expectancy and excess death from heart disease. See Fig. 1 *(32)*. Differences in risk factor profile, access to health care, SES, and health-seeking patterns may account for some of the racial disparity in mortality from heart disease. Two factors are instrumental in improving the heart disease mortality rate in African-American women: (1) physician referral bias must be overcome, and (2) African-American women need to understand that they are vulnerable to heart disease. They must be educated about the risk factors, warning signs, and preventive strategies for heart disease.

REFERENCES

1. Casper ML, Barnet E, Halverson JA, et al. Women and Heart Disease: An Atlas of Racial and Ethnic Disparities in Mortality. Publication of the Center for Disease Control and Prevention and West Virginia University, Morgantown, WV, 2001.
2. Gillum RF, Musilino MA, Madans JH, et al. Coronary heart disease incidence and survival in African-American women and men: The NHANES I epidemiology follow-up study: Ann Intern Med 1997;127:111–118.
3. Gillum RF. Coronary heart disease in black population. I Mortality and morbidity. Am Heart J 1982;104:839–851.
4. Toffler GH, Stone PH, Muller JE, et al. Effects on gender and Race on prognosis after myocardial infarction: adverse prognosis for women, particularly black women. J Am Coll Cardiol 1987;9:473–482.
5. Bransford Tl, Ofili E. The paradox of coronary heart disease in African American women. J Natl Med Assoc 2000;92:327–333.
6. Kumanyika SK. Special Issues regarding obesity in minority population. Ann Inter Med 1993;119:650–654.
7. Johnson JL, et al. Cardiovascular disease risk factors and mortality among black women and white women aged 40–64 in Evans County Georgia. Ann J Epidemio 1986;123:209–220.
8. Winkleby MA, Robinson TN, Sundquist J, et al. Ethnic and socioeconomic differences in cardiovascular disease risk factors: findings for women form the third National Health and Nutrition Examination Survey 1988–1994. J Am Med Assoc 1998;280:356–362.
9. Winkleby MA. Accelerated cardiovascular risk factors in ethnic minority and low socio-economic groups: Ann Epidemiol 1997;7:596–51034–9.
10. Rosenberg L, Palmer JR, Sowmya R, et al. Risk Factors for Coronary Heart Disease in African American Women. Am J Epidemiol 1999;150:904–909.
11. Kannel WB, Gordon T, Schwarttz MJ, et al. Systolic versus diastolic Blood Pressure and risk for coronary heart disease: The Framingham Study. Am J Cardiol 1971;27:335–346.
12. 1997 Heart and Stroke Statistical Update. American Heart Association, Dallas, TX, 1997.
13. Burt VL, Whelan P, Roccella ES, et al. Prevalence of hypertension in the US adult population: Results from the third National Health and Nutrition Examination Survey 1988–1991: Hypertension 1995;25:305–313.

14. Quan A, Kerlikowshe K, Gueyffier F, Boissel JP. Efficacy of treating hypertension in women. J Gen Intern Med 1999;14:718–729.
15. Calle EE, Thun MJ, Petrelli JM, et al. Body mass index and mortality in a prospective cohort of US adults. N Engl J Med 1999;341:1097–1105.
16. US Department of Health and Human Service. Physical Activity and Health: A Report of the Surgeon General. US Department of Health and Human Services, Centers for Disease Control and Prevention, National Center for Chronic Disease Prevention and Health Promotion, Atlanta, GA, 1996.
17. AHA 2000 Heart and Stroke Statistical Update. American Heart Association, Dallas, TX, 1999.
18. Manson JE, Spelsberg A. Risk modification in the diabetic patient. In: Manson JE, Ridker PM, Gaziano JM, Hennekens CH, eds. Prevention of Myocardial Infarction. Oxford university Press, New York, NY, 1996, pp. 241–273.
19. Harris MI, Flegal KM, Cowie CC, et al. Prevalence of diabetes, impaired fasting glucose and impaired glucose tolerance in US adults; The third National Health and Nutrition Examination Survey, 1988–1994. Diabetes Care 1998;21:518–524.
20. Nygard O, Nordrehaug JE, Refsum H, et al. Plasma homocysteine levels and mortality in patients with CAD. N Engl J Med 1997;337:230–236.
21. Gerhard GT, Malinow MR, De Loughery TG, et al. Higher homocysteine concentration and lower folate concentrations in premenopausal black women than in premenopausal white women. Am J Clin Nutr 1999;70:252–260.
22. Langford HG, Oberman A, Borhani NO, et al. Black-white comparison of indices of coronary heart disease and myocardial infarction in the stepped care cohort of the hypertension, detection and follow-up program. Am Heart J 1984;104:707–714.
23. Maynard C, Fisher L, Passamani ER, Pullum T. Blacks in the Coronary Artery Surgery Study: risk factors and coronary artery disease. Circulation 1986;74:64–71.
24. Taillefer R, DePuey EG, Udelson JE, et al. Comparision of Thallium-201 and Tc-99m Sestamibi myocardial perfusion imaging in detection of coronary artery disease in women. J Am Coll Cardiol 1997;29:69–77.
25. Alkeylani A, Miller DD, Shaw LJ, et al. Influence of race on the prediction of cardiac events with stress Tc-99m sestamibi tomographic imaging in patients with stable angina pectoris. Am J Cardiol 1998;81:293–297.
26. Marwick TH, Anderson T, William MJ, et al. Exercise ecchocardiography is an accurate and cost-effective technique for detection of coronary artery disease in women. J Am Coll Cardiol 1995;26:335–341.
27. Peterson ED, Shaw LK, Delong ER, et al. Racial Variation in the use of coronary- revasularization procedures, Are the differences real? Do they matter? N Engl J Med 1997;336:480–486.
28. Laouri M, Kravitz RL, French WJ, et al. Underuse of coronary revascularization procedures: application of a clinical method. J Am Coll Cardiol 1997;29:891–897.
29. Blustein J, Weitzman BC. Access to hospitals with high-technology cardiac services: how is race important? Am J Public Health 1995;85:345–351.
30. Schulman KA, Berlin JA, Harless W, et al. The effect of race and sex on physicians' recommendations for cardiac catheterization. N Engl J Med 1999;340:618–626.
31. Gillum RF, Gillum BS, Francis CK. Coronary revascularization and cardiac catheterization in the United States: trends in racial differences. J Am Coll Cardiol 1997;29:1557–1562.
32. American Heart Association. Heart Disease and Stroke Statistics—2003 Update. Dallas, TX, American Heart Association, 2002.

B. Varying Symptom Presentation in Women

10 Clinical Risk Assessment in Women

Chest Discomfort. Report from the WISE Study

B. Delia Johnson, PhD, Sheryl F. Kelsey, PhD, and C. Noel Bairey Merz, MD

CONTENTS

INTRODUCTION

Chest pain is one of the most common complaints encountered by the emergency physician. Each year, 5.3 million patients appear at US emergency rooms with chest pain *(1)*. More than half of these patients are women *(2)*. The chief clinical concern in evaluation is the possibility of acute coronary syndrome (ACS) and the need to provide quick and appropriate therapy to reduce the risk of death and serious complications *(3)*. Often, coronary angiography and other objective testing is performed only after clinical history, including chest pain evaluation, reveals a reasonable likelihood that a patient might suffer from ACS. For women, such a likelihood is more difficult to assess than in men. This chapter addresses the issues in using chest pain assessment as part of a coronary artery disease (CAD) diagnostic work-up in women. The first part summarizes the available literature. In the second part, the widely used Coronary Artery Surgery Study (CASS) symptom classification is tested in a pilot group of Women's Ischemia Syndrome Evaluation (WISE) study participants to provide preliminary evidence toward the development of a female pattern angina classification.

TYPICAL ANGINA AND CAD IN WOMEN

A systematic chest pain classification was developed in the CASS study in the 1980s as part of CADENZA, a microcomputer program to estimate the probability of CAD in patients. Besides symptom classification, this program also evaluated risk factors, including gender and noninvasive test results. Symptoms were evaluated according to

From: *Contemporary Cardiology: Coronary Disease in Women: Evidence-Based Diagnosis and Treatment*
Edited by: L. J. Shaw and R. F. Redberg © Humana Press Inc., Totowa, NJ

three criteria: is the discomfort (1) substernal, (2) precipitated by physical exertion, (3) relieved within 10 minutes by rest or nitroglycerin. *Typical angina* was defined as the presence of all three-symptom characteristics; *atypical angina* was defined as the presence of any two; *nonanginal discomfort* was defined as the presence of only one; and *asymptomatic* referred to patients without any of these symptom characteristics *(4)*. The investigators found that a probability estimate based on a patient's age, sex, symptom classification, and Framingham risk factors predicted the disease prevalence as accurately as one also based on various combinations of noninvasive test procedures. Even in women, who had a lower CAD incidence than men *(5)*, symptom classification was closely linked with CAD prevalence. Among women, 62% with typical angina had CAD; 40% with atypical angina had CAD; and only 4% with nonanginal pain had CAD *(6)*.

Because of its elegant simplicity and apparently widespread application, this chest pain classification has become the standard in clinical practice. However, subsequent experience has suggested that CAD is not as easy to diagnose in women as it is in men. It is a common observation that women have a different pattern of coronary symptoms than men *(7–10)*. Hence, women with chronic stable angina are more likely than men to experience angina during rest, sleep, or mental stress *(11)*. They often experience their symptoms in locations other than the substernum: lower jaw and teeth, arms, shoulders, back, and epigastrium *(12–14)*. Rather than actual pain, symptoms may include dyspnea, palpitations, presyncope, fatigue, sweating, nausea, or vomiting *(15–18)*. Compared to the highly predictable angina patterns in men, typical angina appears to be far less predictive of CAD in women *(12,19)*. Conversely, the presence of symptoms other than typical angina does not decrease CAD likelihood *(20)*.

Moreover, at follow-up, twice as many women (as men) with normal arteries experience continued chest pain, angina treatments, chest pain-related hospital admissions *(12,21–23)*, and significantly impaired quality of life *(24)*. Women without angiographically significant CAD continue to experience persistent chest pain over time nearly as frequently as women with CAD *(25)*. The concept of gender differences in the association of symptom presentation and CAD is not uniformly accepted. Some authors suggest that there are more similarities than differences between the sexes and that some observed differences may be the result of communication style *(26)*.

A second complication for symptom assessment is that among women clinically referred for coronary angiography, only approx 50% or less are found to have significant coronary artery obstruction when compared to approx 85% of men *(27–30)*. Along with the additional complication of higher false positive-test responses on noninvasive diagnostic tests *(31,32)*, these problems partly explain why women have often received less careful evaluation of their chest pain symptoms and are less likely to undergo coronary angiography and less aggressive treatment *(33–39)*. Noninvasive CAD tests were largely developed and verified in men and may be less robust in women *(40)*, as women have historically been understudied *(41–43)*. When presenting with non-"classic" symptoms, a woman is often not taken seriously and may be sent home without diagnostic assessment *(44)*. An "exaggeratedly emotional presentation style" may reduce her assessed CAD probability *(45)*. Women themselves substantially underestimate their own CAD risk and attribute their symptoms to other possible diseases *(46)*. Thus, they are likely to ignore their atypical symptoms and delay seeking medical care *(47,48)*. As a result, ischemic heart disease is diagnosed less often in women *(44,49)* and at a more advanced disease stage *(50)*. The consequences are enormous. When women develop significant CAD, they typically have greater disease severity and disability than men. Women are more likely to die from an episode of myocardial infarction (MI) than men *(51–53)*. Only recently has angina pectoris been recognized as a serious clinical problem for women *(34,54)*, whereas in fact, coronary heart disease is the leading cause of mortality and leads to serious morbidity and disability in adult US women *(34)*.

MECHANISMS OF NON-CAD CHEST PAIN IN WOMEN

The syndrome of typical anginal symptoms and normal coronary angiograms, often accompanied by positive echocardiogram (ECG) responses to exercise suggestive of ischemia, has been termed *Syndrome X (55,56)*. Early observations have noted that this syndrome predominates in women and that the symptoms can be severe and disabling *(57)*. However, once CAD is ruled out, further physiological studies are rarely carried out in women, and their symptoms are often dismissed as noncardiac *(58,59)*. The search for noncardiac etiologies has focused primarily on gastrointestinal disorders *(60)* and anxiety or panic disorders. However, even if present, the presumed cause-and-effect sequence between chest pain and noncardiac etiologies has been questioned in several studies *(61,62)*. It would not be surprising in a large patient population with severe, debilitating, and persistent symptoms of undetermined etiology to find a high incidence of anxiety, panic disorder, and somaticizing complaints secondary to their unexplained and often untreated symptoms. In many women with Syndrome X, the presence of comorbid conditions does not necessarily obviate the need for more detailed evaluations for myocardial ischemia.

Myocardial ischemia is mediated, to a large degree, by endothelial dysfunction, defined as the disordered response of arteries (macrovascular dysfunction) and arterioles (microvascular dysfunction) to physiological stimuli (exercise, mental stress, acetylcholine, etc.). Recent evidence suggests that much of women's chest discomfort in the absence of CAD may result from a higher prevalence among women of vasospastic *(63)* and microvascular angina *(19)*, resulting from functional abnormalities of the coronary microcirculation during stress *(64,65)*. Such functional abnormalities may include abnormal dilator and exaggerated responses to vasoconstrictors, as well as attenuated changes in coronary blood flow following stress *(19,65)*, as demonstrated in studies of exercise testing, coronary flow reserve *(66)*, and coronary velocity reserve *(67)*. Patients with Syndrome X may present with either typical or atypical angina *(68,69)*. Recent work has provided direct evidence of abnormal metabolic responses to stress that are consistent with abnormal dilator responses of the coronary microvasculature *(70)*. Additionally, studies have indicated that the microvascular impairment in Syndrome X may not just be functional, but may also represent structural changes in the small coronary arteries *(71,72)*. Although current evidence suggests that patients with this syndrome have a relatively low likelihood of adverse outcomes, the prognostic significance for downstream CAD development is as yet poorly understood. However, it is clear that women with vasospastic or microvascular angina can be treated by vasoactive pharmacological agents *(58)*. Therefore, it is important that chest pain evaluation, particularly in women, include microvascular dysfunction analysis after ruling out CAD.

A woman's diagnostic assessment is not complete without consideration of hormonal status. Menopausal status, irrespective of age, is now recognized as a risk factor for CAD *(73)*. Menopause not only alters risk factors, such as lipoprotein profiles *(74)*, but the reduced estrogen levels may also impact the coronary microvasculature *(75)*. The relationship between hormonal status and chest discomfort and the possible role of hormone replacement therapy (HRT) in reducing or even reversing the damaging effects of estrogen loss are currently controversial. Although the Nurses' Health Study and the Lipid Research Clinics Program have demonstrated significant decreases in CAD risk and cardiovascular mortality at follow-up *(76,77)*, more recent prospective placebo-controlled trials have failed to find beneficial effects. For example, the Heart and Estrogen Replacement Study (HERS) has found no reduction in cardiovascular event rates at 4-year follow-up among women with established CAD who received HRT, despite a beneficial effect on lipid profiles *(78)*.

In summary, for many years, chest pain diagnosis in women has followed the male disease model. A comparative female model has not been developed, partly because women's anginal symptoms do not track as easily with CAD and partly because of the traditional lack of appreciation in considering CAD as a serious clinical problem for women. Although cardiovascular disease is the most frequent cause of death among women in the United States and the developed world, women continue to be underdiagnosed and undertreated in comparison to men, and referral tends to be delayed until a later stage in the disease process. As a partial result, women are more likely to die from their first MI. However, even in the absence of significant CAD, women who experience debilitating and frightening symptoms continue to consume large amounts of diagnostic and health care resources and costs. To develop better diagnostic models requires two directions. One is to recognize that, under the current state of knowledge, clinical history alone is inadequate to distinguish cardiac from noncardiac chest pain *(34)*, thus requiring more objective testing in women. Objective testing should also include assessment for microvascular dysfunction, which is often responsible for chest discomfort of noncoronary etiology and can be pharmacologically treated. The second direction is to develop a better assessment instrument for female pattern angina. The following section reports on our ongoing work in the WISE study in seeking to develop such an instrument.

FEMALE PATTERN ANGINA: REPORT FROM THE WISE STUDY

The National Heart, Lung, and Blood Institute (NHLBI) WISE is an ongoing four-center study designed to optimize symptom evaluation and diagnostic testing for ischemic heart disease in women *(79)*. A primary goal has been to improve chest pain symptom modeling. Over the past 3 years, WISE has enrolled nearly 1000 consecutive women with symptoms leading to clinical referral for coronary angiographic evaluation of suspected ischemia. The study has collected the largest contemporary dataset of a unique female cohort. The WISE common core data include demographic and clinical data, psychosocial variables, coronary angiography and ventriculography data, blood determinations, and a variety of noninvasive diagnostic tests.

Prior WISE results have shown that approx 40% of the WISE participants experience chest pain or other symptoms daily or almost daily, and approx 70% experience symptoms at least weekly. Symptom frequency does not differ by severity of CAD, but is associated with significantly lower quality of life *(80)*. Frequency of symptoms at baseline also predicts whether a woman will continue to experience persistent symptoms over time. Other predictors of persistent chest pain (or other symptoms) were pain location (e.g., neck, left arm, but not substernal pain), symptoms waking at night, younger age, and a history of reproductive abnormality *(25)*.

Methods

We are reporting pilot results on 481 women consecutively enrolled in WISE who had complete angiographic, demographic, risk factor, and anginal chest pain evaluation. A subgroup of 435 also completed the WISE symptom questionnaire. In the original CASS study, Diamond et al. *(4)* excluded patients with documented prior CAD, which we attempted to replicate by excluding women who reported a past MI or who had undergone coronary artery bypass grafting (CABG) or percutaneous transluminal coronary angioplasty (PTCA) revascularization procedures. It was believed that symptom descriptions might be influenced by prior knowledge of CAD presence. The WISE sample ranged in age from 27 to 85 years, mean 57±11, and 17% were non-white. Most of the women (79%) listed chest pain as their primary reason for being referred for coronary angiography, although other reasons included abnormal stress test results and shortness of breath. All the women had experienced chest pain or other symptoms in the year prior to WISE enrollment. Angiographic results indicate that 48% of the women had no detectable coronary disease (<20% luminal diameter stenosis), 26% had minimal coronary disease (20 to <50% stenosis), and 26% had significant coronary disease (≥50% stenosis) in one or more epicardial coronary artery. This low CAD incidence in the study population resulted from the exclusion of women with known CAD from the present analysis. Most of the women had multiple cardiac risk factors, such as hypertension, obesity, and diabetes. Most were postmenopausal (74%), and 41% were on HRT at the time of their evaluation.

CORONARY ANGIOGRAPHY

All women received clinically ordered coronary angiograms that were reviewed by a WISE core angiographic laboratory to provide a uniform quantitative and qualitative assessment of the presence, severity, and complexity of epicardial coronary artery stenosis.

CHEST PAIN ASSESSMENT

Most women completed two chest pain symptom questionnaires administered at the same setting. The traditional chest pain assessment questionnaire, validated in large female and male populations for coronary disease prediction *(4)*, was used to classify women's symptoms as typical angina, atypical angina, nonanginal symptoms, and asymptomatic (*see* p. 130). A second questionnaire developed for WISE explored a wide list of other pain symptoms, including location, intensity, duration, remedies, and chest pain triggers.

Results: Anginal Classification

Table 1 summarizes the demographic and risk factor information for the 481 WISE participants, stratified by absence or presence of CAD. Women with CAD were older and postmenopausal and had a higher prevalence of diabetes, hypertension, and dys-

Table 1
Demographics and Risk Factors by Presence of CAD for WISE Women

	No CAD n = 354	CAD n = 127	p*
Age (mean ± SD)	56 ± 10	62 ± 11	<0.0001
Systolic blood pressure (mean ± SD)	135 ± 20	139 ± 22	0.05
Total cholesterol (mean ± SD)	196 ± 44	202 ± 51	0.26
Body mass index (mean ± SD)	29.6 ± 6.6	29.0 ± 5.8	0.38
Diabetes (%)	14	32	<0.0001
Race (non-white) (%)	14	24	0.01
Postmenopausal (%)	72	82	0.02
History of dyslipidemia (%)	43	55	0.02
History of hypertension (%)	52	63	0.02
On HRT (%)	44	33	0.03
Reports high stress last 5 years (%)	36	28	0.10
History of smoking (%)	48	50	0.65
Family CAD history (%)	66	66	0.94

* p-values based on t-tests for continuous variables and chi-squares for frequencies.
SD, standard deviation.

lipidemia than women without CAD. They were also more likely to be non-white and less likely to be on HRT. A more detailed analysis shows a close relationship between CAD and age. When divided into four age categories, the percent of women with CAD was: age less than 45, 10%; 45–55, 19%; 55–65, 25%; and greater than 65, 43%. Of the 22 women age 75 years or older, 68% had CAD. Age has consistently been the strongest CAD predictor in the WISE study.

The percent of women with CAD by anginal classification was less dramatic: 35% for typical angina; 22% for atypical angina; 27% for nonanginal symptoms; and 8% for asymptomatic women. Although decreasing with less typical angina, this trend does not show much diagnostic discrimination, particularly when compared with CASS results (62, 40, and 4%, respectively, for the first three categories). Typical angina had a 35% sensitivity and a 77% specificity suggesting a high rate of false-negatives or an underdiagnosis of women with CAD. It is of note that although the so-called "asymptomatic" women had a very low CAD prevalence, these women were not truly asymptomatic. More than 50% of these women described their symptoms as "discomfort" in the left chest, left shoulder, or left arm. This discomfort most often took the form of chest pressure, tightness, numbness, or shortness of breath, and typically occurred at rest. Although most women described their symptoms as "tolerable," 97% had sought medical care.

We next stratified WISE women by both anginal classification and age according to the CASS categories. Diamond estimated the probability of CAD using Bayes' theorem of conditional probability, calculated separately for men and women with no prior CAD documentation, by age group and anginal class and normalized for Framingham risk factors (81). These probabilities are replicated in Fig. 1 (gray columns) and compared to CAD prevalence in the WISE women, adjusted for diabetes, total cholesterol, smoking, and hypertension (black columns).

First, the results demonstrate the expected increase of CAD prevalence with age. Second, the hypothesized relationship between anginal classification and CAD only

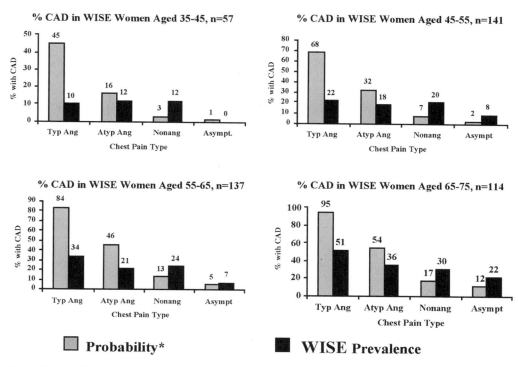

Fig. 1. Probability vs prevalence of coronary artery disease (CAD) by anginal classification and by age. (From ref. *81*.) Typ Ang, typical angina; Atyp Ang, atypical angina; Nonang, nonanginal; Asympt, asymptomatic.

begins to appear in the 55- to 65-year group and becomes more pronounced with increasing age. Finally, in all four age groups, the probability and prevalence slopes consistently cross, such that WISE women with nonanginal chest pain had nearly double the CAD frequency predicted by CASS, despite the overall lower prevalence. The probability and prevalence distributions were significantly different in all age groups (p = 0.0001, using the Jonckheere-Terpstra test). We can conclude that in this pilot group of women with chest pain referred for clinical ischemia evaluation, anginal chest pain evaluation was only a weak CAD predictor, and only among women over 55 years of age. Among younger women, anginal chest pain classification did not track with CAD. These results are consistent with prior work that suggests inherent pathophysiological differences between young men and women that tend to equalize when women lose female hormone protection after menopause *(49,82)*.

Table 2 lists the three variables that underly the anginal classification: substernal pain, effort or stress triggers, and relief with rest or nitroglycerin. These variables were evaluated for all women combined, then for women below and above age 55. Notably, although these variables approached significance in predicting CAD among women above age 55, they did not predict CAD in younger women, with the possible exception of effort or stress triggers. These results confirm the previous findings that the composite CASS anginal symptom classification only predicts CAD in older women.

Table 2
Angina Indicators by Presence of CAD for WISE Women

	No CAD	CAD	p*
All women	n = 354	n = 127	
Pain center chest (substernal) (%)	62	71	0.09
Pain with effort or stress (%)	50	63	0.02
Relief with rest or nitroglycerine (%)	72	80	0.11
Older women (≥55 years)	n = 180	n = 93	
Pain center chest (substernal) (%)	63	74	0.07
Pain with effort or stress (%)	53	63	0.09
Relief with rest or nitroglycerine (%)	67	81	0.02
Younger women (<55 years)	n = 174	n = 34	
Pain center chest (substernal) (%)	61	62	0.98
Pain with effort or stress (%)	48	62	0.15
Relief with rest or nitroglycerine (%)	78	76	0.83

* *p*-values based on chi-squares for frequencies.

Pilot Results from the WISE Chest Pain Questionnaire

Next, we evaluated the relationship of other pain descriptors with CAD (Table 3). Among the 65 discomfort items on this questionnaire, only 8 significantly distinguished among women with and without CAD. Most of these items were negatively associated with CAD, such that the presence of these symptoms tended to indicate CAD absence. Hence, neck pain, weakness, fatigue, palpitations, knife-like pain, sweating, and emotional triggers were significantly less common in women with CAD than in women without CAD. When analyzed by age group, each group emerged with a separate set of significant symptoms. For women above age 55, neck pain was again negatively associated with CAD, whereas upper body exertion and relief with nitroglycerin were positively predictive of CAD. By contrast, younger women with CAD experienced an array of significant symptoms, primarily focused on the arm, shoulder, and hands. For these women, symptom descriptions of heaviness, tightness, numbness, or burning were positively related to CAD, whereas weakness, fatigue, and faintness were negatively related to CAD.

In summary, pilot results from the WISE study confirm published findings that women with CAD experience a wide variety of symptoms. This reality is complicated by a woman's age. In older women, the traditional anginal classifications are moderately predictive of CAD, although not as strongly as prior studies have suggested. WISE has identified additional symptom variables which, when added to the traditional angina questionnaire, might improve prediction for older women. By contrast, traditional angina variables are not CAD predictive in younger women, either individually or combined. Younger women's symptoms seem to focus more on arms, shoulders, hands, have nonspecific triggers or relief sources, with a range of descriptive manifestations. WISE is currently investigating the results' validity against the possibility of type I error (i.e., finding a significant difference between two groups when none, in fact, is present). Such an error is likely when numerous statistical tests find only a few

Table 3
Significant WISE Pain Indicators by Presence of CAD in WISE Women

	No CAD	CAD	p*
All women	n = 337	n = 98	
Location:			
Neck	55	41	0.01
Description:			
Weakness, fatigue	63	47	0.004
Palpitations	62	46	0.006
Sharp knife	28	18	0.04
Sweating	44	33	0.04
Triggers:			
Strong emotion	60	48	0.04
Relief:			
Nitroglycerin	25	38	0.01
Older women (≥55 years)	n = 169	n = 69	
Location:			
Neck	56	35	0.003
Triggers:			
Upper body exertion	29	45	0.02
Relief:			
Nitroglycerin	22	37	0.02
Younger women (<55 years)	n = 168	n = 29	
Location:			
Arm or shoulder	63	86	0.02
Hands	46	69	0.02
Description:			
Weakness/fatigue/faintness	70	38	0.001
Burning	16	38	0.007
Numbness	28	52	0.01
Tightness	61	83	0.02
Heaviness	79	93	0.04

p-values based on chi-squares for frequencies.

significant effects. To verify the results, we are currently testing pilot group results in the larger WISE population and in a non-WISE sample of women clinically referred for coronary angiography.

SUMMARY AND CONCLUSIONS

Review of the extensive research on CAD symptomology literature in women confirms the consensus that women experience CAD differently from men. However, there is very little agreement among studies regarding the specific symptom locations and descriptors, and no attempt has successfully identified a unified female pattern angina classification. The lower CAD incidence in women, particularly younger women, and the wide range of symptom presentations are partly responsible for the belief that including women in clinical investigations would add unnecessary randomness or noise. This would somewhat explain why women have tended to be excluded from prior studies.

The WISE study has developed a large contemporary database on women clinically referred for angiography for ischemia evaluation. One of its aims has been to study CAD symptom presentation in women, and the present report is a first step toward the systematic assessment of female pattern angina. From the outset, WISE has recognized the role of age and reproductive variables in predicting CAD in women *(83)*. The present analysis extends this finding to the role of age in symptom presentation. The results suggest that CAD symptoms become more similar to the male model with increasing age, postmenopause, lending renewed evidence for the role of reproductive hormones in female CAD. Regarding significant variables from the WISE symptom questionnaire, we are currently validating our findings in other populations, with the goal to develop an angina classification that facilitates clinical risk assessment for CAD in all women.

REFERENCES

1. McCaig LF. National hospital ambulatory medical care survey: 1998 emergency department summary. Advance data from vital and health statistics, no. 313. National Center for Health Statistics, Hyattsville, MD: 2000.
2. Burt CW. Summary statistics for acute cardiac ischemia and chest pain visits to the United States EDs, 1995–1996. Am J Emerg Med 1999;17:552–559.
3. Hlatky MA. Evaluation of chest pain in the emergency department. N Engl J Med 1997;337:1687–1689.
4. Diamond GA, Staniloff HM, Forrester JS, Pollock BH. Computer-assisted diagnosis in the noninvasive evaluation of patients with suspected coronary artery disease. J Am Coll Cardiol 1983;1:444–455.
5. Zucker DR, Griffith JL, Beshansky JR, Selker HP. Presentations of acute myocardial infarction in men and women. J Gen Intern Med 1997;12:79–87.
6. Weiner DA, Ryan TJ, McCabe CH, et al. Exercise stress testing: correlations among history of angina, ST-segment response and prevalence of coronary artery disease in the Coronary Artery Surgery Study (CASS). N Engl J Med 1979;301:230–235.
7. DeSanctis RW. Clinical manifestations of coronary artery disease: chest pain in women. In: Wenger NK, SperoffL, Packard B (eds.). Cardiovascular Health and Disease in Women. Le Jacq Communications, Greenwich, CT: 1993, pp. 67–72.
8. Chiamvimonvat V, Sternberg L. Coronary artery disease in women. Canad Fam Phys 1998;44:2709–2717.
9. Sharpe PA, Clark NM, Janz NK. Differences in the impact and management of heart disease between older women and men. Women's Health 1991;17:25–43.
10. Cunningham MA, Lee TH, Cook EF, et al. The effect of gender on the probability of myocardial infarction among emergency department patients with acute chest pain: a report from the Multicenter Chest Pain Study Group. J Gen Intern Med 1989;4:392–398.
11. Pepine CJ, Adams J, Marks RG, et al. Characteristics of a contemporary population with angina pectoris. Am J Cardiol 1994;74:226–231.
12. Sullivan AK, Holdright DR, Wright CA, et al. Chest pain in women: clinical, investigative, and prognostic features. BMJ 1994;308:883–886.
13. Goldberg RJ, O'Donnell C, Yarzebski J, et al. Sex differences in symptom presentation associated with acute myocardial infarction: a population-based perspective. Am Heart J 1998;136:189–195.
14. Penque S, Halm M, Smith M, et al. Women and coronary disease: relationship between descriptors and signs and symptoms and diagnostic and treatment course. Am J Crit Care 1998;7:175–182.
15. Eaker ED, Packard B, Wenger NK, et al. Coronary artery disease in women. Am J Cardiol 1988;61:641–644.
16. Maynard C, Weaver WD. Treatment of women with acute MI: new findings from the MITI registry. J Myocardial Ischemia 1992;4:27–33.

17. Willich SN, Lowell H, Lewis M, et al. Unexplained gender differences in clinical symptoms of acute myocardial infarction. J Am Coll Cardiol 1993;21:238A.
18. Lusiani L, Perrone A, Pesavento R, Conte G. Prevalence, clinical features, and acute course of atypical myocardial infarction. Angiology 1994;45:49–55.
19. Cannon RO III, Camici PG, Epstein SE. Pathopysiological dilemma of syndrome X. Circulation 1992;85:883–892.
20. Douglas PS (ed.). Cardiovascular Health and Disease in Women. W.B. Saunders, Philadelphia, PA: 1993.
21. Van Peski-Oosterbaan AS, Spinhoven P, et al. [Unexplained non-cardiac chest pain; its prevalence and natural course]. Ned Tijdschr Geneeskunde 1998;142:2468–2472.
22. Best RA. Non-cardiac chest pain: a useful physical sign? Heart 1999;81:450–451.
23. Sanders D, Bass C, Mayou RA, et al. Non-cardiac chest pain: why was a brief intervention apparently ineffective? Psychol Med 1997;27:1033–1040.
24. Atienza F, Velasco JA, Brown S, et al. Assessment of quality of life in patients with chest pain and normal coronary arteriogram (syndrome X) using a specific questionnaire. Clin Cardiol 1999;22:283–290.
25. Johnson BD, Bairey Merz CN, Kelsey SF, et al. Persistent chest pain (PCP) in women at six-week follow-up: the NHLBI-sponsored WISE study. J Am Coll Cardiol 2000;(Suppl A):A-546–547.
26. Milner KA, Funk M, Richards S, et al. Gender differences in symptom presentation associated with coronary heart disease. Am J Cardiol 1999;84:396–399.
27. Kennedy JW, Killip T, Fisher LD, et al. The clinical spectrum of coronary artery disease and its surgical and medical management, 1974–1979. The Coronary Artery Surgery Study. Circulation 1982;66(Suppl III):III:16–23.
28. Sharaf BL, Pepine CJ, Reis SE, et al. A detailed angiographic analysis of women presenting with suspected ischemic chest pain: pilot phase data from the NHLBI Women's Ischemia Syndrome Evaluation (WISE) Study Angiographic Core Laboratory. Circulation 1999;100(Suppl)I–185.
29. Lee TH, Cook EF, Weisberg ME, et al. Acute chest pain in the emergency room: identification and examination of low-risk patients. Arch Intern Med 1985;145:65–69.
30. Murabito JM, Anderson KM, Kannel WB, et al. Risk of coronary heart disease in subjects with chest discomfort: the Framingham Heart Study. Am J Med 1990;89:297–302.
31. Shaw LJ, Miller DD, Romeis JC, et al. Gender differences in the noninvasive evaluation and management of patients with suspected coronary artery disease. Ann Intern Med 1994;120:559–566.
32. Kwok YS, Kim C, Grady D, et al. Exercise testing in women to detect coronary artery disease in women: a meta-analysis. Am J Cardiol 1999;83:660–666.
33. Ayanian JZ, Epstein AM. Differences in the use of procedures between women and men hospitalized for coronary heart disease. N Engl J Med 1991;325:221–225.
34. Wenger NK. An update on coronary heart disease in women. Int J Fertil 1998;43:84–90.
35. Douglas PS, Ginsburg GS. Current concepts: the evaluation of chest pain in women. N Engl J Med 1996;334:1311–1315.
36. Healy B. The Yentl syndrome. N Engl J Med 1991;325:274–276.
37. Lehmann JB, Wehner PS, Lehmann CU, Savory LM. Gender bias in the evaluation of chest pain in the emergency department. Am J Cardiol 1996;77:641–644.
38. Heston TF, Lewis LM. Gender bias in acute myocardial infarction. Am J Cardiol 1997;79:844–845.
39. Kim C, Kwok YS, Saha S, Redberg RF. Diagnosis of suspected coronary artery disease in women: a cost-effective analysis. Am Heart J 1999;137:1019–1027.
40. Diamond GA, Forrester JS. Analysis of probability as an aid in the clinical diagnosis of coronary-artery disease. N Engl J Med 1979;300:1350–1358.
41. Gurwitz JH, Col NF, Avron J. The exclusion of the elderly and women from clinical trials in acute myocardial infarction. JAMA 1992;268:1417–1422.
42. Rich-Edwards JW, Manson JE, Hennekens CH, Buring JE. The primary prevention of coronary heart disease in women. N Engl J Med 1995;332:1758–1766.
43. Pinn, VW. Commentary: women, research, and the National Institutes of Health. Am J Prev Med 1992;8:324–327.
44. Peterson ED, Alexander KP. Learning to suspect the unexpected: evaluating women with cardiac syndromes. Am Heart J 1998;136:186–188.
45. Birdwell BG, Herbers JE, Kroenke K. Evaluating chest pain: the patient's presentation style alters the physician's diagnostic approach. Arch Intern Med 1993;153:1991–1995.

46. Pilote L, Hlatky MA. Attitudes of women toward hormone therapy and prevention of hert disease. Am Heart J 1995;129:1237–1238.
47. Johnson JA, King KB. Influence of expectations about symptoms on delay in seeking treatment during myocardial infarction. Am J Crit Care 1995;4:413.
48. Herlitz J, Bang A, Karlson BW, Hartford M. Is there a gender difference in aetiology of chest pain and symptoms associated with acute myocardial infarction? Eur J Emerg Med 1999;6:311–315.
49. Lerner DJ, Kannel WB. Patterns of coronary heart disease morbidity and mortality in the sexes: a 26-year follow-up of the Framingham population. Am Heart J 1986;111:383–390.
50. Khan SS, Nessim S, Gray R, et al. Increased mortality of women in coronary artery bypass surgery: evidence for referral bias. Ann Intern Med 1990;112:561–567.
51. Vaccarino V, Krumholz HM, Berkman LF, Horwitz RI. Sex differences in mortality after myocardial infarction: is there evidence for an increased risk for women? Circulation 1995;91:1861–1871.
52. Malacrida R, Genoni M, Maggioni A, for the Third International Study of Infarct Survival Collaborative Group. A comparison of the early outcome of acute myocardial infarction in women and men. N Engl J Med 1998;338:8–14.
53. Davis KB, Chaitman B, Ryan T, et al. Comparison of 15-year survival for men and women after initial medical or surgical treatment for coronary artery disease: a CASS registry study. J Am Coll Cardiol 1995;25:1000–1009.
54. Wenger NK. Coronary heart disease in women: a "new" problem. Hosp Pract 1992;27:59–62,64,67.
55. Kemp HG, Elliott WC, Gorlin R. The anginal syndrome with normal coronary arteriograms in patients considered to have unmistakable coronary heart disease. Trans Assoc Am Physicians 1967;80:59–70.
56. Kemp HG Jr. Left ventricular function in patients with the anginal syndrome and normal coronary angiograms. Am J Cardiol 1973;32:375–376.
57. Likoff W. Segal BL, Kasparian H. Paradox of normal selective coronary arteriograms in patients considered to have unmistakable coronary heart disease. N Engl J Med 1967;276:1063–1036.
58. Holubkov R, Reis SE. Diagnosis and Treatment of Heart Disease in women. In: Goldman MD, Hatch MC (eds.). Women and Health. Academic Press, San Diego, CA: 2000, pp. 771–781.
59. Sox H. Noninvasive testing in coronary artery disease. Selection of procedures and interpretation of results. Postgrad Med 1983;74:319–336.
60. Jouriles NJ. Atypical chest pain. Emerg Med Clin of North Amer 1998;16:717–740.
61. Frobert O, Funch-Jensen P, Bagger JP. Chest pain and the esophagus. Ann Int Med 1997;126:740–741.
62. Johnson BD, Bairey Merz CN, Matthews K, et al. Persistent chest pain (PCP) and psychological disorders: Cause or effect? The NHLBI-sponsored WISE study. Circulation 2001;104:II–724.
63. Maseri A, Severi S, De Nes M. "Variant" angina. One aspect of a continuous spectrum of vasospastic myocardial ischemia. Am J Cardiol 1978;42:1019–1035.
64. Camici PG, Marraccini P, Lorenzoni R, et al. Coronary hemodynamics and myocardial metabolism in patients with syndrome X: response to pacing stress. J Am Coll Cardiol 1991;17:1461–1470.
65. Chen JW, Lin SJ, Ting CT. Syndrome X: Pathophysiology and clinical management. Chin Med J 1997;60:177–183.
66. Cannon RO, Schenke WH, Quyyumi A. et al. Comparison of exercise testing with studies of coronary flow reserve in patients with microvascular angina. Circulation 1991;83(Suppl III):77–81.
67. Reis SE, Holubkov R, Lee JS, et al. Coronary flow velocity response to adenosine characterizes coronary microvascular function in women with chest pain and no obstructive coronary disease. Results from the pilot phase of the women's ischemia syndrome evaluation (WISE) study. J Am Coll Cardiol 1999;33:1469–1475.
68. Maseri A, Crea F, Kaski JC, Crake T. Mechanism of angina pectoris in syndrome X. J Am Coll Cardiol 1991;17:499–506.
69. Kaski JC, Rosano GC, Collins P, et al. Cardiac syndrome X: clinical characteristics and left ventricular function – long-term follow-up study. J Am Coll Cardiol 1995;25:807–814.
70. Buchthal SD, den Hollander JA, Bairey Merz CN, et al. Abnormal myocardial phosphorus-31 nuclear magnetic resonance spectroscopy in women with chest pain but normal coronary angiograms. N Engl J Med 2000;342:829–835.
71. Mosseri M, Yarom R, Gotsman MS, Hasin Y. Histologic evidence for small vessel coronary disease in patients with angina pectoris and patent large coronary arteries. Circulation 1986;74:964–972.
72. Suzuki H, Takeyama Y, Koba S, et al. Small vessel pathology and coronary hemodynamics in patients with microvascular angina. Int J Cardiol 1994;43:139–150.

73. Second report of the Expert Panel on detection, evaluation, and treatment of high blood cholesterol in adults (Adult Treatment Panel II). Circulation 1994;89:1333–1445.

74. Matthews KA, Meilahn E, Kuller LH, et al. Menopause and risk factors for coronary heart disease. N Engl J Med 1989;321:641–646.

75. Bairey Merz CN, Johnson BD, Sharaf BL, et al. Hypoestrogenemia of hypothalamic origin and coronary artery disease in premenopausal women: A report from the NHLBI-sponsored WISE study. J Am Coll Cardiol 2003;41:413–419.

76. Stampfer MJ, Colditz GA, Willett WC, et al. Postmenopausal estrogen therapy and cardiovascular disease. Ten-year follow-up from the nurses' health Study. N Engl J Med 1991;325:756–762.

77. Bush TL, Barrett-Connor E, Cowan LD, et al. Cardiovascular mortality and noncontraceptive use of estrogen in women: results from the lipid research clinics program follow-up study. Circulation 1987;75:1102–1109.

78. Hulley S, Grady D, Bush T, et al. Randomized trial of estrogen plus progestin for secondary prevention of coronary heart disease in postmenopausal women. JAMA 1998;280:605–613.

79. Bairey Merz CN, Kelsey SF, Pepine CF, et al. The women's ischemia syndrome evauation (WISE) study: protocol design, methodology and feasibility report. J Am Coll Cardiol 1999;33:1453–1461.

80. Olson MB, Bairey Merz CN, Kelsey SF, et al. Quality of life in women with chest pain: the NHLBI-sponsored WISE study. J Am Coll Cardiol 2000;35:554A.

81. Diamond GA, Forrester JS, Hirsch M, et al. Application of conditional probability analysis to the clinical diagnosis of coronary artery disease. J Clin Invest 1980;65:1210–1221.

82. Bairey Merz CN, Kop W, Krantz DS, et al. Cardiovascular stress response and coronary artery disease: evidence of an adverse postmenopausal effect in women. Am Heart J 1998;135:881–887.

83. Bairey Merz CN, Kelsey SF, et al. Women's Ischemia Syndrome Evaluation (WISE): initial report from pilot phase. Circulation 1997;96:I–563.

11

Quality-of-Life Issues for Women With Coronary Disease

John Spertus, MD, MPH, FACC
and Darcy Green Conaway, MD

CONTENTS

INTRODUCTION

Coronary artery disease (CAD) is a chronic condition without a cure. The fundamental goals in treating patients with coronary disease are to maximize their survival duration and to optimize the quality of that survival. Thus, a principal goal in treating patients with heart disease is to alleviate symptoms, improve function, and maximize quality of life. The ways in which a disease manifests itself to patients (i.e., their symptoms, function, and quality of life) is collectively referred to as *health status.*

Developing a chapter on health status assessment in women is particularly challenging because of the limitations in available data. Although clinical trials are currently the best source of health status outcomes data, health status assessment in clinical trials of cardiovascular treatment have been limited in both their frequency and scope. All too often, the endpoints of clinical trials focus on surrogate physiological or anatomical markers of disease state, rather than clinically meaningful outcomes (1), or when outcomes are included, they track only survival or hospitalization events, not health status *(2)*. When clinical trials do include assessments of patients' health status, these are often limited. Although some health status measures, such as the New York Heart Association (NYHA) classification for congestive heart failure (CHF) *(3)* or the Canadian Cardiovascular Society Classification *(4)* of angina have been used, the field of health

From: *Contemporary Cardiology: Coronary Disease in Women: Evidence-Based Diagnosis and Treatment*
Edited by: L. J. Shaw and R. F. Redberg © Humana Press Inc., Totowa, NJ

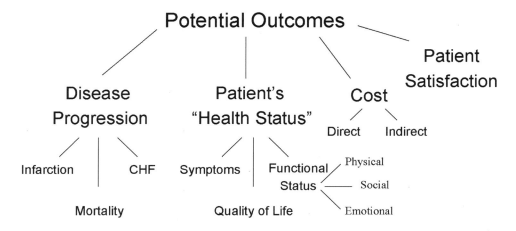

Fig. 1. The spectrum of outcomes in coronary artery disease.

status assessment has matured substantially since the late 1980s *(5,6),* and many of the currently available disease-specific instruments have only become available since the 1990s. Additionally, describing the health status of women with cardiovascular disease (CVD) is problematic because women have been underrepresented in clinical trials, further limiting the availability of health status data in women *(7)*. Finally, essentially no methodological work that qualitatively seeks to differentiate health status acquisition between men and women has been conducted. (The ongoing female-only Women's Ischemia Study Evaluation [WISE] is a notable exception [8]). Despite these readily acknowledged limitations, the import of health status is such that a thoughtful discussion should be attempted. Therefore, this chapter describes the range of health status outcomes, outlines the methods and required attributes in quantifying these outcomes, articulates gender-specific considerations in health status acquisition among women, illustrates what is currently known about female health status outcomes, and suggests recommendations for future researchers interested in advancing the field.

CONCEPTUALIZING HEALTH STATUS AND QUALITY OF LIFE

The nomenclature surrounding health status is confusing. *Health status, quality of life, health-related quality of life,* and other terms are frequently used interchangeably in the literature to describe the ways in which a disease can affect patients. In their review, Gill and Feinstein found that the term *quality of life* was substituted for terms such as health status or functional status, often confusing the meaning of both *(9)*. We refer to *health status* as the way in which a disease manifests itself to patients in their daily lives—their symptoms, ability to function, and quality of life. Figure 1 places health status within the context of other meaningful disease outcomes: further progression of the disease, costs, and satisfaction.

Within the range of health status outcomes, we conceptualize symptoms, functions, and quality of life as unique domains, which allows each domain to be independently quantified and allows the relationships between different domains with other clinical variables and each other to be directly examined. Figure 2 represents a modified version of Wilson and Cleary's model integrating clinical and health status characteristics *(10)*.

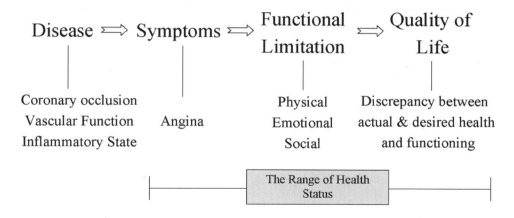

Fig. 2. A taxonomy of health status in coronary artery disease.

Although an underlying disease process precipitated by vascular dysfunction, inflammation, and atherosclerotic plaque deposition, can be the underlying substrate for CAD, these processes are usually hidden from the patient's perspective. We conceptualize health status as being those disease manifestations that are directly perceived by the patient. In this model, symptoms can refer to generic concepts, such as pain, or may focus in particular instruments on those symptoms directly referrable to the disease being studied (e.g., angina). Functional status refers to the physical, emotional, and social consequences of the disease process. It often includes an assessment of routine activities and functions, such as walking or interacting with family *(11)*. The greater the patients' symptoms, the more likely the disease will interfere with their ability to function. Yet, functional status is not necessarily the same as quality of life. Although functional status is often estimated or measured by constructs that are external to the patients themselves, quality of life is not. For example, physical function can be assessed with an exercise test, and social function can be evaluated with a structured interview with family and friends. Quality of life, however, can only be assessed by patients themselves.

Quality of life is a complex concept that can mean different things to different people *(9,12)*. We conceptualize quality of life as representing patients' unique perspectives on whether they are currently living in a meaningful and satisfying way. It is inversely related to the discrepancy between patients' assessments of their current functioning and their desired functioning, such that the larger the gap between current function and how they would like or expect to function, the worse their quality of life. For example, an elderly retired woman with occasional angina that limits her ability to walk more than two blocks may not be particularly bothered by this limitation if her routine daily activities do not exceed her angina threshold. Consequently, she may have a well-preserved quality of life. A 38-year-old manual laborer, on the other hand, might find similar limitations devastating and have a very poor quality of life, despite similar symptoms and functioning in comparison to her senior counterpart. Thus, only through the direct solicitation of patients can the quality of their lives be assessed.

It is important to note that although a direct linear relationship is suggested among the different components of health status in Fig. 2, the true association is much more complex. For example, whereas functional status is depicted as being determined primarily by symptoms, depression—a manifestation of poor mental functioning—is associated with worse symptoms (13) and can even serve as a risk factor for the initial development of CAD (14,15).

QUANTIFYING HEALTH STATUS: TYPES OF INSTRUMENTS AND REQUIRED ATTRIBUTES

A variety of techniques and measures are used to quantify patients' health status (16). The selection of appropriate measures requires an understanding of an intervention's expected benefits, an understanding of the study population, and a clear formulation of what kind of data, potential analyses, and interpretations are desired from the investigation. Three broad classes of patient-centered instruments can be used to assess health status in patients: generic health status measures, disease-specific health status measures, and utilities.

Types of Health Status Measures

GENERIC HEALTH STATUS MEASURES

Generic health status instruments capture patients' perceptions of how their overall health affects their lives. Measured symptoms often include global concepts, such as pain and fatigue, that can be manifestations of multiple disease processes. No attempt is made to attribute which of a patient's comorbidities is responsible for particular symptoms or functional limitations. Consequently, generic measures of health status broadly assess the impact of patients' overall health on their function across various diseases and patient populations. The universal applicability of items addressed by a generic health status measure allows the effects of different treatments or health interventions to be quantified and compared (11,17,18). An advantage of generic health status measures over more focused disease-specific measures is that generic measures can detect the impact of medication's side effects that occur outside of the cardiovascular system. Because generic measures provide a common metric with which to compare the impact of one disease and its treatment with those of another, they are frequently used in population-based health assessments, which allows the health status of a study population to be benchmarked against national norms. Examples of generic health status measures used in CAD include the Short Form (SF)-36 (19), the Sickness Impact Profile (20), and the Duke Activity Status Index (21).

Because these instruments measure overall health status, including the effect of patients' comorbid conditions as well as their CAD, they tend to be less sensitive than disease-specific measures in quantifying the changes in health status realized by interventions directed at only one of a patient's comorbid conditions (5,17,22). For example, a patient with extensive multivessel coronary disease and severe rheumatoid arthritis may have physical function limitations as the result of both angina and joint pain. If successful coronary revascularization is performed, and the patient's angina is completely eliminated, the patient may still be limited by her arthritic pain. A generic health status measure may not detect an improvement after revascularization despite the intervention's success. Consequently, generic measures may fail to capture changes in a particular disease's status, which patients and their physicians might consider to be clinically important.

DISEASE-SPECIFIC HEALTH STATUS MEASURES

Disease-specific measures are designed to assess specific groups or patient populations, often with the goal of focusing on clinically meaningful aspects of the disease being studied *(5,17)*. Such measures can be more responsive to changes in patients' health partly because they highlight more relevant manifestations of the illness and partly because they can tailor their response categories to a more relevant range of function than generic measures *(11)*. This allows disease-specific instruments to tap the areas of life that are most relevant to a specific illness or condition (e.g., CAD), certain patient population (e.g., elderly), area of function (e.g., sleep), or symptoms (e.g., angina) *(5)*. Because these instruments typically address those domains of health that are focused on by clinicians, the domains of disease-specific instruments also tend to be more interpretable than the domains captured by generic measures. For example, the clinical interpretations of "anginal frequency" and the "physical limitations due to angina" are more tangible to clinicians than broad concepts of "emotional role functioning" and "vitality." Hence, disease-specific data are often more "actionable" (i.e., they "make sense" and/or suggest a course of therapeutic intervention) than more abstract generic health status domains.

In CVD patients, disease-specific instruments are more responsive than generic measures to changes in patients' cardiovascular symptoms *(23,24)*, which is particularly important when a therapy is tested in patients with comorbid conditions. In the example of the patient with both severe arthritis and coronary disease as mentioned previously, a disease-specific measure should be able to quantify the improvements in physical functioning gained from the coronary revascularization procedure, whereas a generic measure may not.

UTILITIES

Utilities are used in economic and decision analyses to modify survival duration by the quality of that survival. They seek to represent the sum total of a patient's health status into a single number. By convention, a utility value of 1 is assigned to perfect health, whereas a value of 0 is assigned to death *(25)*.

Defining utilities for patients can be both theoretically and practically challenging. Several techniques have been developed to assist in the acquisition of patients' utilities. The most widely accepted approach is the Standard Gamble because it conforms to the Von Neumann and Morgenstern model for making decisions under uncertain conditions *(26)*. However, recent work has demonstrated that human behavior may not conform to the theoretical models used for the Standard Gamble, and, thus, other approaches to describe health status values have been developed *(27–33)*. The simplest techniques currently used to measure utilities are questionnaires that are weighted by societal preferences in order to derive a utility value. Two of the more prominent examples include the Health Utility Index *(34,35)* and the EuroQOL or EQ-5D *(36)*.

Required Attributes of Health Status Measures

Although researchers would often like to design new instruments for their studies, existing measures should be used whenever possible. The rationale for this approach is that before an instrument can be used, it should be explicitly demonstrated as valid (measure what it is supposed to), reliable (provide reproducible assessments in stable patients over time), responsive (sensitive to clinically important change), and interpretable (understanding of the prognostic implications of score or insights into the clinical significance of changes in score). Furthermore, established metrics enable comparisons of different studies and treatments on the same scale. When selecting a measure for use, a range of design and performance characteristics should be considered.

VALIDITY

Validity refers to the ability of the instrument's domains to measure what they are supposed to. Validity types include content validity, face validity, criterion validity, and construct validity (5). Content validity refers to the extent to which the domains of interest are comprehensively sampled by items or questions in the measure. Content validity may vary by purpose. For example, to assess a population's general health, a generic health status measure (e.g., Sickness Impact Profile) might have good content validity (20). However, it might not have good content validity for a study of coronary disease patients where an angina frequency assessment would be very important. Face validity reflects whether an instrument appears to measure what it is supposed to. Items should be clinically reasonable and have "common sense," often from a clinician's perspective; this determines the face validity of a health status instrument. Criterion validity refers to whether an instrument is measuring what it is intended to by comparing the instrument results with those of a "gold" standard. Because of the highly personal nature of patients' experiences with their illness, identifying criterion standards for comparison are seldom accomplished. In the absence of a criterion standard, the validity of health status measures is often established using the concept of construct validity. Construct validity consists of comparisons between different measures that quantify a similar health status dimension, predicting logical relationships between population measures or characteristics and comparing questionnaire responses with these measures.

RELIABILITY

Reliability can refer to either the internal consistency of a measure or its reproducibility. Internal reliability describes whether or not the instrument items quantify a concept homogeneously, i.e., all the items within a given domain are measuring the same construct. It is usually quantified by examining Chronbach's alpha (range 0–1), where an internally consistent domain is considered to have a value of 0.8 (37). In contrast, reproducibility refers to the consistency of answers over time in stable patients. Guyatt et al. refer to a discriminative health status measure as being reliable if it has a high signal-to-noise ratio (5). That is, the variability in scores between patients (signal) is much greater than the variability within patients (noise). Often the noise is assessed by repeatedly administering the same instrument on different occasions to the same patients during a period where their underlying condition is stable. The test–retest instrument reliability is supported by evidence of a high correlation between scores using Pearson's correlation coefficient, a paired t-test, or the intraclass correlation coefficient (38).

RESPONSIVENESS

In contrast to reliability, responsiveness refers to the sensitivity of changes in instrument scores to reflect changes in clinical status. Responsiveness is the signal in the signal-to-noise ratio, reflecting the magnitude of the score difference in patients who have improved or deteriorated (5). Responsiveness of health status instruments can be measured using the relative efficiency statistic (ratio of paired *t* statistics *[39]*), relative change and its relationship to clinical change as assessed by receiver operating characteristic curves *(40)*, effect sizes *(38,41)*, standard error of measurement *(42,43)*, and responsiveness statistics (ratio of minimal clinically important difference to the variability in stable subjects; *[44,45]*). Some argue that if an instrument is valid and reliable, then it must also be responsive. Yet, because of the difficulty in establishing validity, we believe it is critically important to independently demonstrate the responsiveness of an instrument to change. After all, it is the instrument's responsiveness that is most important in serving as a sensitive endpoint in clinical applications.

INTERPRETABILITY

Interpretability identifies the meaning of a score or change in score. In the case of a discriminative evaluation, interpretability facilitates knowing whether a certain score indicates that a patient is functioning normally or has some degree of impairment in health status. Interpreting discriminative measures is greatly aided with the knowledge of normal reference ranges for clinically significant patient populations. Toward this end, general health status measures, such as the EQ-5D or the SF-36, for which population norms are readily available, can be useful. To facilitate its interpretation, SF-36 developers proposed transformations of scale scores, such that a score of 50 represents the US population norm and 10-point differences represent a standard deviation from that norm *(46)*. An additional aid to the interpretation of a single health status score is whether such a score is prognostically important. For example, recent work with the Seattle Angina Questionnaire demonstrates that those patients scoring in the lowest range of physical function (0–24 on a 100-point scale) have a fourfold risk of dying over the next year when compared with those patients scoring in the highest range (75–100 points), even after controlling for a wide range of clinical and sociodemographic characteristics *(47)*.

For evaluative instruments, interpretability ascertains whether the change in scores represent a trivial, small but important, moderate, or large improvement or deterioration *(5,43)*. This framework focuses on the need to understand whether score changes are clinically meaningful. How many points must a given instrument change for patients or their physicians to validate that their condition has changed? When interpreting changes in scores, it is important to understand the perspective of the analysis. Group changes refer to the mean differences in score for patient groups. The statistical significance of such group changes is highly dependent on the numbers of patients analyzed. For example, with a sufficiently large trial, a group difference in scores of 1 point on a 100-point scale might be statistically significant. Yet, this magnitude of difference may not represent a clinically meaningful difference when changing one response on a single item of a questionnaire might result in a scale score change of 8 points. Clarification of this distinction is particularly important when investigators seek to summarize health status changes by extrapolating mean differences in groups to individual patients.

GENDER-SPECIFIC CONSIDERATIONS WHEN QUANTIFYING HEALTH STATUS

Despite the significant methodological advances that have occurred since the 1980s in quantifying patients' experiences of their illness, a paucity of gender-specific information currently exists on the health status outcomes of women with coronary disease. As future researchers begin to describe female health status outcomes and explore the determinants of such outcomes, several considerations should be entertained. These include the older age of women with coronary disease, the questionnaires' design to avoid gender bias, the assessment timing and the characteristics of women's socioeconomical environment that may underlie many of the perceived differences in observed health status.

Age

In measuring the health status of women with coronary disease, it is important to understand whether observed differences with men are, in fact, the result of gender or whether gender is merely a marker of other sociodemographical and clinical differences that more directly affect health status. Among the important considerations is age, because the onset of coronary disease is often at an older age among women than for men. Women, on average, are affected by coronary disease 10–15 years later in life than men *(48)*, and, consequently, different issues may affect their quality of life. Health status questionnaires may bias patient scores by selecting activities and functions that are not as relevant to an older population as to a younger one. For example, questions about work performance may be less relevant or meaningful to older adults who are more likely to be retired. Additionally, questions about sexual function may be less relevant to older individuals who have a higher likelihood of being widowed or without a partner. Without explicitly using analyses that control for age and its associated characteristics, lower scores for women when compared with men might be incorrectly attributed to their gender rather than their age.

Gender-Neutrality of Questions

In addition, even after controlling for age, the types of activities in the physical function domain of a questionnaire might be culturally less relevant to women than men. For example, physical activity items related to contact sports or manual labor may be less relevant to women than men. Depending on the way the question is framed, negative responses may be interpreted as an inability to perform certain activities, rather than a lack of desire or need to perform them. Although the former scenario suggests poor function, the latter does not necessarily imply the same. Without carefully designed gender-neutral items in a questionnaire, biased results among women may arise.

Timing of Health Status Assessments

Not only is a focus on age and the gender-neutrality of items important, but the timing of health status assessments may artifactually influence results as well. Women may have different recoveries after procedures than their male counterparts *(49)*. If women recover from a procedure more slowly than their male counterparts, then a lower health status may be detected if the assessment is acquired at a point in time when men have maximally recovered and women are still continuing to improve. Sensitivity to this issue is important when designing the follow-up of patients.

Confounding Sociodemographic and Clinical Considerations

Finally, women may have a different social environment than men, with higher stress and depression levels *(50–53)*, different levels and types of social support

(49,54–58), or worse socioeconomic status *(59,60)*, each of which may influence the potential health status benefits of certain treatment strategies. Although only a small number of studies that have tried to reveal what physiological and psychosocial factors impact quality of life in a female cardiac patient *(61)*, if these other variables aren't quantified, then study results might be influenced by unmeasured confounding, rather than a true gender effect. Lacking knowledge of the underlying reason for apparent outcome differences between men and women limits our ability to identify potentially modifiable factors that can improve the women's outcomes with coronary disease.

CURRENT KNOWLEDGE OF HEALTH STATUS IN WOMEN WITH CAD

The number of female myocardial infarction (MI) patients increased from 35% in 1975 to 43% in 1995 *(62)*. Despite this increase, female representation in cardiac clinical trials has not improved as dramatically *(7,63)*, with the result that women remain underrepresented in clinical trials *(64)*. Given that the majority of information regarding patients' health status with CVD comes from clinical trials, little information about women's health status with CVD is available, and the known data may not be sufficiently generalized to the female cardiac population as a whole.

One area that has been addressed is the presentation difference between men and women with CAD. Women experience angina 47% of the time as their initial presentation when compared with 26% of men *(48,65)*. Yet, part of the difficulty in appropriately treating women with chest pain arises from the knowledge that angina is less predictive of CAD in women than men *(66,67)*. Importantly, more than one half of women with ischemic heart disease symptoms have no obstructive CVD at coronary angiography, yet these women frequently have persistent symptom-related disability and consume large amounts of health care resources *(68)*. Many of these women are diagnosed with noncardiac chest pain or Syndrome X (angina, ischemic stress test response, no obstructive CAD; *69*); however, coronary microvascular dysfunction is an alternative mechanism for their symptoms. Findings by Reis and colleagues from the National Heart, Lung, and Blood Institute (NHLBI)-WISE study *(70)* reported coronary microvascular dysfunction (i.e., abnormally attenuated coronary flow velocity reserve) to be present in approx 50% of women with chest pain and no obstructive CAD. Their findings suggest that microvascular dysfunction should be considered as a potential etiology of chest pain, and it is associated with disability in women without obstructive CAD. Future work will be needed to define whether such symptoms are treatable with vasoactive therapies *(70)*.

Generally, however, there is a paucity of information regarding health status in women with CAD in the medical literature. One study by Herlitz et al. examined symptom relief and quality of life 5 years post-CABG in women and men who underwent CABG in Western Sweden *(71)*. This study found that women had a higher 5-year mortality rate (17% vs 13%), but both men and women had significant improvement with respect to symptoms and quality of life. Women were found to experience more symptoms in terms of physical activity, dyspnea, and chest pain both prior to and after CABG, but had more pronounced improvement than men in some aspects. In a recent study examining the recovery of function after bypass surgery, Vaccarino and colleagues demonstrated that women have a worse recovery of physical function 6 weeks after surgery than men, particularly after controlling for baseline function. This effect was independent of age, illness severity, presurgery health status, and other patient characteristics (72).

Moreover, the female social and behavioral determinants of heart disease are essentially unexplored (73). Previous studies have shown that a woman's quality of life is dependent on variables, such as social, mental, and physical activities as well as perceived stress levels (61). Those that have addressed this area suggest that there are five psychosocial domains that contribute to the pathogenesis and expression of coronary disease: depression, anxiety, personality factors/character traits, social isolation, and chronic life stress (74–76). A review by Elliott on the role of psychosocial stress as a risk factor in the etiology of women's coronary disease revealed "some evidence for an etiologic link between psychosocial stress and coronary disease in women" (77). Further supporting the potential confounding nature of these psychosocial characteristics are the baseline data from the Post-CABG Biobehavioral Study, which demonstrated women undergoing CABG to be older, less likely to be high school graduates poorer, less likely to be married (i.e., greater difficulty in performing basic self-care activities), have fewer social activities, and to be more anxious and depressed than men (78). The impact of these adverse factors have not yet been reported from this investigation. Currently, most CAD health status measures do not include such risk factors in their health status assessment, and further work is needed to properly assess the female cardiac patient's overall health status.

"One in ten American women between the ages of 45 and 65 years has some form of coronary heart disease (angina or myocardial infarction)" (78a). Yet, infarcts in women are often not recognized (79), and unrecognized MI, according to the 26-year follow-up of the Framingham heart study, increases the chance of cardiac failure, stroke, and death (79,80). Furthermore, women who sustain MI, both in the United States and worldwide, have a substantial increase in morbidity and mortality, both acutely and following hospital discharge (81,82). Yet, further defining the impact on women in comparison to men and the efficacy of treatment will await future researchers and their commitment to stratifying analyses by gender so that unique features of the impact of cardiac disease on women's health status can be determined.

FUTURE RESEARCH PRIORITIES

As is obvious from the previous section, much work is needed to better understand the health status of women with coronary disease. This can be divided into (1) methodological work to advance our knowledge of the potentially unique impact of coronary disease on women and (2) the acquisition of more data about health status outcomes in general, particularly for women. Regarding the methodological challenges, the following pressing questions can be articulated:

1. *Does coronary disease affect women in the same way that it affects men?* To address this issue, qualitative work is necessary to understand the ways in which coronary disease impacts the symptoms, function, and quality of life of women. Without such work, it will be difficult to confirm that our current techniques for quantifying patient's health status will adequately capture domains that are meaningful to women (i.e., with appropriate content validity). Of course, investigators pursuing these inquiries need to be cognizant

of not creating questionnaires that pose such a response burden on participants that they are impractical for large-scale research projects.

2. *Are there unique psychosocial health status determinants that differentially affect the genders?* To facilitate comparisons between health status outcomes of men and women, it is important to account for important sources of variation that could confound gender comparisons. For example, if depression or social isolation affect men and women differentially and also influence health status outcomes, then these need to be discovered and measured in future observational studies and clinical trials.

3. *Do current health status measures quantify different constructs in men and women?* Factor analysis and other psychometrical explorations to test that current measures are equally applicable and interpretable to both men and women should be conducted.

For practical research priorities, it is critical to have more data on the health status of both men and women in clinical trials and observational research studies. This can be accomplished by the following:

1. *Greater inclusion of women in clinical trials.* It is difficult to describe women's health status without data. Because the greatest source of data comes from clinical trials, the inclusion of greater female proportions will rapidly increase current knowledge. Many of the early cardiovascular trials were in Veteran's hospitals, which is partly the reason for women being essentially excluded from early trials. As a result, the US government has sought to ensure that federally funded clinical research yields adequate high-quality information about heart disease in women. Harris and Douglas *(64)* found that federal efforts to increase women's representation in clinical trials have been moderately successful because of a small number of large single-sex trials involving CAD. There were 398,801 subjects, of which 215,796 were women enrolled in NHLBI-funded CVD studies. The enrollment rate for women was 54%, which exceeds the CVD prevalence in women in the general population (49%). With single-sex trials excluded, the enrollment rate for women was 38% *(64)*.

2. *More robust assessments of health status in clinical trials.* Current clinical trial design often overemphasizes surrogate endpoints and asserts inadequate import to the inclusion of health status outcomes. Yet, the principal goal of therapy is to make patients live longer and feel better through improvement of their health status (minimizing symptoms, improving function, and maximizing quality of life). Although the current trend in clinical trial design is to power trials adequately for mortality endpoints, trialists often fail to include adequate health status assessments. Not only should health status be measured serially throughout a study, but the appropriate baseline characteristics that influence quality of life (depression, social support, income, etc.) should be collected so that observational insights from these trials may be made and appropriate subgroups analyzed with an appropriate focus on the relevant health status outcomes.

CONCLUSION

Patients with CVD need treatment to prolong their survival and improve their health status (alleviate symptoms, maximize function, and improve their quality of life). Current insights into the effect of coronary disease and its treatment on female health status outcomes are limited. Through the use of valid, reliable, responsive, and interpretable health status instruments, much understanding of patients' perception of their disease can be gained and used to improve their outcomes. Addressing research gaps mentioned in this chapter has the potential to greatly enhance our understanding of how women are affected by coronary disease and its treatment and how we may leverage these insights to improve their care and outcomes.

REFERENCES

1. Fleming TR, DeMets DL. Surrogate end points in clinical trials: Are we being misled? Ann Intern Med 1996;125:605–613.
2. Spertus J. Selecting end points in clinical trials: What evidence do we really need to evaluate a new treatment? Am Heart J 2001;142:745–747.
3. The Criteria Committee of the New York Heart Association. Nomenclature and Criteria for Diagnosis. 9th ed. Little, Brown, Boston, MA: 1994.
4. Compeau L. Grading of angina pectoris. Circulation 1975;54:522–523.
5. Guyatt GH, Feeny DH, Patrick DL. Measuring health-related quality of life. Ann Intern Med 1993;118:622–629.
6. Guyatt G, Haynes RB, Jaeschke RZ, et al. Users' guides to the medical literature XII. How to use articles about health-related quality of life. J Am Med Assoc 1997;277:1232–1237.
7. Lee P, Alexander KP, Hammill BG, et al. Representation of elderly persons and women in published randomized trials of acute coronary syndromes. JAMA 2001;286:708–713.
8. Merz CN, Kelsey SF, Pepine CJ, et al. The Women's Ischemia Syndrome Evaluation (WISE) study: protocol design, methodology and feasibility report. J Am Coll Cardiol 1999;33:1453–1461.
9. Gill TM, Feinstein AR. A critical appraisal of the quality of quality-of-life measurements. JAMA 1994;272:619–626.
10. Wilson IB, Cleary PD. Linking clinical variables with health-related quality of life. A conceptual model of patient outcomes. JAMA 1995;273:59–65.
11. Swenson J, Clinch J. Assessment of quality of life in patients with cardiac disease: the role of psychosomatic medicine. J Psychosom Res 2000;48:405–415.
12. Fayers P, Bjordal K. Should quality-of-life needs influence resource allocation? Lancet 2001;357:978.
13. Spertus JA, McDonell M, Woodman CL, Fihn SD. Association between depression and worse disease-specific functional status in outpatients with coronary artery disease. Am Heart J 2000;140:105–110.
14. Ford DE, Mead LA, Chang PP, et al. Depression is a risk factor for coronary artery disease in men: the precursors study. Arch Intern Med 1998;158:1422–1426.
15. Ariyo AA, Haan M, Taugen CM, et al. Depressive symptoms and risks of coronary heart disease and mortality in elderly Americans. Cardiovascular Health Study Collaborative Research Group. Circulation 2000;102:1773–1779.
16. Testa MA, Simonson DC. Assessment of Quality of Life Outcomes. N Engl J Med 1996;334:835–840.
17. Patrick D, Deyo R. Generic and disease-specific measures in assessing health status and quality of life. Med Care 1989;27:S217–S232.
18. Dempster M, Donnelly M. Measuring the health related quality of life of people with ischaemic heart disease. Heart 2000;83:641–644.
19. Stewart A, Hays R, Ware J. The MOS short form general health survey: reliability and validity in a patient population. Med Care 1988;26:724–735.
20. Bergner M, Bobbitt RA, Carter WS, Glson BS. The Sickness Impact Profile: development and final revision of a health status measure. Med Care 1981;19:787–805.
21. Hlatky M, Boineau RE, Higginbotham MB, et al. A brief self-administered questionnaire to determine functional capacity (the Duke Activity Status Index). Am J Cardiol 1989;64:651–654.
22. Spertus J, Winder JA, Dewhurst TA, et al. Monitoring the quality of life in patients with coronary artery disease. Am J Cardiol 1994;74:1240–1244.
23. Green C, Porter CB, BresnahanDR, Spertus JA. Development and evaluation of the Kansas City Cardiomyopathy Questionnaire: a new health status measure for heart failure. J Am Coll Cardiol 2000;35:1245–1255.
24. Spertus J, Winder JA, Dewhurst TA, et al. Development and evaluation of the Seattle Angina Questionnaire: a new functional status measure for coronary artery disease. J Am Coll Cardiol 1995;25:333–341.
25. Torrance GW. Utility approach to measuring health-related quality of life. J Chronic Dis 1987;40:593–603.
26. Von Neumann J, Morgenstern O. Theory of Games and Economic Behaviour. Princeton University Press, Princeton, NJ: 1994.

27. Wu G. The strengths and limitations of expected utility theory. Med Decis Making 1996;16:9–10.
28. Torrance GW. Measurement of health state utilities for economic appraisal: A review. J Health Econ 1986;5:1–30.
29. Douard J. Is risk neutrality rational? Med Decis Making 1996;16:10–11.
30. Cohen BJ. Reply: Utilitarianism, risk aversion, and expected utility. Med Decis Making 1996;16:14.
31. Cohen BJ. Is expected utility theory mornative for medical decision making? Med Decis Making 1996;16:1–6.
32. Baron J. Why expected utility theory is normative, but not prescriptive. Med Decis Making 1996;16:7–9.
33. Eeckhoudt L. Expected utility theory–Is it normative or simply "practical"? Med Decis Making 1996;16:12–13.
34. Torrance GW, Furlons W, Feeny D, Boyle M. Multi-attribute preference functions. Health utilities index. Pharmacoeconomics 1995;7:503–520.
35. Feeny D, Furlons W, Boyle M, Torrance GW. Multi-attribute health status classification systems: Health utilities index. Pharmaco economics 1995;7:490–502.
36. Kind P. The EuroQoL instrument: An index of health-related quality of life. In: Spilker B. (ed.). Quality of Life and Pharnacoeconomis in Clinical Trials. Lippincott-Raven, Philadelphia, PA: 1996, pp. 191–201.
37. Nunnally JC, Bernstein IH. Psychometric Theory. 3rd ed. McGraw-Hill, New York, NY: 1994, p. 752.
38. Deyo RA, Diehr P, Patrick DL. Reproducibility and responsiveness of health status measures. Statistics and strategies for evaluation. Control Clin Trials 1991;12(4 Suppl):142S–158S.
39. Bombardier C, Raboud J. A comparison of health-related quality-of-life measures for rheumatoid arthritis research. The Auranofin Cooperating Group. Control Clin Trials 1991;12(4 Suppl):243S–256S.
40. Deyo RA, Centor RM. Assessing the responsiveness of functional scales to clinical change: an analogy to diagnostic test performance. J Chronic Dis 1986;39:897–906.
41. Katz JN, Laisou MG, Phillips CB, et al. Comparative measurement sensitivity of short and longer health status instruments. Med Care 1992;30:917–925.
42. Wyrwich KW, Nienaber NA, Tierney WM, Wolinsky FD. Linking clinical relevance and statistical significance in evaluating intra-individual changes in health-related quality of life. Med Care 1999;37:469–478.
43. Guyatt GH, Osoba D, Wu AW, et al. Methods to explain the clinical significance of health status measures. Mayo Clin Proc 2002;77:371–383.
44. Guyatt GH, Kirshner B, Jaeschke R. Measuring health status: what are the necessary measurement properties? J Clin Epidemiol 1992;45:1341–1345.
45. Guyatt G, Walter S, Norman G. Measuring change over time: assessing the usefulness of evaluative instruments. J Chronic Dis 1987;40:171–178.
46. Ware J, Jr., Kosinski M, Keller SD. A 12-Item Short-Form Health Survey: construction of scales and preliminary tests of reliability and validity. Med Care 1996;34:220–233.
47. Spertus JA, Jones P, McDonell M, et al. Health status predicts long-term outcome in outpatients with coronary disease. Circulation 2002;106(1):43-49.
48. Silberberg J. Better coronary risk assessment in women. Lancet 1999;353:1637–1638.
49. King KM. Gender and short-term recovery from cardiac surgery. Nurs Res 2000;49:29–36.
50. Hallman T, Burell G, Setterlind S, et al. Psychosocial risk factors for coronary heart disease, their importance compared with other risk factors and gender differences in sensitivity. J Cardiovasc Risk 2001;8:39–49.
51. Allen J, Markovitz J, Jacobs DR Jr, Knox SS. Social support and health behavior in hostile black and white men and women in CARDIA. Coronary Artery Risk Development in Young Adults. Psychosom Med 2001;63:609–618.
52. Mendes de Leon CF, Pilillo V, Czajkowski S, et al. Psychosocial characteristics after acute myocardial infarction: the ENRICHD pilot study. Enhancing Recovery in Coronary Heart Disease. J Cardiopulm Rehabil 2001;21:353–362.
53. Panagiotakos DB, Pitsavos C, Chrysohoou C, et al. Risk stratification of coronary heart disease through established and emerging lifestyle factors in a Mediterranean population: CARDIO2000 epidemiological study. J Cardiovasc Risk 2001;8:329–335.
54. Eaker ED. Psychosocial factors in the epidemiology of coronary heart disease in women. Psychiatr Clin North Am 1989;12:167–173.

55. Brezinka V, Kittel F. Psychosocial factors of coronary heart disease in women: a review. Soc Sci Med 1996;42:1351–1365.
56. Con AH, Linden W, Thompson JM, Ignaszewski A. The psychology of men and women recovering from coronary artery bypass surgery. J Cardiopulm Rehabil 1999;19:152–161.
57. King KM, Koop PM. The influence of the cardiac surgery patient's sex and age on care-giving received. Soc Sci Med 1999;48:1735–1742.
58. Barefoot JC, Brummett BH, Clapp-Channing NE, et al. Moderators of the effect of social support on depressive symptoms in cardiac patients. Am J Cardiol 2000;86:438–442.
59. Ancona C, Agabiti N, Forastiere F, et al. Coronary artery bypass graft surgery: socioeconomic inequalities in access and in 30 day mortality. A population-based study in Rome, Italy. J Epidemiol Community Health 2000;54:930–935.
60. Andersson P, Leppert J. Men of low socio-economic and educational level possess pronounced deficient knowledge about the risk factors related to coronary heart disease. J Cardiovasc Risk 2001;8:371–377.
61. Janz NK, Janevic MR, Dodge JA, et al. Factors influencing quality of life in older women with heart disease. Med Care 2001;39:588–598.
62. Goldberg R, Yarzebski J, Lessard D, Gore JM. A two-decades (1975–1995) Long experience in the incidence, in-hospital and long-term case-fatality rates of acute myocardial infarction: a community-wide perspective. J Am Coll Cardiol 1999;33:1533–1539.
63. Gurwitz J, Col N, Avorn J. The exclusion of the elderly and women from clinical trials in acute myocardial infarction. JAMA 1992;268:1417–1422.
64. Harris DJ, Douglas PS. Enrollment of women in cardiovascular clinical trials funded by the National Heart, Lung, and Blood Institute. N Engl J Med 2000;343:475–480.
65. Flavell C. Women and coronary heart disease. Prog Cardiovasc Nurs 1994;9:18–27.
66. Diamond G, Forrester J. Analysis of probability as an aid in the clinical diagnosis of coronary-artery disease. N Engl J Med 1979;300:1350–1358.
67. Kim C, Kwok YS, Saha L, Pedberg RF. Diagnosis of suspected coronary artery disease in women: A cost-effectiveness analysis. Am Heart J 1999;137:1019–1027.
68. Merz N, Johnson BD, Kelsey PSF, et al. Diagnostic, prognostic, and cost assessment of coronary artery disease in women. Am J Manag Care 2001;7:959–965.
69. Kemp H, Elliott W, Gorlin R. The anginal syndrome with normal coronary arteriography. Trans Assoc Am Physicians 1967;80:59–70.
70. Reis S, Holubkov R, Conrad Smith HJ, et al. Coronary microvascular dysfunction is highly prevalent in women with chest pain in the absence of coronary artery disease: Results from the NHLBI WISE study. Am Heart J 2001;141:735–741.
71. Herlitz J, Wiklund I, Sioland H, et al. Relief of symptoms and improvement of health-related quality of life five years after coronary artery bypass graft in women and men. Clin Cardiol 2001;24:385–392.
72. Vaccarino V, Lin ZQ, Kasl SV, et al. Gender differences in recovery after coronary artery bypass surgery. J Am Coll Cardiol 2003;41(2):307–314.
73. Clarke S. Women's health. Factors linking women and CHD. Nursing Times 1995;91:29–31.
74. Rozanski A, Blumenthal J, Kaplan J. Impact of psychological factors on the pathogenesis of cardiovascular disease and implications for therapy. Circulation 1999;101:E177–E178.
75. Rutledge T, Reis SE, Olsm M, et al. Psychosocial variables are associated with atherosclerosis risk factors among women with chest pain: the WISE study. Psychosom Med 2001;63:282–288.
76. Haynes S, Feinleib M. Women, work and coronary heart disease: prospective findings from the Framingham heart study. Am J Public Health 1980;70:133–141.
77. Elliott S. Psychosocial stress, women and heart health: A critical review. Soc Sci Med 1995;40:105–115.
78. Czajkowski SM, Terrin M, Lindguist R, et al. Comparison of preoperative characteristics of men and women undergoing coronary artery bypass grafting (the Post Coronary Artery Bypass Graft [CABG] Biobehavioral Study). Am J Cardiol 1997;79:1017–1024.
78a. US Public Health Service and Department. Women's Health. Washington, DC: Author, 1996.
79. Evanoski C. Myocardial infarction, the number one killer of women. Crit Care Nurs Clin North Am 1997;9:489–496.
80. Lerner D, Kannel W. Patterns of coronary heart disease morbidity and mortality in the sexes: a 26-year follow-up of the Framingham population. Am Heart J 1986;111:383–390.

81. Greenland P, Reicher-Reiss H, Goldbourt U, Behar S. In-hospital and 1-year mortality in 1,524 women after myocardial infarction. Comparison with 4,315 men. Circulation 1991;83:484–491.
82. Tofler G, Stone PH, Muller JE, et al. Effects of gender and race on prognosis after myocardial infarction: adverse prognosis for women, particularly black women. J Am Coll Cardiol 1987;9:473–482.

C. Choosing the Best Diagnostic Test for Women

12 Should All Women With Suspected Coronary Disease Undergo Stress Cardiac Imaging?

Anthony P. Morise, MD

Contents

INTRODUCTION

Whether all women with suspected coronary disease should undergo stress cardiac imaging is an important and challenging question. It is important because women comprise more than 50% of our population, and coronary disease is the leading cause of death in women. It is challenging because, although the response seems obvious to many physicians, as evidenced by their practice patterns, the role and value of the treadmill exercise electrocardiogram (ECG) in women is clouded by misconceptions concerning the test's performance characteristics and the overwhelming concern to avoid a false-positive study. The brief answer to the above question is "no." The following discussion supports this answer.

ACCURACY OF THE EXERCISE ECG IN WOMEN

Prior to exploring how to select women for exercise ECG, discussing the exercise ECG's accuracy in women is appropriate because it lays the foundation for what is later discussed. It is my belief that the single most important concern for most physicians regarding exercise ECG application to women, and the reason why it is underutilized in women in comparison to men, is the fear of the false-positive ST segment response (i.e., poor specificity).

From: *Contemporary Cardiology: Coronary Disease in Women: Evidence-Based Diagnosis and Treatment*
Edited by: L. J. Shaw and R. F. Redberg © Humana Press Inc., Totowa, NJ

Sensitivity and Specificity

Both the sensitivity and specificity of the exercise ECG in women are well documented to be lower than the respective values in men. In a 1999 meta-analysis, Kwok et al. reported an exercise ECG sensitivity of 61% and a 69% specificity for women without prior coronary disease *(1)*. Ten years earlier, Gianrossi et al. had performed a similar meta-analysis in studies where the majority of the patients considered were men *(2)*. The study reported a 67% sensitivity and a 72% specificity. A comparison of these performance characteristics suggests that both are lower in women.

However, both meta-analyses used studies affected by referral bias (i.e., the preferential patient referral with positive exercise tests to coronary angiography). A prior study from my laboratory found that, when sensitivity and specificity were statistically adjusted for referral bias, sensitivity was in the 40–50% range, and specificity was in the 80–90% range for both men and women *(3)*. These findings were distinctly different from both the unadjusted accuracy results in that study and the meta-analyses. Froelicher et al. later confirmed this observation in a male Veterans Affairs (VA) population by reporting that when an attempt was made to prospectively minimize referral bias, sensitivity was 45% and specificity was 85% *(4)*.

In a subsequent analysis, using the same studies from the meta-analysis of Gianrossi et al. and Froelicher et al. found a relationship between both sensitivity and specificity, along with the frequency of a positive exercise ST-segment response *(5)*. They considered the frequency of a positive test to be a surrogate marker for referral bias. This relationship suggests that referral bias should lead to an overestimation of sensitivity and an underestimation of specificity, exactly as predicted by the prior studies.

Unfortunately, a female study comparable to the Froelicher et al. study *(4)* does not exist and is unlikely to be accomplished in the foreseeable future. Nevertheless, data from our prior report suggests the following conclusions concerning referral bias in women *(3)*. First, even after adjustment for referral bias, sensitivity and specificity are still lower in women in comparison to men. Second, the referral bias effects were similar in men and women, suggesting that referral bias is not an explanation for the male and female differences.

Many reasons have been proposed for the lower accuracy of exercise testing in women. As stated earlier, referral bias is not likely a factor. The lower sensitivity has been attributed to a lower prevalence and severity of coronary disease in women, that is, lower disease frequency and multivessel disease frequency makes it difficult to find those individual women with disease. Lower exercise capacity and a lower ECG voltage have also been proposed as reasons for lower sensitivity. Lower specificity has been most recently attributed to hormonal differences between men and women.

Hormonal Effects on Accuracy

Because of its structural similarity to digitalis, a well-documented producer of false-positive exercise tests, estrogen has been assumed to be the source of false-positive exercise tests or the lower female specificity. The first clinical evaluation of this hypothesis was by Jaffe *(6)*, who evaluated 33 men and 18 women that had abnormal ECGs prior to any medication. He found that the immediate postexercise ECGs (Masters test) revealed further hormone associated worsening of the ST-segment response in 90% of the subjects, irrespective of the estrogen replacement type they received (i.e., conjugated or synthetic estrogens or a combination of estrogen and progestin. A more recent study by Rosano et al. *(7)* investigated 11 postmenopausal women with coronary atherosclerosis and abnormal exercise ST-segment responses and found a different result from Jaffe. They found that sublingual estradiol reduced the ST-segment response to exercise. In 109 women with normal coronary angiograms *(8)*, my laboratory found an independent association between a positive exercise ST-segment response and the presence of estrogen replacement therapy (ERT) at the time of the exercise test. However, no such association was found for premenopausal women. We later reported that unselected postmenopausal women on ERT during the time of the exercise test had a significantly lower specificity than premenopausal women, as well as postmenopausal women not receiving ERT *(9)*. In fact, the specificity in the premenopausal women was not different than the male specificity.

As a follow-up, our group later reported that in 385 women on either ERT or no medication at all, progestin with estrogen (but not estrogen alone) was an independent predictor of a positive exercise ST-segment response *(10)*. This would be consistent with data from monkeys, indicating that medroxyprogesterone diminishes the estrogen effect on endothelium-dependent coronary vasodilation *(11)*, along with two human female studies *(12,13)*. Very recently, Rovang et al. *(14)* published the results of a prospective study in 47 postmenopausal women with normal exercise echocardiograms. They noted that 20% of these women converted from a normal to an abnormal exercise ST-segment response while receiving ERT.

What can be concluded from the available data concerning ERT and the exercise ECG? First, pharmacological ERT seems to have a specificity effect on the ST-segment response to exercise. Second, in women with coronary disease, estrogen has an antiischemic effect on exercise-induced ST-segment changes, consistent with accumulating evidence that estradiol potentiates endothelium-dependent coronary vasodilation in women *(15,16)*. This effect is counteracted by synthetic progestins. Therefore, from currently available literature, it is possible that ERT may have a dual effect on the accuracy of the exercise ST-segment response. There is potential for estrogen to decrease sensitivity through a tendency to reduce ischemia and, conversely, for progestin to decrease specificity through a tendency to promote ischemia.

Other Accuracy Considerations

Prior to a change in discussion, several other factors regarding accuracy are significant. Although sensitivity and specificity are the accepted standards for defining a test's performance characteristics, they do not represent how well the test answers clinically relevant questions. For example, specificity asks the following question: "How likely is it that a patient without a disease will have a negative test?" This is not a clinically relevant question. The relevant question would be: "How likely is it that a patient with a negative test will have no disease?" Here is the essence of negative predictive value. Its converse positive predictive value asks, "How likely is it that a patient with a positive test will have disease?" Unfortunately, unlike sensitivity and specificity, predictive value varies according to disease prevalence or pretest probability. However, if pretest probability is accounted for, then predictive value becomes very important in interpreting the test results and determining the test's usefulness in individual patient decisions.

The performance characteristics of sensitivity and specificity reflect accuracy using only one variable, namely, ST-segment changes. Obviously, the exercise test interpretation should incorporate more than simply ST-segment depression. When incorporated into multivariable models, exercise ECG variables, including ST-segment change, have incremental diagnostic value over clinical female variables (e.g., age, symptoms, and risk factors) *(17,18)*. Despite the lower sensitivity and specificity of ST-segment depression in women, when considered with clinical variables, these models have equivalent diagnostic value in men and women, which serves as a basis for the subsequent discussion of exercise test multivariable scores.

CANDIDATES FOR STRESS IMAGING AS INITIAL TEST

There are female groups for whom initial stress cardiac imaging is preferred over the simple treadmill exercise ECG. Women who cannot exercise need pharmacological stress imaging simply because pharmacological stress ECG as its own option does not exist. This constitutes 30–40% of women who present with suspected coronary disease.

Similarly, women with uninterpretable ECGs as defined by the American College of Cardiology/American Heart Association (ACC/AHA) guidelines (complete left-bundle branch block, Wolff-Parkinson-White syndrome, electronically paced rhythm, and ST-segment depression ≥ 1 mm) constitute 1–2% of women able to exercise. These women should undergo initial exercise imaging.

Women with other specific electrocardiographic abnormalities not previously mentioned require further explanation. Those with minor ST-segment depression (<1 mm) do not require imaging (2–3%). Those with right-bundle branch block (1–2%) also do not require imaging, although the right-sided precordial leads (V1–V3), which often manifest a false-positive ST-segment response, should be ignored. Those women receiving digitalis preparations; those with voltage criteria for left ventricular hypertrophy, but < 1 mm ST-segment depression; or those with lateral lead T-wave inversions without ST-segment depression all have reliable negative ST-segment responses. The problem exists in the frequent positive ST-segment responses. Until further studies clarify this situation, women with any of these three scenarios (5–7%) should likely undergo initial stress imaging. The approx 60% of remaining women with suspected CAD are potential candidates for initial exercise ECG.

SELECTING WOMEN FOR EXERCISE ECG AS THE INITIAL TEST

ACC/AHA Guidelines

Guidelines published in 1986 classified the use of the exercise ECG in women for diagnostic purposes as Class II *(19)*. In other words, there was a divergence of opinion regarding the value and appropriateness of the test. As a comparison, exercise ECG's use in men was classified as Class I (i.e., consensus agreement that it was indicated).

The next revision to the guidelines, which did not appear until 1997 *(20)*, explicitly stated that, despite the greater frequency of false-positive tests, there are "currently insufficient data to justify routine stress imaging tests as the initial test for CAD in women." This is a significant change from the previous guidelines. Additionally, these guidelines emphasize that women as well as men with suspected coronary disease symptoms and an intermediate pretest probability of CAD have a Class I indication. On the other hand, women and men with a low- or high-pretest probability have a Class IIb indication (i.e., its usefulness is less well-established by evidence or opinion). Although not a ringing endorsement as with the intermediate-pretest probability women, nevertheless, it is not a Class III indication (i.e., general agreement that exercise testing is ineffective). In lieu of randomized studies that assess health outcomes for diagnostic tests, these indications were based primarily on the potential effect of the exercise ECG's result on diagnostic outcome.

Intermediate probability patients were assigned a Class I indication because of the well-established Bayesian principle that populations with an intermediate disease prevalence will have the greater diagnostic impact or incremental value from a test result. A recently published study (21) has demonstrated that the incremental value of exercise ECG in intermediate probability patients is quite substantial. In contrast, it was difficult to document significant incremental value for the exercise test in the low- and high-pretest probability groups. Does this mean that there is no value to perform this test in all low or high probability patients? The short answer is "no." The extensive answer is developed in the following section.

Estimating Pretest Probability

For most clinicians, the problem has been how to most effectively apply the exercise ECG, particularly for women. Until this time, most have chosen to solve this dilemma by using exercise imaging. The ACC/AHA guidelines suggest to start with pretest probability, recommending the Diamond-Forrester method, which incorporates age, sex, and symptoms to estimate low-, intermediate-, or high-pretest probability status. This familiar and validated method requires a table to translate clinical variables into probability groups.

Another method to estimate pretest probability allows for the consideration of other risk factors, including diabetes, estrogen status, and others, as well as age, sex, and symptoms (22,23). This pretest score could be memorized and calculated while a history is being taken. The point total of 0–24 is well-calibrated with coronary disease prevalence (i.e., low scores mean low prevalence, high scores mean high prevalence, etc.) and compares well with the Diamond-Forrester method for grouping patients into low-, intermediate-, and high-pretest probability groups (24).

Test Characteristics

Once the pretest probability group is determined, the clinician must decide if the exercise ECG provides an adequate response as to whether coronary disease is likely to be present or not. Because noninvasive tests do not provide complete assurance that a negative or positive test result is true, the principles of probability analysis can be used as a guide.

Figure 1 is a scatter plot of data from more than 2500 women from West Virginia University School of Medicine. Plotted is the probability of coronary disease after an exercise ECG (postexercise test probability) as a function of the coronary disease pretest probability. These pre- and postexercise test probabilities were calculated from previously published and validated equations (18,22). They incorporate many standard clinical and exercise test variables, such as ST-segment depression, ST-segment slope, and peak exercise heart rate. The diagonal line ascending from the point of origin represents the line of identity where the exercise test results did not change a woman's

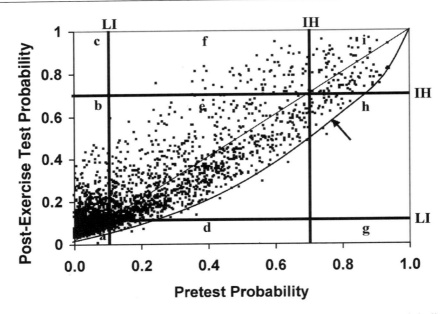

Fig. 1. Scatter plot of pretest probability vs postexercise test probability. Diagonal straight line represents line of identity. Curved line delineated by arrow represents the lowest border of the scatter plot. Dark horizontal and vertical lines represent the borders of the low to intermediate (LI) and intermediate to high (IH) probability zones for both pretest and posttest probability. These four lines divide plot into a grid of nine sections labeled a through i. See text for further discussion.

probability. Points that fall below this line represent women whose test results lowered their disease probability. Conversely, points that are above this line represent women whose test results raised their probability of disease. The outer edges of this plot represent the extreme negative and positive test results. Particularly, the lower edge (drawn with arrow) represents the lowest attainable probability from the exercise ECG for any level of pretest probability, which is a reflection of the negative predictive value. This curve, ascending gradually from left to right, suggests that as pretest probability increases, negative predictive value decreases (i.e., the lowest attainable posttest probability rises). A prior study has confirmed this association *(21)*.

The reason for emphasis on negative predictive value should be clear. For most screening tests, results are reported as positive or negative because of the selection of a cutpoint with a defined sensitivity and specificity. For a screening test to have clinical value, it should have a high-negative predictive value. High-positive predictive value is good, but false-positives are generally dealt with effectively by ordering another test. This is a manageable situation as long as the frequency of false-positive studies is not very high. Anything other than a low false-negative rate (or high-negative predictive value) is unacceptable, resulting from the fact that, because consideration of the disease-of-inerest's presence will generally cease, an unacceptable number of diseased patients will be missed when the false-negative rate is not low. Therefore, a negative screening result should have accurate meaning with a high degree of confidence.

Returning to Fig. 1, darker straight lines mark the respective borders between low- and intermediate-probability zones and intermediate- and high-probability zones for both pretest (vertical lines) and postexercise test (horizontal lines) probability. The intermediate-to-high probability border of 0.70 was selected as suggested by a prior cost-effectiveness analysis *(25)*. The low-to-intermediate probability border of 0.10 was suggested by Diamond et al. *(26)* The resultant grid has nine sections that represent different ranges of pre- and postexercise test probability, each with different clinical implications.

Test Selection

Given that the ACC/AHA guidelines suggest that *intermediate-pretest probability* patients have a Class I indication for exercise ECG, this group is considered first (sections d, e, and f in Fig. 1). Approximately one-third of women who present for diagnostic exercise testing will have an intermediate-pretest probability *(21)*. Those high-posttest probability women (section f), should be considered to have coronary disease and rightfully referred for angiography. For those in sections d and e, the management is less straightforward. As reported previously *(21)*, the negative predictive value in intermediate-pretest probability women is between 70 and 80%, which is unacceptably low. This same report also indicates that negative predictive value varies within the intermediate-pretest probability group, such that it falls as pretest probability increases within the intermediate-pretest probability range. The curved line in Fig. 1 is also consistent with this. According to Fig. 1, only those women with a pretest probability between 10 and 25% had any chance of having a posttest probability below 10%. Therefore, for these women at the lower end of the intermediate-pretest group, initial exercise ECG might be appropriate because of the acceptable negative predictive value. However, women in the upper two-thirds of the intermediate group might need a different initial strategy with better negative predictive value (e.g., exercise imaging). Those women who fall into section d have a low posttest probability and should have their chest pain evaluation consider diagnoses other than coronary disease. Given that a large percentage of intermediate-pretest probability women end up in section e (i.e., intermediate-posttest probability), an initial strategy of exercise imaging plus exercise ECG may be appropriate. However, further studies are needed to resolve this question, as well as the optimal approach to intermediate-pretest probability women.

Next, consider the *high-pretest probability* group (sections g, h, and i in Fig. 1), categorized by the ACC/AHA guidelines as having a Class IIb indication for exercise ECG. Approximately 5–10% of women who present for diagnostic exercise testing will have a high-pretest probability *(21)*. As with section f noted earlier, those women falling into section i (high-posttest probability) should be considered for coronary angiography. However, the more important question is whether exercise ECG should be performed at all in high-pretest probability women. First, no woman in this cohort was transformed from high-pretest to low-posttest probability. Second, prior studies have demonstrated that the negative predictive value in high-pretest probability women is extremely poor (30–40%; *21*), which is suggested by the curve in Fig. 1. Third, the frequency of negative exercise ECGs in this same group is not small (40–50%). In other words, if high-pretest probability women have little chance of being categorized as having a low-postexercise test probability and a large frequency of potentially false-negative tests, why should exercise testing be performed at all? Because of these considerations, from a practical standpoint, one can make a case for a strategy of initial coronary angiography prior to any exercise testing consideration. This is supported by two cost-effectiveness analyses

(25,27). On the contrary, it has been suggested that initial exercise testing be considered as a means of risk-stratifying these patients into medical and revascularization therapy groups, assuming that coronary disease is present and that the principal issue is disease severity *(28,29)*. This approach could have merit in the appropriate clinical setting, but it needs to be validated in a prospective trial.

Finally, consider the *low-pretest probability* group (sections a, b, and c in Fig. 1), also categorized by the ACC/AHA guidelines as having a Class IIb indication for exercise ECG. More than one-half of women who present for diagnostic exercise testing will have a low-pretest probability *(21)*. As can be seen in section c, no patient in this cohort was transformed from low-pretest to high-posttest probability, which directly addresses the low-positive predictive value in low-pretest probability women. It should also be noted that a very large percentage of low-pretest probability women are concentrated in section a. Prior studies indicate that 85% of low-pretest probability women will have a negative exercise ECG *(21)*, being consistent with this distribution in section a. These women are unlikely to have coronary disease that provides explanation of their symptoms. Section b likely represents the 15% of low-pretest probability women with an abnormal exercise ECG, who would be candidates for follow-up exercise imaging to resolve whether their abnormal exercise ECG response is a false-positive.

Suggestions concerning how to evaluate women with a low-pretest probability of coronary disease vary from no cardiac testing *(29)*, to exercise echocardiography *(27)*, to exercise ECG *(21,28,30)*. A recent AHA Science Advisory recommended exercise ECG in low-risk/low-likelihood patients presenting to chest pain centers *(31)*. My strategy is similar to the strategy proposed by Shaw et al. *(30)*. Without prospective trials, it is not possible to state which approach would be the most effective.

Likely, some combination of all three approaches has merit. From Fig. 1, it is difficult to clarify which women begin and end in section a. These are the women least likely to benefit from screening stress testing. This point is discussed in the next section when considering exercise test scores. In considering exercise echocardiography, it is likely that the associated negative predictive value would be very high (>95%). However, exercise ECG also has a very high-negative predictive value (>95%) in low-pretest probability women *(21)*. Those low-probability women with abnormal exercise ECGs would be candidates for either exercise echocardiography or nuclear perfusion imaging. When negative predictive value is very high, a negative test result can be reassuring to both physicians and patients that the coronary disease probability is very low. Unfortunately, this type of value is difficult to measure. Suffice it to say, a randomized trial would be of great value.

Exercise Test Scores

Presently, methods to estimate postexercise test probability, as displayed in Fig. 1, are not user-friendly. The ACC/AHA guidelines urge physicians to use "more than just the ST-segment in interpreting the exercise test..." They suggest several multivariable equations, but concede that their use is limited.

A simple user-friendly exercise test score that is comparable to the pretest score mentioned previously has been developed for use in women *(32)*. A similar but separate score has also been developed for men *(33)*. These scores are presently undergoing validation to assure their accuracy in other populations. The scores include both clinical and treadmill test variables specific to women and men. The exercise test

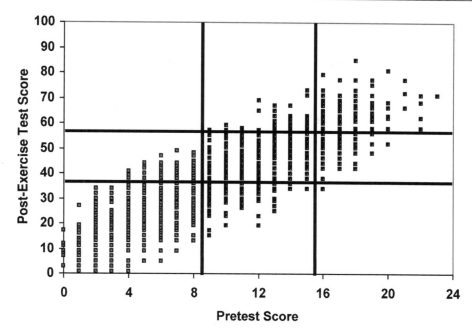

Fig. 2. Scatter plot of pretest score vs exercise test score. As in Fig. 1, dark horizontal and vertical lines represent the borders of the low-to-intermediate and intermediate-to-high probability zones for both pretest and posttest probability. These four lines divide plot into a grid of nine sections. See text for further discussion.

variables included in the scores for men and women are the same, but they are weighted differently.

Figure 2 is a plot using data from the same women in Fig. 1. However, instead of plotting posttest probability as a function of pretest probability, exercise test score is plotted as a function of pretest score. This scatter plot approximates the visual probability distribution shown in Fig. 1. Similar to Fig. 1, pre- and posttest cutpoints separating low from intermediate and intermediate from high probability women are superimposed. The true impact of this approach awaits further studies, but the potential for its use is apparent in this figure. For example, women with a pretest score of 3 or less should not undergo exercise testing at all. They have no chance of being transformed to a higher probability group. Similarly, women with pretest scores of 14 or higher have a very low chance of ending up in the low posttest probability group. Further discussion of this method is forthcoming following validation studies.

WISE Study

The National Heart, Lung, and Blood Institute (NHLBI)-sponsored Women's Ischemia Syndrome Evaluation (WISE) study *(34)* is a multicentered study with goals that are threefold: (1) optimize symptom evaluation and diagnostic testing for ischemic heart disease; (2) explore mechanisms for symptoms and myocardial ischemia in the absence of epicardial coronary artery stenosis; and (3) evaluate the reproductive hormone influence on symptoms and diagnostic test responses. This important study addresses issues that focus on how best to evaluate women with suspected coronary disease. This ongoing study has already borne fruit *(35)*, and I anticipate more reports in the future that address its stated goals. Additionally, the clinical syndrome presently called *microvascular angina,* an important cause of chest pain in women, will come under intense scrutiny *(36)*.

THE NEED FOR TRIALS

At several points in this discussion, I have suggested the need for prospective trials. In undertaking these trials, it is crucial to the field that the following principles be steadfastly applied.

First, women (and men) should be initially stratified into low-, intermediate-, and high-pretest probability groups using a method that is both accurate and easy to use. Using a method that clinicians are unlikely to embrace is futile.

Second, randomization of the proposed competing strategies where potential equipoise exists should be undertaken within each pretest probability group. Depending on potential enrollment, some limit to the number of different strategies within a pretest probability group may have to be imposed.

Third, in the interest of fairness, each competing technology should be given the opportunity to employ its best and most currently applicable techniques. Multipartisan cooperation among all of the disciplines ensures that each has equal input into how the trials are conducted. Because each technology is continually improving, strategies should allow for the consideration of these improvements as they become available, which would reflect the best practice available. Candidate technologies would include exercise ECG, exercise echocardiography, exercise nuclear imaging, electron beam computed tomography for coronary calcium, and coronary angiography. Also, magnetic resonance imaging and computed tomography angiography are future potential candidates.

Finally, this field requires evidence-based approaches that should consider a variety of outcomes to answer the questions of those with varying perspectives. Until the appropriate studies are completed, this field will consist of diverse, somewhat overlapping, and somewhat discordant guidelines that reflect the biases of their creators. Both the clinician and patient will be left to wonder what is best for them.

SUMMARY

Again, the question is asked whether all women with suspected coronary disease should undergo stress cardiac imaging. As previously stated, although exercise ECG is less accurate in women than in men, when considered in the context of pretest clinical data, the accuracy, incremental value, and utility in women is similar to men. For diagnostic purposes, the exercise ECG is most useful as an initial test in low- and selected intermediate-pretest probability women with interpretable resting ECGs. This constitutes approx 60–70% of women who can exercise and have interpretable ECGs. Management decisions following exercise ECG should be based on either a multivariable score or positive/negative test results in the context of pretest probability. Given the present economical landscape, the simple, inexpensive, and readily available exercise ECG (when properly used and interpreted) has the potential to perform as a gatekeeper to the use of exercise imaging in many women. Only properly designed trials will settle the debate over the best approach to women with suspected coronary disease.

REFERENCES

1. Kwok Y, Kim C, Grady D, et al. Meta-analysis of exercise testing to detect coronary artery disease in women. Am J Cardiol 1999;83:660–666.
2. 2.Gianrossi R, Detrano R, Lehmann K, et al. Exercise-induced ST depression in the diagnosis of coronary artery disease: a meta-analysis. Circulation 1989;80:87–98.
3. Morise AP, Diamond GA. Comparison of the sensitivity and specificity of exercise electrocardiography in biased and unbiased populations of men and women. Am Heart J 1995;130:741–747.
4. Froelicher VF, Lehmann KG, Thmas R, et al. The electrocardiographic exercise test in a population with reduced work-up bias: diagnostic performance, computerized interpretation, and multivariable prediction. Ann Intern Med 1998;128:965–974.
5. Froelicher VF, Fearon WF, Ferguson CM, et al. Lessons learned from studies of the standard exercise ECG test. Chest 1999;116:1442–1451.
6. Jaffe MD. Effect of oestrogens on postexercise ECG. Br Heart J 1977;38:1299–1303.
7. Rosano GMC, Sarrel PM, Poole-Wilson PA. Beneficial effect of oestrogen on exercise-induced myocardial ischemia in women with coronary artery disease. Lancet 1993;342:133–136.
8. Morise AP, Dalal JN, Duval RD. Frequency of oral estrogen replacement therapy in women with normal and abnormal exercise electrocardiograms and normal coronary arteries by angiogram. Am J Cardiol 1993;72:1197–1199.
9. Morise AP, Beto R. The specificity of exercise ECG in women grouped by estrogen status. Int J Cardiol 1997;60:55–65.
10. Morise AP. Progestin therapy as a variable auxillary to established predictors of positive exercise tests in women. J Noninvasive Cardiol 1997;1:27–32.
11. Williams JK, Honore EK, Washburn SA, et al. Effects of hormone replacement therapy on reactivity of atherosclerotic coronary arteries in cynomolgus monkeys. J Am Coll Cardiol 1994;24:1757–1761.
12. Sorensen KE, Dorup I, Hermann AP, et al. Combined hormone replacement therapy does not protect women against the age-related decline in endothelium-dependent vasomotor function. Circulation 1998;97:1234–1238.
13. Rosano G, Rosano GMC, Sarrel PM, et al. Medroxyprogesterone but not natural progesterone reverses the ebenficial effect of estradiol 17-beta upon exercise-induced myocardial ischemia. Circulation 1996;94:I-18.
14. Rovang KS, Arouni AJ, Mohiuddin SM, et al. Effect of estrogen on exercise electrocardiograms in healthy postmenopausal women. Am J Cardiol 2000;86:477–479.
15. Gilligan DM, Badar DM, Panza JA, et al. Acute vascular effects of estrogen in postmenopausal women. Circulation 1994;90:786–791.
16. Leiberman EH, Gerhard MD, Uehata A, et al. Estrogen improves endothelium-dependent flow-mediated vasodilation in postmenopausal women. Ann Intern Med 1994;121:936–941.
17. Morise AP, Dalal JN, Duval RD. Value of a simple measure of estrogen status for improving the diagnosis of coronary artery disease in women. Am J Med 1993;94:491–496.
18. Morise AP, Diamond GA, Detrano R, et al. Incremental value of exercise ECG and thallium-201 testing I in men and women for the presence and extent of coronary artery disease. Am Heart J 1995;130:267–276.
19. Schlant RC, Blomqvist CG, Brandenburg RO, et al. Guidelines for exercise testing: a report of the joint American College of Cardiology/American Heart Association task force on assessment of cardiovascular procedures (subcommittee on exercise testing). Circulation 1986;74:653A–667A.
20. Gibbons RJ, Balady GJ, Beasley JW, et al. ACC/AHA guidelines for exercise testing: a report of the American College of Cardiology/American Heart Association Task Force on Practice Guidelines (Committee on Exercise Testing). J Am Coll Cardiol 1997;30:260–315.
21. Morise AP. Are the ACC/AHA guidelines for exercise testing for suspected coronary disease correct? Chest 2000;118:535–541.
22. Morise AP, Haddad WJ, Beckner D. Development and validation of a clinical score to estimate the probability of coronary artery disease in men and women presenting with suspected coronary disease. Am J Med 1997;102:350–356.
23. Morise AP, Haddad WJ. Validation of estrogen status as an independent predictor of coronary artery disease presence and extent in women. J Cardiovasc Risk 1997;3:507–511.
24. Morise AP. Comparison of the Diamond-Forrester method and a new score to estimate the pretest probability of coronary disease before exercise testing. Am Heart J 1999;138;740–745.

25. Patterson RE, Eisner RL, Horowitz SF. Comparison of cost-effectiveness and utility of exercise ECG, single photon emission computed tomography, positron emission tomography, and coronary angiography for diagnosis of coronary artery disease. Circulation 1995;91:54–65.

26. Diamond GA, Forrester JS, Hirsch M, et al. Application of conditional probability analysis to the clinical diagnosis of coronary artery disease. J Clin Invest 1980:65:1210–1221.

27. Kim C, Kwok YS, Saha S, Redberg R. Diagnosis of suspected coronary artery disease in women: a cost-effectiveness analysis. Am Heart J 1999;137:1019–1027.

28. Hachamovitch R, Berman DS, Kiat H, et al. Exercise myocardial perfusion SPECT in patients without known coronary artery disease: incremental prognostic value and use in risk stratification. Circulation 1996;93:905–914.

29. Douglas PS, Ginsburg GS. The evaluation of chest pain in women. N Engl J Med 1996;334:1311–1315.

30. Shaw LJ, Hachamovitch R, Redberg RF. Current evidence on diagnostic testing in women with suspected coronary artery disease. Cardiol Rev 2000;8:65–74.

31. Stein RA, Chaitman BR, Balady GJ, et al. Safety and utility of exercise testing in emergency room chest pain centers. Circulation 2000;102:1463–1467.

32. Morise AP, Lauer MS, Froelicher VF. Development and validation of a simple exercise test score for use in women with symptoms of suspected coronary artery disease. Am Heart J 2002;144:818–825.

33. Raxwal VK, Shetler K, Morise AP, et al. Simple treadmill score to diagnose coronary disease. Chest 2001;119:1933–1940.

34. Bairey Merz CN, Kelsey SF, Pepine CJ, et al. The Women's Ischemia Syndrome Evaluation (WISE) study: protocol, design, methodology and feasibility report. J Am Coll Cardiol 1999;33:1453–1461.

35. Lewis JF, Lang L, McGorray S, et al. Dobutamine stress echocardiography in women with chest pain: pilot phase data from the National Heart, Lung and Blood Institute Women's Ischemia Syndrome Evaluation (WISE). J Am Coll Cardiol 1999;33:1462–1468.

36. Reis SE, Holubkov R, Lee JS, et al. Coronary flow velocity response to adenosine characterizes coronary microvascular function in women with chest pain and no obstructive coronary disease. Results from the pilot phase of the Women's Ischemia Syndrome Evaluation (WISE) Study. J Am Coll Cardiol 1999;33:1469–1475.

13 State-of-the-Art Diagnostic Testing in Women
A Research Update

Leslee J. Shaw, PhD, B. Delia Johnson, PhD, Sharon Mulvagh, MD, Jennifer H. Mieres, MD, Rita F. Redberg, MD, FACC, and C. Noel Bairey Merz, MD

CONTENTS

BACKGROUND
GENDER DIFFERENCES IN NONINVASIVE DIAGNOSTIC TESTING
    FOR CORONARY ARTERY DISEASE
ASSESSING PRETEST RISK OF CORONARY ARTERY DISEASE
ASYMPTOMATIC SCREENING
DIAGNOSTIC TESTING FOR THE EVALUATION OF SYMPTOMATIC
    WOMEN
NEW HORIZONS FOR CARDIOVASCULAR IMAGING FOR WOMEN
RECOMMENDATIONS FOR DIAGNOSTIC TESTING IN WOMEN
CONCLUSIONS
REFERENCES

BACKGROUND

Despite advances in the diagnosis and management of cardiovascular disease (CVD), nearly 250,000 female lives are claimed each year *(1)*. Research continues to report underrecognition, underdiagnosis, and undertreatment of coronary disease in women causative to higher CVD mortality *(2-9)*. Nonspecific symptoms, such as generalized malaise, fatigue, and dyspnea in women are imprecise and ineffective discriminators of disease *(10)*. Older age of presentation and delays in atypical symptom recognition contribute to a greater morbidity and mortality for the female patient *(11)*. Screening of the asymptomatic woman is a topic of much interest because the initial presentation of sudden cardiac death occurs more frequently in women (63%) than in men (50%) *(1)*.

From: *Contemporary Cardiology: Coronary Disease in Women: Evidence-Based Diagnosis and Treatment*
Edited by: L. J. Shaw and R. F. Redberg © Humana Press Inc., Totowa, NJ

One key to affecting significant changes in cardiovascular mortality for women is the appropriate use of highly accurate diagnostic tests that result in early and effective treatment, improved outcomes for at-risk women, and lower costs for end-stage health care. This chapter aims to put forth a synopsis of available evidence on diagnostic testing in women.

GENDER DIFFERENCES IN NONINVASIVE DIAGNOSTIC TESTING FOR CORONARY ARTERY DISEASE

A large body of evidence suggests that there is a diminished diagnostic accuracy for an array of cardiac noninvasive tests for women (12–13). Reduced specificity has been noted for exercise electrocardiography (ECG) (due to lower ECG voltage, hormonal factors, functional capacity, to name a few), and for the lower energy isotope thallium (Tl)-201 imaging (owing to breast artifact) (14,15). A reduced sensitivity has been noted in female populations with single-vessel coronary disease who undergo both ECG and single photon emission computed tomography (SPECT) imaging. Technical considerations as well as inappropriate patient selection are contributing factors to differences in diagnostic accuracy. However, a major consideration in evaluating diagnostic accuracy is the problem of verification or work-up bias that precludes calculation of the "true" sensitivity and specificity (16). As catheterization is largely performed in patients with provocative ischemia and women are largely under "cathed," diagnostic sensitivity will be miscalculated. Conversely, the estimation of specificity should include clinical follow-up for several years posttest in order to capture the true false negative rate. Additionally, prior reports have noted a more protracted work-up time for women, such that, during the episode of care, angiography for suspected myocardial ischemia may be undertaken as much as 1 year following initial presentation and, often, after an array of other tests are performed (2). Although diagnostic accuracy has known limitations in women, a number of recent reports have noted a gender-neutral ability to risk stratify patients (17–19). There is a growing body of evidence on the prognostic value of noninvasive testing techniques. As such, this is the primary focus of this chapter.

ASSESSING PRETEST RISK OF CORONARY ARTERY DISEASE

Evaluation of Asymptomatic Women

A new paradigm is unfolding where screening is being undertaken in asymptomatic individuals and was the subject matter of the 34th Bethesda Conference on atherosclerotic imaging (20). The rationale for screening is based on the frequent initial presentation of acute myocardial infarction (MI) and sudden cardiac death in previously asymptomatic individuals. Thus, additional population-based risk reduction is considered one option for the detection of subclinical (or presymptomatic) disease.

The aggregation and detection of high risk may be accomplished by integrating a number of traditional risk factors, including age, systolic blood pressure, cholesterol, and gender, into an estimated coronary heart disease risk (21–23). Risk scores have been put forth by the European Society of Cardiology (23), the American Heart Association's (AHA) Prevention V conference (22), and the National Heart Lung and Blood Institute's (NHLBI) National Cholesterol Education Program (NCEP) Adult Treatment Panel III (21). The latter risk score is based on the Framingham study (including offspring). For example, based on the NCEP risk calculator, individuals may have a calculated risk that is low, intermediate, or high, which corresponds to their 10-year risk of "hard" cardiac events (including cardiac death or nonfatal MI). Currently, the AHA Prevention V conference defines subgroupings of risk using this 10-year estimate of cardiac death or nonfatal MI *(22)*. Low risk is defined as an annualized risk of death or infarction less than <0.6%. Intermediate and high risk are defined as a risk of death or infarction of 0.6–2%, and greater than 2%, respectively, per year. A high-risk individual is one whose event risk is equivalent to that of a person with established coronary disease and, most recently, this also includes diabetics. Diabetes is now considered a coronary heart disease risk equivalent because of the lengthy delays to disease diagnosis and the frequency with which macrovascular disease is present. Clinicians can download a program from the NIH-NHLBI website for easy calculation of these risk subsets *(21)*.

Based on the 34th Bethesda Conference, screening would be considered for individuals who are at intermediate risk *(20)*. However, generally speaking, an asymptomatic individual with more than one risk factor is at intermediate risk and, although this remains controversial, may be considered a candidate for screening. The ensuing value of a screening test is to then further risk stratify patients as posttest low or high risk.

Evaluation of Symptomatic Women

The selection and referral of appropriate at-risk symptomatic women remains one of the greatest challenges facing clinicians. The American College of Cardiology (ACC)/AHA guidelines for exercise testing suggest that symptomatic patients with an intermediate pretest likelihood of coronary disease are candidates for exercise testing *(24)*. Additionally, serial testing of patients with established coronary disease with a new onset or medically refractory stable symptoms is also recommended *(24)*. Recent evidence from the NIH-NHLBI-sponsored Women's Ischemia Syndrome Evaluation (WISE; *see* Chapter 10 for further details) study reveals that the most common symptoms associated and with coronary disease in women are jaw pain, dyspnea, nausea, dizziness, weakness, fatigue. Often, these symptoms are triggered by strong emotions (*see* Chapter 10). Evidence suggests that women presenting with atypical symptoms have a lower likelihood of obstructive coronary disease *(25-26)*. As such, a compendium of data supports the concept that symptoms are a less than efficient guide to optimal test selection in women. It seems practical that physicians should allow greater latitude in defining symptoms for the female patient and be more inquisitive during the physical examination for changes in perceived well-being or a diminished ability to perform routine activities of daily living (*see* Chapter 8).

An evolving concept arising out of the ACC/AHA guidelines for exercise testing revolves around the inclusion of estimated physical work capacity during the patient's pretest evaluation. Performing routine household activities requires approximately 4 metabolic equivalents (METs) of work *(24)*. Thus, physicians at the time of symptom evaluation should include some estimate of functional capacity. As patients do tailor their physical capabilities to their symptoms, an evolving pattern of lowered functional capacity with increasing symptom frequency may ensue, thus, creating the perception of a more "atypical" symptom presentation. However, the estimation of physical work capacity may also serve as a guide for the type of exercise protocol (e.g., the more aggressive Bruce or less aggressive Asymptomatic Cardiac Ischemia Pilot (ACIP) protocol). Self-reported questionnaires, like the 12-item Duke Activity Status Index

(DASI), are available to estimate peak oxygen consumption values (divide by 3.5 to estimate METs) to assist the clinician in determining a woman's abilities to perform routine activities of daily living *(27)*.

The compilation of risk, including age, traditional cardiac risk factors, and symptoms is aided by the availability of a number of multivariable risk predictions models *(28)*. For symptomatic presentation, the secondary prevention Bethesda Conference has published a number of gender-based algorithms for estimating major adverse cardiac event risk *(28)*. The use of risk-prediction models will aid the clinician in defining intermediate- as compared with low- to high-risk women.

A woman with typical exertional angina generally has an intermediate-high pretest probability of coronary disease (i.e., probability ≥15%) *(26)*. For those women with atypical or nonanginal symptoms, concomitant risk factors increase the likelihood of disease. Patients with diabetes are more often asymptomatic due to neuropathy and are considered high risk according to the most recent NCEP consensus document, with an expected 2% annualized risk of cardiac death or MI *(21)*.

Current evidence does not support testing women with a low likelihood of coronary disease (i.e., probability <15%). False positives test results will occur more often when testing low-risk patients consequently, driving up costs of care *(26)*. The greatest incremental value for testing is in women whose pretest risk is considered to be intermediate *(24,26,28,29)*. The ensuing results of ischemia testing would risk stratify women with negative results to a low posttest risk and those with abnormal results to a higher posttest risk of disease (depending on the extent and severity of abnormalities). That is, following the results of a test in an intermediate-risk woman, the test results may shift posttest risk to a lower (i.e., negative test) or higher (i.e., positive test) risk group. Many physicians also consider testing higher risk women as the extent and severity of ischemia and localization of abnormalities can aid in ensuing decisions regarding medical and surgical options.

Role of Hormones in Risk Assessment

The incidence of coronary disease is decidedly diminished in the premenopausal woman due to endogenous estrogen. As women enter the perimenopausal phase (i.e., fourth decade of life), there is a gradual loss of estrogen. By the time a woman reaches the age of 55 years, she is considered postmenopausal and her estrogen levels are nearly one-tenth that of her premenopausal state (*see also* Chapter 21).

For the premenopausal woman, endogenous estrogen has a digoxin-like effect that may precipitate ST segment depression, resulting in a false positive stress ECG *(17,30)*. Physicians testing premenopausal women with chest pain or established coronary disease should note the stage of a woman's menstrual cycle. An unfolding body of evidence suggests that stress testing during a woman's mid-cycle, when estrogen levels are highest, may be associated with less inducible ischemia and a lower frequency of chest pain symptoms *(31–33)*. As such, in order to optimize test accuracy, it would be preferable for a premenopausal woman to undergo stress testing in the late stages of the luteal phase (~12 days postovulation) or during menses when estradiol levels are lowest. It also seems reasonable for a clinician to query women as to symptom fluctuations occurring with her menstrual cycle. The documentation of a woman with a history of polycystic ovary syndrome would be of additional importance as she is at increased risk of coronary disease with an increased link to obesity, central obesity, insulin resistance, and diabetes *(34)*.

A number of studies have noted that coronary disease may be masked for the woman taking hormone replacement therapy (HRT) owing to its vasodilatory action, resulting in a reduced frequency of chest pain and ischemia as well as improved exercise tolerance *(35-37)*. Because of the adverse risk associated with HRT, as noted in the Heart and Estrogen/Progestin Replacement Study (HERS) and the Women's Health Initiative (WHI) trials *(see also* Chapter 21), it is likely that fewer women will be presenting for evaluation with concomitant estrogen or combination progestin use *(38-39)*. However, should they be referred for testing, clinicians should note that an increased risk of major adverse cardiovascular events (especially thromboembolic events) has been reported for women with and without a prior history of coronary disease. This increased risk is correlated with an increase in inflammatory markers (i.e., C-reactive protein) that has been reported for women taking HRT but not with the newer Selective Estrogen Receptor Modulators *(see also* Chapter 21). Increasing inflammation is corroborated by the fact that most of the excess risk, as recently reported in the WHI, was in nonfatal MI *(40)*. It is likely that the ischemic event risk for women using HRT may be estimated by provocative stress testing. This latter point is further supported by the increased thromboembolic risk that occurs early after treatment initiation (i.e., in the first year) and the body of evidence supporting near-term event prediction by imaging modalities, such as echocardiography or SPECT imaging (discussed later in this chapter).

Of the cohorts of women enrolled in randomized trials such as HERS or WHI, those who will remain on HRT include women with moderate-severe vasomotor symptoms. Women who receive a benefit from treatment may also be suboptimal testing candidates due to the vasodilatory effects of HRT. Clinicians should further inquire as to the type and severity of symptoms and consider the fact that false negative results may occur; that is, latent coronary disease may be masked due to an HRT-induced coronary vasodilation.

ASYMPTOMATIC SCREENING

For asymptomatic women, the current public health challenge is the identification of high-risk subsets that may be at risk for sudden cardiac death or acute MI. Because of the greater frequency of presentation without prior symptoms, it may be possible to prescreen patients using an array of tests that detect subclinical disease, which might result in life-saving care *(20)*. A number of atherosclerotic imaging modalities have been advocated for the evaluation of cardiovascular screening in asymptomatic individuals including ankle brachial index, brachial reactivity, coronary calcium, and carotid intima-media thickness (IMT). Although the added value of screening asymptomatics has been inconsistently reported, atherosclerotic imaging modalities, such as coronary calcium, have been shown to provide information independent of traditional risk factors *(20,41)* *(see also* Chapter 5).

Because of differences in the onset of disease, artery size, as well as the prevalence of traditional risk parameters, a number of reports have identified gender differences in the detection and accuracy of atherosclerotic imaging measurements *(42-46)*. For example, the results of brachial reactivity testing require gender adjustment as women have a greater vasodilator response than men *(20)*. In general, the overall prevalence of imaging abnormalities is lower and lags approximately 10 years in female populations when compared with men, similar to the prevalence of the disease *(47-48)*. Despite this, recent evidence from the Atherosclerosis Risk in Communities (ARIC) Study reported that carotid IMT was a stronger predictor of stroke in women than in men *(46)*. That is, using Cox proportional hazards models, the hazard ratios for a mean IMT value of 1 mm or greater was 8.5 for women (95% confidence interval [CI]: 3.5- 20.7) and 3.6 for men (95% CI: 1.5-9.2). Similarly, owing to small artery size, a given amount of coronary calcification encumbers a greater extent of the myocardium and has been associated with worsening survival for women as compared with men *(47)*. These latter results call for imaging scoring systems tailored for women and for more aggressive treatment of women who have evidence of subclinical disease on a screening examination.

Inflammatory markers have been suggested to be useful prognostic markers. *(48-50)*. High sensitivity C-reactive protein (HsCRP) is an acute phase reactant and has been reported to correlate with an increased risk of MI and stroke (*see also* Chapter 4). With regard to atherosclerotic imaging, however, there is a reported lack of association between HsCRP and coronary calcium in postmenopausal women *(51)*. It is likely that coronary calcium is not a good predictor of acute ischemic events due to the fact that calcification does not correlate with functional coronary stenosis, flow-limiting disease, or to plaque vulnerability *(41,52-54)* but rather may provide a measure of the global burden of atherosclerosis *(47)*.

For coronary calcium, there are remaining challenges in risk thresholds where published reports have noted anything from detectable calcium to calcium scores greater than 680 as being high risk *(20,41)*. However, our group has recently published data revealing that 5-year survival exceeds 99% for women and men with a low-risk calcium score of less than 10 *(47)*. Survival decrementally worsens for women with increasingly higher calcium scores (Fig. 1). As previously noted, due to small artery size, any given amount of calcium is associated with worsening survival in women as compared with men; as such lower thresholds of risk may be required for women (*see* Fig. 1).

Recommendations for Cardiovascular Risk Screening in Women

Based on existing evidence, we have formulated a preliminary management strategy for the evaluation of intermediate-risk asymptomatic women (Fig. 2). This strategy includes an estimation of global risk in all women and their perimenopausal years, with exception to include women with risk factors (at any age). Arguments may also be put forth that women with metabolic syndrome or polycystic ovary syndromes should have a multifactorial risk assessment performed (at a minimum) and considered as candidates for screening. Despite the lower prevalence of disease in younger women, the European Society of Cardiology is expected to soon recommend predicting risk at age 60 years for a given risk assessment. That is, for a 40-year-old woman with multiple risk factors, estimation of risk should be calculated as if she were 60 years of age *(55)*.

A woman whose calcium score exceeds 400 has an annualized risk of death of 2% and should be considered to be at high risk. A follow-up ischemia test should be considered *(56)*. Retesting may be considered for women with a score ranging from 100 to less than 400, where rates of progression greater than 15% are associated with an increased risk of nonfatal MI *(57)*. Aggressive risk factor management should be

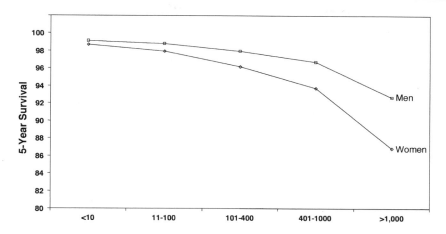

Fig. 1. Five-year all-cause survival in 4191 intermediate-risk, asymptomatic women and 6186 intermediate-risk, asymptomatic men by electron beam tomography coronary calcium score. (From ref. *47*.)

undertaken in women with evidence of atherosclerosis on screening. In two prior reports, the use of statin therapy has been associated with a lack of progression in the calcium volume score *(58-59)*.

DIAGNOSTIC TESTING FOR THE EVALUATION OF SYMPTOMATIC WOMEN

Exercise Electrocardiography

The exercise ECG (*see also* Chapter 12) has been part of the testing armamentarium for coronary disease for many decades with a wealth of available gender-specific data. Based on the ACC/AHA guidelines for stable angina, women are candidates for the exercise ECG if they have a normal resting 12-lead ECG (i.e., no resting ST-T wave changes precluding interpretation of peak exertional changes) and have sufficient physical work capacity to attain maximal levels of exercise (*see also* Chapter 14) *(29)*.

The exercise ECG has been reported to have a lower diagnostic accuracy in women *(14,15)* Several reviews on the diagnostic sensitivity and specificity have revealed lower accuracy of 1 mm or more of ST segment depression for women compared to men with an average sensitivity and specificity for the exercise ECG of 61 and 69% *(12-15)*. The lower diagnostic accuracy of the exercise ECG may in part result from the fact that disease prevalence is less or that women are older and have higher rates of functional impairment leading to a diminished exercise capacity, an inability to attain maximal stress, and provoke ischemia. Additional critical factors that have been reported to affect test accuracy in women include resting ST-T wave changes, lower ECG voltage, and hormonal factors (endogenous estrogen in premenopausal women and the use of HRT in older women).

A major key to enhanced accuracy of the exercise ECG is to include other factors than ST segment depression when interpreting the test. The integration of parameters such as the simple Δ ST/heart rate index or the Duke treadmill score (defined as exercise time - [5 x ST deviation] - [4 x chest pain {1 = non limiting, 2 = limiting}] dramatically improves the diagnostic and prognostic accuracy of testing in women *(19,60)*.

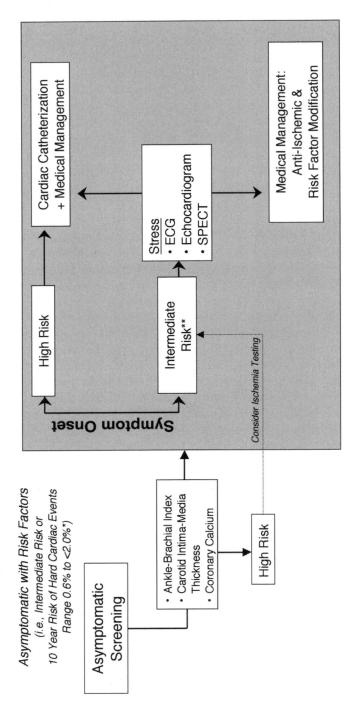

Fig. 2. New paradigm for testing at-risk asymptomatic and symptomatic women.

*10-year risk of cardiac death or nonfatal myocardial infarction may be estimated by the National Cholesterol Education Program Adult Treatment Panel III risk calculator (www.nhlbi.nih.gov/guidelines/).

**Use risk-prediction algorithms for symptomatic women (e.g., American College of Cardiology / American Heart Association's stable angina guidelines).

ECG=Electrocardiogram

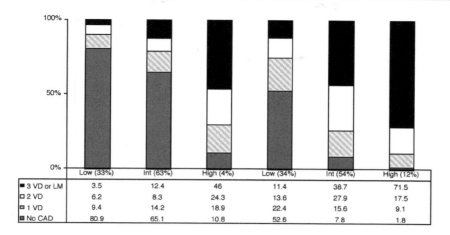

	Low (33%)	Int (63%)	High (4%)	Low (34%)	Int (54%)	High (12%)
■ 3 VD or LM	3.5	12.4	46	11.4	38.7	71.5
▫ 2 VD	6.2	8.3	24.3	13.6	27.9	17.5
▫ 1 VD	9.4	14.2	18.9	22.4	15.6	9.1
▨ No CAD	80.9	65.1	10.8	52.6	7.8	1.8

Fig. 3. Prevalence of significant and severe coronary disease by the Duke treadmill score risk groups in 976 women and 2249 men. Int, intermediate Duke treadmill score; VD, vessel disease; LM, left main; CAD, coronary artery disease.

Although the accuracy of routine treadmill testing is discussed in Chapter 12, the estimated rate of significant and severe coronary disease for women and men by the Duke treadmill score risk groups is depicted in Fig. 3 *(19)*. As noted, higher rates of obstructive and severe coronary disease are reported in women and men with high-risk Duke treadmill scores; although the rates in women generally lag that of their male counterparts. Similarly, for women, 5-year survival exceeds 97% for a low-risk and is less than 90% for a high-risk Duke treadmill score *(19)*. Women may then proceed to subsequent cardiac imaging when their Duke treadmill score is intermediate risk. Additionally, those at high risk may be considered candidates for either an imaging test or coronary angiography; depending on the clinical scenario.

Physicians should consider simple factors such as total exercise time and heart rate recovery (at 1 or 2 minutes postexercise) as major predictors of adverse prognosis *(61)*. Following maximal exercise, in the recovery phase, there is a reactivation of cardiac vagal tone. A decrease in heart rate of less than 44 beats at 2 minutes into recovery is associated with a nearly threefold increased hazard for death *(62)*. Heart rate recovery has been related to heart rate variability and has also been correlated with insulin resistance *(63)*; with an abnormal heart rate recovery being more common among those individuals with impaired fasting glucose *(64)*.

Another simple measure that is also one of our strongest prognosticators is physical work capacity or exercise duration on a bicycle ergometer or treadmill (*see also* Chapters 8 and 12) *(24)*. Of note, women have generally worse functional capacity, engage less often in leisure-time activities, and have more functional decline during their menopausal years. Lower exercise times (on average 5-7 minutes) challenge the ability to provoke a central myocardial stress and an abundance of literature supports that fact that women who exercise less than 5 METs are at increased risk of worsening prognosis *(24)*.

One method to estimate maximal oxygen consumption (METs x 3.5) is to use the Duke Activity Status Index (DASI) *(65)*. This may aid in identifying women incapable of performing a minimum of 5 METs of exercise who then should be referred for pharmacologic stress testing *(24,29)*. Although maximal stress may be defined by achieving 85% or greater of predicted maximal heart rate, care should be taken when interpreting a woman's heart rate response. For deconditioned patients, an exaggerated response to physical work may result in marked increases in heart rate. Thus, the test should be continued until maximal symptom-limited exercise capacity is achieved.

These latter simple measures provide an abundance of data on risk assessment and should be included in every physician's interpretation of the exercise ECG. Although a woman may exhibit no ST segment changes, evidence of functional impairment or impaired heart rate responses may aid in identifying at-risk women. Additional risk markers that may be of added diagnostic and prognostic value include an impaired blood pressure response to exercise, as well as the presence and frequency of premature ventricular contractions and more serious ventricular arrhythmias *(24)*. One factor, exercise-induced chest pain, however, has shown to be poorly predictive of disease and outcome for women *(19)*.

Candidates for Cardiac Imaging

Current evidence and medical society guidelines recommend cardiac imaging for women whose resting 12-lead ECG is abnormal (defined as resting ST-T wave changes that would interfere with discerning exercise-induced changes) and for those women with an indeterminate or intermediate risk exercise ECG. Additional candidates, as previously stated, include the large proportion of women with functional impairment, encompassing approximately 25–40% of women referred to imaging laboratories. Diabetic women are another cohort that may be considered as candidates for imaging. Recently, the American Society of Nuclear Cardiology has published an algorithm of candidates for testing and is reasonable to use for referral to both echocardiographic and nuclear imaging (*see* Fig. 4) *(13)*.

Gated Myocardial Perfusion SPECT

Gated myocardial perfusion SPECT is a nuclear-based technique that provides a combination of risk parameters that aid in the detection of disease and risk in women including regional perfusion deficits, global and regional ventricular function, and left ventricular volumes *(66)*. Of the imaging modalities, SPECT stress imaging is the most commonly performed in the United States, undertaken in approximately 7 million patients every year. Nuclear imaging has been reported to have technical limitations in women *(13)*, including the false positive results due to breast attenuation, small left ventricular chamber size, and a higher prevalence of single vessel disease. *(13)*. For example, the accuracy of Tl-201 SPECT imaging was reduced in patients with small hearts, more commonly seen in women than men, *(13)*. When using Tl-201 as the radioisotope in women, false positive test results may be the result of soft-tissue (breast) attenuation in the anterior and antero-lateral segments *(13)*.

Despite these limitations, recent updates to stress myocardial perfusion imaging have resulted in substantial improvements in the accuracy of testing *(67)*. For women, the lower energy isotope Tl-201 is now largely supplanted by the use of technetium-based imaging agents that improve accuracy, particularly when performing gated

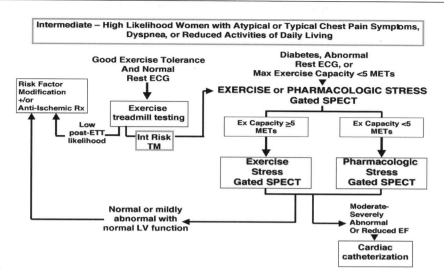

Fig. 4. Candidates for cardiac imaging based on the American Society of Nuclear Cardiology guidelines for the evaluation of women with suspected coronary disease symptoms.
Rx, therapy; TM, treadmill; ETT, exercise tolerance testing; ECG, electrocardiogram; METs, metabolic equivalents; EF, ejection fraction. (From ref. *13*.)

SPECT imaging (where a post-stress ejection fraction is obtained) *(67)*. In a small, randomized trial comparing the diagnostic accuracy of Tl-201 with gated Tc-99m sestamibi SPECT in women, test specificity was improved dramatically from 67% for Tl-201 to 92% for gated Tc-99m sestamibi SPECT *(67)*. The higher count profile that is exhibited with Tc-99m sestamibi results in an enhanced image quality and improved accuracy for women *(13,67)*. Amanullah and colleagues reported on 130 women undergoing adenosine Tc-99m sestamibi SPECT revealing that a moderate to severely abnormal perfusion scan (i.e., summed stress score >8) was associated with a sensitivity and specificity of 91 and 70% for the detection of multivessel coronary disease *(68)*.

Reports from several large samples have noted that for both Tc-99m sestamibi (rest and exercise) and for dual isotope (i.e., Tl-201 at rest and Tc-99m at stress) myocardial perfusion SPECT, there is an added incremental prognostic value of myocardial perfusion data as compared to clinical and exercise variables in women *(69-71)*. From a recent multicenter registry of 3402 women with stable chest pain symptoms, risk stratification was similar by gender (Fig. 5A; *[71]*). By the number of vascular territories with ischemia, 3-year survival ranged from 98.5 to 85% for none to three vascular territories, respectively *(71)*.

Additional prognostic variables that may be derived from SPECT imaging include an immediate post-stress ejection fraction of less than 45%, end systolic volume greater than 70 mL, transient ischemic dilation, and increased lung uptake of Tl-201 *(72)*.

Exercise Echocardiography

Stress echocardiography is another common noninvasive test. A number of reports have examined both the diagnostic and prognostic accuracy of stress echocardiogra-

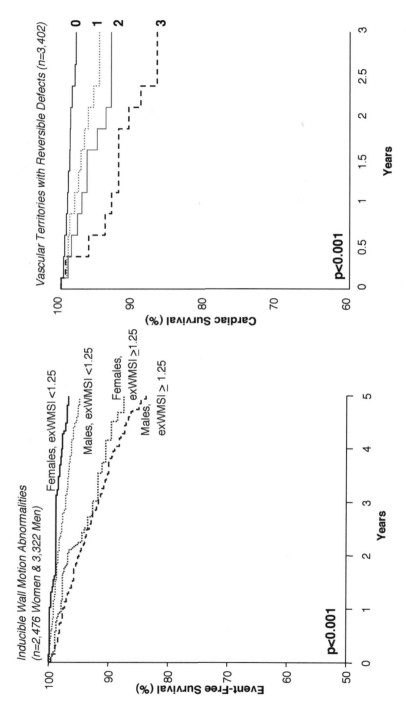

Fig. 5. Risk stratification with exercise echocardiography (**A**) and myocardial perfusion SPECT (**B**) in symptomatic women. WMSI, sum of segmental scores/number of segments visualized (i.e., new or worsening abnormalities). (From ref. *18*.)

Table 1
Meta-Analysis of the Diagnostic Accuracy of Exercise Electrocardiography (ECG),
Echocardiogram, and Tl-201 Perfusion Imaging (including planar and SPECT)

Imaging modality	No. of studies	N	Sensitivity	Specificity
Exercise ECG	20	3,874	61	69
Tl-201 Perfusion	5	842	78	64
Exercise Echocardiogram	3	296	86	79

phy echo in women *(15,18,73-75)*. Overall advantages to the use of exercise echo are the lack of ionizing radiation, the portability, and lower cost of the equipment allowing for greater use and affordability in the outpatient setting, and an increased ability to image cardiac structures and function. The evaluation of valve disease is particularly helpful for women with chest pain whose differential diagnosis includes mitral valve prolapse. Table 1 reports data from a meta-analysis comparing the diagnostic accuracy of stress ECG, echocardiography, and Tl-201 imaging *(15)*. Given the fact that inducible wall motion abnormalities appear later on in the ischemic cascade, there is greater test specificity with echocardiography when compared to SPECT imaging. However, intermediate stenosis that may cause flow limitations and perfusion deficits on SPECT may be less detectable with wall motion techniques. Consequently, there is a lower accuracy for detection of 50-70% lesions and those with single-vessel coronary disease *(73)*.

Regarding prognosis, recent evidence supports the use of stress echocardiographic techniques for the estimation of event-free survival in women *(18)*. A report from the Mayo Clinic concerning 2476 women revealed that event-free survival was 97% for women with no inducible wall motion abnormalities as compared with 88% for those with a wall motion score index of 1.25 or more (defined as the sum of segmental scores/number of segments visualized with new or worsening abnormalities) (Fig. 5A; *[18,21]*).

There are several intravenous contrast agents that are approved for left ventricular opacification and endocardial border delineation with echocardiography. In the clinical setting, quick delineation of immediate post-stress wall motion changes may be enhanced by the use of myocardial contrast agents, such as Optison™ or Definity™. The use of contrast agents clinically results in enhanced image appearance, improved diagnostic feasibility, and interpretation, especially in technically difficult patents including obese women and those with lung disease whose acoustic window may be suboptimal. Additionally, there is ongoing research for the use of myocardial contrast agents in the delineation of regional myocardial perfusion with echocardiographic techniques. Thus, in the future, we would hope for both echocardiographic and SPECT techniques to optimally provide information on global and regional function as well as regional perfusion thus providing equivalent risk markers on which to optimally guide decision making.

Candidates for Pharmacologic Imaging

Approximately 25–40% of patients who are referred for cardiac imaging for the evaluation of known or suspected coronary artery disease (CAD) are candidates for pharmacologic stress imaging. Because women are generally older when they present with CAD and have a higher incidence of decreased exercise capacity, many with known or suspected CAD are not able to complete a symptom-limited exercise protocol and are therefore candidates for pharmacologic stress testing *(29)*. Functional impairment may be defined as incapable of performing 5 METs of exercise (or less than stage 1 of the Bruce protocol) *(24)*.

Either with dobutamine echocardiography or dipyridamole or adenosine vasodilator SPECT stress, the interpretation of wall motion abnormalities and perfusion deficits is generally similar to that applied with exercise (and was described previously) *(66,75)*. A second generation of vasodilator agents (a 2α receptor antagonists) that are more cardio-specific (i.e., with minimal systemic effects—blood pressure and reduced side-effect profile) are under development. Importantly, there is a reduced risk of bronchospasm and, therefore, patients who are currently contraindicated to receive dipyridamole or adenosine may be eligible for vasodilator stress with one of the three agents now in Phase III clinical trials.

Cardiovascular Magnetic Resonance Imaging

Perhaps no other imaging modality is undergoing such rapid development as that of cardiovascular magnetic resonance imaging (CMR) *(76)*. CMR has many features making it suitable for evaluating patients with a wide range of cardiovascular diseases including fast examination times, excellent tissue characterization (high soft-tissue contrast), three-dimensional volumetric acquisition/display, and the ability to quantify blood flow *(76)*. Furthermore, CMR is attractive because it does not require the use of ionizing radiation nor are contrast agents nephrotoxic. CMR is capable of yielding superior temporal and spatial resolution and may image the great vessels, congenital abnormalities, valvular heart disease, pericardial disease, as well as left ventricular mass and function, perfusion, wall thickness, and myocardial perfusion and blood flow (including contrast-enhanced differentiation of subendocardial and epicardial flow) *(76-82)*. However, CMR is not widely available, the equipment is expensive, and currently there are few outcomes studies utilizing the technique.

MR perfusion for the diagnosis of CAD has not been extensively studied in women, but the overall sensitivity and specificity values are in the 70 to 80% range *(76,78)*. Interestingly, CMR is capable of separating subendocardial from epicardial perfusion deficits *(77)*. A recent report from the Royal Brompton Hospital in London revealed that women with syndrome X (chest pain, evidence of provocative ischemia, and nonobstructive coronary disease) have subendocardial ischemia noted with MR perfusion imaging *(77)*. One of the benefits of MR perfusion estimates is that absolute reductions in perfusion may be determined. This is compared to the fact that SPECT determines regional deficits in perfusion by normalizing the myocardium and therefore assesses relative perfusion. Recently, data from the WISE study indicated that the provocation of perfusion ischemia is reliant on an adequate hyperemic response to stress *(83)*. Additionally, with the three dimensionality of CMR, wall motion abnormalities may be superior to other modalities and detect coronary disease in 74% of patients with less extensive (i.e., single-vessel) disease *(78)*.

MR angiography (MRA) has been shown in preliminary reports to have a similar diagnostic accuracy when compared to invasive cardiac catheterization *(80)*. Imaging is currently most reliable for proximal stenosis (in particular, left anterior descending),

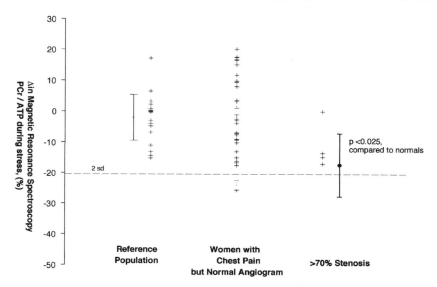

Fig. 6. Handgrip stress magnetic resonance spectroscopy: a reduced phosphocreatine/adenosine triphosphate (ATP) ratio is noted in approximately one-third of women with nonobstructive coronary disease.

although this modality still requires substantial validation. Despite this, women may benefit from initial screening with MRA. Approximately half of women undergo diagnostic coronary angiography, which, owing to its invasive nature, carries a slight, but notable, risk of complication *(11, 80)*.

In women with normal coronaries, recent evidence has identified a unique imaging method using P31 MR spectroscopy to identify alterations in high-energy phosphates *(81)*. A reduction in phosphocreatine/adenosine triphosphate (PCr/ATP) provides a measure of metabolic dysfunction representing myocardial ischemia. Figure 6 reveals that a reduced PCr/ATP ratio of 20% or less is noted in one-third of women with normal coronaries *(81)*. A recent update from this investigative group reveals that women with abnormal P31 MR spectroscopy are at increased risk of major adverse cardiac events, in particular a substantially higher rate of acute coronary syndromes (at 2 years of follow-up) *(82)*. It appears that although survival may be excellent in women with nonobstructive coronary disease, a subset of patients may have microvascular disease precipitating metabolic dysfunction and leading to continuing symptoms and unstable angina. However, longer term follow-up and validation of these results is required to clearly establish the relationship between major adverse cardiac events and P31 spectroscopic results.

NEW HORIZONS FOR CARDIOVASCULAR IMAGING FOR WOMEN

Although we have discussed a number of imaging modalities that are under development, it is noteworthy to identify a few additional developments in imaging that may provide a potential value in the assessment of at-risk women. Computed tomographic methods assessing angiographic (CTA) extent and severity of disease is currently undergoing rapid development and testing. It appears that CTA may also provide promise in a noninvasive assessment of coronary disease in women, similar to MRA.

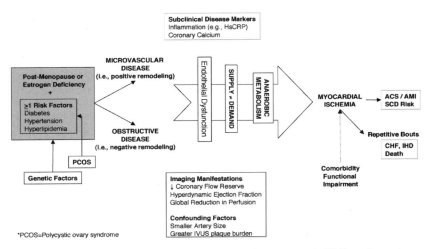

Fig. 7. Schematic of myocardial ischemia in symptomatic women. PCOS, polycystic ovary syndrome.

Historic assessments of prognosis with cardiac imaging modalities have been limited to the estimation of ischemic events including cardiac death or nonfatal MI. Increasing evidence, in particular with CT and MR methods, visualize the importance of aortic, carotid, and peripheral atherosclerosis. In the future, more reports will be available on the detection of coronary and noncoronary atherosclerosis and its association with the global CVD burden.

Increasing evidence suggests that the risk of CVD is multifactorial with new standards of assessment including integrated risk-factor scores *(21,28,30)*. In general, imaging markers have not been well integrated into laboratory and other historical parameters. Given the increased complexity in the diagnosis and assessment of risk in women, new research must aim at integrating historical, hormonal, traditional, and emerging risk markers along with cardiovascular imaging data in the assessment of major adverse cardiac outcomes in sufficiently large female samples.

Figure 7 provides a detail of the current understanding of the complexity for assessing atherosclerotic imaging modalities in women. In this proposed model, estrogen deficiency (e.g., postmenopause) has been shown to exhibit a number of effects on the vasculature that may affect imaging results. The combination of estrogen loss in the setting of traditional cardiac risk factors (including emerging risk markers such as HsCRP) is associated with alterations in (1) myocardial blood flow and coronary flow reserve noted during angiography, SPECT, CMR, or PET imaging; (2) greater deposition of atheromatous disease noted during intravascular ultrasound, carotid IMT, and retinography; (3) hyperdynamic left ventricular function noted with echocardiographic and SPECT techniques; and (4) smaller artery size noted during cardiac catheterization. Generally, the result of this is believed to be a greater burden of microvascular disease. The ensuing sequelae of a stress-induced mismatch between blood supply and myocardial oxygen demand results in a shift toward a greater reliance on anaerobic metabolism (as supported by the WISE MR spectroscopy data) and documentation of myocardial ischemia with an array of noninvasive tests (described herein).

The potential role each of these interactive forces plays on clinical outcome is also summarized in this figure. The smaller size of coronary arteries contributes to a greater atherosclerotic burden in the setting of any given amount of disease (including coronary calcification). These data are further supported by evidence that retinal artery narrowing is associated with an increased risk of coronary heart disease death or nonfatal MI in women but not in men *(84)*. Additionally, even in the setting of nonobstructive coronary disease, women with evidence of provocative ischemia (which may be subendocardial or microvascular) are potentially at increased risk for major adverse cardiac events that include unstable angina, MI, and sudden cardiac death. Repetitive bouts of ischemia, left untreated, could result in MI leading to left ventricular dysfunction predisposing a woman to heart failure and cardiac death.

To further speculate, the higher rate of recurrent and persistent symptoms may suggest that our current treatment paradigm may be less effective in this cohort of effected women. As such, future research should focus on the development of better imaging tools to estimate vascular function and metabolism as well as treatments effective at ameliorating provocative ischemia and symptoms in women.

RECOMMENDATIONS FOR DIAGNOSTIC TESTING IN WOMEN

For enhanced care of at-risk women, a careful clinical history should not only include the nature, type, and quality of cardiac symptoms and cardiac risk factors, but also a woman's relevant reproductive history including use of HRT, prior diagnosis of polycystic ovary syndrome, and stage of her menstrual cycle (for those younger females). Asymptomatic women who have one or more risk factors are generally at intermediate risk and may be candidates for cardiovascular screening including the use of inflammatory markers or imaging (e.g., coronary calcium). For the symptomatic women, clinicians should carefully consider two critical factors—functional capacity and hormonal factors-when deciding on a choice of tests. Although care should be taken when interpreting negative test results in the setting of HRT use, testing of premenopausal women should optimize the lowest estrogen level so that provocative ischemia may be elicited.

Additionally, women who are incapable of exercising to 5 METs should be considered candidates for pharmacologic stress testing. Use of the DASI can be applied in the pretesting setting to provide insight into activities of daily living *(65)*. This being said, simple measures such as functional capacity or heart rate responses to stress remain valuable prognosticators.

For women with a normal resting ECG and good exercise tolerance, a routine exercise treadmill test is currently indicated for the evaluation of suspected myocardial ischemia. The interpretation of the exercise test should consider more than the interpretation of ST segment changes including exercise capacity and heart rate changes. A number of risk scores are available to aid in the integration of several treadmill test parameters (e.g., Duke treadmill score). Figure 4 reviews current indications for cardiac imaging; most commonly including stress echocardiography or SPECT imaging. Cardiac imaging, using stress echocardiographic and SPECT techniques, should optimally include measures of left ventricular function and extent and severity of provocative ischemia noted by regional wall motion and/or perfusion abnormalities to aid in optimal posttest decision making.

The intensity of posttest management is then graded to increasing risk as noted during testing. Those at highest posttest risk should be considered candidates for coronary angiography. Intermediate stress test results should prompt both risk factor modification and anti-ischemic therapy for the control of symptoms. Women with an indeterminant exercise ECG should be referred to cardiac imaging. Additionally, repeat testing on medications may allow the clinician to measure the effectiveness of therapy. Low-risk patients require no additional follow-up testing (unless clinical status worsens) with management including treating risk factors to current goals as well as control of symptoms. However, care should be taken in evaluating a lack of provocative ischemia, in particular for women with submaximal levels of exercise. It is also possible that for women with nonobstructive coronary disease that subendocardial ischemia during exercise may not elicit ST segment changes or wall motion abnormalities but may only be detected by CMR techniques.

CONCLUSIONS\

The current paradigm of diagnostic testing requires substantial variation when applied to the female patient. The multifactorial role of reproductive hormones on the vascular system has yet to be fully appreciated. The interaction of small artery size with the effects of traditional risk factors (e.g., hypercholesterolemia) on artery responsiveness leading to microvascular disease is a sizeable problem for symptomatic women. Evidence of inflammation and atherosclerosis may ensue. Thus, even in the absence of obstructive coronary disease, the risk in postmenopausal women with risk factors may be underappreciated.

For women whose symptomatology is more nonspecific, there may be much more of a "blurring" between the classification of symptomatic and asymptomatic status. This may be particularly true for women with functional impairment. Extreme care should be employed in the selection of stress testing and in interpretation of test results for the work-up of symptomatic women. Consideration of hormonal status and functional impairment are critical factors to minimizing both false negative and positive test results. The intensity of posttest management should be directly proportional to the extent and severity of inducible ischemia and consideration of left ventricular function.

An abundance of evidence suggests that women are less often counseled for risk factor control, less often receive effective diagnostic tests that may lead to underuse of optimal medical and surgical therapies, and furthermore, evidence of ischemia is more often left untreated (2–9). Certainly, the complexity of management that is required for the female patient has yet to be fully assimilated into clinical guidelines and into every day clinical practice. However, current data suggest that women could benefit from risk stratification with the use of an array of commonly used noninvasive cardiac tests. Local expertise should guide the use of commonly employed echocardiographic or nuclear-based techniques. It is likely that a greater use of testing in women may result in earlier diagnosis and improved outcome for women thus, potentially impacting upon on population mortality statistics, and perhaps, realizing the dramatic declines in cardiovascular mortality noted for men.

References

1. American Heart Association. Heart and Stroke facts: 2002 statistical supplement, AHA, Dallas, 2002.
2. Shaw LJ, Miller DD, Romeis JC, et al. Gender differences in the noninvasive evaluation and management of patients with suspected coronary artery disease. Ann Int Med 1994;120:559-556.

3. Tobin JN, Wassertheil-Smoller S, Wexler JP, et al. Sex bias in considering coronary bypass surgery. Ann Int Med 1987;107:19-25.
4. Douglas PS, Ginsburg GS. The evaluation of chest pain in women. N Engl J Med 1996;334:1311-1315.
5. Steingart RM, Packer M, Hamm P, et al. Sex differences in the management of coronary artery disease. Survival and Ventricular Enlargement Investigators. N Engl J Med 1991;325:226-230.
6. Kilaru PK, Kelly RF, Calvin JE, et al. Utilization of Coronary angiography and revascularization after acute myocardial infarction in men and women risk stratified by the American College of Cardiology/ American Heart association guidelines. J Am Coll Cardiol 2000;35:974-979.
7. Hochleitner M. Coronary heart disease: Sexual bias in referral for coronary angiogram. How does it work in a state- run health system ? J Wom Health Gend Based Med 2000;9:29-34.
8. Wong CC, Froelicher ES, Bacchetti P et al. Influence of gender on cardiovascular mortality in acute myocardial infarction patients with high indication for coronary angiography. Circulation 1997;96:II-51-57.
9. Mosca L, Grundy SM, Judelson D, et al. Guide to Preventive Cardiology for Women. AHA/ACC Scientific Statement Concensus Panel Statement. Circulation 1999;99(18):2480-2484.
10. Merz CN, Kelsey SF, Pepine CJ, et al. The Women's ischemia syndrome evaluation (WISE) study: protocol design, methodology and feasibility report. J Am Coll Cardiol 1999;33:1453-1461.
11. Merz NB, Johnson BD, Kelsey PSF, et al. Diagnostic, prognostic, and cost assessment of coronary artery disease in women. Am J Managed Care 2001;7(10):959-965.
12. Shaw LJ, Peterson ED, Johnson LL. Non-invasive stress testing. In: Charney P, ed. Coronary Artery Disease in Women: What all Physicians Need to Know. American College of Physician's Women's Health Series, Philadelphia, PA, 1999, pp. 327-350.
13. Mieres JH, Shaw LJ, Hendel RC, Miller DD, et al. American Society of Nuclear Cardiology: task force on women and coronary artery disease. J Nucl Cardiol 2003;10:95-101.
14. Hlatky MA, Pryor DB, Harrel FE Jr., et al. Factors affecting sensitivity and specificity of exercise electrocardiography: Multivariable analysis. Am J Med 1984;77:64-71
15. Kwok YS, Kim C, Grady D, et al. Meta-analysis of exercise testing to detect coronary artery disease in women. Am J Cardiol 1999;83:660-666.
16. Cecil MP, Kosinski AS, Jones MT, et al. The importance of work-up (verification) bias correction in assessing the accuracy of SPECT thallium-201 testing for the diagnosis of coronary artery disease. J Clin Epidemiol 1996;49:735-742.
17. Marwick T, Shaw L, Lauer M, et al. The noninvasive prediction of cardiac mortality in men and women with known or suspected coronary artery disease. Am J Med 1999;106:172-178.
18. Arruda-Olson AM, Juracan EM, Mahoney DW, et al. Prognostic value of exercise echocardiography in 5,798 patients: is there a gender difference? J Am Coll Cardiol 2002;39(4):625-631.
19. Alexander KP, Shaw LJ, Delong ER, et al. Value of exercise treadmill testing in women. J Am Coll Cardiol 1998;32:1657-1664.
20. Redberg RF, Vogel RA, Criqui MH, et al. What is the spectrum of current and emerging techniques for the measurement of atherosclerosis? J Am Coll Cardiol 2003;41:1886-1898.
21. www.nhlbi.nih.gov/guidelines/cholesterol/index.htm, access date: July 2003.
22. Greenland P, Abrams J, Aurigemma GP, et al. Prevention Conference V: Beyond secondary prevention: Identifying the high-risk patient for primary prevention: Noninvasive tests of atherosclerotic burden. Circulation 2000;101:E12-E15.
23. Conroy RM, Pyorala K, Fitzgerald AP, et al. Estimation of ten-year risk of fatal cardiovascular disease in Europe: the SCORE project. Eur Heart J 2003;24:987-1003.
24. Gibbons RJ, Balady, GJ, Bricker, JT, et al. ACC/AHA 2002 Guideline Update for Exercise Testing—Summary Article. J Am Coll Cardiol 2002;106:1883-1892.
25. Douglas PS. Coronary artery disease in women. In: Braunwald E, Zipes DP, Libby P, eds. Heart Disease—A Textbook of Cardiovascular Medicine. 6th ed. Saunders Philadelphia, PA, 2001, pp. 2038-2051.
26. Diamond GA, Forrester JS. Analysis of probability as an aid in the clinical diagnosis of coronary-artery disease. N Engl J Med 1987;300:1350-1358.
27. Hlatky MA, Boineau RE, Higginbotham MB, et al. A brief self-administered questionnaire to determine functional capacity (The Duke activity status index). Am J Cardiol 1989;64:651-644.
28. Califf RM, Armstrong PW, Carver JR, et al. 27th Bethesda Conference: Matching the intensity of risk factor management with the hazard for coronary disease events. Task Force 5. Stratification of patients into high, medium and low risk subgroups for purposes of risk factor management. J Am Coll Cardol 1996;27:1007-1019.

29. http://www.acc.org/clinical/guidelines/stable/stable_clean.pdf, access date: July 2003.
30. Morise AP, Dalal JN, Duval RD. value of a simple measure of estrogen status for improving the diagnosis of coronary artery disease in women. Am J Med 1993;94:491-496.
31. Kawano H, Motoyama T, Ohgushi K et al. Menstrual cyclic variation of myocardial Ishemia in premenopausal women with variant angina. Ann Int Med 2001;135:977-981.
32. Kawano H, Motoyama T, Hirai N, et al. Estradiol supplementation suppresses hyperventilation-induced attacks in postmenopausal women with variant angina. J Am Coll Cardiol 2001;37:735-740.
33. Schulman SP, Thiemann DR, Ouyang P, et al. Effects of acute hormone therapy on recurrent ischemia in postmenopausal women with unstable angina. J Am Coll Cardiol 2002;39:231-237.
34. Lord J, Wilkin T. Polycystic ovary syndrome and fat distribution: the central issue? Hum Fertil (Camb) 2002;5:67-71.
35. Rosano GM, Webb CM, Chierchia S, et al. Natural progesterone, but not medroxyprogesterone acetate, enhances the beneficial effect of estrogen on exercise-induced myocardial ischemia in postmenopausal women. J Am Coll Cardiol 2000;36:2154-2159.
36. Morise AP, Dalal JN, Duval RD. Frequency of oral estrogen replacement therapy in women with normal and abnormal exercise electrocardiograms and normal coronary arteries by angiogram. Am J Cardiol 1993;72:1197-1199.
37. Morise AP, Haddad WJ. Validation of estrogen status as an independent predictor of coronary artery disease presence and extent in women. J Cardiov Risk 1996;3:507-511.
38. Hulley S, Grady D, Bush T, et al. Randomized trial of estrogen plus progestin for secondary prevention of coronary heart disease in postmenopausal women. Heart and Estrogen/progestin Replacement Study (HERS) Research Group. J Am Med Assoc 1998;280:605-613.
39. Writing Group for the Women's Health Initiative Investigators. Risks and benefits of estrogen plus progestin in healthy postmenopausal women. J Am Med Assoc 2002;288:321-333.
40. Cushman M, Legault C, Barrett-Connor E, et al. Effect of postmenopausal hormones on inflammation-sensitive proteins: the Postmenopausal Estrogen/Progestin Interventions (PEPI) Study. Circulation 1999;100:717-722.
41. O'Rourke RA, Brundage BH, Froelicher VF, et al. American College of Cardiology/American Heart Association Expert Consensus Document on electron-beam computed tomography for the diagnosis and prognosis of coronary artery disease. J Am Coll Cardiol 2000; 36:326-340.
42. Hecht HS, Superko HR. Electron beam tomography and National Cholesterol Education Program guidelines in asymptomatic women. J Am Coll Cardiol 2001;37:1506-1511.
43. Newman AB, Naydeck BL, Sutton-Tyrrell K, et al. Coronary artery calcification in older adults to age 99: prevalence and risk factors. Circulation 2001;104:2679-2684.
44. Hoff JA, Chomka EV, Krainik AJ, et al. Age and gender distributions of coronary artery calcium detected by electron beam tomography in 35,246 adults. Am J Cardiol 2001;87:1335-1339.
45. Wong ND, Kouwabunpat D, Vo AN, et al. Coronary calcium and atherosclerosis by ultrafast computed tomography in asymptomatic men and women: relation to age and risk factors. Am Heart J 1994;127:422-430.
46. Chambless LE, Folsom AR, Clegg LX, et al. Carotid wall thickness is predictive of incident clinical stroke: the Atherosclerosis Risk in Communities (ARIC) study. Am J Epidemiol 2000;151:478-487.
47. Shaw LJ, Raggi P, Schisterman E, et al. Prognostic value of cardiac risk factors and coronary artery calcium screening for all-cause mortality. Radiology 2003; access date: July 17, 2003 http://www.rsna-jls.org.
48. Ridker PM, Buring JE, Shih J, et al. Prospective study of C-reactive protein and the risk of future cardiovascular events among apparently healthy women. Circulation 1998;98:731-733.
49. Ridker PM, Glynn RJ, Hennekens CH. C-reactive protein adds to the predictive value of total and HDL cholesterol in determining risk of first myocardial infarction. Circulation 1998;97:2007-2011.
50. Ridker PM, Hennekens CH, Buring JE, et al. C-reactive protein and other markers of inflammation in the prediction of cardiovascular disease in women. New Engl J Med 2000;342:836-843.
51. Redberg RF, Rifai N, Gee L, et al. Lack of association of C-reactive protein and coronary calcium by electron beam computed tomography in postmenopausal women: implications for coronary artery disease screening. J Am Coll Cardiol 2000;36:39-43.
52. Falk E, Fuster V. Athrogenesis and its determinants. In: Fuster V, Alexander RW, O'Rourke RA, eds. Hurst's The Heart, 10th Edition. McGraw Hill, New York:2001:1065-1094.
53. Shemesh J, Stroh CI, Tenenbaum A, et al. Comparison of coronary calcium in stable angina pectoris and in first acute myocardial infarction utilizing double helical computerized tomography. Am J Cardiol 1998;81:271-275.

54. Detrano RC, Wong ND, Doherty TM, et al. Coronary calcium does not accurately predict near-term future coronary events in high-risk adults. Circulation 1999;99:2633-2638.
55. http://www.escardio.org, access date: July 17, 2003.
56. He ZX, Hedrick TD, Pratt CM, et al. Severity of coronary artery calcification by electron beam computed tomography predicts silent myocardial ischemia. Circulation 2000;101:244-251.
57. Raggi P, Cooil B, Shaw LJ, et al. Progression of coronary calcification on serial electron beam tomography scanning is greater in patients with future myocardial infarction. Am J Cardiol (in press).
58. Achenbach S, Ropers D, Pohle K, et al. Influence of lipid-lowering therapy on the progression of coronary artery calcification: A prospective evaluation. Circulation 2002;106:1077-1082.
59. Callister TQ, Raggi P, Cooil B, et al. Effect of HMG-CoA reductase inhibitors on coronary artery disease as assessed by electron-beam computed tomography. New Engl J Med 1998;339:1972-1978.
60. Okin PM, Kligfield PM. Gender-specific criteria and performance of the exercise electrocardiogram. Circulation 1995;92:1209-1216.
61. Lauer MS, Froelicher V. Abnormal heart-rate recovery after exercise. Lancet 2002;360:1176-1177.
62. Shetler K, Marcus R, Froelicher VF, et al . Heart rate recovery: validation and methodologic issues. J Am Coll Cardiol 2001;38:1980-1987.
63. Lind L, Andren B. Heart rate recovery after exercise is related to the insulin resistance syndrome and heart rate variability in elderly men. Am Heart J 2002;144:580-582.
64. Panzer C, Lauer MS, Brieke A, et al. Association of fasting plasma glucose with heart rate recovery in healthy adults: a population-based study. Diabetes 2002;51:803-807.
65. von Dras DD, Siegler IC, Williams RB, et al. Surrogate assessment of coronary artery disease patients' functional capacity. Soc Sci Med 1997;44:1491-1502.
66. Berman DS, Shaw LJ, Germano G. Nuclear cardiology. In: Fuster V, Alexander RW, O'Rourke RA, eds. Hurst's The Heart 10th Edition. McGraw Hill, New York 2001, pp. 525-556.
67. Taillefer R, DePuey EG, Udelson JE, et al. Comparative diagnostic accuracy of Tl-201 and Tc-99m sestamibi SPECT imaging (perfusion and ECG gated SPECT) in detecting coronary artery disease in women. J Am Coll Cardiol 1997,29:69-77.
68. Amanullah AM, Berman DS, Hachamovitch R, et al. Identification of severe or extensive coronary artery disease in women by adenosine technetium-99m seatamibi SPECT. Am J Cardiol 1997;80:132-137.
69. Travin M, Duca M, Kline G, et al. Relation of gender to physician use of test results and prognostic value of technetium-99m myocardial single-photon emission computed tomography scintigraphy. Am Heart J 1997;134:78-82.
70. Hachamovitch R, Berman D, Kiat H, et al. Effective risk stratification using exercise myocardial perfusion single-photon emission computed tomography SPECT in women: gender-related differences in prognostic nuclear testing. J Am Coll Cardiol 1996;28:24-44.
71. Marwick TH, Shaw LJ, Lauer MS, et al. The noninvasive prediction of cardiac mortality in men and women with known or suspected coronary artery disease. Economics of Noninvasive Diagnosis (END) Study Group. Am J Med 1999;106:172-178.
72. Sharir T, Germano G, Kavanagh PB, et al. Incremental prognostic value of post-stress left ventricular ejection fraction and volume by gated myocardial perfusion single photon emission computed tomography. Circulation 1999;100:1035-1042.
73. Williams MJ, Marwick TH, O'Gorman D, et al. Comparison of exercise echocardiography with an exercise score to diagnose coronary artery disease in women. Am J Cardiol 1994;74:435-8.
74. Marwick TH, Anderson T, Williams MJ, et al. Exercise echocardiography is an accurate and cost-efficient technique for detection of coronary artery disease in women. J Am Coll Cardiol 1995;26:335-341.
75. Kim C, Kwok YS, Heagerty P, et al. Pharmacologic stress testing for coronary disease diagnosis: A meta-analysis. Am Heart J 2001; 142:934-944.
76. Pohost GM, Biederman RW, Doyle M. Cardiovascular magnetic resonance imaging and spectroscopy in the new millennium. Curr Probl Cardiol 2000;25:525-620.
77. Panting JR, Gatehouse PD, Yang GZ, et al. Abnormal subendocardial perfusion in cardiac syndrome X detected by cardiovascular magnetic resonance imaging. New Engl J Med 2002;346:1948-1953.
78. Keijer JT, van Rossum AC, van Eenige MJ, et al. Magnetic resonance imaging of regional perfusion in patients with single-vessel coronary artery disease. J Magn Reson Imaging 2000;11:607-615.
79. Nagel E, Lehmkuhl HB, Bocksch W, et al. Noninvasive diagnosis of ischemia-induced wall motion abnormalities with the use of high-dose dobutamine stress MRI: comparison with dobutamine stress echocardiography. Circulation 1999;99:763-770.

80. Kim WY, Danias PG, Stuber M, et al. Coronary magnetic resonance angiography for the detection of coronary stenoses. New Engl J Med 2001;345:863-869.

81. Buchthal SD, Den Hollander JA, Hee-Won K, et al. Metabolic evidence of myocardial ischemia by 31-P NMR spectroscopy in women with chest pain by no significant coronary stenoses: pilot phase results from The NHLBI WISE Study." New Engl J Med 2000;342:829-835.

82. Pohost GM, Buchthal SD, Johnson BD, et al. Abnormal 31P NMR stress test is predictive of myocardial events: A report from the NIH-NHLBI sponsored women's ischemia syndrome evaluation (WISE). J Am Coll Cardiol 2002;39:455A.

83. Doyle M, Fuisz A, Kortright E, et al. The impact of myocardial blood flow reserve on the detection of coronary artery disease by perfusion imaging methods: An NHLBI WISE study. J Cardiovasc Magn Reson (in press).

84. Wong TY, Klein R, Sharrett AR, et al. Retinal arteriolar narrowing is related to risk of coronary heart disease in women, but not men: The Atherosclerosis Risk in Communities Study. J Am Med Assoc 2002; 287:1153-1159.

III Management of Coronary Disease in Women

A. Evaluation of Stable Chest Pain Syndromes in Women

14 Treatment Strategies for Women With Stable Angina

Paul R. Casperson, PhD, Leslee J. Shaw, PhD, and Robert A. O'Rourke, MD

CONTENTS

CARDIOVASCULAR MORBIDITY AND MORTALITY

Recent evidence suggests that cardiovascular disease (CVD) mortality has been reduced 35–50% owing, in large part, to significant improvements in the management of coronary artery disease (CAD). However, CAD remains the single most important cause of morbidity and mortality in most Westernized countries for both women and men alike. Generally, the prevalence of coronary disease increases by age and varies by gender. The age-adjusted death rate per 100,000 for major CVDs in 1999 was 414.8 for men and 300.3 for women *(1)*. However, for patients with CAD, the case fatality rate for CVD is higher for women than men *(2)*. Since 1984, 50,000 more women on average have died each year than men.

For the nearly 8 million Americans evaluated with stable chest pain symptoms, an array of medical and surgical therapies have been highly effective in reducing the risk of major adverse cardiac events.

Gender Differences in Symptom Presentation

Although Chapter 10 by Johnson and colleagues from the National Institutes of Health-National Heart, Lung, and Blood Institute's (NIH-NHLBI) Women's Ischemia Syndrome Evaluation (WISE) covers this topic in detail, a brief explanation of the differences in the relative importance of risk factors and in symptom presentation between genders should be noted. Although common signs and symptoms in both males and females include chest pain, fatigue, rest pain, shortness of breath, and weakness *(3)*, angina pec-

From: *Contemporary Cardiology: Coronary Disease in Women: Evidence-Based Diagnosis and Treatment*
Edited by: L. J. Shaw and R. F. Redberg © Humana Press Inc., Totowa, NJ

toris is the most common initial and subsequent clinical presentation of CAD in women; men are more likely to present with a myocardial infarction (MI) or sudden coronary death *(4)*. However, this picture is complicated, as women with chest pain have a lower CAD probability than men (Table 1), largely because women of all ages are less likely to have triple-vessel and left-main CAD than men *(5)*. The second most frequent CAD sign and symptom, in addition to chest pain, is dizziness for women and arm pain for men. Milder symptoms, including appetite loss, dyspnea (especially in elderly women), and back pain without accompanying chest pain, generally occur more often in women.

Approaches for Diagnosing Coronary Heart Disease (CHD) in Women

The recent American College of Cardiology/American Heart Association (ACC/AHA) 2002 Guideline Update *(6)* provides a detailed approach for the gender evaluation with stable chest pain symptoms. A careful medical history and physical exam can provide the key elements to determine CAD likelihood. As presented in Table 1, the likelihood of significant obstructive coronary disease is variable by the type of chest pain symptoms, including noncardiac chest pain, atypical angina, or typical angina. For those who manifest chest pain symptoms, typical angina is defined as having *all three* of the following characteristics: (1) substernal chest discomfort (almost never a sharp or stabbing pain) with a *quality* characterized by patients as "squeezing," "grip-like," "pressure-like," "suffocating" and "heavy," unchanging with position or respiration, and a *duration* of anginal episodes that typically last minutes (a fleeting discomfort or a dull ache lasting for hours is unlikely to be angina); (2) provoked by exertion or emotional stress; and (3) relieved by rest or nitroglycerin. Atypical angina meets two of the previous characteristics, whereas noncardiac chest pain meets one or none of the typical anginal characteristics. However, the symptoms that women experience often differ from those "classic" symptoms (substernal crushing chest pain radiating to the left arm) typically perceived by men. In women, the pain may be: (1) centered in the chest with or without radiation down one or both arms; (2) located in the ear, jaw, or neck region; or (3) located in the back or shoulder region *(6)*. Other reported symptoms are diaphoresis, light-headedness, shortness of breath, nausea, and vomiting; these symptoms may or may not accompany chest pain or discomfort *(3)*.

As women present later in life and are more often functionally impaired, their frequency of nonexertional symptoms is higher than that of their male counterparts *(7)*. Additionally, for elderly women, shortness of breath is more often the initial presenting symptom for acute MI (AMI). As such, the differential presentation of an at- risk symptomatic woman provides a unique diagnostic challenge. In Chapter 10, investigators from the NIH-NHLBI-sponsored WISE study provide us with insight into the typical symptomatology in approx 1000 women *(8)*.

Functional impairment and other comorbidities and risk factors increase the risk in any patient. Table 2 details the range in disease likelihood for low- to high-risk patients. For low-risk young women, CAD likelihood is exceedingly low. With increasing age, particularly in the postmenopausal age groups, likelihood increases dramatically. The combination of advanced age, typical angina symptoms, and additional risk factors (increasing a woman to a high-risk category) sharply increases disease risk to the range of 60–80%.

Women are also more likely to have a greater degree of comorbidity, which contributes to an increasing complication risk during the acute symptoms evaluation. Although age is perhaps one of the greatest prognosticators and, for women, provides a great deal of infor-

Table 1
Pretest CAD Likelihood in Symptomatic Patients According to Age and Sex*
(Combined Diamond/Forrester and CASS Data)

Age years	Nonanginal chest pain		Atypical angina		Typical angina	
	Men	Women	Men	Women	Men	Women
30–39	4	2	34	12	76	26
40–49	13	3	51	22	87	55
50–59	20	7	65	31	93	73
60–69	27	14	72	51	94	86

* Each value represents the percent with significant CAD on catheterization. CASS, Coronary Artery Surgery Study.

Source: refs. *38,42.*

Table 2
Comparing Pretest CAD Likelihoods in Low-Risk Symptomatic Patients
With High-Risk Symptomatic Patients—Duke Database

Age years	Nonanginal chest pain		Atypical angina		Typical angina	
	Men	Women	Men	Women	Men	Women
35	3–35	1–19	8–59	2–39	30–88	10–78
45	9–47	2–22	21–70	5–43	51–92	20–79
55	23–59	4–25	45–79	10–47	80–95	38–82
65	49–69	9–29	71–86	20–51	93–97	56–84

Each value represents the percent with significant CAD. The first is the percentage for a low-risk, mid-decade patient without diabetes, smoking, or hyperlipidemia. The second is that of the same age patient with diabetes, smoking, and hyperlipidemia. Both high- and low-risk patients have normal resting ECGs. If ST-T-wave changes or Q waves would have been present, the CAD likelihood would be higher in each entry of the table.

Source: ref. *41.*

mation as to coronary disease likelihood, recent evidence from the National Registry of Myocardial Infarction (i.e., NRMI-3) database by Vaccarino and colleagues suggests that younger women who present with an AMI have a risk of dying that is, on average, 22% higher than that of their elderly female counterparts per decade of decreasing age *(9,10)*. The authors' rationale for this risk increase was related to differences in medical history, the MI severity, and early management variability in presenting women as it impacts clinical outcomes. Figure 1 provides a depiction of the adjusted odds ratios for death by age groups. For men, the 1- and 2-year post-MI mortality was 25% and 20%, respectively, in comparison to 38% and 29% for post-MI women.

Noninvasive Diagnostic Tests for Women With Symptoms of Stable Angina

Figure 2 provides an algorithm for the work-up of women presenting with stable angina and an intermediate-to-high CAD probability based on the results of the medical and physical history. For women with stable symptoms, the preferred management approach is to perform a noninvasive stress test to assess the severity of the residual

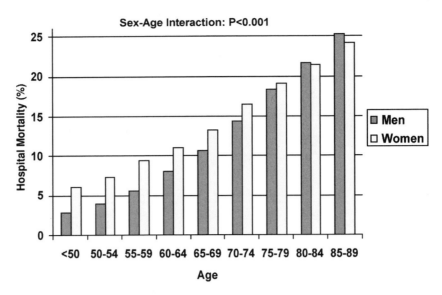

Fig. 1. Hospital mortality rates by sex and age (unadjusted). (From ref. *10.*)

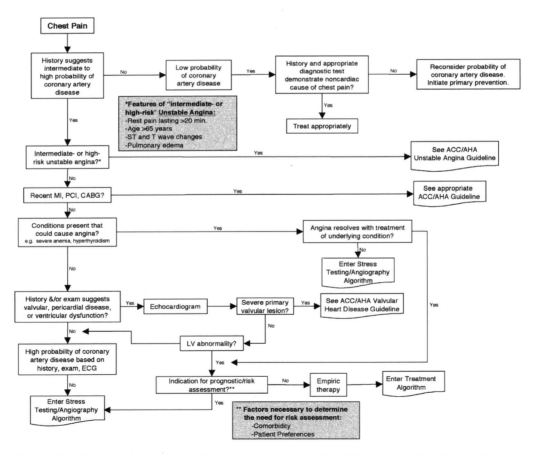

Fig. 2. Algorithm for the work-up of women presenting with stable angina and an intermediate-to-high CAD probability based on results of medical and physical history. (From ref. *6.*)

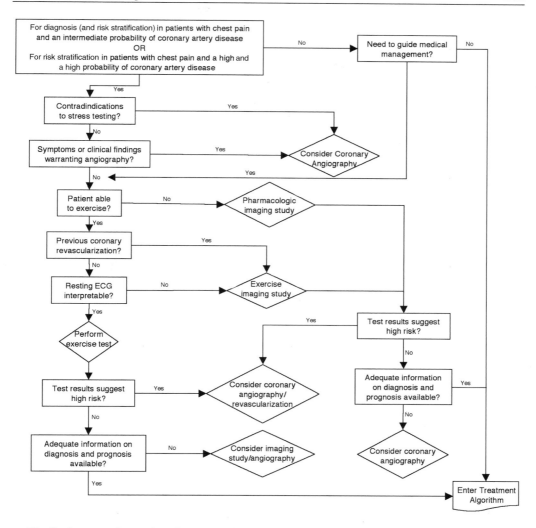

Fig. 3. Stress testing and angiography algorithm for the management of chronic stable angina. (From ref. *6*.)

ischemia. Although specific exceptions were allowed, the AHA/ACC Task Force recommended that standard exercise testing be used in the initial female evaluation (Fig. 3).

Generally, the pretest CAD probability is lower for women, especially for premenopausal women, with a subsequent greater number of false-positives. As a result, an exercise electrocardiogram (ECG) is a less sensitive diagnostic test for women than men, and perhaps less specific as well *(6)*. The ACC/AHA Chronic Stable Angina Guidelines present several reasons for this observation that compare diagnoses in gender, including criteria differences for defining coronary disease; differences in the prevalence of multivessel disease and prior MI; criteria differences for ST-segment positivity; differences in exercise type; the inability of many women to exercise to maximum aerobic capacity; greater prevalence of mitral valve prolapse and Syndrome X in women; microvascular function differences (leading perhaps to coronary spasm); and, possibly, hormonal differences *(6)*.

However, despite its limitations, it is better to perform exercise testing before stress imaging, as the combination of a low pretest CAD probability and a negative stress ECG will be sufficient to rule out a coronary disease diagnosis, obviating the need for stress imaging (6). The best candidates for an exercise ECG include those women who are capable of maximal exertional stress (or approx 5 metabolic equivalents [METs] or higher). If the woman has severe functional impairment, peripheral arterial disease, or orthopedic limitations, then either dobutamine stress echocardiography or vasodilator stress signal photon emission tomography (SPECT) imaging is an excellent option. Additional candidates for cardiac imaging include those women with an abnormal rest ECG, defined as significant ST-T wave changes that preclude adequate interpretation of any changes during maximal exercise.

Although ^{201}Tl SPECT and ^{99m}Tc sestamibi SPECT imaging have a similar sensitivity for stenosis detection greater than or equal to 70% (84.3% and 80.4%, respectively), ^{99m}Tc sestamibi SPECT imaging has superior specificity (84.4% vs 67.2%). ECG-gated ^{99m}Tc sestamibi SPECT imaging has been shown to provide even greater specificity (92.2%), as well as artifact reduction caused by breast attenuation present when ^{201}Tl SPECT imaging is used (11). Stress echocardiology can also be used to avoid breast artifacts; however, echocardiography loses efficacy when used for obese patients. For elderly patients and those unable to exercise at the required level, pharmacological stress is an appropriate alternative for both myocardial imaging and echocardiology.

INVASIVE DIAGNOSTIC TESTS FOR WOMEN WITH SYMPTOMS OF STABLE ANGINA

Coronary angiography use as a diagnostic tool may be indicated if a patient's risk factors, medical history, and clinical presentation are consistent with an intermediate-to-high CAD probability. The conditions necessary for recommending a diagnostic angiogram are presented in Fig. 3.

If a patient's symptoms are definitive for CAD, a diagnostic angiogram would help define the patient's coronary anatomy and the amount of myocardium at risk. However, if more information is needed before a diagnosis can be made, it is preferable to proceed with noninvasive testing first, starting with an ECG (despite the limitations previously noted), proceeding to an exercise imaging study (myocardial perfusion imaging or electrocardiography) if the ECG is ambiguous. Pharmacological stress should be used if the patient is unable to exercise. If the patient is not at high risk for a cardiac event, and if noninvasive testing has provided sufficient information for diagnosis, an angiogram can be postponed until its need becomes evident in the future.

Much was written about the gender bias issue in the referral for angiography in the first half of the 1990s, and most observers reported that after age adjustment, women were still less likely to be referred for a diagnostic angiogram, pecutaneous coronary intervention (PCI), or coronary artery bypass grafting (CABG). More recent reviews have indicated a continuation of lower female referral rates for diagnostic angiography (12). However, once referred, they are generally as likely as men to receive a revascularization procedure (13).

For high-risk women, with either a high coronary disease probability or with unstable symptoms (e.g., increasing chest pain frequency in the proceeding 6 weeks of eval-

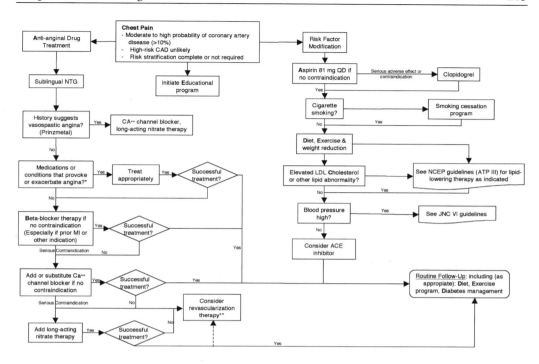

Fig. 4. Treatment.

uation, rest angina, etc.), the decision to perform diagnostic coronary angiography is supported by an abundance of evidence *(6)*. However, coronary angiography may not be an option for women who are not good candidates for revascularization, especially elderly women. For those patients and symptomatic women with an intermediate risk of coronary disease, the decision to perform diagnostic testing, including exercise echocardiography or myocardial perfusion imaging, is part of the standard work-up. Subsequent management ensues for women who undergo noninvasive testing based on the extent and severity of abnormalities detected during testing.

Risk Factor Management and Anti-Ischemic Therapies for Stable Chest Pain

Recently, there has been a revolution in the medical therapies for CAD management. Current medical therapy should conform to updated ACC/AHA Treatment Guidelines (Table 3, Fig. 4, and refs. *14–17*). Optimal management is both aggressive and multifaceted, targeted to achieve stabilization of existing atherosclerotic plaque and reduce future risk of ischemic events. The guidelines provide a consistent therapeutic approach with the understanding that a particular drug (or drugs) may be administered for more than one purpose. The therapy goals are, of course, to keep patients as symptom-free as possible within their individual tolerance for medication and to configure prophylactic therapy targeted to abolish ischemia and aggressively treat all abnormal cardiac risk factors (Tables 4–6). A recent paper by Ridker et al., based on data from the 27,939 participants in the Women's Health Study, suggests a potential role of C-reactive protein in predicting cardiovascular events *(18)*.

Table 3
Anti-Ischemic Therapy for Patients With Stable CAD

		LVEF > 40%	LVEF < 40%
Recommendation	Secondary prevention	*Q Wave AMI* Long-acting metoprolol *Non Q Wave AMI* Diltiazem or long-acting metoprolol +/– ACE inhibitor	ACE inhibitor (lisinopril) Long-acting metoprolol (if tolerated)
Guidelines	Symptomatic ischemia	*Maximize existing drug therapy* Amlodipine Long-acting metoprolol Isosorbide 5-mononitrate	*Maximize existing drug therapy* Amlodipine Long-acting metoprolol Isosorbide 5-mononitrate
	Silent ischemia	Amlodipine Long-acting metoprolol Isosorbide 5-mononitrate	Amlodipine Long-acting metoprolol Isosorbide 5-mononitrate
	Diabetics	ACE inhibitor recommended for all diabetics	

Table 4
Goals for Risk Factor Management in Symptomatic Women

Risk Factor	*Goal*	
Smoking	Cessation	
Total dietary fat	<30% calories	
Saturated fat	<7% calories	
Dietary cholesterol	<200 mg/day	
LDL cholesterol (primary goal)	60–85 mg/dL (1.56–2.21 mmol/L)	
HDL cholesterol (secondary goal)	≥40 mg/dL (1.04 mmol/L)	
Triglycerides (TG) (secondary goal)	<150 mg/dL (1.69 mmol/L)	
Physical activity	30–45 minutes of moderate intensity activity 5 times/week supplemented by an increase in daily lifestyle activities	
Body weight by body mass index (BMI) Desirable <25 Overweight 25.0–29.9 Obese >30.0	Initial BMI 25–27.5 27.5 27.5	Weight loss goal BMI <25 10% Relative weight loss 10% Relative weight loss
Blood pressure	<130/85 mmHg	
Diabetes	HbA1c < 7.0%	

Table 5
Recommendations for Risk Intervention

Risk intervention	Recommendations
Smoking: goal complete cessation	Strongly encourage patient and family to stop smoking. Provide counselling, nicotine replacement, and formal cessation programs as appropriate.
Lipid management: Primary goal LDL<100 mg/dL Secondary goals HDL>35 mg/dL; TG<200 mg/dL	Start AHA Step II Diet in all patients: ≤30% fat, <7% saturated fat, <200 mg/dL cholesterol. Assess fasting lipid profile. In post-MI patients, lipid profile may take 4–6 weeks to stabilize. Add drug therapy according to the following guide:

LDL<100 mg/dL	LDL 100–130 mg/dL	LDL>130 mg/dL	HDL<35 mg/dL
No drug therapy	Consider adding drug therapy to diet as follows:	Add drug therapy to diet as follows:	Emphasize weight management and physical activity. Advise smoking cessation. If needed to achieve LDL goals, consider niacin, statin, fibrate.

Suggested drug therapy

TG <200 mg/dL	TG 200–400 mg/dL	TG >400 mg/dL
Statin Resin Niacin	Statin Niacin	Consider combined drug therapy (niacin, fibrate, statin)

If LDL goal not achieved, consider combination therapy.

Risk intervention	Recommendations
Physical activity: Minimum goal 30 minutes 3–4 times/week	Assess risk, preferably with exercise test, to guide prescription. Encourage minimum of 30–60 minutes of moderate-intensity activity 3 or 4 times weekly (walking, jogging, cycling, or other aerobic activity) supplemented by an increase in daily lifestyle activities (eg, walking breaks at work, using stairs, gardening, household work). Maximum benefit 5–6 hours a week. Advise medically supervised programs for moderate- to high-risk patients.
Weight management:	Start intensive diet and appropriate physical activity intervention, as outlined above, in patients >120% of ideal weight for height. Particularly emphasize need for weight loss in patients with hypertension, elevated triglycerides, or elevated glucose levels.
Antiplatelet agents/anticoagulants:	Start aspirin 80 to 325 mg/d if not contraindicated. Consider clopidogrel as an alternative if aspirin contraindicated. Manage warfarin to international normalized ratio=2 to 3.5 for post-MI patients not able to take aspirin or clopidogrel.
ACE inhibitors post-MI:	Start early post-MI in stable high-risk patients (anterior MI, previous MI, Killip class II [S₃ gallop, rates, radiographic CHF]). Continue indefinitely for all with LV dysfunction (EF ≤ 40) or symptoms of failure. Use as needed to manage blood pressure or symptoms in all other patients.
Beta-blockers:	Start in most post-MI patients (arrhythmia, LV dysfunction, inducible ischemia) at 5–28 days. Continue 6 months minimum. Observe usual contraindications. Use as needed to manage angina, rhythm, or blood pressure in all other patients.
Estrogens:	Consider estrogen replacement in all postmenopausal women. Individualize recommendation consistent with other health risks.
Blood pressure control:* Goal ≤ 130/85 mmHg	Initiate lifestyle modification—weight control, physical activity, alcohol moderation, and moderate sodium restriction—in all patients with blood pressure >130 mmHg systolic or 85 mmHg diastolic (drug therapy of diabetes, renal failure or heart failure). Add blood pressure medication, individualized to other patient requirements and characteristics (i.e. age, race, need for drugs with specific benefits) if blood pressure ≥ 140 mmHg systolic or ≥90 mmHg diastolic.

(From ref. 6.)

Table 6
Guide to Lipid Management of High-Risk Patients With Stable Chest Pain

Primary goal	LDL 60–85 mg/dL (1.55–2.20 mmol/L)

Initiating therapy
For subjects on statins other than simvastatin:

LDL (mg/dL)	Initial therapy
<60 (1.55 mmol/L)	Back titrate to simvastatin at equivalent 1/2 dose
50–85 (1.29–2.20 mmol/L)	Simvastatin at equivalent dose
>85 (2.20 mmol/L)	Simvastatin dose at one step higher than current equivalent

For subjects not on any lipid medication at baseline:

LDL (mg/dL)	Initial therapy
<100 (2.59 mmol/L)	Simvastatin 10 mg qhs
100–129 (2.59–3.36 mmol/L)	Simvastatin 20 mg qhs
>130 (3.36 mmol/L)	Simvastatin 40 mg qhs

Titrating therapy

LDL > 85 mg/dL (2.20 mmol/L)	Double dose every 4–6 weeks until LDL < 85mg/dL
LDL < 50 mg/dL (1.29 mmol/L)	Back titrate to previous dose
LDL > 85mg/dL (2.20 mmol/L)*	Add bile acid binding resin and titrate, as necessary

Secondary goals	HDL	≥ 40 mg/dL (1.04 mmol/L)
	Triglycerides	< 150mg/dL (1.69 mmol/L)

* On Simvastatin 80 mg.
Based on the Courage trial.

All patients with coronary disease and chest pain symptoms (female and male) should receive antithrombotic therapy with aspirin (enteric coated) 80–325 mg/day *(19)*. In the case of an aspirin allergy, clopidogrel 75 mg/day may be prescribed. For patients undergoing PCI, aspirin plus clopidogrel will be used in accordance with accepted practice. For patients with stable Canadian Cardiovascular Society (CCS) class I-III angina, anti-ischemic therapy is outlined in Table 3.

In a recent study, the ability of beta-blockers to prolong life after AMI infarction was demonstrated conclusively *(20)*. Angiotensin-converting enzyme (ACE) inhibitors also improve survival rates in several ways, including modulation of the renin angiotensin system and beneficial vascular remodeling effects *(21,22)*, and numerous clinical trials have confirmed the important role of aggressive lipid-lowering and antiplatelet therapy along with optimal blood pressure control to reduce the progression of coronary heart disease (CHD) *(22–27)*. ACE inhibitors are indicated for all patients with a depressed systolic function (<40%) regardless the cause (e.g., prior MI, congestive heart failure [CHF], etc.) and all diabetics (type 1 and type 2, with or without a depressed left ventricular [LV] function) unless contraindicated by a severely repressed renal function *(6)*.

Optimal medical management goals for both genders with stable chest pain symptoms are detailed in Table 4. These goals include risk factor treatment based on the sixth report of the Joint National Committee on Prevention, Detection, Evaluation, and Treatment of High Blood Pressure (JNC-VI) and National Cholesterol Education Program Adult Treatment Program (NCEP ATP-III) (Table 5). Although this algorithm suggests the use of hormone replacement therapy (HRT), recent evidence from the

Women's Health Initiative trial has removed opposed-estrogen therapy as a secondary preventive treatment for women with established coronary disease. In Chapter 21, Dr. Nanette Wenger provides a detailed evaluation of HRT use.

The current standard for antihypertensive therapy is to achieve and maintain a target blood pressure (BP) of 130/85 mmHg or lower (17). If therapy is needed, an ACE inhibitor will be considered for first-line therapy, although a beta-blocker without intrinsic sympathetic activity (ISA), amlodipine, angiotensin II receptor blocker, or a diuretic may be used. Within each treatment class, attempts should be made to maximize dosages, as tolerated clinically, to achieve and maintain the desired treatment targets before adding a second or third agent.

Epidemiological data reveal that women over the age of 55 years are more likely to have high blood cholesterol than men in the same age groups. Prior to menopause, the cardioprotective effects of endogenous estrogen result in higher high-density lipoprotein (HDL) levels. Consequently, lower HDL cholesterol values are more predictive of CAD in women (28). It has long been known that hypertriglyceridemia is a risk factor for coronary disease in women, but not in men (29). Recent treatment guidelines have been released by the NCEP ATP III (15). This report reiterates that for patients with CHD, LDL remains the primary therapy target, with a goal of less than 100 mg/dL (2.59 mmol/L). The Health Protection Study (30) recently reported finding beneficial effects to lowering LDL cholesterol to less than or equal to 85 mg/dL (2.20 mmol/L). In ATP III, the definition of low HDL was revised to less than 50 mg/dL (1.30 mmol/L) for women; low HDL for men was changed to below 40 mg/dL (1.04 mmol/L), up from the level of less than 35 mg/dL (0.91 mmol/L) used in the first two ATP reports. ATP III does not explicitly specify a goal for raising HDL. The definition of normal triglycerides was revised to less than 150 mg/dL (1.70 mmol/L), decreased from the definition of less than 200 mg/dL (2.26 mmol/L) used in the ATP II report. The new report defines triglycerides of 150–199 mg/dL (1.70–2.25 mmol/L) as borderline high, 200–499 mg/dL (2.26–5.64 mmol/L) as high, and greater than or equal to 500 mg/dL (5.65 mmol/L) as very high.

Substantial evidence is available on the lipid-lowering therapies' effectiveness for women and men (Figs. 5 and 6). In the Scandinavian Simvastatin Survival Study (4S), 4444 patients with an established CHD diagnosis or stable angina symptoms were enrolled, treated with simvastatin, and followed for the occurrence of major cardiovascular events for 5 years. From the 4S study, a 26% reduction in total cholesterol was observed for women; a rate similar to the overall treatment effect in this study cohort. Additional reductions in LDL cholesterol and triglycerides were 37% and 16%, respectively. A comparison of the survival benefit of simvastatin treatment is noted in Fig. 6, where both women and men enrolled in the 4S study had a substantial reduction in major CHD events in the 6 years following therapy initiation. LaRosa et al. (31) performed a meta-analysis of five statin trials including a subset analysis for women and the elderly (Fig. 7). Because of the inclusion of fewer women, the confidence intervals for a treatment effect were larger. However, there is a similar trend in effectiveness for women.

Another major development was announced with the release of the new NCEP III guidelines: diabetes should now be considered a coronary disease risk equivalent. Other high-risk groups include those with peripheral arterial disease or significant carotid stenosis. As such, lipid management goals for diabetics should be similar to those of patients with established coronary disease (Table 4). Subsequent management

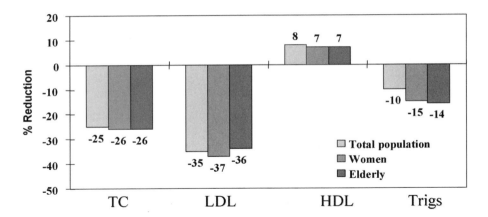

Fig. 5. Mean between-treatment group differences (percent change from baseline) for serum lipids in 4S subpopulations. (From ref. *63.*)

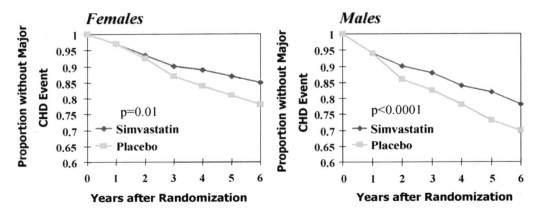

Fig. 6. Kaplan-Meier survival curves for women and men in the 4S trial: subset analysis of major coronary events for women and the elderly in five statin trials. (From ref. *63.*)

of diabetics is perhaps even more critical for risk reduction in women; largely in part because it has long been known that the mortality risk for diabetic women is substantially greater (as much as threefold higher) than that of nondiabetic women *(32,33).* This is particularly true for insulin-dependent diabetics. The goal for diabetes management in the Clinical Outcomes Using Revascularization and Aggressive Drug Evaluation (COURAGE) trial patients is to maintain fasting blood glucose levels between 80 and 126 mg/dL and HbA1C levels less than 7% (Table 6). These guidelines are in accord with published recommendations of the American Diabetes Association and the Diabetes Control and Complications Trial (DCCT) Consensus Report *(34,35).*

CORONARY ANGIOGRAPHY AND REVASCULARIZATION

Women with chest pain and evidence of provocative ischemia have a lower frequency of obstructive coronary disease than men *(36,37).* As many as half of all

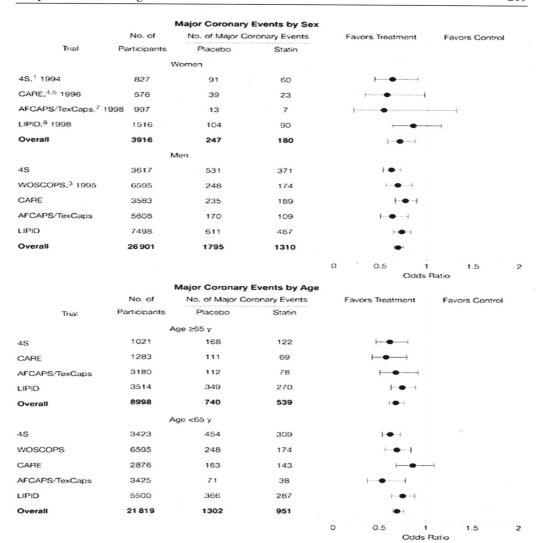

Fig. 7. Relative odds of major coronary events associated with statin treatment from individual trials and overall by sex and age. Error bars indicate 95% confidence intervals. (From ref. *31*.)

women with chest pain undergoing diagnostic cardiac catheterization have less than 70% coronary stenosis *(37).* Recent evidence from the WISE trial (Chapter 13) suggests that of the women without significant coronary disease, microvascular disease may be precipitating ischemia. ACE inhibitor management has been shown to reduce ischemia frequency in this population *(38).*

Since the early 1970s, numerous large-scale clinical trials have established the respective roles of PCI and CABG in patients with stable and unstable CAD. Several factors contribute to women's increased risk of complications during their hospital stay and for up to 30 days after hospital discharge. In addition to their older age of presentation and greater risk factor frequency, women have a greater degree of acuity on presentation, smaller body size, and arterial size that contribute in some cases to lower rates of procedural success, a greater need for recurrent intervention, and less symptom relief *(39–42)*. It should be noted that numerous reports have shown high rates of procedural success for women; rates in the range of 90–95% *(39–42)*.

PCI is recommended for a proximal coronary artery stenosis that jeopardizes a large myocardium area, which may result in severe inducible ischemia and also angina refractory treatment to medical therapy *(1)*. Catheter-based techniques utilizing coronary stents have likewise improved the procedural success rate of coronary interventions and reduced complications (e.g., restenosis). The recent evaluation of drug-eluding stents may provide an additional reduction in restenosis rates. In a recent report by Kastrati and colleagues, the 30-day event rate for women and men undergoing PCI was 3.1% vs 1.8% ($p = 0.02$; *42*). However, long-term outcome was similar at 1-year (men = 6.0%, women = 5.8%, $p = 0.77$). These results reveal that the presentation of new onset and acute disease is driving near-term complications *(43)*. In a recent report in 118,548 patients undergoing PCI, women who underwent coronary stenting had higher rates of same-admission mortality and urgent CABG when compared with men *(44)*. Upon event-free survival through hospitalization, the overall therapeutic PCI benefit for women is equivalent to that of men.

CABG surgery is considered the treatment of choice for patients with significant obstruction of the left-main coronary artery, as well as for those with triple-vessel CAD and LV systolic dysfunction. Women who undergo CABG generally have less symptomatic relief than men *(45)*. This has been related to smaller-diameter vessels and more incomplete revascularization. In a recent study conducted in Western Sweden, women had more symptoms (dyspnea and chest pain) and physical limitations prior to and up to 5-year post-CABG than men *(45)*. In a recent review from the New York state database of 19,224 patients undergoing CABG, smaller female body surface area resulted in a lesser degree of revascularization *(46)*. Women also had a lower rate of internal mammary artery use. In conjunction with advanced age and greater comorbidity, these factors predispose women to higher in-hospital mortality. Similar results were noted in the Society of Thoracic Surgeons (STS) database of 441,542 patients *(47)*. Despite differences in near-term outcomes, female sex is not associated with late morbidity and mortality following CABG *(48)*.

Off-pump bypass surgery, in preliminary studies, has not resulted in a dramatic improvement in in-hospital outcomes for women, owing largely to advanced age and greater comorbidities *(49)*. Recently, fast-track recovery programs have been used to promote the early discharge of patients post-CABG. Early extubation is possible in more men than women (74% vs 64%, $p = 0.03$; *50*). Generally, women have a longer recovery interval compared to men, which is a reflection of their higher preoperative risk profile *(51)*. Although lower participation rates have been noted, women who participate in cardiovascular rehabilitation programs have a definite improvement in health-related quality of life and social functioning *(52)*.

Postprocedure Management of Recurring Symptoms

Because women have less symptom relief, new, worsening, or "breakthrough" angina may still be a problem even after coronary revascularization. Guidance for this situation is currently under investigation in the COURAGE trial. The COURAGE trial is enrolling 2546 patients with mild-to-moderate CAD randomized to optimal medical therapy when compared to PCI plus optimal medical management. In the case of women with a angina deterioration, the following recommendations have been put forth:

1. In all patients whose angina deteriorates to CCS class II–III angina, medical therapy will be intensified; if the patient stabilizes to CCS class I–II, medical therapy will be continued indefinitely.
2. If symptoms do not stabilize or progress after 6–8 weeks of maximum medical therapy, it is recommended that patients undergo stress testing with ECG-gated SPECT sestamibi myocardial perfusion imaging. If there is a high-risk result (LV ejection fraction [EF] <35% or severe reversible ischemia), the patient should undergo catheterization and revascularization as clinically indicated.

If a patient destabilizes after being randomized to PCI plus intensive medical therapy, the following guidelines are recommended:

1. For patients with CCS class I–II, and no evidence of spontaneous ischemic ECG changes at rest, a repeat stress test (exercise or pharmacological) with ECG-gated SPECT sestamibi imaging is recommended. If perfusion imaging shows moderate-to-severe evidence of inducible ischemia or worsening LV function, including evidence of severe dysfunction (i.e., EF <35%), the patient should undergo repeat coronary angiography.
2. If the patient is CCS class III–IV after maximizing medical therapy, repeat cardiac angiography and/or PCI should be performed.

Gender Bias in Treatment

Despite the abundance of clinical evidence that supports a substantial therapeutic benefit for an array of medical therapies, several studies have documented underuse of aspirin, beta-blockers, heparin, statins, and thrombolytics in women *(53)*. In a recent study using the National Ambulatory Medical Care Survey in Outpatients (1980–1996), overall aspirin use for patients with an established CAD diagnosis was 26% lower for women. Albeit, aspirin use was inadequate for both genders, helping 29% of men and 21% of women *(54)*. Additionally, women are less often counseled about nutrition, exercise, and weight control *(28)*.

In a patient cohort presenting with stable symptoms and undergoing noninvasive assessment for provocative ischemia, women were 25% less likely to have any additional work-up following an abnormal noninvasive test *(55)*. The lack of follow-up in this female cohort, including lower rates of coronary revascularization, precipitated a greater number of cardiac deaths or MIs. More recent data reveal an underutilization of exercise treadmill testing and cardiac catheterization in women when compared with men *(56,57)*. More than 90% of women who met ACC/AHA class I criteria for cardiac catheterization did not undergo angiography *(56)*. Also, in higher risk patients, women were less likely to be offered CABG following AMI *(58)*.

CONCLUSION

Certainly, one should consider whether differential (nonspecific) presentation in conjunction with undertreatment has contributed to the higher case fatality rate of women. A substantial amount of evidence suggests that on diagnosis, the initiation of life-saving therapies can provide considerable benefit to women. Early and aggressive management has been shown to lower risk and result in a reduced need for repeat intervention *(59–62)*. For these reasons, we believe that although there are many differences in presentation, degrees of comorbidity, onset age, and other factors that may contribute to differential clinical outcomes, current treatment regimens applied consistently for both genders can be effective in reducing the risk of major adverse cardiac events in women and men alike.

REFERENCES

1. Ryan TJ, Bauman WB, Kennedy JW, et al. Guidelines for percutaneous transluminal coronary angioplasty: a report of the American Heart Association/American College of Cardiology Task Force on Assessment of Diagnostic and Therapeutic Cardiovascular Procedures (Committee on Percutaneous Transluminal Coronary Angioplasty). Circulation 1993;88:2987–3007.
2. Anonymous. AHA medical/scientific statement. 1994 revisions to classification of functional capacity and objective assessment of patients with diseases of the heart. Circulation 1994;90:644–465.
3. Penque S, Halm M, Smith M, et al. Women and coronary disease: relationship between descriptors of signs and symptoms and diagnostic and treatment course. Am J Crit Care 1998;7:175–82.
4. Lerner DJ, Kennel WB. Patterns of coronary heart disease morbidity and mortality in the sexes: a 26-year follow-up of the Framingham population. Am Heart J 1986;111:383–390.
5. Wenger NK. Clinical characteristics of coronary heart disease in women: emphasis on gender differences. Cardiovasc Res 2002;53:558–567.
6. Gibbons RJ, Abrams J, Chatterjee K, et al. ACC/AHA 2002 Guideline Update for the Management of Patients with Chronic Stable Angina: A Report of the American College of Cardiology/American Heart Association Task Force on Practice Guidelines (Committee to Update the 1999 Guidelines for the Management of Patients with Chronic Stable Angina), 2002.
7. Milner KA, Funk M, Richards S. Gender differences in symptom presentation associated with coronary artery disease. Am J Cardiol 1999;84:396–399.
8. Merz CN, Kelsey SF, Pepine CJ, et al. The Women's Ischemia Syndrome Evaluation (WISE) study: protocol design, methodology and feasibility report. J Am Coll Cardiol 1999;33:1453–1461.
9. Vaccarino V, Krumholz HM, Yarzebski J, et al. Sex differences in 2-year mortality after hospital discharge for myocardial infarction. Ann Intern Med 2001;134:173–181.
10. Vaccarino V, Parsons L, Every NR. Sex-based differences in early mortality after myocardial infarction. National Registry of Myocardial Infarction 2 Participants. N Engl J Med;1999;341:217–225.
11. Taillefer R, DePuey EG, et al. Comparative diagnostic accuracy of Tl-201 and Tc-99m sestamibi SPECT imaging (perfusion and ECG-gated SPECT) in detecting coronary artery disease in women. J Am Coll Cardiol 1997;29:69–77.
12. Garg PP, Landrum MB, Normand SL, et al. Understanding individual and small area variation in the underuse of coronary angiography following acute myocardial infarction. Med Care 2002;40:614–626.
13. Bell MR, Berger PB, Holmes DR Jr, et al. Referral for coronary artery revascularization procedures after diagnostic coronary angiography: evidence for gender bias? J Am Coll Cardiol 1995;25:1650–1655.
14. Smith SC, Blair S, Bonow R, et al. AHA/ACC consensus statement on preventing heart attack and death in patients with atherosclerotic cardiovascular disease: 2001 update. Circulation 2001;104:1577–1579.
15. Adult Treatment Panel III. Executive summary of the third report of National Cholesterol Education Program (NCEP) Expert Panel on detection, evaluation, and treatment of high blood cholesterol in adults. JAMA 2001;285:2486–2497.
16. Smith SC, Blair SN, Criqui MH, et al. Preventing heart attack and death in patients with coronary disease. Circulation 1995;92:2–4.
17. The Sixth Report of the Joint National Committee on Prevention, Detection, Evaluation, and Treatment of High Blood Pressure. November, 1997. NIH Publication 98-4080.
18. Ridker PM, Rifai N, Rose L, et al. Comparison of C-reactive protein and low-density lipoprotein cholesterol levels in the prediction of first cardiovascular events. N Engl J Med 2002;347:1557–1565.
19. Yusuf S, Wittes J, Friedman L. Overview of results of randomized clinical trials in heart disease 1. Treatments following myocardial infarction. JAMA 1988;260:2088–2093.

20. Beta Blocker Heart Attack Trial Research Group. A randomized trial of propanolol in patients with acute myocardial infarction. JAMA 1982;247:1707–1714.
21. Pfeiffer MA, Braunwald E, Moye LA, et al. Effect of captopril on mortality and morbidity in patients with left ventricular dysfunction after myocardial infarction: results of the survival and ventricular enlargement trial. N Engl J Med 1992;327:669–677.
22. The SOLVD investigators. Effect of angiotensin converting enzyme inhibitor enalapril on survival in patients with reduced left ventricular ejection fraction and congestive heart failure. N Engl J Med 1991;325:293–302.
23. Brown BG, Zhao X-Q, Sacco DE, et al. Lipid lowering and plaque regression; new insights into prevention of plaque disruption and clinical events in coronary disease Circulation 1993;87:1781–1791.
24. Blankenhom DH, Azen SP, Dramsch D, et al. Coronary angiographic changes with lovastatin therapy: The Monitored Atherosclerosis Regression Study (MARS). Ann Int Med 1993;119:969–976.
25. Waters D, Higginson L, Gladstone P, et al. Effect of monotherapy with an HMG-CoA reductase inhibitor on the progression of coronary atherosclerosis as assessed by serial quantitative arteriography: the Canadian Coronary Atherosclerosis Intervention Trial. Circulation 1994;89:959–968.
26. Waters D, Craven TE, Lesperance J. Prognostic significance of progression of coronary atherosclerosis. Circulation 1993;87:1067–1075.
27. Scandinavian Simvastatin Survival Study Group. Randomized trial of cholesterol lowering in 4,444 patients with coronary heart disease: the Scandinavian Simvastatin Survival Study (4S). Lancet 1994;344:1383–1389.
28. Mosca L, Grundy SM, Judelson D, et al. Guide to Preventive Cardiology for Women: AHA/ACC Scientific Statement: Consensus Panel Statement. Circulation 1999;99:2480–2484.
29. Castelli WP. Cholesterol and lipids in the risk of coronary artery disease – the Framingham Heart Study. Can J Cardiol 1988(4 Suppl A):5A–10A.
30. Heart Protection Study Collaborative Group. MRC/BHF Heart Protection Study of cholesterol lowering with simvastatin in 20,536 high-risk individuals: a randomized placebo-controlled trial. Lancet 2002;360:7–22.
31. LaRosa JC, He J, Vupputuri S. Effect of statins on risk of coronary disease: a meta-analysis of randomized controlled trials. JAMA 1999;282:2340–2346.
32. Barrett-Connor E, Stuenkel CA. Questions of life and death in old age. JAMA 1998;279:622–623.
33. Geiss LS, in National Diabetes Data Group (U.S.). Diabetes in America, 2nd ed. National Institutes of Health, National Institute of Diabetes and Digestive and Kidney Diseases: 1995, pp. 233–257.
34. American Diabetes Association: Standards of medical care for patients with diabetes mellitus (Position Statement). Diabetes Care 1997;20(Suppl 1);S5–S13.
35. DCCT Research Group. The effect of intensive diabetes treatment on the development and progression of long-term complications in insulin-dependent diabetes mellitus: The Diabetes Control and Complications Trial. N Engl J Med 1993;329:977–986.
36. Shaw RE, Anderson HV, Brindis RG, et al. Development of a risk adjustment mortality model using the American College of Cardiology-National Cardiovascular Data Registry (ACC-NCDR) experience: 1998–2000. J Am Coll Cardiol 2002;39:1104–1112.
37. Shaw LJ, Heller GV, Travin MI, et al. Cost analysis of diagnostic testing for coronary artery disease in women with stable chest pain. Economics of Noninvasive Diagnosis (END) Study Group. J Nucl Cardiol 1999;6:559–569.
38. Sawada SG, Lewis SJ, Foltz J, et al. Usefulness of rest and low-dose dobutamine wall motion scores in predicting survival and benefit from revascularization in patients with ischemic cardiomyopathy. Am J Cardiol 2002;89:811–816.
39. Ahmed JM, Dangas G, Lansky AJ, et al. Influence of gender on early and one-year clinical outcomes after saphenous vein graft stenting. Am J Cardiol 2001;87:401–405.
40. Cho L, Marso SP, Bhatt DL, Topol EJ. Optimizing percutaneous coronary revascularization in diabetic women: analysis from the EPISTENT trial. Journal of Womens Health Gender-Based Med 2000;9:741–746.
41. Mehilli J, Kastrati A, Dirschinger J, et al. Differences in prognostic factors and outcomes between women and men undergoing coronary artery stenting. JAMA 2000;284:1799–1805.
42. Pepine CJ, Handberg EM. The vascular biology of hypertension and atherosclerosis and intervention with calcium antagonists and angiotensin-converting enzyme inhibitors. Clin Cardiol 2001;24(11 Suppl):V1–V5.

43. van Domburg RT, Foley DP, de Feyter PJ, et al. Long-term clinical outcome after balloon angioplasty: identification of a population at low risk of recurrent events during 17 years of follow-up. Eur Heart J 2001;22:934–941.
44. Watanabe CT, Maynard C, Ritchie JL. Comparison of short-term outcomes following coronary artery stenting in men versus women. Am J Cardiol 2001;88:848–852.
45. Herlitz J, Wiklund I, Sjorland H, et al. Relief of symptoms and improvement of health related quality of life five years after coronary artery bypass in women and men. Clin Cardiol 2001;24:385–392.
46. Williams MR, Choudri AF, Morales DL, et al. Gender differences in patients undergoing coronary bypass surgery, from a mandatory statewide database. J Gend Specif Med 2000;3:41–48.
47. Hartz RS, Rao AV, Plomondon ME, et al. Effects of race, with or without gender, on operative mortality after coronary artery bypass grafting: a study using The Society of Thoracic Surgeons National Database. Ann Thorac Surg 2001;71:512–520.
48. Brandrup-Wognsen G, Berggren H, Hartford M, et al. Female sex is associated with increased mortality and morbidity early, but not late, after coronary bypass grafting. Eur Heart J 1996;17:1426–1431.
49. Capdeville M, Chamogeogarkis T, Lee JH. Effect of gender on outcomes of beating heart operations. Ann Thorac Surg 2001;72:S1022–S1025.
50. Capdeville M, Lee JH, Taylor AL. Effect of gender on fast-track recovery after coronary artery bypass graft surgery. J Cardiothorac Vasc Anesth 2001;15:146–151.
51. Ott RA, Gutfinger DE, Alimadadian H, et al. Conventional coronary artery bypass grafting: why women take longer to recover. J Cardiovasc Surg (Torino) 2001;42:311–315.
52. Simchen E, Naveh I, Zitser-Gurevich Y, et al. Is participation in cardiac rehabilatation programs associated with better quality of life and return to work after coronary bypass operations? The Israeli CABG Study. Isr Med Assoc J 2001;3:399–403.
53. Shaw LJ, Tarkington L, Callister J, et al. The HCA National Disease Management Program for coronary disease detection and treatment in women. Am J Manag Care 2001;7 Spec No:SP25–SP30.
54. Stafford RS. Aspirin use is low among United States outpatients with coronary artery disease. Circulation 2000;101:1097–1101.
55. Shaw LJ, Miller DD, Romeis JC, et al. Gender differences in the noninvasive evaluation and management of patients with suspected coronary artery disease. Ann Intern Med 1994;120:559–566.
56. Bowling A, Bond M, McKee D, et al. Equity in access to exercise tolerance testing, coronary angiography, and coronary artery bypass grafting by age, sex and clinical indications. Heart 2001;85:680–686.
57. Battleman DS, Callahan M. Gender differences in utilization of exercise treadmill testing: a claims based analysis. J Healthc Qual 2001;23:38–41.
58. Watson RE, Stein AD, Dwamena FC, et al. Do race and gender influence the use of invasive procedures? J Gen Intern Med 2001;16:227–234.
59. Lagerqvist B, Safstrom K, Stahle E, et al. FRISC II Study Group Investigators. Is early invasive treatment of unstable coronary artery disease equally effective for both women and men? J Am Coll Cardiol 2001;38:41–48.
60. Bedinghaus J, Leshan L, Diehr S. Coronary artery disease prevention: what's different for women? Am Fam Physician 2001;63:1290,1292.
61. Welty FK. Cardiovascular disease and dyslipidemia in women. Arch Intern Med 2001;161:514–522.
62. Keller KB, Lemberg L. Gender differences in acute coronary events. Am J Crit Care 2000;9:207–209.
63. Miettinen T, Pyorala K, Olsson A, et al. Cholesterol lowering therapy in women and elderly patients with myocardial infarction or angina pectoris: findings from the Scandinavian Simvastatin Survival Study (4S). Circulation 1997;96:4211–4218.

15 Improving the Diagnosis and Management of Women With Coronary Disease in Primary Care Settings

Kimberly J. Rask, MD, PhD

CONTENTS

SCOPE OF THE PROBLEM

Coronary heart disease (CHD) is the single leading cause of death among American women. In 1997, all cardiovascular diseases (CVD) combined claimed the lives of more than 502,938 women. In the same year, 450,172 men died from these diseases *(1)*. Following a myocardial infarction (MI), 42% of women die when compared with 24% of men *(1)*. During the first 6 years after a heart attack, the rate of having a second attack is 33% for women and 21% for men. In addition, two-thirds of women who experience sudden death from coronary artery disease (CAD) have no known disease in comparison to only one-half of similar deaths in men *(2)*.

MODIFIABLE RISK FACTORS

Although men and women share many risk factors, disturbing trends exist in the prevalence of risk factors in women *(2)*. Tobacco use remains the leading cause of CHD in women and, although the US prevalence of women smokers is declining, this

From: *Contemporary Cardiology: Coronary Disease in Women: Evidence-Based Diagnosis and Treatment*
Edited by: L. J. Shaw and R. F. Redberg © Humana Press Inc., Totowa, NJ

decline is less for women than for men *(2)*. Obesity remains a significant CVD risk factor, yet the percent of obese American women increased over the past 15 years from 16.5% to 24.9% *(3)*. Increased serum cholesterol is also a risk factor for CHD in both men and women, yet from 1980 to 1991, more than the half of women above age 55 had elevated lipid levels *(2)*.

MANAGEMENT OF WOMEN WITH CHD

CHD evaluation and management in women is more challenging, resulting from sex-based differences in the clinical presentation of ischemic heart disease and the accuracy of diagnostic testing *(2)*. Additionally, women's mortality following an MI is three times that of men and may account for disparities in the use of diagnostic and therapeutic procedures *(4)*. Results from the Myocardial Infarction Triage and Intervention (MITI) registry suggest that sex-based differences in mortality after an MI are associated with a lower likelihood of women receiving cardiac catheterization, angioplasty, thrombolysis, or coronary bypass surgery *(5)*. Numerous studies have shown that women undergo fewer diagnostic and treatment procedures, although some fail to find a sex-related bias after adjusting for cofounders *(6–13)*. Gender-based differences in pharmocological therapy have also been documented. Despite clear indications, several authors have reported a decreased use of beta-blockers, angiotensin-converting enzyme (ACE) inhibitors, and cholesterol-lowering medication *(7,8,14)*.

PHYSICIAN PRACTICE VARIATION

Wide variations in physician care patterns have been recognized across a range of clinical conditions *(15)*. A large body of evidence also demonstrates performance gaps between generally accepted care guidelines and the actual care delivered *(16,17)*. Studies suggest that an average of 17 years is necessary for research evidence to reach clinical practice *(18,19)*. Optimizing the diagnosis and management of coronary disease requires a concerted effort to overcome the barriers that prevent new scientific knowledge being translated into improved clinical care. The practice of true evidence-based medicine requires health care professionals to have a balanced knowledge of basic science advances, clinical technology assessment, disease epidemiology, and clinical decision making *(20)*. Primary care physicians typically spend most of their professional time caring for and managing patients with a broad array of clinical syndromes and multiple comorbidities. Over the past two decades, the number of clinical trials in cardiology alone has increased fivefold *(18,19)*. Primary care practitioners are generally ill-prepared to efficiently absorb and act on this accelerating volume of new information. As a result, timely, usable, and easily accessible practice guidelines are crucial in order to bring high-quality information within the busy practitioner's grasp. This chapter reviews the evidence regarding effective implementation of clinical guidelines and highlights the most promising approaches to promote evidence-based clinical practice in primary care settings.

CHANGING PHYSICIAN PRACTICES

The resistance of clinical practice to change is a longstanding problem. Most physicians treat patients according to their personal medical knowledge and individual clini-

Table 1
Strategies for Changing Physician Practice

Education
    Continuing medical education
    Academic detailing
Administrative restrictions
    Precertification
    Drug formularies
Financial incentives
    Quality bonuses
    Capitated payments for ancillary services
Performance feedback
    Physician profiling
    Quality report cards
Health system redesign
    Automated prompts
    Condition-specific mini-clinics

cal experiences. These heuristics vary from practitioner to practitioner, perhaps accounting for much of the clinical practice variations. Such variations, as well as sub-optimal practice evidence, have led to several efforts to change physician practice. There are five general methods of changing physician practices: education, administrative restrictions, financial incentives, performance feedback, and health system redesign (*see* Table 1).

A systematic review found that continuing medical education (CME) courses of 1 day or less have little impact on changing practice *(21)*. Opinion leaders and academic detailing tended to have a more positive effect *(21)*. Clinical opinion leaders can be powerful champions for guidelines. Academic detailing is based on pharmaceutical detailing and involves short one-on-one conversations where the "detailer" provides information and attempts to persuade the "detailee" to change behavior. Education in the form of clinical practice guidelines has gained popularity as a means of influencing physician's practice. However, there is general awareness that dissemination alone has little measurable impact on guideline implementation *(22)*.

Another alternative is to mandate change through administrative restrictions. Although interventions designed to restrict physician practice are widely used, they can be costly, burdensome, and unpopular. Financial incentives and penalties have been shown to produce change, but are more effective when applied to salaried physicians or physicians providing care to insured patients under one managed care plan.

Feedback, providing physicians with information as to how their practice compares with that of their peers, has been demonstrated as successful when accompanied by timely and relevant information, appearing more successful for out-patient than for in-patient services *(23)*. Feedback has also been an effective intervention when accompanied by a practice-reinforcing strategy (e.g., a reminder system) or an intervention that focuses on the health delivery system as a target for change as opposed to focusing on physician behavior alone *(24)*. Physician support is crucial to successful health care quality improvement. Physician profiling can be useful to flag.potential problems, serve as a catalyst for positive change, and foster an awareness of the accountability to which physicians are held. However, a recent review found that physician profiling alone had minimal impact on the clinical procedure utilization (25–27).

PRACTICE GUIDELINES

Practice guidelines are guides for physician decision making in the ambulatory care setting. In contrast, Clinical pathways tend to be procedure-oriented and used primarily in the in-patient setting. Practice guidelines can include recommendations for disease diagnosis, treatment, health maintenance, primary prevention, patient education, and self-management. (Published guidelines often exceed 30 pages in length.) Ideally, key points are extracted and presented in an annotated algorithm, which can graphically represent the thinking process that physicians follow in patient management. Algorithms consist of a set of boxes containing either "yes or no" questions that are user friendly and efficient discriminators (28). The efficiency of a given question or characteristic to separate patients into clinically meaningful subgroups depends largely in part on the variable's sensitivity, specificity, and predictive power.

Algorithms that include both diagnostic and treatment modalities are referred to as management algorithms. Their primary function is to identify patients who do or do not stand to benefit from a particular diagnostic or treatment strategy. Algorithms are easily computerized and can be linked to clinical information systems. Medical specialty societies, physician groups, pharmaceutical companies, and others have produced more than 1500 sets of clinical guidelines (29).

The design and development of good clinical practice guidelines has become a science. This design includes a methodology that bases the guideline on best available evidence, using tools for comprehensive multilingual literature to search and summarize data that enables grading both the evidence and practical recommendations (30). Clinical practice guidelines can usefully digest vast amounts of evidence regarding important clinical problems into a readily useable format. Unfortunately, the rapid proliferation of guidelines has not been matched by the consistent use of sound guideline development methods (31). Even the most straightforward guidelines may be produced by more than one organization, where conflicting recommendations exist. Many guidelines offer thorough reviews and carefully worded consensus statements from expert panels that are not helpful to practicing physicians (32). Positions are usually reached through consensus rather than decision analysis or vote. Therefore, the final recommendations tend to classify a minority of interventions as "inappropriate" or "always indicated" and leave large clinical gaps for which the use of an intervention is neither inappropriate nor unequivocally appropriate.

USING CLINICAL GUIDELINES TO CHANGE PRACTICE

Despite the appeal of evidence-based health care, the current challenge is how best to disseminate and implement guidelines in a way that leads to measurable improvements in the quality of care delivered. Clinical guidelines' dissemination implies a systematic process to confirm that the guideline reaches the clinician, and the clinician learns and uses it. The incorporation of new treatment recommendations into general practice is commonly delayed by slow dissemination of the recommendations and by the medical community's reluctance to accept them. Traditionally, it was assumed that

Preawareness—> Awareness—> Agreement—> Adoption—> Adherence

Fig. 1. Model of the cognitive steps physicians make in adhering to clinical guidelines.

information synthesized and disseminated by respected national authorities reliably led to change in physician clinical behavior. However, research has demonstrated that dissemination alone has little measurable effect on guideline physicians implementation *(23)*. Dissemination may increase knowledge and modify attitudes, but it has little influence on behavior and consequent outcomes. A systematic review of the effects of clinical practice guidelines on patient outcomes in primary care found little evidence that guidelines improved patient outcomes *(33)*.

Newer behavioral models postulate a more complex sequential process to guideline adherence (*see* Fig. 1; *34*). Physicians initially unaware of a specific guideline must first become aware of it (awareness), then intellectually agree with it (agreement), then decide to follow it in their practice (adoption), and finally succeed in following it at the appropriate times (adherence). Progression along the path to adherence can stop at any point for a variety of reasons. Efforts to improve guideline compliance may be better targeted by understanding where failure occurs in the progression from preawareness to adherence, as well as by identifying the physicians, practice settings, and situations for which progression at each step is less likely *(34)*.

There are three general strategies for implementing clinical guidelines: continuous quality improvement (CQI), academic detailing, and re-engineering. CQI is also known as total-quality management, requiring a systematic internal operation examination of the organization and focusing on the identity and implementation in improving overall performance. It is a participative systematical approach to changing practice patterns. The evidence that CQI interventions improve primary care delivery according to clinical guidelines is disappointing *(26,27,35–37)*.

As previously discussed, academic detailing focuses on physician behavior change. A key or influential decision maker is recruited to provide group and one-on-one consultation with peers. Academic detailing is best at illustrating that the new guideline is an improvement over existing processes. It is less likely to be successful when the guideline is complex or when an organizational change, rather than physician-specific, is required *(21)*. Academic detailing has been successful in the hospital setting, but is less well-studied in out-patient settings.

Re-engineering is a top-down rethinking and redesign of fundamental care delivery processes. It requires the buy-in of top-level administration and is not likely to succeed if there is no awareness in the organization of a performance gap and a major opportunity for improvement. Because of the uniqueness of each health care organization or practice, it is unlikely that case reports of re-engineering successes are generalizable across primary care settings.

SUCCESSFUL STRATEGIES FOR CHANGING PRACTICE

Changing clinical practice is complex. The implementation and facilitation of change is most likely to succeed if careful consideration is given to a combination of implementation tools that meet the unique educational, practice, and system characteristics of the target audience (*see* Table 2).

Table 2
Examples of Factors That Can Facilitate or Hinder Guideline Adherence

Guideline characteristics
    Complexity
    Source
    Evidence base
Patient characteristics
    Health care beliefs
    Insurance coverage
    Comorbidities
Physician characteristics
    Awareness of performance gap
    Specialty training
    Degree of involvement in guideline implementation
Practice characteristics
    Practice size
    Group practice style
    Delegation of patient care tasks
    Appointment availability
Organizational factors
    Automated clinical information systems
    Staff and professional development programs
    Administrative commitment and reinforcement
Environmental factors
    Geographical accessibility
    Health care payor policies

What do physicians say that they want? Clinicians are interested in credible guidelines endorsed by respected colleagues and professional organizations *(38)*. They want information presented concisely with evidence synopses and patient benefit quantifications that are likely to accrue. As previously stated, however, knowledge is necessary, but not sufficient to ensure the adoption of evidence-based practice. The practice environment and incentives for change are critical. Rather than try to make individual physician behavior comply with guidelines, leaders should affect organizational policies that ensure physician compliance.

Clinical decision support for providers is likely to be most valued by primary care physicians. The key to success is simplicity; one-page summaries, evidence tables, reminders, and algorithms have been well received. Many practice guidelines define descriptor variables in general or nonspecific terms, e.g., "increased risk" or "abnormal." Qualitative descriptors defeat an algorithm's usefulness for clinicians who face a decision in how to manage a particular patient. For example, quantitative information about threshold values is key. Algorithms result in faster learning, higher retention, and better compliance with established practice standards *(39)*. An additional benefit to algorithms is that they are readily translatable into computerized formats, thus facilitating clinical decision support.

Patient-specific clinical decision support is one of the most promising strategies for quality improvement. Computerized decision support systems may assist the physician by (1) providing ready access to appropriate knowledge or protocols, (2) involving patients in the decision-making process, and (3) providing a rational aid to the diagnosis or probable outcome based on patient-specific data *(40)*. An example of the latter system is the cardiovascular risk calculator, which determines an individual's risk of a cardiovascular event based on the Framingham data.

Prompting physicians leads to significant health maintenance improvements *(18,19)*. Traditional prompting tools include checklists attached to patient charts, tagged notes, prompting stickers, and patient-carried prompting cards. The beneficial effect of prompting is extinguished soon after the prompting is discontinued; thus, physicians need a low-cost and sustainable prompting strategy. One such strategy may be to use automated analyses of patient-specific diagnostic or treatment information. Existing examples include drug interaction alerts and preventive care reminders. In order to realize the full potential of this technology, computerized databases need to be linked, and patient-specific information should be provided to the clinician with clinical decision making, which is generally during the time of care delivery.

In an effort to narrow the gap between current practice and the best evidence, online medical information retrieval systems are increasingly available, particularly on the Internet. However, research has shown that information systems are not well integrated into clinical practice *(41–43)*. In a recent study, Hersh *(41)* showed that, whereas the average physician has an unmet information need in two out of every three patient encounters, on-line retrieval systems are only used a few times per month. One promising strategy is to provide physicians with access to current treatment guidelines on wireless handheld devices. Wireless systems have an advantage over office-based computers as they can be integrated more seamlessly into clinical settings. By allowing for access to clinical information at the point of care, physicians may retrieve and use the guideline information on a more consistent basis during the patient encounter.

WOMEN'S HEALTH IMPLICATIONS

Despite the prevalence of heart disease in women and the evidence that hyperlipidemic women are likely to benefit from lipid-lowering therapy, several studies have shown that treatment patterns are suboptimal. The Prospective Randomized Evaluation of the Vascular Effects of Norvase Trial found that almost half of women with arteriographically demonstrated CAD had elevated low-density lipoprotein (LDL) cholesterol levels throughout follow-up *(44)*. Baseline lipid management in the Heart and Estrogen Progestin Replacement Study (HERS), a cohort of 2763 women with clearly defined CHD, showed similar results *(14)*. More than half of the postmenopausal women were not taking any lipid-lowering agents. Those taking medication were either not adherent or did not have their dosage titrated to achieve recommended treatment goals. As a result, 91% were not at goal as defined by the 1993 National Cholesterol Education Program-Adult Treatment Panel (NCEP-ATTP) treatment goals. Given that the entire study population were volunteers, it is possible that the cohort was healthier and more health-conscious than the general population. In addition, lipid management may be more favorable in the cohort than in usual clinical practice. Similar findings have been reported for other preventive cardiac therapies. The use of established therapies, such as aspirin, beta-blockers, and ACE inhibitors following MI is low for women as well as men *(8,45,46)*.

Primary prevention begins with young adults, taking advantage of routine care and "well visits." Primary care providers that assess primary prevention programs for female patients should use well visits to briefly inquire about menstrual history, smoking history, physical activity, and diabetes symptoms. The physical examination should include body weight, height, and blood pressure, and the laboratory evaluation should include total and high-density lipoprotein cholesterol. Identification is the first step in risk factor modification. Once identified, women need active management of all modifiable risk factors.

Why haven't clinically proven prevention strategies been more widely adopted for women with heart disease? Many studies have found that women with coronary disease also carry diagnoses of diabetes, hypertension, and congestive heart failure. Some evidence suggests that women are more likely than men to have these comorbid conditions *(47)*. The presence of comorbid diseases may lead primary care physicians to be more reluctant in offering diagnostic or therapeutic options, despite their proven clinical effectiveness. Additionally, the later CAD onset in women may affect both patients' and providers' perceptions of heart disease. This delay may also contribute to the less aggressive diagnosis and treatment in women *(48)*.

The fragmented organizational structure of primary care services in our country and the traditional independence of individual practitioners means that there is no "one size fits all" solution. Usable, timely, and easily accessible practice guidelines are necessary to place high-quality evidence-based clinical information into the grasp of busy practitioners. Facilitating change in primary care practices is most likely to succeed if careful consideration is given to the unique characteristics of out-patient primary care practices as opposed to hospital-based specialty practices. Explicit and concise guidelines and algorithms are needed to aid decision making, and these guidelines must accommodate the range of patients seen by primary care providers. Clinical practice guidelines need to acknowledge the prevalence of comorbid conditions and provide recommended diagnostic or therapeutic options given the most common comorbidities.

One successful example of this strategy is the National Heart, Lung, and Blood Institute hypertension guideline that classifies patients into several risk groups based on both blood pressure level and coexisting diseases *(49)*. The guideline offers specific treatment recommendations and goals for patients with coexisting diseases. However, previously indicated physician knowledge is necessary, but not sufficient, to ensure evidence-based practice. Improved accessibility of clinical information should be accompanied by organizational changes that facilitate the conversion of new knowledge into improved clinical practice. Patient-specific clinical decision support, including automated reminders and prompts, seem to be the most promising strategy.

The overwhelming evidence suggests that women face a disparity in coronary disease evaluation and treatment. Primary care physicians play an important role in the identification and treatment of risk factors and comorbidities. The integration of these proven therapies into the routine care of all heart disease patients requires identifying and overcoming the current optimal treatment barriers.

REFERENCES

1. American Heart Association: Women, Heart Disease and Stroke Statistics. The American Heart Association National Center, Dallas, TX: 2000.
2. Mosca L, Manson JE, Sutherland SE, et al. Cardiovascular disease in women: A statement for healthcare professionals from the American Heart Association. Circulation 1997;96:2468–2482.
3. Bray GA. Obesity: A time bomb to be defused. Lancet 1998;352:160–161.

4. Cariou A, Himbert D, Golmanrd JL. Sex-related differences in eligibility for reperfusion therapy and in-hospital outcome after acute myocardial infarction. Eur Heart J 1997;18:1583.
5. Kaski JC, Rosano GC, Collins P, et al. Cardiac Syndrome X: Clinical characteristics and left ventricular function. J Am Coll Cardiol 1995;25:807–814.
6. Ayanian JZ, Epstein AM. Differences in the use of procedures between women and men hospitalized for coronary heart disease. N Engl J Med 1991;325:221–225.
7. Becker RC, Terrin M, Ross R, et al. Comparison of clinical outcomes for men and women after acute myocardial infarction. Ann Intern Med 1994;120:638–645.
8. Chandra NC, Ziegelstein R, Rogers WJ, et al. Observations of the treatment of women in the United States with myocardial infarction. Arch Intern Med 1998;158:981–988.
9. Jenkins JS, Flaker GC, Nolte B, et al. Causes of higher in-hospital mortality in women than in men after acute myocardial infarction. Am J Cardiol 1994;73:319–322.
10. Johnson PA, Goldman L, Orav EJ, et al. Gender differences in the management of acute chest pain: Support for the "Yentl Syndrome." J Gen Intern Med 1996;11:209–217.
11. Kostis JB, Wilson AC, O'Dowd K, et al. Sex differences in the management and long-term outcome of acute myocardial infarction. A statewide study. MIDAS Study Group. Circulation 1994;90:1715–1730.
12. Maynard C, Beshansky JR, Griffith JL, Selker, HP. Influence of sex on the use of cardiac procedures in patients presenting to the emergency department. Circulation 1996;94(9 Suppl):II93–II98.
13. Stone PH, Thompson B, Anderson HV, et al. Influence of race, sex, and age on management of unstable angina and non-Q-wave myocardial infarction: The TIMI III registry. JAMA 1996;275:1104–1112.
14. Schrott HG, Bittner V, Vittinghoff E, et al. Adherence to national cholesterol education program treatment goals in postmenopausal women with heart disease. JAMA 1997;277:1281–1321.
15. Chassin MR, Brook RH, Park RE, et al. Variation in the use of medical and surgical services by the Medicare population. N Eng J Med 1986;314:285–290.
16. Chassin MR, Hannan EL, DeBuono BA. Benefits and hazards of reporting medical outcomes publicly. New Eng J Med 1996;334:394–398.
17. Ellerbeck EF, Jencks SF, Radford MJ, et al. Quality of care for Medicare patients with acute myocardial infarction. JAMA 1995;273:1509–1514.
18. Balas EA, Weingarten S, Garb CT, et al. Improving preventive care by prompting physicians. Arch Intern Med 2000;160:301–308.
19. Balas EA, Boren SA. Managing Clinical Knowledge for Health Care Improvement. Yearbook of Medical Informatics. Center for Health Care Quality, University of Missouri, Columbia, MO: 2000, pp. 65–70.
20. Sackett DL. Applying overviews and meta-analysis at the bedside. J Clin Epidem 1995;48:61–66.
21. Davis DA, Thompson MA, Oxman AD, Hayes BR. Changing physician performance: A systematic review of the effects of continuing medical education strategies. JAMA 1995;274:700–705.
22. Eisenberg JM. Using clinical guidelines: Impact on public policy, clinical policy, and individual care decisions. In: National Quality of Care Forum. Bridging the Gap Between Theory and Practice: Exploring Clinical Practice Guidelines. Hospital Research and Education Trust, Chicago, IL: 1993.
23. Greco PJ, Eisenberg JM. Changing physician practices. N Engl J Med 1993;329:1270–1273.
24. Restuccia JD. The effect of concurrent feedback in reducing inappropriate hospital utilization. Med Care 1982;20:42–62.
25. Balas EA, Boren SA, Brown GD, et al. Effect of physician profiling on utilization: Meta-analysis of randomized clinical trails. J Gen Intern Med 1996;11:584–590.
26. Rask KJ, Kohler SK, Wells KJ, Diamond CC. Performance feedback to improve women's health screening in primary care practices. Unpublished manuscript, 2002.
27. Rask KJ, Kohler SA, Wells KJ, et al. Improving the care provided to diabetic patients in a primary care practice. J Clin Outcomes Manage 2001;8:23–29.
28. Margolis CZ, Sokol N, Susskind O, et al. Proposal for clinical algorithm standards. Med Decis Making 1992;12:149–154.
29. Granata AV, Hillman AL. Competing practice guidelines: Using cost-effectiveness analysis to make optimal decisions. Ann Intern Med 1998;128:56–63.
30. Margolis CZ. Clinical practice guidelines: Methodological considerations. Inter J Qual Health Care 1997;9:303–306.
31. Woolf SH. Practice guidelines: a new reality in medicine. III. Impact on patient care. Arch Intern Med 1993;153:2646–2655.

32. Lee T. Beyond Guidelines: Can general internists show the (critical) paths. J Gen Intern Med 1996;11:174–175.

33. Worrall G, Freake D, Kelland J, et al. Care of patients with type II diabetes: A study of family physicians' compliance with clinical practice guidelines. J Fam Pract 1997;44:374–381.

34. Pathman DE, Konrad TR, Freed GL, et al. The awareness-to-adherence model of the steps to clinical guideline compliance. Med Care 1996;34:873–888.

35. Goldberg HI, Wagner EH, Fihn SD, et al. A randomized controlled trial of CQI teams and academic detailing: Can they alter compliance with guidelines? Jt Comm J Qual Improv 1998;24:130–142.

36. Solberg LI, Kottke TE, Brekke ML. Will primary care clinics organize themselves to improve the delivery of preventive services? A randomized controlled trial. Prev Med 1998;27:623–631.

37. Solberg LI, Kottke TE, Brekke ML, et al. Failure of a continuous quality improvement intervention to increase the delivery of preventive services: A randomized trial. Effec Clin Pract 2000;3:105–115.

38. Hayward RS, Wilson MC, Tunis SR, et al. Practice guidelines: what are internists looking for? J Gen Intern Med 1996;11:176–178.

39. Sox HC. Quality of patient care by nurse practitioners and physician's assistants: A ten year prospective. Ann Intern Med 1979;91:449–468.

40. Delaney BC, Fitzmaurice DA, Riaz A, Hobbs FD. Can computerized decision support systems deliver improved quality in primary care? BMJ 1999;319:1–3.

41. Hersh W. A world of knowledge at your fingertips: The promise, reality, and future directions of on-line information retrieval. Acad Med 1999;74:240–243.

42. Grol R, Zwaard A, Mokkink H, et al. Dissemination of guidelines: which sources do physicians use in order to be informed? Internat J Qual Health Care 1998;10:135–140.

43. Stolte JJ, Ash J, Chin H. The dissemination of clinical practice guidelines over an intranet: an evaluation. Proc AMIA Symp 1999:960–964.

44. Miller M, Byington R, Hunninghake D, et al. Sex bias and underutilization of lipid-lowering therapy in patients with coronary artery disease at academic medical centers in the United States and Canada. Arch Intern Med 2000;160:343–347.

45. Bowker TJ, Clayton TC, Ingham J, et al. A British Cardiac Society survey of the potential for the secondary prevention of coronary disease: ASPIRE (Action on Secondary Prevention through Intervention to Reduce Events). Heart 1996;75:334–342.

46. Scheifer S, Escarce JJ, Schulman DA. Race and sex differences in the management of coronary artery disease. Am Heart J 2000;139:848–857.

47. Frishman W, Gomberg-Maitland M, Hirsh H, et al. Differences between male and female patients with regard to baseline demographics and clinical outcomes in the Asymptomatic Cardiac Ischemia Pilot (ACIP) trial. Clin Cardiol 1998;21:184–190.

48. Heim LJ, Brunsell SC. Heart disease in women. Prim Care 2000;27:741–766;vii.

49. National Heart, Lung, and Blood Institute. Cholesterol Lowering in the Patient with Coronary Heart Disease: Physician Monograph. National Heart, Lung, and Blood Institute; NIH publication 97-3794, Bethesda, MD: September 1997.

B. Evaluation of Acute Ischemic Syndromes in Women

16 Evaluation of Acute Chest Pain in Women

Andra L. Blomkalns, MD, W. Brian Gibler, MD, and L. Kristin Newby, MD

CONTENTS

INTRODUCTION: DEFINING THE PROBLEM

Coronary artery disease (CAD) is the leading cause of mortality among North American women, claiming nearly 500,000 lives each year. Cardiovascular disease (CVD) also ranks first among all disease categories in women for hospital discharges. In an attempt to combat this dominant cause of death, approx 2.5 million women are hospitalized annually for the evaluation of possible cardiovascular illness, but fewer than 40% of these patients are ultimately found to have a cardiac etiology of their symptoms *(1,2)*. Current evaluation practices lack both the sensitivity to appropriately identify female patients at risk for acute coronary syndrome (ACS) and the specificity to avoid unnecessary in-patient hospitalization. Additionally, the present medicolegal climate exerts tremendous pressure on physicians to both accurately and efficiently evaluate all patients with chest discomfort.

Why does correct CAD and ACS diagnosis continue to be elusive in the female population? There are several important explanations and even more that have yet to be studied. First, women with ACS present differently than men. Second, current clinical standards may not appropriately or effectively evaluate women. This chapter outlines and reviews classic and current literature that illustrates appropriate evaluation of women who present with possible ACS, highlighting important gender differences.

BACKGROUND

The underlying risk of CAD at presentation with chest discomfort is heavily influenced by the patient's sex and age. Epidemiological data from the Framingham Heart

From: *Contemporary Cardiology: Coronary Disease in Women: Evidence-Based Diagnosis and Treatment*
Edited by: L. J. Shaw and R. F. Redberg © Humana Press Inc., Totowa, NJ

Study shows that women have first CAD diagnosis approx 10 years later than men, but elderly women have rates similar to age-matched male counterparts *(3)*. Knowing that CAD prevalence in elderly women is equal to that of men does not solve the evaluation problem. Pope et al. found that in patients with acute ischemic syndromes, women below the age of 55 were most likely to be discharged from the emergency department *(4)*. To make this issue more challenging, women are more likely to experience clinically "silent" myocardial infarctions (MI), where nearly half of all MIs in women are clinically unrecognized *(3,5)*. Even women themselves tend to attribute potential ACS symptoms to other causes *(6)*. Perhaps partly attributable to these characteristics, both invasive and noninvasive chest discomfort evaluation are often delayed in women *(7–9)*.

To compound this problem, when women are referred for testing, many are not found to have significant CAD even when presenting with typical anginal symptoms. In a study of 1000 women below 50 years old undergoing angiography, only half of those thought to have typical anginal symptoms had significant CAD *(10)*, which implies that traditional methods and protocols to evaluate chest discomfort may not be sufficient in the female population.

Even if CAD and ACS are correctly diagnosed in female patients, there are continued obstacles in further evaluation and treatment. Female patient management with unstable angina or non-Q-wave MI tends to be less aggressive *(11)*. Women with known CAD and ongoing symptoms of angina pectoris are still considerably less likely than men to undergo cardiac catheterization or revascularization procedures *(12)*. In patients with known CAD, women generally have a worse initial prognosis after medical therapy, angioplasty, and bypass surgery than their male counterparts *(13–15)*. However, long-term survival outcomes may not necessarily be compromised *(16)*.

Overall, the methods for evaluating chest pain and possible ACS have progressed in recent years. Only a decade ago, patients with symptoms suspicious for ACS were admitted to a coronary care unit to "rule out" acute myocardial infarction (AMI), a process that may have taken several days. Sophisticated diagnostic technologies and increasing financial pressures have condensed current evaluation to as little as several hours in the emergency department setting from the previous duration in the hospital setting. Technological advances have allowed rapid serial cardiac marker determination and diagnostic testing in the setting of chest pain evaluation units (CPUs).

In these units, accelerated protocols that involve serial electrocardiogram (ECG) acquisition, serial cardiac marker determination, and diagnostic testing efficiently and cost-effectively evaluate patients with a low-to-moderate likelihood of cardiac chest pain *(17–20)*. Current protocols vary from various institutions, but most incorporate serial ECGs and cardiac markers over a period of 6 to 12 hours followed by a testing type, such as an exercise ECG (exercise treadmill testing [ETT]), rest or stress radionulcide imaging, or echocardiography. However, current chest pain evaluation protocols may not properly evaluate certain populations, particularly women.

Tailoring medical evaluation and treatment to specific populations and genders is not a new concept. For instance, abdominal pain etiologies are vastly different in women, even when accounting for differences in reproductive organs. Certain races and ethnic groups are predisposed to particular disease processes: African-American patients are linked to sickle cell disease, Native Americans to biliary tract disease, and Asians to hepatic and gastric carcinomas. Continued study and further experience with

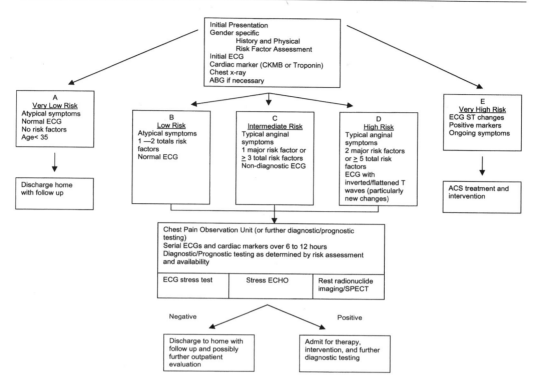

Fig. 1. Suggested approach to the evaluation of women with symptoms consistent with possible acute coronary syndrome.

CPUs will assist in understanding gender-specific issues in the presentation, evaluation, and treatment of women with chest discomfort.

RISK STRATIFICATION

When evaluating female patients (or any patient) with chest discomfort, the presence or absence of numerous factors lead to an overall assessment of ACS risk or likelihood. These factors are derived from an initial goal-directed evaluation to determine the diagnoses at highest likelihood followed by more specific studies to narrow the possible diagnoses. For potential ACS patients, these may include cardiac risk factor assessment, physical examination, ECG, determination of cardiac markers, and, ultimately, diagnostic and prognostic testing. In aggregate, the results from these assessments can be used to assign a patient to a particular risk stratum and help guide further disposition and therapy. Risk stratification places a patient on a continuum, and regardless how low a patient's risk may seem, the risk is never zero for any individual. Each of these evaluation components are discussed in the following subsections. One helpful approach may be to categorize patients into subsets of five-risk strata (A–E), thereby guiding appropriate and timely evaluation. A representative flowchart is presented in Fig. 1.

Table 1
Likelihood That Signs and Symptoms Represent an ACS Secondary to CAD

Feature	High likelihood	Intermediate likelihood	Low likelihood
	Any of the following:	Absence of high-likeli-hood features and presence of any of the following:	Absence of high- or intermediate-likeli-hood features but may have:
History	Chest or left arm pain or discomfort as chief symptom reproducing prior documented angina Known history of CAD, including MI	Chest or left arm pain or discomfort as chief symptom Age > 70 years Male sex Deabetes mellitus	Probable ischemic symptoms in absence of any of the intermediate likelihood characteristics Recent cocaine use
Examination	Transient magnetic resonance hypotension, diaphoresis, pulmonary edema, or rales	Extracardiac vascular disease	Chest discomfort reproduced by palpation
ECG	New, or presumably new, transient ST-segment deviation ($\geq$0.05 mV) or T-wave inversion ($\geq$0.2 mV) with symptoms	Fixed Q waves Abnormal ST segments or T waves not documented to be new	T-wave flattening or inversion in leads with dominant R-waves Normal ECG
Cardiac markers	Elevated cardiac TnI, TnT, or CK-MB	Normal	Normal

Source: ref. 97.

Initial Evaluation

All patients who present with acute nontraumatic chest discomfort should be evaluated for potential ACS. The differential diagnosis of acute chest discomfort is vast and can involve many different organ systems. Aside from ACS, the differential diagnosis includes pulmonary embolism, aortic dissection, pericarditis, musculoskeletal chest pain, gastroesophageal reflux disease, and pleurisy. A careful history and physical examination combined with appropriate preliminary diagnostic studies (e.g., ECG, chest radiograph, and/or arterial blood gas) are essential. Tables 1 and 2 show how information from the initial history, physical examination, and ECG may be helpful in determining both the probability of underlying CAD in a patient with chest pain and estimating that patient's qualitative risk. Further laboratory evaluation and diagnostic testing should be guided by this initial assessment.

Table 2
Estimation of Short-Term Risk of Death or Nonfatal MI in Patients With Unstable Angina

Feature	High risk	Intermediate risk	Low risk
	At least one of the following features must be present	No high-risk feature but must have one of the following	No high- or interme-diate-risk feature but may have any of the following features
History	Accelerating tempo of ischemic symp-toms in preceding 48 h	Prior MI, peripheral or cerebrovascular disease, or CABG, prior aspirin use	
Character of pain	Prolonged ongoing (>20 min) rest pain	Prolonged (>20 min) rest angina, now resolved, with moderate or high CAD likelihood Rest angina (<20 min) or relieved with rest or NTG	New onset CCS Class III or IV angina in the past 2 weeks without prolonged (>20 min) rest pain, but with moderate or high CAD likeli-hood (see Table 1)
Clinical findings	Pulmonary edema, most likely owing ischemia New or worsening magnetic reso-nance murmur S3 or new/worsening rales Hypotension, bradycardia, or tachycardia Age >75 years		Age > 70 years
ECG	Angina at rest with transient ST-seg-ment changes (>0.05 mV) Bundle-branch block, new or presumed new Sustained ventricular tachycardia		T-wave inversions (>0.2 mV) Patho-logical Q wave Normal or unchanged ECG during an episode of chest discomfort
Cardiac markers	Markedly elevated (e.g., TnT or TnI >0.1ng/mL)	Slightly elevated (e.g., TnT > 0.01, but <0.1 ng/mL)	Normal

Adapted from ref. 97.

Risk Factor Assessment

Traditional risk factors, such as age, gender, diabetes, smoking, hyperlipidemia, and family history, were originally identified from studies in predominantly male populations *(5,21)*. The postmenopausal state is an additional high morbidity risk factor specific to women *(22)*.

Age, sex, and menopausal status are significant factors in the evaluation of acute chest pain in women. The Acute Coronary Ischemia–Time Insensitive Predictive Instrument database demonstrated an overall AMI prevalence twofold higher in males in all age groups *(23)*. However, CAD incidence although lower in age-matched males than in young and middle-aged women, increases significantly after 45 years of age and equals that of males after age 75 *(3)*.

Diabetes is one of the most significant risk factors in the assessment of potential CAD in women and seems to differentially affect women. Among genders evaluated for symptomatic CAD, women are more likely to have diabetes, and diabetic women have significantly higher mortality rates from CAD than their nondiabetic female counterparts, as well as diabetic or nondiabetic men *(24,25)*. The diabetes effect is believed to be primarily because of its effect on lipid levels and blood pressure, and it negates the protective effect of hormonal status.

Smoking as few as one to four cigarettes per day is associated with up to a four times greater CAD risk *(26)*. The impact of this largely modifiable risk factor is similar in women and men, exceeding that of family history, obesity, sedentary lifestyle, and even age. Smoking cessation results in a return to baseline risk level in as little as 3 years.

Hyperlipidemia ranks similar to smoking in its overall contribution to CAD. As with other risk factors, there are gender differences in lipid assessment. In males, elevated low-density lipoprotein (LDL) levels are associated with an increased CAD risk. In contrast, female high-risk parameters include decreased high-density lipoproteins (HDL) and high triglyceride levels (TG, *27–29*).

Hypertension commonly affects men and women greater than age 65. Both diastolic and systolic hypertension has been associated with an increased CAD risk *(30)*. The immediate hypertension assessment in the acute setting may be unreliable owing to anxiety or pain. A history of hypertension or an extremely elevated pressure should be considered in risk factor assessment.

The postmenopausal state is associated with a decrease in endogenous estrogen production and an increase in CAD incidence. Estrogen likely exerts its effect by altering blood pressure, insulin sensitivity, coagulation, atherogenesis, platelet aggregation, and vasomotor tone *(31–33)*. Postulations of estrogen's protective effects have been largely based on epidemiological studies *(24,34)*. With opposed or unopposed estrogen, observational studies indicated that hormone replacement therapy (HRT) was associated with a 70–90% decline in death or the composite of death and MI among postmenopausal women, with its greatest effects in those with known CAD *(35–39)*. Conversely, the Heart and Estrogen Progestin Replacement Study (HERS), a randomized trial of HRT vs placebo, found no overall HRT effect for secondary CAD prevention in postmenopausal women *(40,41)*. However, although the exact effects of the loss of endogenous estrogen production remains unclear, and the role of HRT is in question, postmenopausal status should still be considered a major risk factor in the evaluation of women with possible ACS.

Table 3
Risk Factor Assessment for Women With Potential CAD

Minor risk factors	Intermediate risk factors	Major risk factors
Sedentary lifestyle	Lipid abnormalities*	Diabetes
Obesity	Hypertension	Postmenopausal state without
Family history	Smoking	estrogen replacement therapy
Age > 65 years		

* Particularly decreased HDL and increased triglycerides. (Adapted from ref. *22.*)

Many cardiac risk factors are interdependent, which can make the assessment of their individual contribution to risk difficult to determine. For instance, HRT can improve many lipid parameters, but at the same time, can increase triglycerides and enhance thrombosis. Diabetes indirectly increases serum lipids. Both smoking and the postmenopausal state are associated with a rise in vascular reactivity. The interactions are complex and certainly not mutually exclusive.

Clinicians that evaluate women with ACS symptoms should carefully screen for all previously mentioned risk factors. This information should be used to help assess the chance that a woman presenting with chest discomfort has underlying CAD, but should not be used to rule in or rule out an ACS diagnosis (Table 3).

Clinical Features

Recent work suggests that significant differences may exist in ACS presentation between genders *(42–44)*. Women often present atypically, making their initial evaluation more difficult. Atypical presentations generally refer to the signs and symptoms that differ from what is traditionally known as the male presentation of ACS. Current knowledge suggests the classic textbook listing of substernal pressing chest pain that radiates down the left arm, associated with nausea and diaphoresis, might need to be revisited when assessing female patients. A modified listing may be more appropriate in female patient assessment (Table 4).

Chest pain is considered to be the classic presenting ACS symptom; however, data from the Framingham study indicate that although women have chest pain more frequently, this pain rarely resulted in AMI *(45)*. The Coronary Artery Surgery Study (CASS) showed that half of all women undergoing cardiac catheterization for angina symptoms and presumptive CAD did not have significant obstruction *(46)*. Yet, other studies have shown that the predictive value of anginal chest pain does increase with age *(3)*.

Despite the abundant data that proves chest pain is not a reliable predictor for ACS, chest discomfort remains the most common symptom among women with AMI as in men as well *(47)*. However, women may both describe and perceive their chest pain differently. Goldberg et al. surveyed symptoms from a group of 550 women with validated AMI and compared them with a similar male cohort, finding that women were more likely to complain of associated neck pain, back pain, jaw pain, or nausea. Conversely, men were more likely to complain of diaphoresis. Differing pain presentations and descriptions in women have been noted in other studies, indicating a higher pain likelihood in the lower jaw and teeth, both arms, shoulders, back, and epigastrium *(48,49)*. In other studies, women more often tended to have less classic ACS presentations, such as

Table 4
Atypical Presenting Signs and Symptoms of ACS in Women

Neck or jaw pain
Pain in teeth
Back pain
Shoulder pain
Nausea
Epigastric discomfort or abdominal pain
Palpitations
Dyspnea
Presyncope
Pain in both arms
Loss of appetite
Orthopnea, paroxysmal nocturnal

Source: refs. 3,47–53.

abdominal pain, paroxysmal nocturnal dyspnea, or congestive heart failure (CHF; 3,50,51,52). In a small study evaluating the symptoms between genders with MI diagnosis Penque et al. demonstrated that women more often reported appetite loss, paroxysmal nocturnal dyspnea, and back pain (53). CHF signs and symptoms are more highly associated with an increased AMI probability in women (23). As is similarly the case with men, CHF findings should be considered a high-risk marker when evaluating the female population. The clinical implications in evaluating women with symptoms suggestive of ACS require the baseline understanding that women with AMI or ACS may present differently than men (Table 4).

Cardiac Markers

Over the last three decades, several generations of cardiac markers have evolved for myocardial necrosis identification. Current evaluation protocols most commonly include myoglobin, creatine kinase (CK/CKMB), and the cardiac troponins I and T (cTnI and cTnT). MI was previously defined by the World Health Organization as the combination of two of three characteristics: typical symptoms (i.e., chest discomfort), enzyme rise, and a typical ECG pattern that involves Q-wave development . More recently, a consensus document of The Joint European Society of Cardiology and American College of Cardiology (ACC) has proposed AMI redefinition using markers as the following: typical rise and fall of biochemical markers (troponin or CK-MB) in the presence of ischemic symptoms, development of pathological Q-waves on ECG, ECG evidence of acute ischemia (ST-segment elevation or depression), or coronary artery intervention (54). In situations where laboratory turn-around time is slow (>60 minutes), point-of-care testing (POCT) may be necessary to maximize the utility of these tests. Currently, these markers can aid in real-time AMI diagnosis and also in risk stratification of patients being evaluated for possible ACS (55–57).

Myoglobin is a heme protein present in both skeletal and cardiac muscle, making it less specific in potential cardiac injury evaluation. Myoglobin's advantage lies in its early release kinetics with elevations as early as 1 hour after symptom onset, which makes it useful within the first 3–4 hours following onset (58). Less of an advantage is its rapid kidney clearance and return to baseline levels within 6–12 hours *(59,60)*. Thus, it may be false-negative in patients who present later in the course of their acute episode. Generally, myoglobin use should be combined with a more specific later marker, such as CKMB or a troponin *(61)*.

Creatine kinase and its MB fraction have been the gold standards for the AMI diagnosis. CK plasma levels rise approx 6 hours after symptom onset and persist over a 24–36-hour period. Serial determinations result in a sensitivity and specificity for AMI of 92% and 98%, respectively *(62)*. Rapid and frequent serial determinations have been used to aid in patient diagnosis in the emergency department. Gibler et al. showed that serial CKMB measurements over 3 hours in patients with nondiagnostic ECGs presenting to the emergency department had an approx 80% sensitivity *(63)*. Early CKMB determinations have also been shown to have prognostic value in admitted patients with symptoms for AMI, but nondiagnostic ECGs *(64)*.

Troponins are structural proteins of troponin–tropomyosin complex of cardiac myocytes and are virtually undetectable in the serum under normal circumstances. They have been shown to be both sensitive and specific for evaluation of myocardial cell necrosis *(55,65)*. Cardiac TnT and TnI have variable expressions in different circumstances, but largely manifest similar release kinetics and diagnostic information. These proteins are released after cardiac muscle injury in a similar pattern to CKMB, persisting in the serum for up to 10 days. In a study of 338 patients by Katus et al., cTnT diagnostic sensitivity and specificity was 100% and 78%, respectively *(62)*. In a study of 383 CPU patients, Newby et al. determined that cTnT identified more patients with myocardial necrosis and multivessel CAD than CKMB. Additionally, cTnT positivity identified a population with high long-term mortality risk *(66)*. Several other studies have suggested that the troponins may not only be more sensitive markers for myocardial damage, but also useful in risk stratification in patients with potential ACS *(56,57,67–69)*.

As a general rule, a single-marker level determination is insufficient to effectively evaluate and risk stratify patients presenting with acute symptoms. Serial determinations, usually over 6–12 hours, are typically required. There is no current data to suggest that cardiac marker release, kinetics, and clinical utility are different between men and women. Consideration of marker attributes and kinetics should help guide appropriate choices in individual patients.

Diagnostic and Prognostic Testing

Diagnostic testing is helpful in risk stratification, prognosis, and to determine appropriate treatment for patients with potential ACS. Most of the current knowledge available in this area comes from male studies. Noninvasive tests are sometimes known to be less sensitive and specific in women, perhaps leading to misdiagnosis and incorrect treatment *(5,70)*.

Electrocardiographic stress testing or ETT, although frequently used in evaluation protocols, is believed to be less sensitive and specific in women than in men. According to some authors, this may be the result of lower exercise tolerance and inability to achieve target heart rates *(71)*. More prevalent baseline ECG changes, such as repolarization abnormalities, mitral valve prolapse, and estrogen-mediated digoxin-like effect, may also contribute to a decrease in specificity *(72)*. Conversely, other authors believe that exercise-based tests do indeed have comparable diagnostic accuracy for women

Table 5
Pretest and Posttest Probability of Significant CAD: History and Exercise Resting Results

Age (years)	History of angina	Risk factors	Sex	Pretest CAD probability	CAD probability: ETT+	CAD probability: ETT–
45	Atypical	None	Male	30%	65%	13%
45	Atypical	None	Female	5%	20%	2%
55	Typical	Smoker	Male	85%	96%	33%
55	Typical	Smoker	Female	55%	84%	30%

Source: ref. 5.

and men when corrected for variables that contribute to false-positive testing *(73,74)*. For women with typical angina symptoms and a normal ECG, exercise electrocardiographic testing is still recommended *(73,75)*. The reasons for the relative inaccuracy and conflicting ETT data in diagnosing women with potential CAD presently remains unclear. However, a major attributing factor may simply be the lower pretest CAD likelihood in women (Table 5).

Despite these conflicting views regarding ETT in women, its use as a prognostic indicator has been well-studied, and the results are more reassuring. Mark et al. developed a treadmill exercise index that predicted outcomes equally well in both genders *(76)*. When combined with serial marker determination and serial ECGs, exercise ECG testing has proven clinical value in diagnostic algorithms as evident in two large studies *(17,77)*. Negative exercise testing has also accurately identified patients at low prognostic risk in the CPU setting after a negative accelerated protocol *(78)*. A recent report from the American Heart Association (AHA) Science Advisory concluded that exercise ECG is safe and cost-effective in diagnostic risk stratification of selected low-risk patients with chest pain *(79)*.

Radionuclide imaging is an indirect visualization technique that has improved sensitivity and specificity over ETT. Previously, this modality's diagnostic accuracy was limited in women partially because of the presence of breast attenuation artifacts *(80,81)*. Limitations of emergency department radionuclide imaging include time, cost, and availability. Despite these initial obstacles, more chest pain evaluation protocols include radionuclide imaging as part of their testing regime.

Newer higher energy radionuclides, such as technetium-99m sestamibi and technetium-99m tetrofosmin, are replacing thallium, which results in less tissue attenuation. Other advantages of these newer agents include the better ability to assess ECG-gated wall motion to more accurately identify areas of decreased perfusion. Sestamibi imaging has been shown to have a significantly higher CAD specificity in women when compared with thallium studies *(82)*.

Rest single photon emission computed tomography (SPECT) has been used with great success in a variety of clinical arenas. Tatum and colleagues reported 93% sensitivity for diagnosing AMI when evaluating patients with early SPECT and serial cardiac marker analysis *(83)*. SPECT has also been shown to be an effective and safe risk stratification tool in patients who present to the emergency department with chest discomfort. A normal study indicates low risk for subsequent adverse cardiac events *(84–87)*.

Radionuclide imaging can be combined with exercise and pharmacological stressors to improve the diagnostic accuracy. Amanullah et al. concluded that adenosine Tc-99m sestamibi SPECT had a high sensitivity and specificity for CAD detection in women, regardless of presenting symptoms (93% and 83%, respectively; *88*). However, data extrapolation from women in the acute setting to those with low-to-moderate risk is difficult and should be done with caution. Geleijnse et al. demonstrated that normal dobutamine-atropine stress sestamibi scintigraphy was associated with excellent prognosis in women with stable chest pain syndromes. No major cardiac events were observed among the study subjects, even those with a high-pretest CAD likelihood (*89*).

Transthoracic echocardiography has been used with success in the evaluation of acute chest pain patients (*90,91*). Overall, the sensitivity and specificity of echocardiography is most reliable when performed during the chest pain episode. One of the major limitations of this modality is the necessity of immediate trained personnel to obtain and interpret the study.

Pharmacological or exercise stress echocardiography has also been shown to be an effective tool in the noninvasive evaluation among women with chest pain and unknown CAD. This modality improves the sensitivity and specificity over exercise ECG testing that approaches the diagnostic accuracy of radionulcide imaging (*92*). Stress echocardiography has important prognostic implications as well. In one study, the 3-year survival rate for patients with positive and negative evaluations was 99.5% and 69.5%, respectively, considering hard cardiac events of death or infarction (*93*). Likely the most pronounced modality weaknesses are operator dependence in obtaining quality images and the need for having operator availability 24 hours per day.

Cardiac catheterization is reserved for those patients in which other diagnostic modalities are inconclusive or for higher risk patients. As previously noted, women tend to be referred less often for angiography and generally tend to have a worse early prognosis following surgical or interventional therapies (*13–15*). However, long-term outcomes are similar (*16*). Because overall diagnostic testing appears to be less accurate in women, the angiography threshold may need to be lower (*94*).

The ultimate choice of diagnostic and prognostic testing largely depends on institutional resources and expertise. Figure 1 provides a flow diagram for suggested evaluation of women who present with acute chest pain. Evaluation should be based on an overall risk assessment, with diagnostic testing being reserved for those in the intermediate categories.

TREATMENT AND DISPOSITION

Although few studies address gender-specific ACS treatment, current evidence suggests that men and women should be treated similarly (*5,95*). Every patient with a suspected ACS should receive an aspirin. Nitroglycerin is indicated in the absence of severe bradycardia or hypotension. Oxygen use is most valuable for patients with overt pulmonary congestion or oxygen saturations less than 90%. Heparin, beta-blockers, and glycoprotein IIb/IIIa antagonists should also be given when indicated. Thrombolysis is indicated in the AMI setting when immediate percutaneous transluminal coronary angioplasty (PTCA) is unavailable or delayed. Rescue catheterization might then be reserved for patients with persistent pain or lack of postthrombolytic reperfusion (*96*).

The ideal evaluation protocol for chest discomfort evaluation in women is both theoretical and controversial. In summary, symptoms consistent with angina (whether typical or atypical) in a patient with known or unknown CAD warrants further evaluation. It may be helpful to divide patients into the risk categories described in Fig. 1. Very high-risk (E) patients for ACS should be admitted for further urgent evaluation and treatment. Very low-risk patients (A) can be safely discharged with appropriate outpatient follow-up. Intermediate-risk patients (B–D) need further acute evaluation for appropriate disposition, ideally in a CPU environment, or if not available, as an inpatient.

CONCLUSION

The evaluation of acute chest pain in women has certain gender-specific differences. The clinician should recognize that women have different symptom presentations, risk factor profiles, and different needs in terms of diagnostic, prognostic, and provocative testing. An understanding of these differences is necessary to further reduce the morbidity and mortality associated with this increasingly prevalent disease in the female population.

REFERENCES

1. Murphy SL. Deaths: Final data for 1998. Natl Vital Stat Rep 2000;48:1–105.
2. American Heart Association. 1997 Heart and Stroke Facts: Statistical Update. American Heart Association, Dallas, TX: 1997.
3. Lerner DJ, Kannel WB. Patterns of coronary heart disease morbidity and mortality in the sexes: a 26-year follow-up of the Framingham population. Am Heart J 1986;111:383–390.
4. Pope JH, Aufderheide TP, Ruthazer R, et al. Missed diagnoses of acute cardiac ischemia in the emergency department. N Engl J Med 2000;342:1163–1170.
5. Fetters JK, Peterson ED, Shaw LJ, et al. Sex-specific differences in coronary artery disease risk factors, evaluation, and treatment: have they been adequately evaluated? Am Heart J 1996;131:796–813.
6. Pilote L, Hlatky MA. Attitudes of women toward hormone therapy and prevention of heart disease. Am Heart J 1995;129:1237–1238.
7. Johnson PA, Goldman L, Orav EJ, et al. Gender differences in the management of acute chest pain. Support for the "Yentl syndrome". J Gen Intern Med 1996;11:209–217.
8. Steingart RM, Packer M, Hamm P, et al. Sex differences in the management of coronary artery disease. Survival and Ventricular Enlargement Investigators. N Engl J Med 1991;325:226–230.
9. Ayanian JZ, Epstein AM. Differences in the use of procedures between women and men hospitalized for coronary heart disease. N Engl J Med 1991;325:221–225.
10. Welch CC, Proudfit WL, Sheldon WC. Coronary arteriographic findings in 1000 women under age 50. Am J Cardiol 1975;35:211–215.
11. Stone PH, Thompson B, Anderson HV, et al. Influence of race, sex, and age on management of unstable angina and non-Q-wave myocardial infarction: The TIMI III registry. JAMA 1996;275:1104–1112.
12. Maynard C, Beshansky JR, Griffith JL, Selker HP. Influence of sex on the use of cardiac procedures in patients presenting to the emergency department. A prospective multicenter study. Circulation 1996;94(9 Suppl):II93–II98.
13. Vaccarino V, Krumholz HM, Berkman LF, Horwitz RI. Sex differences in mortality after myocardial infarction. Is there evidence for an increased risk for women? Circulation 1995;91:1861–1871.
14. Malacrida R, Genoni M, Maggioni AP, et al. A comparison of the early outcome of acute myocardial infarction in women and men. The Third International Study of Infarct Survival Collaborative Group. N Engl J Med 1998;338:8–14.
15. Davis KB, Chaitman B, Ryan T, et al. Comparison of 15-year survival for men and women after initial medical or surgical treatment for coronary artery disease: a CASS registry study. Coronary Artery Surgery Study. J Am Coll Cardiol 1995;25:1000–1009.

16. Bickell NA, Pieper KS, Lee KL, et al. Referral patterns for coronary artery disease treatment: gender bias or good clinical judgment? Ann Intern Med 1992;116:791–797.

17. Farkouh ME, Smars PA, Reeder GS, et al. A clinical trial of a chest-pain observation unit for patients with unstable angina. Chest Pain Evaluation in the Emergency Room (CHEER) Investigators. N Engl J Med 1998;339:1882–1888.

18. Roberts RR, Zalenski RJ, Mensah EK, et al. Costs of an emergency department-based accelerated diagnostic protocol vs hospitalization in patients with chest pain: a randomized controlled trial. JAMA 1997;278:1670–1676.

19. Gomez MA, Anderson JL, Karagounis LA, et al. An emergency department-based protocol for rapidly ruling out myocardial ischemia reduces hospital time and expense: results of a randomized study (ROMIO). J Am Coll Cardiol 1996;28:25–33.

20. Storrow AB, Gibler WB. Chest pain centers: diagnosis of acute coronary syndromes. Ann Emerg Med 2000;35:449–461.

21. Wenger NK, Speroff L, Packard B. Cardiovascular health and disease in women. N Engl J Med 1993;329:247–256.

22. Douglas PS, Ginsburg GS. The evaluation of chest pain in women. N Engl J Med 1996;334:1311–1315.

23. Zucker DR, Griffith JL, Beshansky JR, Selker HP. Presentations of acute myocardial infarction in men and women. J Gen Intern Med 1997;12:79–87.

24. Kannel WB, Hjortland MC, McNamara PM, Gordon T. Menopause and risk of cardiovascular disease: the Framingham study. Ann Intern Med 1976;85:447–452.

25. Granger CB, Califf RM, Young S, et al. Outcome of patients with diabetes mellitus and acute myocardial infarction treated with thrombolytic agents. The Thrombolysis and Angioplasty in Myocardial Infarction (TAMI) Study Group. J Am Coll Cardiol 1993;21:920–925.

26. Willett WC, Green A, Stampfer MJ, et al. Relative and absolute excess risks of coronary heart disease among women who smoke cigarettes. N Engl J Med 1987;317:1303–1309.

27. Rich-Edwards JW, Manson JE, Hennekens CH, Buring JE. The primary prevention of coronary heart disease in women. N Engl J Med 1995;332:1758–1766.

28. Sempos CT, Cleeman JI, Carroll MD, et al. Prevalence of high blood cholesterol among US adults. An update based on guidelines from the second report of the National Cholesterol Education Program Adult Treatment Panel. JAMA 1993;269:3009–3014.

29. LaRosa JC. Triglycerides and coronary risk in women and the elderly. Arch Intern Med 1997;157:961–968.

30. Cornoni-Huntley J, LaCroix AZ, Havlik RJ. Race and sex differentials in the impact of hypertension in the United States. The National Health and Nutrition Examination Survey I Epidemiologic Follow-up Study. Arch Intern Med 1989;149:780–788.

31. Peterson LR. Estrogen replacement therapy and coronary artery disease. Curr Opin Cardiol 1998;13:223–231.

32. Bairey Merz CN, Kop W, Krantz DS, et al. Cardiovascular stress response and coronary artery disease: evidence of an adverse postmenopausal effect in women. Am Heart J 1998;135:881–887.

33. Miller VM. Gender and vascular reactivity. Lupus 1999;8:409–415.

34. Grady D, Rubin SM, Petitti DB, et al. Hormone therapy to prevent disease and prolong life in postmenopausal women. Ann Intern Med 1992;117:1016–1037.

35. Bush TL. Evidence for primary and secondary prevention of coronary artery disease in women taking oestrogen replacement therapy. Eur Heart J 1996;17(Suppl D):9–14.

36. Sullivan JM, Vander ZR, Lemp GF, et al. Postmenopausal estrogen use and coronary atherosclerosis. Ann Intern Med 1988;108:358–363.

37. Forrester JS, Merz CN, Bush TL, et al. 27th Bethesda Conference: matching the intensity of risk factor management with the hazard for coronary disease events. Task Force 4. Efficacy of risk factor management. J Am Coll Cardiol 1996;27:991–1006.

38. Grodstein F, Stampfer MJ, Colditz GA, et al. Postmenopausal hormone therapy and mortality. N Engl J Med 1997;336:1769–1775.

39. Grodstein F, Stampfer MJ, Manson JE, et al. Postmenopausal estrogen and progestin use and the risk of cardiovascular disease [published erratum appears in N Engl J Med 1996 Oct 31;335(18):1406]. N Engl J Med 1996;335:453–461.

40. Seed M. Hormone replacement therapy and cardiovascular disease. Curr Opin Lipidol 1999;10:581–587.

41. Herrington DM. The HERS trial results: paradigms lost? Heart and Estrogen/progestin Replacement Study. Ann Intern Med 1999;131:463–466.

42. Roger VL, Farkouh ME, Weston SA, et al. Sex differences in evaluation and outcome of unstable angina. JAMA 2000;283:646–652.

43. Reunanen A, Suhonen O, Aromaa A, et al. Incidence of different manifestations of coronary heart disease in middle-aged Finnish men and women. Acta Med Scand 1985;218:19–26.

44. Pepine CJ, Abrams J, Marks RG, et al. Characteristics of a contemporary population with angina pectoris. TIDES Investigators. Am J Cardiol 1994;74:226–231.

45. Colditz GA, Willett WC, Stampfer MJ, et al. Menopause and the risk of coronary heart disease in women. N Engl J Med 1987;316:1105–1110.

46. Kannel WB, Feinleib M. Natural history of angina pectoris in the Framingham study. Prognosis and survival. Am J Cardiol 1972;29:154–163.

47. Goldberg RJ, O'Donnell C, Yarzebski J, et al. Sex differences in symptom presentation associated with acute myocardial infarction: a population-based perspective. Am Heart J 1998;136:189–195.

48. Everts B, Karlson BW, Wahrborg P, et al. Localization of pain in suspected acute myocardial infarction in relation to final diagnosis, age and sex, and site and type of infarction [published erratum appears in Heart Lung 1997 May-Jun;26(3):176]. Heart Lung 1996;25:430–437.

49. Sullivan AK, Holdright DR, Wright CA, et al. Chest pain in women: clinical, investigative, and prognostic features. BMJ 1994;308:883–886.

50. Kannel WB, Abbott RD. Incidence and prognosis of unrecognized myocardial infarction. An update on the Framingham study. N Engl J Med 1984;311:1144–1147.

51. Fiebach NH, Viscoli CM, Horwitz RI. Differences between women and men in survival after myocardial infarction. Biology or methodology? JAMA 1990;263:1092–1096.

52. Dittrich H, Gilpin E, Nicod P, et al. Acute myocardial infarction in women: influence of gender on mortality and prognostic variables. Am J Cardiol 1988;62:1–7.

53. Penque S, Halm M, Smith M, et al. Women and coronary disease: relationship between descriptors of signs and symptoms and diagnostic and treatment course. Am J Crit Care 1998;7:175–182.

54. Myocardial infarction redefined—a consensus document of The Joint European Society of Cardiology/American College of Cardiology Committee for the redefinition of myocardial infarction. J Am Coll Cardiol 2000;36:959–969.

55. Hamm CW, Goldmann BU, Heeschen C, et al. Emergency room triage of patients with acute chest pain by means of rapid testing for cardiac troponin T or troponin I. N Engl J Med 1997;337:1648–1653.

56. Ohman EM, Armstrong PW, Christenson RH, et al. Cardiac troponin T levels for risk stratification in acute myocardial ischemia. GUSTO IIA Investigators. N Engl J Med 1996;335:1333–1341.

57. Antman EM, Tanasijevic MJ, Thompson B, et al. Cardiac-specific troponin I levels to predict the risk of mortality in patients with acute coronary syndromes. N Engl J Med 1996;335:1342–1349.

58. Vaidya HC. Myoglobin. Lab Med 1992;23:306–310.

59. Brogan GX, Jr., Friedman S, McCuskey C, et al. Evaluation of a new rapid quantitative immunoassay for serum myoglobin versus CK-MB for ruling out acute myocardial infarction in the emergency department. Ann Emerg Med 1994;24:665–671.

60. Tucker JF, Collins RA, Anderson AJ, et al. Value of serial myoglobin levels in the early diagnosis of patients admitted for acute myocardial infarction. Ann Emerg Med 1994;24:704–708.

61. Storrow AB, Gibler WB. The role of cardiac markers in the emergency department. Clin Chim Acta 1999;284:187–196.

62. Katus HA, Remppis A, Neumann FJ, et al. Diagnostic efficiency of troponin T measurements in acute myocardial infarction. Circulation 1991;83:902–912.

63. Gibler WB, Young GP, Hedges JR, et al. Acute myocardial infarction in chest pain patients with nondiagnostic ECGs: serial CK-MB sampling in the emergency department. The Emergency Medicine Cardiac Research Group. Ann Emerg Med 1992;21:504–512.

64. Hoekstra JW, Hedges JR, Gibler WB, et al. Emergency department CK-MB: a predictor of ischemic complications. National cooperative CK-MB project group. Acad Emerg Med 1994;1:17–27.

65. Hamm CW, Ravkilde J, Gerhardt W, et al. The prognostic value of serum troponin T in unstable angina. N Engl J Med 1992;327:146–150.

66. Newby LK, Kaplan AL, Granger BB, et al. Comparison of cardiac troponin T versus creatine kinase-MB for risk stratification in a chest pain evaluation unit. Am J Cardiol 2000;85:801–805.

67. Polanczyk CA, Lee TH, Cook EF, et al. Cardiac troponin I as a predictor of major cardiac events in emergency department patients with acute chest pain. J Am Coll Cardiol 1998;32:8–14.
68. Ravkilde J, Nissen H, Horder M, Thygesen K. Independent prognostic value of serum creatine kinase isoenzyme MB mass, cardiac troponin T and myosin light chain levels in suspected acute myocardial infarction. Analysis of 28 months of follow-up in 196 patients. J Am Coll Cardiol 1995;25:574–581.
69. Lindahl B, Venge P, Wallentin L. Relation between troponin T and the risk of subsequent cardiac events in unstable coronary artery disease. The FRISC study group. Circulation 1996;93:1651–1657.
70. Hung J, Chaitman BR, Lam J, et al. Noninvasive diagnostic test choices for the evaluation of coronary artery disease in women: a multivariate comparison of cardiac fluoroscopy, exercise electrocardiography and exercise thallium myocardial perfusion scintigraphy. J Am Coll Cardiol 1984;4:8–16.
71. Cerqueira MD. Diagnostic testing strategies for coronary artery disease: special issues related to gender. Am J Cardiol 1995;75:52D–60D.
72. Sketch MH, Mohiuddin SM, Lynch JD, et al. Significant sex differences in the correlation of electrocardiographic exercise testing and coronary arteriograms. Am J Cardiol 1975;36:169–173.
73. Weiner DA, Ryan TJ, McCabe CH, et al. Exercise stress testing. Correlations among history of angina, ST- segment response and prevalence of coronary-artery disease in the Coronary Artery Aurgery Study (CASS). N Engl J Med 1979;301:230–235.
74. Melin JA, Wijns W, Vanbutsele RJ, et al. Alternative diagnostic strategies for coronary artery disease in women: demonstration of the usefulness and efficiency of probability analysis. Circulation 1985;71:535–542.
75. Hlatky MA, Pryor DB, Harrell FE, Jr., et al. Factors affecting sensitivity and specificity of exercise electrocardiography. Multivariable analysis. Am J Med 1984;77:64–71.
76. Mark DB, Shaw L, Harrell FE, Jr., et al. Prognostic value of a treadmill exercise score in outpatients with suspected coronary artery disease. N Engl J Med 1991;325:849–853.
77. Zalenski RJ, McCarren M, Roberts R, et al. An evaluation of a chest pain diagnostic protocol to exclude acute cardiac ischemia in the emergency department. Arch Intern Med 1997;157:1085–1091.
78. Lewis WR, Amsterdam EA. Chest pain emergency units. Curr Opin Cardiol 1999;14:321–328.
79. Stein RA, Chaitman BR, Balady GJ, et al. Safety and utility of exercise testing in emergency room chest pain centers: An advisory from the Committee on Exercise, Rehabilitation, and Prevention, Council on Clinical Cardiology, American Heart Association. Circulation 2000;102:1463–1467.
80. Manglos SH, Thomas FD, Gagne GM, Hellwig BJ. Phantom study of breast tissue attenuation in myocardial imaging. J Nucl Med 1993;34:992–996.
81. Friedman TD, Greene AC, Iskandrian AS, Hakki AH, Kane SA, Segal BL. Exercise thallium-201 myocardial scintigraphy in women: correlation with coronary arteriography. Am J Cardiol 1982;49:1632–1637.
82. Taillefer R, DePuey EG, Udelson JE, et al. Comparative diagnostic accuracy of Tl-201 and Tc-99m sestamibi SPECT imaging (perfusion and ECG-gated SPECT) in detecting coronary artery disease in women. J Am Coll Cardiol 1997;29:69–77.
83. Tatum JL, Jesse RL, Kontos MC, et al. Comprehensive strategy for the evaluation and triage of the chest pain patient. Ann Emerg Med 1997;29:116–125.
84. Hilton TC, Thompson RC, Williams HJ, et al. Technetium-99m sestamibi myocardial perfusion imaging in the emergency room evaluation of chest pain. J Am Coll Cardiol 1994;23:1016–1022.
85. Gregoire J, Theroux P. Detection and assessment of unstable angina using myocardial perfusion imaging: comparison between technetium-99m sestamibi SPECT and 12-lead electrocardiogram. Am J Cardiol 1990;66:42E–46E.
86. Beller GA. Acute radionuclide perfusion imaging for evaluation of chest pain in the emergency department: need for a large clinical trial. J Nucl Cardiol 1996;3:546–549.
87. Varetto T, Cantalupi D, Altieri A, Orlandi C. Emergency room technetium-99m sestamibi imaging to rule out acute myocardial ischemic events in patients with nondiagnostic electrocardiograms. J Am Coll Cardiol 1993;22:1804–1808.
88. Amanullah AM, Kiat H, Friedman JD, Berman DS. Adenosine technetium-99m sestamibi myocardial perfusion SPECT in women: diagnostic efficacy in detection of coronary artery disease. J Am Coll Cardiol 1996;27:803–809.
89. Geleijnse ML, Elhendy A, van Domburg RT, et al. Prognostic significance of normal dobutamine-atropine stress sestamibi scintigraphy in women with chest pain. Am J Cardiol 1996;77:1057–1061.
90. Kontos MC, Arrowood JA, Paulsen WH, Nixon JV. Early echocardiography can predict cardiac events in emergency department patients with chest pain. Ann Emerg Med 1998;31:550–557.

91. Levitt MA, Promes SB, Bullock S, et al. Combined cardiac marker approach with adjunct two-dimensional echocardiography to diagnose acute myocardial infarction in the emergency department. Ann Emerg Med 1996;27:1–7.
92. Marcovitz PA, Armstrong WF. Accuracy of dobutamine stress echocardiography in detecting coronary artery disease. Am J Cardiol 1992;69:1269–1273.
93. Cortigiani L, Dodi C, Paolini EA, Bernardi D, Bruno G, Nannini E. Prognostic value of pharmacological stress echocardiography in women with chest pain and unknown coronary artery disease. J Am Coll Cardiol 1998;32:1975–1981.
94. Chiamvimonvat V, Sternberg L. Coronary artery disease in women. Can Fam Physician 1998;44:2709–2717.
95. Braunwald E, Antman EM, Beasley JW, et al. ACC/AHA guidelines for the management of patients with unstable angina and non-ST-segment elevation myocardial infarction: executive summary and recommendations. A report of the American College of Cardiology/American Heart Association task force on practice guidelines (committee on the management of patients with unstable angina). Circulation 2000;102:1193–1209.
96. Ryan TJ, Antman EM, Brooks NH, et al. 1999 update: ACC/AHA guidelines for the management of patients with acute myocardial infarction. A report of the American College of Cardiology/American Heart Association Task Force on Practice Guidelines (Committee on Management of Acute Myocardial Infarction). J Am Coll Cardiol 1999;34:890–911.
97. Braunwald E, Mark DB, Jones RH. Unstable angina: diagnosis and management. AHCPR Practice Guideline no. 10, AHCPR Publication no. 94-0602. Agency for Health Care Policy and Research and the National Heart, Lung, and Blood Institute, US Public Health Service, US Department of Health and Human Services, Rockville, MD: 1994.

17 Acute Ischemic Syndromes

Differences in Presentation and Treatment in Women

Jane A. Leopold, MD and Alice K. Jacobs, MD

CONTENTS

INTRODUCTION

Cardiovascular disease (CVD) remains the leading cause of mortality for women in the United States. Although the incidence of coronary heart disease (CHD) increases with age in women, the clinical presentation of the disease lags 10 years behind that in men. In fact, one out of five women have some form of CVD and since 1984, the number of CVD deaths for females has exceeded those for males (1). Additionally, recent studies have suggested a difference between women and men regarding the natural history of coronary artery disease (CAD) and acute coronary syndromes (ACS) that cannot be attributed to age alone (2–4). Based on these observations and an increased focus on the management of women with heart disease, gender-based differences in patients who present with ACS are under active investigation. Therefore, the goal of this chapter is to briefly review the clinical presentation, evaluation, and medical and revascularization therapy of women with ACS.

From: *Contemporary Cardiology: Coronary Disease in Women: Evidence-Based Diagnosis and Treatment*
Edited by: L. J. Shaw and R. F. Redberg © Humana Press Inc., Totowa, NJ

Table 1
The Age-Specific Incidence Rates of Coronary Disease in Women[a]

Age (years)		
	1980–1982	*1992–1994*
< 49	25	13
50–54	103	53
55–59	177	149
	1982–1984	*1992–1994*
60–64	242	212
	1986–1988	*1992–1994*
≥ 65	422	244

[a] All rates are expressed as cases per 100,000 people-years.
Source: ref. *5.*

Cardiovascular mortality in women has declined over time as evidenced by the Nurses' Health Study, which demonstrated a 31% decrease in the incidence of CHD in women from the period of 1980–1982 to 1992–1994 (Table 1); however, this decline rate was less than that observed for men and the risk of death, reinfarction, and congestive heart failure (CHF) following a nonfatal myocardial infarction (MI) remained significantly higher in women *(5).* In addition, gender-based differences in cardiovascular mortality vary according to age. Among patients less than 50 years of age, the mortality rate for women is twice that for men, whereas after age 74, there is no significant difference in cardiovascular mortality rates between men and women *(3).*

Although the lifetime risk of developing ACS after age 40 is 49% for men and only 32% for women; women are more likely to experience significant morbidity and mortality associated with an ACS (Fig. 1). In part, this is due to the observation that women have MIs at older ages than men and are more likely to die or have a second presentation with an ACS within 1 year of the index event. African-American women are at a particularly high risk for adverse events associated with an ACS; mortality data from 1998 revealed that cardiovascular deaths for African-American females were 400.7 per 1000 compared to 294.9 per 1000 for white females *(1).*

CLINICAL PRESENTATION

Whereas almost two-thirds of men present with an acute ST-segment elevation, MI, or sudden cardiac death as the first manifestation of atherosclerotic CHD, more than 50% of women have a chest pain syndrome as their initial symptom *(6);* however, establishing the diagnosis of ischemic heart disease in women remains problematic owing to a high prevalence of chest pain in women in the absence of a significant epicardial coronary artery stenosis.

Historically, the Coronary Artery Surgery Study (CASS) revealed that chest pain is neither sensitive nor specific in predicting CAD presence in women. The presence of a significant epicardial coronary stenosis, defined as more than 70% stenosis, was found in 70% of women classified as having definite angina when compared to only 36% of women with probable angina. Only 6% of women who were believed to have noncardiac chest pain had significant CAD. In contrast, men in these categories had documented CAD rates of 93%, 66%, and 14%, respectively *(7).*

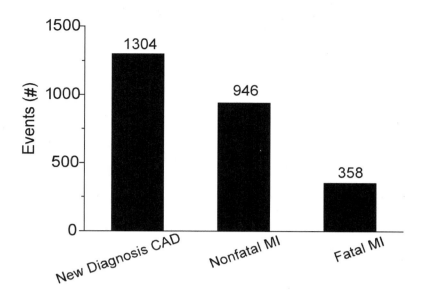

Fig. 1. Trends in the CHD incidence in women. The Nurses' Health Study followed 85,941 women age 34–59 years old without any prior cardiac disease and documented newly diagnosed CHD between the years 1980 and 1994. CAD, coronary artery disease; MI, myocardial infarction *(5)*.

Women with ACSs often present for evaluation with symptom patterns that differ from their male counterparts and are more likely than men to report differences in chest pain quality and frequency. Review of initial symptoms in a series of patients diagnosed with ACSs during hospitalization revealed that chest pain was the most common symptom reported by both men and women; however, women were more likely than men to present with mid-back pain, nausea and/or vomiting, dyspnea, palpitations, and indigestion *(8,9)*. Similarly, among patients presenting with an acute ST-segment elevation MI, men were significantly less likely to complain of neck, back, or jaw pain, and nausea than women *(10)*. Additionally, women were more likely than men to report chest pain during daily activities, but not during physical activity, and when challenged with mental stressors *(11)*.

CLINICAL CHARACTERISTICS AT PRESENTATION

Women who present with ACSs, including unstable angina, non-ST-segment elevation MI and ST-segment elevation MI, are often older than their male counterparts with a higher rate of hypertension, diabetes mellitus, hypercholesterolemia, tobacco use, obesity, and a prior CHF history *(2–4,12)*. These observations were confirmed in the Global Use of Strategies to Open Occluded Arteries in Acute Coronary Syndromes II (GUSTO-II ACS) Study. This trial enrolled 3662 women and 8480 men who presented with ACS. Women who presented with unstable angina were found to be older than men (median age 68 vs 64 years, $p < 0.001$) and had a higher incidence of CHD risk factors including hypertension (57 vs 45%, $p < 0.001$), diabetes mellitus (23 vs 17%, $p < 0.001$), hypercholesterolemia (47 vs 39%, $p < 0.001$), and a history of CHF (10.2 vs 6.1%, $p < 0.001$). Interestingly, in this trial, women were less likely to be current or for-

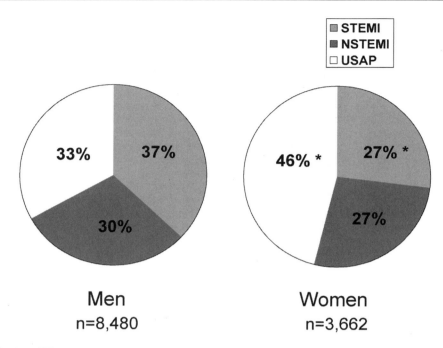

Fig. 2. Sex differences in presentation with ACS. Among ACS patients, men are more likely to present with an ST- segment elevation MI and Non ST-segment elevation MI than women. By contrast, women are more likely to present with unstable angina. STEMI, ST-segment elevation MI; NSTEMI, Non-ST-segment elevation myocardial infarction; USAP, unstable angina. *$p < 0.001$ vs men *(4)*.

mer smokers when compared to men (38 vs 74%, $p < 0.001$), and were less likely to have had a prior MI (27 vs 38%, $p < 0.001$), prior angioplasty (11.8 vs 14.4%, $p < 0.01$), or prior coronary artery bypass surgery (CABG; 9.2 vs 16.6%, $p < 0.001$). Similar results were seen in women who presented with a non-ST-segment or ST-segment MI *(4)*.

The clinical characteristics at presentation in women who present with an ST segment elevation MI were examined further in the National Registry of Myocardial Infarction-2 (NRMI-2) database. A total of 155,565 women and 229,313 men, age 30–89 years, were enrolled in the NRMI-2 database between 1994 and 1998. Women who presented with an ST segment MI were older (72 vs 66 years, $p < 0.001$) and had a higher mortality rate during hospitalization (16.7 vs 11.5%, odds ratio [OR] 1.54, 95% CI, 1.51,1.57). When evaluated by age groups, women age 30–59 years were more likely to have diabetes (OR 2.14), hypertension (OR 1.45), history of CHF (OR 1.95), and history of previous stroke (OR 1.73) than their male counterparts, but no significant differences were apparent in the older age groups. At all ages, women were less likely than men to have had a prior MI and percutaneous or surgical revascularization procedure *(3)*.

GENDER AND TYPE OF ACS AT PRESENTATION

The GUSTO-II ACS Study additionally classified patients according to clinical syndrome at presentation and enrolled 4131 patients with ST-segment elevation MI and

8011 patients with non-ST-segment elevation MI or unstable angina (Fig. 2). Interestingly, fewer women than men presented with ST-segment MI (27 vs 37%, $p < 0.001$), and for the remainder of the patients with non-ST-segment MI unstable angina, approx 37% of women had an infarction when compared to 48% of men. Furthermore, examination of the baseline clinical characteristics of patients who presented with an acute ST-segment elevation MI revealed that female gender was an independent predictor of the absence of ST-segment elevation at presentation. Conversely, among patients that presented with non-ST-segment MI, women were more likely than men to present with unstable angina *(4)*.

PREHOSPITAL EVALUATION OF CHEST PAIN

It has been suggested that there is a gender-based bias in the prehospital evaluation of ACS patients. In a series of 1306 men and 965 women who presented to the Emergency Department with an ACS between 1985 and 1992 in Olmsted County, MN, women were older and less likely to have typical chest pain symptoms. They were also less likely to undergo both noninvasive and invasive diagnostic cardiac procedures. In contrast, male sex was associated with a 24% increase in the use of cardiac procedures, yet, despite this utilization of resources, men had an increased risk of major adverse cardiac events in comparison to women *(13)*. In a similar study, women were less likely to receive a 12-lead EKG and be treated with aspirin than men with analogous symptoms *(14)*. Interestingly, in a survey of 10,689 patients seeking medical attention at an Emergency Department for chest pain evaluation, ACS patients were more likely not to be hospitalized if they were women less than 55 years of age (OR for discharge 6.7; 95% CI, 1.4–32.5), nonwhite (OR 2.2; 1.1–4.3), reported shortness of breath as their chief symptom (OR 2.7; 1.1–6.5), or had a normal or nondiagnostic electrocardiogram (ECG; OR 3.3; 1.7–6.3; *15*).

NONINVASIVE EVALUATION

The most widely employed and studied diagnostic modality for CHD diagnosis in patients that present with ACSs is the exercise treadmill test. Generally, the exercise treadmill test has been reported to have a lower diagnostic accuracy in women than men. In fact, meta-analysis has demonstrated a significantly lower specificity of ST-segment depression on treadmill tests in women when compared to men *(16)*, and, contrary to what is observed in men, resting ST-segment abnormalities in women do not predict exercise stress test outcome independent of other clinical risk factors for CHD *(17)*. The addition of the Duke Treadmill Score, a weighted index that combines treadmill time, exercise-induced anginal symptoms, and ST-segment deviation, to interpretation of exercise treadmill tests has been shown to improve diagnostic accuracy and is performed better in women than men for excluding CHD *(16)*. In fact, a low exercise capacity, one component of the Duke Treadmill Score, has been shown to predict angiographically significant epicardial coronary disease in women *(18)*. For women, a low-risk Duke Treadmill Score is associated with a 97% 5-year survival, with approx 80% of these patients having no evidence of angiographically detectable epicardial coronary artery disease (CAD). Women with high-risk Duke Treadmill Scores have multivessel disease confirmed in 70% of patients at angiography; however, because of early intervention, the 5-year survival rate is 90% *(19)*.

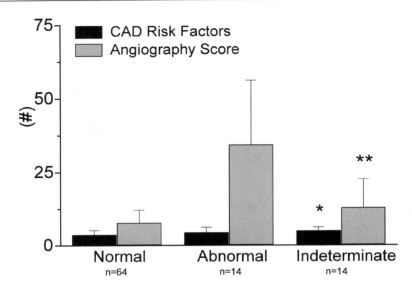

Fig. 3. Dobutamine stress echocardiography and CAD in women. A dobutamine stress echocardiography protocol reliably determines significant CAD in women who present with chest pain and have suspected epicardial coronary stenoses. In fact, although number of risk factors does not correlate with study outcome, women with abnormal studies are more likely to have a higher (more disease) angiography score. CAD, coronary artery disease. $*p < 0.009$, $**p < 0.0001$ (22).

Myocardial perfusion imaging has improved the diagnostic accuracy of noninvasive stress testing in ACS patients and increased sensitivity to 84–90% and 75–87% specificity in women, yet may still be limited in patients that are obese or have large breasts (20). A recent study of 3213 women and 5458 men who underwent exercise treadmill stress testing with myocardial perfusion imaging demonstrated that more women than men had a false-positive test, whereas the false-negative rate was significantly lower in women than men. In fact, women who underwent stress testing with imaging had a lower test sensitivity and positive predictive value, but higher test specificity, negative predictive value, and accuracy in comparison to men (21).

Exercise and pharmacological stress echocardiography have been increasingly utilized as diagnostic and prognostic modalities in women with ACS. In one study of 92 women with chest pain or symptoms suggestive of myocardial ischemia, 78 women had normal left ventricular (LV) wall motion at baseline and during peak dobutamine infusion while the remaining 14 women had wall-motion abnormalities during dobutamine infusion (Fig. 3). Coronary angiography revealed that 25 women had greater than or equal to 50% stenosis, 10 of whom had abnormal dobutamine studies, yielding a 40% and 60% sensitivity for multivessel disease, whereas specificity was determined to be 81% (22).

To examine the prognostic significance of pharmacological stress echocardiography, 456 women who underwent stress testing with dipyridamole or dobutamine were followed for a mean of 32 months. In this study, 51 patients had a positive stress test and, over the study period, 23 cardiac events occurred. Echocardiographical evidence of ischemia was found to be the only death and MI predictor (OR 27.5; 95% confi-

Table 2
Gender Differences in Number of Vessels Diseased in Patients Who Present With ACS

Number of vessels diseased	Men (n = 2,879) (#, %)	Women (n = 1,276) (#, %)
0	275 (10)	293 (23)
1	873 (30)	364 (29)
2	836 (29)	299 (23)
3	895 (31)	320 (25)

Source: ref *4.*

dence interval [CI], 6.5–111.5). Three-year survival for women with a negative stress test was 99.5% when compared to 69.5% for women with a positive stress test *(23).*

CORONARY ANGIOGRAPHY

Among women referred for coronary angiography, the magnitude and frequency of anginal-type chest pain classified as an ACS, yet occurs in the absence of a significant coronary artery stenosis, is of practical importance but remains largely unexplained. It has been shown that women are five times as likely as men to have normal coronary angiograms at catheterization *(24,25).* Although this suggests that women are being referred inappropriately for catheterization, it may be that chest pain in women results from nonobstructive or nonepicardial CAD. In fact, women with unstable angina that had cardiac catheterization as part of the GUSTO-II ACS trial were more likely to have no significant CAD than their male counterparts (30.5 vs 13.9%, $p < 0.001$), as were women who presented with a non-ST-segment elevation MI (Table 2). Numerous clinical syndromes have been implicated in this phenomenon, including mitral valve prolapse, vasospastic angina, microvascular endothelial dysfunction *(26)* as well as hypothyroidism, neuromuscular disorders, hemachromatosis, and tacchyarrhythmias are associated with cardiomyopathy *(27).* In one study of 48 women with chest pain and angiographically normal coronary arteries, approx 60% had abnormal flow velocity response to intracoronary adenosine, which indicates an abnormal coronary microcirculation *(28).* This was confirmed in a larger study that further demonstrated that neither CAD risk factors nor hormone levels predicted coronary microvascular dysfunction (Table 3; *29).* Intravascular evaluation to examine subangiographic atheroma has provided some additional insight. In a small trial, subangiographic disease (intimal thickness > 0.3 mm) was detected in patients by intravascular ultrasound. However, the presence of these luminal irregularities did not correlate with endothelial dysfunction *(30).*

Women who are found to have significant or multivessel epicardial CAD by angiography present with the same degree of disease as men pertaining to lesion severity and distribution *(24,25),* including the prevalence of left-main and three-vessel disease *(31).* In fact, over a 16-year period, there was no significant gender related difference observed with respect to the degree and localization of coronary lesions in patients with angiographically documented CAD. Notably, there was a significant shift from the diagnosis of multivessel disease toward the diagnosis of single-vessel disease in both men and women, indicating that over time, cardiac catheterization had become

Table 3
Risk Factors for Impaired Coronary Flow Reserve for Women With Chest Pain
and Normal Coronary Angiograms

Risk Factor	Odds ratio	95% Confidence interval	P
Current tobacco use	0.78	(0.35–1.73)	NS
Hypertension	1.39	(0.74–2.6)	NS
Diabetes mellitus	1.27	(0.56–2.92)	NS
Hyperlipidemia	1.27	(0.66–2.45)	NS
Current hormone replacement therapy	0.44	(0.22–0.91)	0.026

Source: ref. 29.

increasingly utilized in a wider patient subset earlier in the course of their disease. As to subsequent management, there was no difference following angiography regarding referral for percutaneous or surgical revascularization procedures (32).

CORONARY ANGIOPLASTY

Clinical, Angiographic, and Procedural Characteristics

Women who are offered percutaneous coronary revascularization procedures as a therapeutic modality often have clinical characteristics that are associated with an increased risk of major adverse events. For example, women tend to be older and have a higher prevalence of diabetes mellitus, hypertension, and hypercholesterolemia in comparison to men. Fewer women have had a prior MI or have evidence of LV dysfunction when compared to men, yet women tend to have more CHF episodes (33–36), which has been attributed to an increased prevalence of diastolic dysfunction (37,38). Additionally, women are more likely to be considered suboptimal candidates for surgical revascularization owing to more significant comorbid disease than men.

At catheterization, women have smaller diameter coronary arteries, yet coronary lesion morphology and distribution is similar to that in men, and women tend to have more ostial lesions and calcified lesions (33). The implications of small-vessel size were evaluated in a large contemporary series. In 2306 patients undergoing percutaneous revascularization, patients were divided into groups with reference vessel diameters less than or equal to 2.5 mm or more than 2.5 mm. Patients with smaller vessels were more often female, older, and more likely to have multivessel disease or a type C lesion at angiography. Smaller vessel size and lesion morphology significantly influenced device utilization. In contrast to stents (18.5% vs 41.9%) and directional atherectomy (3.7% vs 13.5%), balloon angioplasty (73% vs 50%) and rotational atherectomy (16.1% vs 8.3%) were used more frequently in smaller vessels. This was associated with an increase in major adverse cardiac events, occurring more often in patients with small, as opposed to large, vessels (39).

It has been suggested in some series that women who undergo contemporary revascularization procedures are at higher risk for procedural complications. This poor outcome has been partly attributed to an increased susceptibility to plaque disruption during the procedure. In fact, women who underwent angioplasty had similar procedural success rates as men; however, there was a significant increase in plaque dissection incidence during intervention, with a consequent increased need for unplanned coronary stent placement (70.4 vs 52.2%, $p < 0.05$) to achieve an adequate final result. Despite stent placement, coronary artery dissection was associated with an increased risk of complications during the procedure *(40)*.

Acute and Long-Term Outcome

Historically, women undergoing coronary angioplasty were reported to have a lower procedural success rate than men *(41)*. However, recent studies have demonstrated a similar angiographic outcome, incidence of periprocedural MI, and need for emergent CABG in women compared to men *(33,42)*. Despite improvements in the procedural success rate for women, in-hospital mortality remains significantly higher, and in some studies, an independent gender effect on acute mortality following coronary angioplasty persists after adjustment for baseline differences in clinical and angiographic characteristics *(33,35)*. Although there is no clear etiology for this mortality increase, both small-vessel caliber and hypertensive heart disease have been implicated. It has also been suggested that women poorly tolerate periods of transient ischemia during angioplasty, which results in a higher incidence of periprocedural CHF and pulmonary edema *(42,43)*. In fact, CHF has been shown to be a gender-independent predictor of mortality in patients undergoing coronary angioplasty *(33,35)*.

Interestingly, it has been shown that women manifest different autonomic and hemodynamic responses to abrupt coronary occlusion than men. In a series of 140 men and 65 women undergoing single-vessel percutaneous coronary intervention (PCI), total occlusion of a coronary vessel was associated with more pronounced ST-segment changes and chest pain in women than men. There was also a higher incidence of significant bradycardia (31% vs 13%) or a heart rate increase variability (25% vs 11%), accompanied by a decrease in blood pressure observed in women when compared to men *(44)*.

In the New Approaches to Coronary Intervention (NACI) Registry, women undergoing percutaneous revascularization with new devices had a higher risk clinical profile, yet, when compared to men, a similar procedural success rate with final percent diameter stenosis and Thrombolysis in Myocardial Infarction (TIMI) flow grade (Fig. 4). However, women did experience a higher percentage of periprocedural complications, including coronary artery dissection, need for vascular access repair, hypotension, and transfusion. There was no significant gender-based difference in the rate of in-hospital death, ST-elevation MI and emergent CABG, and gender was not found to be an independent predictor of major adverse cardiac events. At 1-year follow-up, more women than men reported an improvement in their anginal symptoms (70% vs 62%), and fewer women than men required repeat revascularization (32% vs 36%) *(45)*. Furthermore, the outcome of coronary angioplasty in women has improved *(46)*, and these benefits may be realized as much as 5 years after percutaneous revascularization, as demonstrated in the Bypass Angioplasty Revascularization (BARI) trial. At an average of 5.4 year follow-up, mortality rates were similar between gender (12.8% vs 12.0%, respectively) and after adjustment for baseline differences, women had a significantly lower risk of death *(42)*.

Unstable Angina/Non-ST-Segment MI

Women who present with unstable angina/non-ST-segment MI that are managed by percutaneous revascularization procedures are consistently older and have an increased

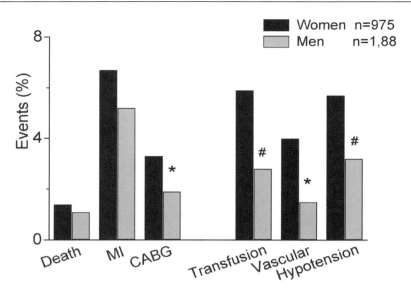

Fig. 4. Influence of gender on in-hospital and procedural outcomes in patients treated in the new device era. In the New Approaches to Coronary Intervention (NACI) Registry, women had a higher rate of procedural complications and were more likely to require CABG surgery than men. MI, myocardial infarction; CABG, coronary artery bypass grafting. $*p < 0.05$, $\# p < 0.01$ *(45)*.

hypertension incidence with a preserved LV ejection fraction (EF) when compared with their male counterparts. Interestingly, as demonstrated in the TIMI-IIIB trial, women who presented with unstable angina were less likely to have significant obstructive epicardial CAD than men at angiography, yet the 42-day rate of death and MI remained similar *(12)*. Similarly, in the Global Unstable Angina Registry and Treatment Evaluation (GUARANTEE) Registry, coronary angiography revealed less severe CAD in women, and, in fact, women were more likely than men to have insignificant CAD at angiography (25% vs 14%, $p = 0.0001$; *47*).

In women with significant CAD who undergo percutaneous revascularization procedures prior to hospital discharge, there are conflicting data regarding outcome and survival. In one report, 941 women who required percutaneous coronary revascularization procedures for management of an ACS had similar success, in-hospital mortality, and emergency CABG rates as men. During a mean 4-year follow-up, overall survival was comparable between women and men. Although the occurrence of severe angina was higher in women than in men during this time, women were less likely to undergo CABG revascularization procedures *(48)*.

Conversely, several studies have demonstrated a significant increase in mortality for women who presented with unstable angina when compared to men. In one study of 101 women who presented with a non-ST-segment elevation MI (Table 4) that had a percutaneous revascularization procedure predischarge, angioplasty was equally successful in women and men with fewer lesions dilated per patient in women (1.38 vs 1.51, $p < 0.04$). In-hospital major adverse cardiac events were similar between men and women, although there was a trend toward a higher in-hospital death rate in women (4% vs 1%, $p = 0.058$), and at 1-year follow-up, women had a significantly worse survival rate than men (89% vs 95%, $p < 0.04$). CABG was performed less commonly in

Table 4
Influence of Gender on Outcome in Patients With Non-ST-Segment Elevation MI Undergoing
Percutaneous Revascularization Prior to Discharge

	Women (n = 101)	Men (n = 275)	P
Age (years)	68 ± 10	61 ± 11	< 0.001
Hypertension (%)	67	51	< 0.01
LVEF (%)	50 ± 10	47 ± 11	< 0.001
Procedural success (%)	96	97	NS
No. lesions dilated	1.38	1.51	< 0.04
In-hospital mortality (%)	4	1	0.058
1-year survival (%)	89	95	< 0.04

Source: ref. 49.

women by the end of 1 year than in men, whereas the rate of repeat percutaneous revascularization procedures was similar *(49)*. Other investigators have reported in-hospital mortality rates up to three times higher for women than men (9.3 vs 3.0%), and, when assessed using a logistic regression model, the association between gender and mortality was not significantly altered when corrected for age, ST-segment EKG changes, and CAD risk factors *(50)*.

MI

Historically, several studies have documented a worse prognosis for women post-MI than men in both the pre- and pharmacological reperfusion era *(51)*. In-hospital mortality in the Multicenter Investigation of the Limitation of Infarct Size (MILIS) trial was 13% in women in comparison to 7% in men, and cumulative mortality at 4 years was 36% in women and 21% in men. Even after adjustment for advanced age, women continued to have a worse prognosis following an acute ST-segment elevation MI *(51)*. In the thrombolytic era, women with AMI treated with these agents were found to have similar 90-minute patency rates, EF, and regional ventricular function when compared to men, yet 30-day mortality rates were significantly higher (13.1% vs 4.8%, $p < 0.0001$), which suggests a gender-based influence on mortality *(52)*.

Some of these early observed differences in outcome may actually reflect differences in the utilization of percutaneous revascularization procedures in women in comparison with men. In the Myocardial Infarction Triage and Intervention (MITI) Registry, women were half as likely to undergo acute coronary angiography or angioplasty as men and had twice the in-hospital mortality *(53)*. Similarly, in the Atherosclerosis Risk in Communities (ARIC) study, women hospitalized for MI were less likely to undergo percutaneous revascularization, suggesting that the observed gender difference in mortality may be associated with a decreased likelihood of women being referred for acute interventions *(54)*. Review of 1737 patients admitted to a cardiac intensive care unit with AMI diagnosis revealed that women took longer to seek medical attention, and, once evaluated, were less likely to receive immediate aspirin therapy (88 vs 91%, $p < 0.03$) and had longer door-to-needle times for thrombolytic therapy administration (90 vs 78 minutes, $p < 0.004$) in comparison to men. This was associated with a decreased 30-day survival for women when compared to men (78 vs 88%), which persisted following adjustment for age, racial group, and diabetes *(55)*.

Table 5
Influence of Age and Gender on Diagnostic Catheterization
Rates Post-MI

Age (years)	Women (%)	Men (%)
65–69	56.1	60.4
70–74	50.3	55.4
75–79	40.3	45.0
80–84	24.7	29.8
≥ 85	8.5	11.8

Interestingly, the Cooperative Cardiovascular Project, which reviewed records from 138,956 Medicare beneficiaries (49% of them women) admitted with an acute MI (AMI) in 1994 or 1995, revealed that women of all age groups were less likely to be referred for coronary angiography than men (Table 5). This was especially noted in women age 85 years or older. Therapeutic interventions were less frequently offered to women. In fact, women were less likely than men to be administered thrombolytic agents within 60 minutes or receive aspirin within the first 24 hours of admission. Yet, despite these differences in treatment, 30-day mortality rates between gender were similar (56).

Compared with men, women are at an increased risk for early and late morbidity and mortality post-AMI. Aggressive pharmacological reperfusion therapies with thrombolytic agents have reduced in-hospital mortality by 25–30%; however, women are more likely than men to have a contraindication to thrombolysis (43 vs 29%, $p < 0.02$; 57). Therefore, to overcome the limitations associated with thrombolytic agents, mechanical reperfusion by primary angioplasty has been advocated as a therapeutic intervention.

Primary Angioplasty

Percutaneous revascularization strategies to restore coronary patency during AMI without prior or concomitant thrombolytic therapy, or primary angioplasty, has been shown to result in a higher infarct-related artery patency rate (58), smaller enzymatic infarct size, preservation of LV function and a better clinical outcome in comparison to thrombolytic therapy (59,60). Additionally, it has been suggested by pooled analysis of early clinical trials that primary angioplasty additionally offers a cardiovascular morbidity and mortality benefit to patients. This analysis demonstrated a 44% reduction in mortality during hospitalization (OR 0.56, CI 0.53–0.94) and a 9% reduction in mortality at 1-year follow-up (61). Yet, despite the apparent survival benefit, and because women have been reported to be more likely than men to accept elective catheterization (62), women are also more likely to refuse emergent cardiac catheterization during AMI as a therapeutic modality (63).

Women who present with an acute ST-segment elevation MI comprise a higher risk patient population when compared to men. For example, in The Primary Angioplasty in Myocardial Infarction (PAMI) trial, which compared primary angioplasty with tissue-type plasminogen activator, women were older (65.7 vs 57.7 years, $p < 0.0001$) and presented later after symptom onset than their male counterparts (229 vs 174 minutes, $p = 0.0004$). The in-hospital mortality for women was 3.3-fold higher than men (9.3%

vs 2.8%, $p = 0.0005$; *64*). This gender-specific increase could not be explained by differences in infarct location or hemodynamic status at presentation. Women were less likely than men to have an angioplasty performed because of a greater likelihood of a noncritical stenosis in the infarct artery, and conversely, a higher surgical disease prevalence. In women that did undergo percutaneous revascularization, the in-hospital mortality rate was not significantly different in comparison to men (4.0% vs 2.1%). In fact, percutaneous revascularization and younger age were independent predictors of in-hospital survival in women. Importantly, intracranial hemorrhage occurred in 5.3% of women treated with a thrombolytic agent when compared with 0.7% men ($p = 0.037$), yet, there was no increase in bleeding events, with primary angioplasty, regardless of gender. These observations suggest that primary angioplasty improves women's survival, such that it is comparable to men and reduces the risk of cerebrovascular hemorrhage associated with thrombolytic therapy *(64,65)*.

One potential reason that women with AMI may have a worse prognosis than men is that they tend to present for treatment much later after symptom onset. To determine the influence of late presentation on the efficacy of primary angioplasty, a study of 496 patients who underwent primary angioplasty for AMI specifically evaluated outcome in patients treated between 6 and 24 hours. Significantly, these patients were more often female. Primary angioplasty performed that followed late presentation was often less successful in comparison to patients with early presentation, resulting in a greater reduction of LV function. Patients treated late following presentation were also more likely to have reocclusion of the infarct artery, repeat MI and a significantly higher mortality rate at 6 months *(66)*.

As coronary stents are increasingly used in primary revascularization procedures, the Stent-PAMI trial compared coronary stent implantation with balloon angioplasty for AMI treatment. At 6-month follow-up, fewer patients in the stent group than in the angioplasty group had angina (11.3% vs 16.9%, $p = 0.02$) or needed target-vessel revascularization because of ischemia (7.7% vs 17%, $p < 0.001$). The combined primary endpoint of death, reinfarction, disabling stroke, or target-vessel revascularization from ischemia occurred in fewer patients in the stent group than in the angioplasty group (12.6% vs 20.1%, $p < 0.01$; *67*). Women enrolled in this trial were older (66 +/– 12 vs 58 +/– 12 yr, $p < 0.0001$), had a higher incidence of hypertension, hypercholesterolemia, diabetes, and a smaller size infarct-related artery when compared to men. Although core laboratory analysis revealed that TIMI-3 flow tended to be restored in a greater percentage of women than men (94% vs 90.0%, $p = 0.07$), women had increased rates of 6-month mortality (7.9% vs 2.0%, $p = 0.0002$), reinfarction (6.4% vs 2.7%, $p = 0.01$), and stroke (2.0% vs 0.3%, $p = 0.01$), with similar rates of late target-vessel revascularization. This suggests that women undergoing mechanical reperfusion in the stent era remain at high risk for adverse events *(68)*. These observations were confirmed in a study of 230 women and 789 men who underwent primary angioplasty or stent placement between 1995 and 1999 (Fig. 5). Women in this study had a higher rate of nonfatal reinfarction (3 vs 1%, $p < 0.01$) and mortality (12 vs 7%, $p < 0.03$) at 6-month follow-up. Despite these findings, multivariate analysis revealed that gender was not an independent mortality predictor *(69)*.

It has also been suggested that women tend to have a poor outcome even when anticoagulant or antiplatelet agents are used in conjunction with primary angioplasty. A pooled analysis of women enrolled in the GUSTO IIb trial (primary angioplasty vs

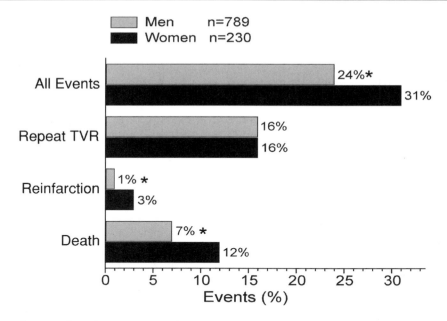

Fig. 5. Influence of gender on outcome following primary angioplasty. In patients with an acute ST-segment MI treated with primary angioplasty and/or coronary stent placement, women are more likely to have a major adverse event than men. TVR, target-vessel revascularization. *$p < 0.05$ (69).

accelerated tissue plasminogen activator (t-PA) and heparin vs hirudin in a factorial design) or the ReoPro and Primary Percutaneous Transluminal Coronary Angioplasty [PTCA] Organization and Randomized Trial (RAPPORT) (abciximab vs placebo in primary angioplasty) demonstrated that women treated with anticoagulant or antiplatelet agents had a significant increase in the risk of death (42% vs 25%, $p = 0.02$) as well as a trend toward a combined endpoint of death or recurrent MI (34% vs 25%, $p = 0.08$) compared to women treated with placebo. Moreover, increased age was found to be associated with a higher mortality rate and independent predictor of mortality and repeat infarction at 30 days (70).

CARDIOGENIC SHOCK

Cardiogenic shock, recognized clinically as systemic hypotension, accompanied by end-organ hypoperfusion and elevated cardiac filling pressures, complicates AMI in 5–15% of patients (71). Patients who present with or develop cardiogenic shock tend to be older, have more CHD risk factors, are more likely to have had a prior MI and preexisting LV dysfunction, CABG surgery, and importantly, are more likely to be women (72).

To determine the role of mechanical reperfusion therapies in the treatment of cardiogenic shock, the SHOCK (SHould we emergently revascularize Occluded Coronary arteries for cardiogenic shocK) trial was conducted (73,74). This multicenter trial randomized 302 patients with AMI complicated by shock because of LV dysfunction confirmed by both clinical and hemodynamic criteria and assigned approx 37% of women to revascularization and 27% to medical therapy. There was no significant difference in

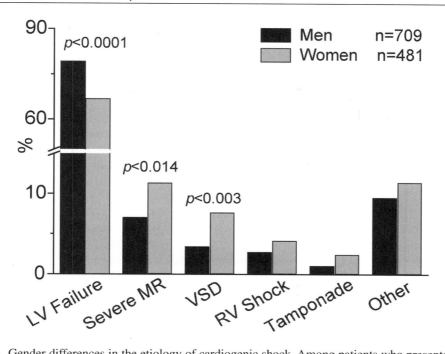

Fig. 6. Gender differences in the etiology of cardiogenic shock. Among patients who presented with or developed cardiogenic shock complicating an AMI, women were less likely than men to present with LV failure yet more likely to have shock owing to a mechanical complication. MR, mitral regurgitation; VSD, ventricular septal defect; RV, right ventricle *(78)*.

30-day mortality between treatment groups (46.7% vs 56.0%), yet by 6 months, there was a survival benefit for patients who underwent revascularization procedures. Of note, age was shown to influence percutaneous revascularization outcome, such that at both 30 days and 6 months, patients 75 years or age or older had a worse outcome if they underwent any (percutaneous or surgical) revascularization procedure *(73)*. As women who present with acute ST-elevation MI and develop cardiogenic shock are often older, these findings suggest that revascularization procedures may not improve mortality and, in fact, may predict a worse outcome in this subset of women.

Importantly, a total of 1107 patients were screened for the SHOCK trial and deemed ineligible and therefore entered into a registry. Women accounted for approx 40% of SHOCK Registry patients and had similar cardiogenic shock rates owing to LV failure as men; however, women were more likely to have mechanical complications, including acute severe mitral regurgitation *(75)*, ventricular septal rupture *(76)*, or isolated right ventricular shock *(77)*, than men (Fig. 6; *78*). Of these diagnoses, shock owing to ventricular septal rupture was associated with a significant increase in mortality compared to shock secondary to LV dysfunction *(77)*. Interestingly, among 884 patients with predominant shock because of LV dysfunction, there was no significant mortality difference between women and men, albeit the mortality rate for the entire cohort was high (61%; *78*). Notably, women entered in the Registry had a higher diabetes incidence than women in the trial, and angiographic data revealed that these patients had significantly more two- and three-vessel disease, yet the revascularization rate (combined percutaneous and surgical) for these patients was lower than that for nondiabetic patients with single-vessel disease *(79)*.

GLYCOPROTEIN IIB/IIIA RECEPTOR ANTAGONISTS

Platelet aggregation and thrombus formation have been implicated in ACS pathophysiology and have been shown to complicate percutaneous revascularization procedures. Although aspirin has been utilized as the primary antiplatelet agent, a meta-analysis of randomized trials of aspirin therapy revealed that despite a 25% reduction in cardiac event risk, only one-third of postmenopausal women were taking aspirin daily, and the majority of these women were doing so for primary prevention *(80,81)*. Additionally, it has been revealed that women are less likely to receive aspirin on hospital admission or to be discharged on aspirin than their male counterparts *(82)*. Based on these observations, inhibitors of the glycoprotein IIb/IIIa receptor, a receptor on the platelet surface that mediates platelet aggregation, have been developed and have demonstrated efficacy in clinical trials in the medical stabilization of ACS patients *(83)*. As it has been suggested that there is a gender-based difference in platelet function, and women are believed to have hyper-reactive platelets, therefore, it follows that women may receive greater benefit from glycoprotein IIb/IIIa receptor antagonist administration *(84)*.

To evaluate the role of glycoprotein IIb/IIIa receptor antagonists in the initial medical management of ACS patients, the Platelet Receptor Inhibition in Ischemic Syndrome Management in Patients Limited by Unstable Signs and Symptoms (PRISM-PLUS) trial randomized 1915 patients with ACS to tirofiban or placebo and, for patients treated with tirofiban when compared to placebo, demonstrated a 32% reduction in the composite endpoint of death, MI, refractory ischemia or rehospitalization for recurrent ischemia, at 7 days, a 22% reduction at 30 days, and a 19% decrease at 6 months. Tirofiban-treated women had a 30% reduction in 7-day event that was similar to the 27% reduction observed in men *(85)*. Interestingly, when the glycoprotein IIb/IIIa antagonist eptifibatide was utilized in a similar population of women in the Platelet Glycoprotein IIb/IIIa in Unstable Angina: Receptor Suppression Using Integrilin Therapy (PURSUIT) trial, these benefits were not as readily recognized. This study randomized 10,948 patients who presented with an ACS to an eptifibatide or placebo infusion. Eptifibatide treatment was associated with a significant reduction in the incidence of MI and treatment effect consistently favored eptifibatide in all major subgroups except women (OR for women, 1.10; 95% CI, 0.91–1.34); however, trial data review revealed that there was a geographical disparity in outcomes, and for women in North America, there was a benefit associated with treatment with eptifibatide (incidence of the composite endpoint: among men, 16.2% in the placebo group vs 12.4% in the eptifibatide group; $p = 0.006$; among women, 12.9% vs 10.6%, respectively; $p = 0.19$; *86)*.

Glycoprotein IIb/IIIa antagonists have also demonstrated therapeutic efficacy as adjunctive agents for percutaneous revascularization procedures. In women with ACS that underwent PCI and were treated with abciximab in the Evaluation of Platelet IIb/IIIa Inhibition for Prevention of Ischemic Complications (EPIC), Evaluation of PTCA to Improve Long-term Outcome with Abciximab GP IIb/IIIa Receptor Blockade (EPILOG), and Evaluation of Platelet IIb/IIIa Inhibition for Stenting (EPISTENT) trials, there was a significant reduction in the primary endpoint of death, MI, or urgent revascularization at 30 days (12.7% to 6.5%, $p < 0.001$). This decrease persisted at 6 months (16.0% vs 9.9%, $p < 0.001$) and at 1 year, there was a mortality reduction from 4% to 2.5% for abciximab-treated women *(87)*. In the EPISTENT trial, women treated with abciximab who underwent balloon angioplasty fared better than if a stent was placed without abciximab therapy (5.1% vs 11.7% event rate, $p < 0.0021$), a finding that contrasted the observation in men *(88)*. At 1-year follow-up, abciximab and stent placement resulted in a lower mortality rate than either coronary stent placement or abciximab alone (placebo plus stent, 2.4%, abciximab plus PTCA, 2.1%, abciximab plus stent, 1.0%; *89*).

Of note, diabetic women, a high-risk subset of women, appeared to benefit significantly from abciximab administration during percutaneous revascularization procedures. Although there were no differences in outcome noted at 30 days or 6 months, at 1 year there was a significant reduction in the combined endpoint of death, MI or target-vessel revascularization in women treated with abciximab who had a stent placed or underwent balloon angioplasty (13.3% vs 28.9% vs 34.5%, $p = 0.02$ for stent-stent comparison and $p = 0.09$ for stent-abciximab and balloon-abciximab comparison). This benefit resulted from a significant reduction in 1 year target-vessel revascularization rates, which were reduced from 21.1% in stent-placebo and 26.7% in balloon-abciximab to 4.5% in stent-abciximab $p = 0.02$ for stent-stent comparison and $p = 0.004$ for stent-abciximab and balloon-abciximab comparison; *90*). Consequently, abciximab did not increase major bleeding events, but there was an increase in minor bleeding events (4.7% vs 6.7%), and, in fact, female gender, abciximab use, and age above 70 years were independent predictors of an increased bleeding risk *(90)*.

Women treated with eptifibatide during percutaneous coronary revascularization procedures had a significant reduction in the rate of death, MI, urgent revascularization, or bailout stent placement (11.6% to 9.1% $p = 0.04$), which was not associated with a significant increase in bleeding *(91)*. To extend these observations to contemporary percutaneous revascularization procedures, the Enhanced Suppression of the Platelet IIb/IIIa Receptor with Integrelin Therapy (ESPRIT) trial was conducted to evaluate the eptifibatide's efficacy with stent implantation. The ESPRIT trial enrolled 2064 patients and demonstrated a 37% relative reduction in the combined endpoint of death, MI, and urgent target vessel revascularization at 48 hours, and a 36% relative reduction at 30 days. Subgroup analysis revealed that women treated with eptifibatide had a 58% relative reduction in events when compared with women treated with placebo, thereby demonstrating that women benefited significantly from eptifibatide administration as an adjunct to coronary stent placement *(92–97)*.

These studies suggest that women with ACS who undergo percutaneous revascularization procedures, particularly diabetic women, will benefit from the administration of a glycoprotein IIb/IIIa receptor antagonist; however, the risk-benefit profile regarding bleeding complications may ultimately determine the use of one of these glycoprotein IIb/IIIa receptor antagonists, as well as the choice of agent.

SURGICAL REVASCULARIZATION

Advances in surgical techniques and myocardial protection have increased the availability of surgical revascularization procedures for women with ACS found to have coronary anatomy that warrants surgical intervention. In spite of these advances, surgical mortality rates have been notably consistent over the past 20 years, and in-hospital

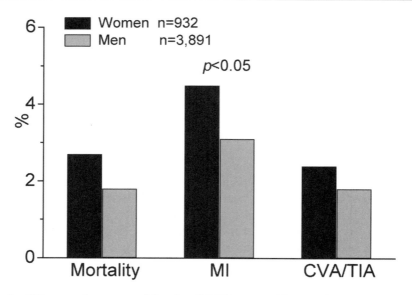

Fig. 7. Gender differences in outcome following CABG surgery. Women who undergo contemporary CABG surgery procedures do so with a similar mortality outcome as men; however, women are more likely to have a MI than their male counterparts. MI, myocardial infarction; CVA/TIA, cerebrovascular accident/transient ischemic attack *(102)*.

mortality rates for women are often two to three times higher than for men. This discrepancy in outcomes is only partially explained by older age and higher risk profiles, and, indeed, has been attributed to greater technical difficulty associated with female operation as well as the increased frequency of urgent or emergent female procedures *(98,99)*.

These observations have been confirmed in a more recent retrospective study of 4823 patients, including 932 women, undergoing CABG, which revealed significant gender-related differences in morbidity and mortality (Fig. 7). In this study, women who underwent CABG surgery were older had a smaller mean body surface area, and a higher prevalence of diabetes, hypertension, peripheral vascular disease, CHF, history of percutaneous revascularization procedures, New York Health Association class III or IV angina, and preoperative intra-aortic balloon pump usage than men. During surgery, women had fewer bypass grafts constructed than men and were less likely to have internal mammary artery grafting, multiple arterial conduits, or coronary endarterectomy performed. The early mortality rate in women in this series was 2.7% vs 1.8% in men ($p = 0.09$), and women were more likely to have a perioperative MI (4.5% vs 3.1% $p < 0.05$). Interestingly, after other risk factor adjustment, female gender was not an independent predictor of early mortality, but it was a weak independent predictor for the composite endpoint of death, perioperative MI, intra-aortic balloon pump placement, or cerebrovascular accident (8.55 vs 5.9%; OR, 1.30; 95% CI, 0.99–1.68; $p = 0.05$). Recurrent anginal symptoms occurred more frequently in female than male patients (15.2% +/– 4% vs 8.5% +/– 2% at 60 months, $p = 0.001$), but did not result in an increase in repeat percutaneous or surgical revascularization procedures *(100)*.

In women, surgical myocardial revascularization has increasingly been performed utilizing an off-pump (without cardiopulmonary bypass) technique. In a series of patients considered appropriate for off-pump revascularization procedures, the mortality for women was lower in comparison to women who underwent traditional surgical revascularization procedures, despite an older age and higher incidence of diabetes. In fact, the mortality rate for operations in women without cardiopulmonary bypass dropped to the mortality rate typically seen in men. This was associated with a shorter hospital length of stay and a lower incidence of transient ischemic attacks, cerebrovascular accidents, postoperative bleeding complications, and blood transfusions. However, these favorable outcomes in women may reflect patient selection and require further study *(101)*.

CONCLUSION

In patients with symptomatic CHD and acute ischemic syndromes, several gender-based differences in clinical presentation, evaluation, treatment strategies, and outcome have been well-documented. Women have consistently been shown to be older, with more high-risk clinical features and comorbid disease than their male counterparts. Additionally, noninvasive and invasive testing often poorly diagnose the etiology of chest pain owing to the high chest pain prevalence in the absence of a fixed epicardial coronary artery stenosis. Women who are found to have obstructive CAD often have more high-risk angiographic features than men. Based on these observations, women with ACS undergo coronary revascularization procedures with a higher risk for adverse outcomes; however, recent advances in device application, adjunctive therapies, and surgical technique suggest that coronary revascularization strategies are safe and effective.

REFERENCES

1. American Heart Association. 2001 Heart and Stroke Statistical Update. American Heart Association, Dallas, TX: 2001.
2. Wexler LF. Studies of acute coronary syndromes in women—lessons for everyone. N Engl J Med 1999;341:275–276.
3. Vaccarino V, Parsons L, Every NR, et al. Sex-based differences in early mortality after myocardial infarction. National Registry of Myocardial Infarction 2 Participants. N Engl J Med 1999;341:217–225.
4. Hochman JS, Tamis JE, Thompson TD, et al. Sex, clinical presentation, and outcome in patients with acute coronary syndromes. Global use of strategies to open occluded coronary arteries in acute coronary syndromes IIb investigators. N Engl J Med 1999;341:226–232.
5. Hu FB, Stampfer MJ, Manson JE, et al. Trends in the incidence of coronary heart disease and changes in diet and lifestyle in women. N Engl J Med 2000;343:530–537.
6. Lerner DJ, Kannel WB. Patterns of coronary heart disease morbidity and mortality in the sexes: a 26-year follow-up of the Framingham population. Am Heart J 1986;111:383–390.
7. Chaitman BR, Bourassa MG, Davis K, et al. Angiographic prevalence of high-risk coronary artery disease in patient subsets (CASS). Circulation 1981;64:360–367.
8. Milner KA, Funk M, Richards S, et al. Gender differences in symptom presentation associated with coronary heart disease. Am J Cardiol 1999;84:396–399.
9. Goldberg R, Goff D, Cooper L, et al. Age and sex differences in presentation of symptoms among patients with acute coronary disease: the REACT Trial. Rapid Early Action for Coronary Treatment. Coron Artery Dis 2000;11:399–407.
10. Goldberg RJ, O'Donnell C, Yarzebski J, et al. Sex differences in symptom presentation associated with acute myocardial infarction: a population-based perspective. Am Heart J 1998;136:189–195.
11. Sheps DS, Kaufmann PG, Sheffield D, et al. Sex differences in chest pain in patients with documented coronary artery disease and exercise-induced ischemia: Results from the PIMI study. Am Heart J 2001;142:864–871.

12. Hochman JS, McCabe CH, Stone PH, et al. Outcome and profile of women and men presenting with acute coronary syndromes: a report from TIMI IIIB. TIMI Investigators. Thrombolysis in Myocardial Infarction. J Am Coll Cardiol 1997;30:141–148.

13. Roger VL, Farkouch ME, Weston SA, et al. Sex differences in evaluation and outcome ofunstable angina. JAMA 2000;283:646–652.

14. Rothrock SG, Brandt P, Godfrey B, et al. Is there gender bias in the prehospital management of patients with acute chest pain? Prehosp Emerg Care 2001;5:331–334.

15. Pope JH, Aufdeheide TP, Ruthuzer R, et al. Missed diagnoses of acute cardiac ischemia in the emergency department. N Engl J Med 2000;342:1163–1170.

16. Alexander KP, Shaw LJ, Shaw LK, et al. Value of exercise treadmill testing in women. J Am Coll Cardiol 1998;32:1657–1664.

17. Elhendy A, van Domburg RT, Bax JJ, Raelandt JR. Gender differences in the relation between ST-T-wave abnormalities at baseline electrocardiogram and stress myocardial perfusion abnormalities in patients with suspected coronary artery disease. Am J Cardiol 1999;84:865–869.

18. Al-Khalili F, Svane B, Wamala SP, et al. Clinical importance of risk factors and exercise testing for prediction of significant coronary artery stenosis in women recovering from unstable coronary artery disease: the Stockholm Female Coronary Risk Study. Am Heart J 2000;139:971–978.

19. Shaw LJ, Hachamovitch R, Redberg RF. Current evidence on diagnostic testing in women with suspected coronary artery disease: choosing the appropriate test. Cardiol Rev 2000;8:65–74.

20. Judelson DR. Examining the Gender Bias in Evaluating Coronary Disease in Women. Medscape Womens Health 1997;2:5.

21. Miller TD, Roger VL, Milavetz JJ, et al. Assessment of the exercise electrocardiogram in women versus men using tomographic myocardial perfusion imaging as the reference standard. Am J Cardiol 2001;87:868–873.

22. Lewis JF, Lin L, McGorray S, et al. Dobutamine stress echocardiography in women with chest pain. Pilot phase data from the National Heart, Lung and Blood Institute Women's Ischemia Syndrome Evaluation (WISE). J Am Coll Cardiol 1999;33:1462–1468.

23. Cortigiani L, Dodi C, Paolini EA, et al. Prognostic value of pharmacological stress echocardiography in women with chest pain and unknown coronary artery disease. J Am Coll Cardiol 1998;32:1975–1981.

24. Jong P, Mohammed S, Sternberg L. Sex differences in the features of coronary artery disease of patients undergoing coronary angiography [published erratum appears in Can J Cardiol 1996 Sep; 12(9): 781]. Can J Cardiol 1996;12:671–677.

25. Sullivan AK, Holdright DR, Wright CA, et al. Chest pain in women: clinical, investigative, and prognostic features. BMJ 1994;308:883–886.

26. Douglas PS, Ginsburg GS. The evaluation of chest pain in women. N Engl J Med 1996;334:1311–1315.

27. Molzer G, Finsterer J, Krugluger W, et al. Possible causes of symptoms in suspected coronary heart disease but normal angiograms. Clin Cardiol 2001;24:307–312.

28. Reis SE, Holubkov R, Lee JS, et al. Coronary flow velocity response to adenosine characterizes coronary microvascular function in women with chest pain and no obstructive coronary disease. Results from the pilot phase of the Women's Ischemia Syndrome Evaluation (WISE) study. J Am Coll Cardiol 1999;33:1469–1475.

29. Reis SE, Holubkov R, Conrad Smith AJ, et al. Coronary microvascular dysfunction is highly prevalent in women with chest pain in the absence of coronary artery disease: results from the NHLBI WISE study. Am Heart J 2001;141:735–741.

30. Cox ID, Clague JR, Bagger JP, et al. Endothelial dysfunction, subangiographic atheroma, and unstable symptoms in patients with chest pain and normal coronary arteriograms. Clin Cardiol 2000;23:645–652.

31. Bernstein SJ, Hilborne LH, Leape LL, et al. The appropriateness of use of cardiovascular procedures in women and men. Arch Intern Med 1994;154:2759–2765.

32. Roeters van Lennep JE, Zwinderman AH, Roeters van Lennep HW, et al. Gender differences in diagnosis and treatment of coronary artery disease from 1981 to 1997. No evidence for the Yentl syndrome. Eur Heart J 2000;21:911–918.

33. Kelsey SF, James M, Holubkov AL, et al. Results of percutaneous transluminal coronary angioplasty in women. 1985–1986 National Heart, Lung, and Blood Institute's Coronary Angioplasty Registry. Circulation 1993;87:720–727.

34. Bell MR, Holmes DR Jr, Berger PP, et al. The changing in-hospital mortality of women undergoing percutaneous transluminal coronary angioplasty. JAMA 1993;269:2091–2095.

35. Malenka DJ, O'Connor GT, Quinton H, et al. Differences in outcomes between women and men associated with percutaneous transluminal coronary angioplasty. A regional prospective study of 13,061 procedures. Northern New England Cardiovascular Disease Study Group. Circulation 1996;94(9 Suppl):II99–II104.

36. Welty FK, Mittleman MA, Healy RW, et al. Similar results of percutaneous transluminal coronary angioplasty for women and men with postmyocardial infarction ischemia. J Am Coll Cardiol 1994;23:35–39.

37. Mendes LA, Davidoff R, Cuppies LA, et al. Congestive heart failure in patients with coronary artery disease: the gender paradox. Am Heart J 1997;132:207–212.

38. Mendes LA, Davidoff R, Capples LA, et al. The gender paradox. Rev Port Cardiol 1999;18(Suppl 3):III21–III24.

39. Schunkert H, Harrell L, Palacios IF. Implications of small reference vessel diameter in patients undergoing percutaneous coronary revascularization. J Am Coll Cardiol 1999;34:40–48.

40. Carcagni A, Camellini M, Maiello L, et al. Percutaneous transluminal coronary revascularization in women: higher risk of dissection and need for stenting. Ital Heart J 2000;1:536–541.

41. Cowley MJ, Mullin SM, Kelsey SF, et al. Sex differences in early and long-term results of coronary angioplasty in the NHLBI PTCA Registry. Circulation 1985;71:90–97.

42. Jacobs AK, Kelsey SF, Brooks MM, et al. Better outcome for women compared with men undergoing coronary revascularization: a report from the bypass angioplasty revascularization investigation (BARI). Circulation 1998;98:1279–1285.

43. Greenberg MA, Mueller HS. Why the excess mortality in women after PTCA? [editorial; comment]. Circulation 1993;87:1030–1032.

44. Airaksinen KE, Ikaheimo MJ, Linnaluoto M, et al. Gender difference in autonomic and hemodynamic reactions to abrupt coronary occlusion. J Am Coll Cardiol 1998;31:301–306.

45. Robertson T, Kennard ED, Menta S, et al. Influence of gender on in-hospital clinical and angiographic outcomes and on one-year follow-up in the New Approaches to Coronary Intervention (NACI) registry. Am J Cardiol 1997;80:26K–39K.

46. Jacobs AK, Kelsey SF, Yen W, et al. Documentation of decline in morbidity in women undergoing coronary angioplasty (a report from the 1993–94 NHLBI Percutaneous Transluminal Coronary Angioplasty Registry). National Heart, Lung, and Blood Institute. Am J Cardiol 1997;80:979–984.

47. Scirica BM, Moliterno DJ, Every NR, et al. Differences between men and women in the management of unstable angina pectoris (The GUARANTEE Registry). The GUARANTEE Investigators. Am J Cardiol 1999;84:1145–1150.

48. Keelan ET, Nunez BD, Grill DE, et al. Comparison of immediate and long-term outcome of coronary angioplasty performed for unstable angina and rest pain in men and women. Mayo Clin Proc 1997;72:5–12.

49. Gowda MS, Vacek JL, Hallas D. Gender-related risk factors and outcomes for non-Q wave myocardial infarction patients receiving in-hospital PTCA. J Invasive Cardiol 1999;11:121–126.

50. Passos LC, Lopes AA, Costa U, et al. Difference in the in-hospital mortality of unstable angina pectoris between men and women. Arq Bras Cardiol 1999;72:669–676.

51. Tofler GH, Stone PH, Muller JB, Braunwald E. Mortality for women after acute myocardial infarction: MILIS Study Group. Am J Cardiol 1989;64:256.

52. Woodfield SL, Lundergoin CF, Reiner JS, et al. Gender and acute myocardial infarction: is there a different response to thrombolysis? J Am Coll Cardiol 1997;29:35–42.

53. Kudenchuk PJ, Maynard C, Martin JS, et al. Comparison of presentation, treatment, and outcome of acute myocardial infarction in men versus women (the Myocardial Infarction Triage and Intervention Registry). Am J Cardiol 1996;78:9–14.

54. Weitzman S, Cooper L, Chambless L, et al. Gender, racial, and geographic differences in the performance of cardiac diagnostic and therapeutic procedures for hospitalized acute myocardial infarction in four states. Am J Cardiol 1997;79:722–726.

55. Barakat K, Wilkinson P, Suliman A, et al. Acute myocardial infarction in women: contribution of treatment variables to adverse outcome. Am Heart J 2000;140:740–746.

56. Gan SC, Beaver SK, Houck PM, et al. Treatment of acute myocardial infarction and 30-day mortality among women and men. N Engl J Med 2000;343:8–15.

57. Cariou A, Himbert D, Golmard JL, et al. Sex-related differences in eligibility for reperfusion therapy and in- hospital outcome after acute myocardial infarction. Eur Heart J 1997;18:1583–1589.

58. Grines CL. Should thrombolysis or primary angioplasty be the treatment of choice for acute myocardial infarction? Primary angioplasty – the strategy of choice. N Engl J Med 1996;335:1313–1317.

59. Grines CL, Browne KF, Marco J, et al. A comparison of immediate angioplasty with thrombolytic therapy for acute myocardial infarction. The Primary Angioplasty in Myocardial Infarction Study Group. N Engl J Med 1993;328:673–679.

60. Zijlstra F, de Boer MJ, Hoomtje JC, et al. A comparison of immediate coronary angioplasty with intravenous streptokinase in acute myocardial infarction. N Engl J Med 1993;328:680–684.

61. Michels KB, Yusuf S. Does PTCA in acute myocardial infarction affect mortality and reinfarction rates? A quantitative overview (meta-analysis) of the randomized clinical trials. Circulation 1995;91:476–485.

62. Saha S, Stettin GD, Redberg RF. Gender and willingness to undergo invasive cardiac procedures. J Gen Intern Med 1999;14:122–125.

63. Rathore SS, Weinfurt KP, Oetgen WJ, et al. Refusal of Catheterization During Acute Myocardial Infarction: Influence of Patient Characteristics. J Am Coll Cardiol 1999;33:356A.

64. Stone GW, Grines CL, Browne KF, et al. Predictors of in-hospital and 6-month outcome after acute myocardial infarction in the reperfusion era: the Primary Angioplasty in Myocardial Infarction (PAMI) trail. J Am Coll Cardiol 1995;25:370–377.

65. Stone GW, Grines CL, Browne KF, et al. Influence of acute myocardial infarction location on in-hospital and late outcome after primary percutaneous transluminal coronary angioplasty versus tissue plasminogen activator therapy. Am J Cardiol 1996;78:19–25.

66. van't Hof AW, Liem A, Suryapranta H, et al. Clinical presentation and outcome of patients with early, intermediate and late reperfusion therapy by primary coronary angioplasty for acute myocardial infarction. Eur Heart J 1998;19:118–123.

67. Grines CL, Cox DA, Stone GW, et al. Coronary angioplasty with or without stent implantation for acute myocardial infarction. Stent Primary Angioplasty in Myocardial Infarction Study Group. N Engl J Med 1999;341:1949–1956.

68. Stone GW, Macrovitz P, Lansky AJ, et al. Differential effects of stenting and angioplasty in women versus men undergoing a primary mechanical reperfusion strategy in acute myocardial infarction– The PAMI Stent Randomized Trial. J Amer Coll Card 1999;33:357A.

69. Antoniucci D, Valente R, Moschi G, et al. Sex-based differences in clinical and angiographic outcomes after primary angioplasty or stenting for acute myocardial infarction. Am J Cardiol 2001;87:289–293.

70. Brener SJ, Ellis SG, Sapp SK, et al. Predictors of death and reinfarction at 30 days after primary angioplasty: the GUSTO IIb and RAPPORT trials. Am Heart J 2000;139:476–481.

71. Wong SC, Sanborn T, Sleeper LA, et al. Angiographic findings and clinical correlates in patients with cardiogenic shock complicating acute myocardial infarction: a report from the SHOCK Trial Registry. SHould we emergently revascularize Occluded Coronaries for cardiogenic shocK? J Am Coll Cardiol 2000;36(3 Suppl A):1077–1083.

72. Berger PB, Tuttle RH, Holmes DR Jr, et al. One-year survival among patients with acute myocardial infarction complicated by cardiogenic shock, and its relation to early revascularization: results from the GUSTO-I trial. Circulation 1999;99:873–878.

73. Hochman JS, Sleeper LA, Webb JG, et al. Early revascularization in acute myocardial infarction complicated by cardiogenic shock. SHOCK Investigators. Should we emergently revascularize occluded coronaries for cardiogenic shock. N Engl J Med 1999;341:625–634.

74. Hochman JS, Sleeper LA, Godfrey Z, et al. SHould we emergently revascularize Occluded Coronaries for cardiogenic shocK: an international randomized trial of emergency PTCA/CABG-trial design. The SHOCK Trial Study Group. Am Heart J 1999;137:313–321.

75. Thompson CR, Buller CE, Sleeper LA, et al. Cardiogenic shock due to acute severe mitral regurgitation complicating acute myocardial infarction: a report from the SHOCK Trial Registry. SHould we use emergently revascularize Occluded Coronaries in cardiogenic shocK? J Am Coll Cardiol 2000;36(3 Suppl A):1104–1109.

76. Menon V, White H, Le Jerntel T, et al. The clinical profile of patients with suspected cardiogenic shock due to predominant left ventricular failure: a report from the SHOCK Trial Registry. SHould we emergently revascularize Occluded Coronaries in cardiogenic shocK? J Am Coll Cardiol 2000;36(3 Suppl A):1071–1076.

77. Hochman JS, Buller CE, Sleeper LA, et al. Cardiogenic shock complicating acute myocardial infarction—etiologies, management and outcome: a report from the SHOCK Trial Registry. SHould we emergently revascularize Occluded Coronaries for cardiogenic shocK? J Am Coll Cardiol 2000;36(3 Suppl A):1063–1070.

78. Wong SC, Sleeper LA, Monrad ES, et al. Absence of gender differences in clinical outcomes in patients with cardiogenic shock complicating acute myocardial infarction. A report from the SHOCK Trial Registry. J Am Coll Cardiol 2001;38:1395–1401.

79. Shindler DM, Palmeri ST, Antonelli TA, et al. Diabetes mellitus in cardiogenic shock complicating acute myocardial infarction: a report from the SHOCK Trial Registry. SHould we emergently revascularize Occluded Coronaries for cardiogenic shocK? J Am Coll Cardiol 2000;36(3 Suppl A):1097–1103.

80. Collaborative overview of randomised trials of antiplatelet therapy—II: Maintenance of vascular graft or arterial patency by antiplatelet therapy. Antiplatelet Trialists' Collaboration. BMJ 1994;308:159–168.

81. Lawlor DA, Bedford C, Taylor M, Ebrahim S. Aspirin use for the prevention of cardiovascular disease: the British Women's Heart and Health Study. Br J Gen Pract 2001;51:743–745.

82. Becker RC, Burns M, Gore JM, et al. Early and pre-discharge aspirin administration among patients with acute myocardial infarction: current clinical practice and trends in the United States. J Thromb Thrombolysis 2000;9:207–215.

83. Kong DF, Califf RM, Miller DP, et al. Clinical outcomes of therapeutic agents that block the platelet glycoprotein IIb/IIIa integrin in ischemic heart disease. Circulation 1998;98:2829–2835.

84. Goldschmidt-Clermont PJ, Schulman SP, Bray PF, et al. Refining the treatment of women with unstable angina—a randomized, double-blind, comparative safety and efficacy evaluation of Integrelin versus aspirin in the management of unstable angina. Clin Cardiol 1996;19:869–874.

85. Inhibition of the platelet glycoprotein IIb/IIIa receptor with tirofiban in unstable angina and non-Q-wave myocardial infarction. Platelet Receptor Inhibition in Ischemic Syndrome Management in Patients Limited by Unstable Signs and Symptoms (PRISM-PLUS) Study Investigators. N Engl J Med 1998;338:1488–1497.

86. Inhibition of platelet glycoprotein IIb/IIIa with eptifibatide in patients with acute coronary syndromes. The PURSUIT Trial Investigators. Platelet Glycoprotein IIb/IIIa in Unstable Angina: Receptor Suppression Using Integrilin Therapy. N Engl J Med 1998;339:436–443.

87. Cho L., Topol EJ, Balog C, et al. Clinical benefit of glycoprotein IIb/IIIa blockade with Abciximab is independent of gender: pooled analysis from EPIC, EPILOG and EPISTENT trials. Evaluation of 7E3 for the Prevention of Ischemic Complications. Evaluation in Percutaneous Transluminal Coronary Angioplasty to Improve Long-Term Outcome with Abciximab GP IIb/IIIa blockade. Evaluation of Platelet IIb/IIIa Inhibitor for Stent. J Am Coll Cardiol 2000;36:381–386.

88. Randomised placebo-controlled and balloon-angioplasty-controlled trial to assess safety of coronary stenting with use of platelet glycoprotein- IIb/IIIa blockade. The EPISTENT Investigators. Evaluation of Platelet IIb/IIIa Inhibitor for Stenting. Lancet 1998;352:87–92.

89. Topol EJ, Mark DB, Lincoff AM, et al. Outcomes at 1 year and economic implications of platelet glycoprotein IIb/IIIa blockade in patients undergoing coronary stenting: results from a multicentre randomised trial. EPISTENT Investigators. Evaluation of Platelet IIb/IIIa Inhibitor for Stenting. [published erratum appears in Lancet 2000 Mar 25;355(9209):1104]. Lancet 1999;354:2019–2024.

90. Cho L, Marco SP, Bhatt DL, Topol EJ. Optimizing percutaneous coronary revascularization in diabetic women: analysis from the EPISTENT trial [In Process Citation]. J Womens Health Gend Based Med 2000;9:741–746.

91. Randomised placebo-controlled trial of effect of eptifibatide on complications of percutaneous coronary intervention: IMPACT-II. Integrilin to Minimise Platelet Aggregation and Coronary Thrombosis-II. Lancet 1997;349:1422–1428.

92. Blankenship JC, Sigmon KN, Pieper KS, et al. Effect of eptifibatide on angiographic complications during percutaneous coronary intervention in the IMPACT- (integrilin to minimize platelet aggregation and coronary thrombosis) II Trial. Am J Cardiol 2001;88:969–973.

93. Tcheng JE, Talley JD, O'Shea JC, et al. Clinical pharmacology of higher dose eptifibatide in percutaneous coronary intervention (the PRIDE study). Am J Cardiol 2001;88:1097–1102.

94. Blankenship JC, Tasissa G, O'Shea JC, et al. Effect of glycoprotein IIb/IIIa receptor inhibition on angiographic complications during percutaneous coronary intervention in the ESPRIT trial. J Am Coll Cardiol 2001;38:653–658.

95. O'Shea JC, Hafley GE, Greenberg S, et al. Platelet glycoprotein IIb/IIIa integrin blockade with eptifibatide in coronary stent intervention: the ESPRIT trial: a randomized controlled trial. JAMA 2001;285:2468–2473.

96. O'Shea JC, Tcheng JE. Eptifibatide in Percutaneous Coronary Intervention: The ESPRIT Trial Results. Curr Interv Cardiol Rep 2001;3:62–68.

97. Kleiman NS, Califf RM. Results from late-breaking clinical trials sessions at ACCIS 2000 and ACC 2000. American College of Cardiology. J Am Coll Cardiol 2000;6:310–325.

98. Weintraub WS, Wenger NK, Jones EL, et al. Changing clinical characteristics of coronary surgery patients. Differences between men and women. Circulation 1993;88:II79–II86.

99. O'Connor GT, Morton JR, Diehl MJ, et al. Differences between men and women in hospital mortality associated with coronary artery bypass graft surgery. The Northern New England Cardiovascular Disease Study Group. Circulation 1993;88:2104–2110.

100. Abramov D, Tamariz MG, Fremes SE, et al. Trends in coronary artery bypass surgery results: a recent, 9-year study. Ann Thorac Surg 2000;70:84–90.

101. Petro KR, Dullum MK, Garcia JM, et al. Minimally invasive coronary revascularization in women: A safe approach for a high-risk group. Heart Surg Forum 2000;3:41–46.

102. Abramov D, Tamariz MG, Sever JY, et al. The influence of gender on the outcome of coronary artery bypass surgery. Ann Thorac Surg 2000;70:800–806.

C. Variations in Therapeutic Effectiveness in Women

18 Effectiveness of Coronary Revascularization
Gender and Racial Differences

Christi Deaton, PhD, RN, FAHA,
Cherie L. Kunik, MSN, RN, CS,
and Eric Peterson, MD, FACC

CONTENTS

INTRODUCTION

This chapter reviews the gender differences in coronary revascularization, including percutaneous coronary intervention (PCI) and coronary artery bypass surgery (CABG). Briefly highlighted are racial differences in PCI and CABG, particularly as they interact with gender comparison. This chapter also covers issues regarding access to coronary revascularization, safety procedures (morbidity and mortality), and effectiveness (influence on survival and functional outcomes). However, it is necessary to point out some of the major challenges in this field, including an overall underrepresentation of women and minorities in clinical research, as well as certain factors that confound gender and racial studies.

LIMITATIONS IN STUDY REPRESENTATION

Determining the effectiveness of coronary revascularization by gender and race is a daunting task for several reasons. Because there are generally fewer data on women and racial/ethnic minorities, comparisons by race and gender are often hindered by small samples of these subgroups. A recent review of female enrollment in federally

From: *Contemporary Cardiology: Coronary Disease in Women: Evidence-Based Diagnosis and Treatment*
Edited by: L. J. Shaw and R. F. Redberg © Humana Press Inc., Totowa, NJ

funded cardiovascular clinical trials noted that women were still underenrolled when single-sex studies were excluded. The enrollment rate for women in trials of coronary artery disease (CAD) had increased over time, being proportional to disease prevalence among women. However, subgroup analyses with large enough samples of women to detect sex-related differences were performed infrequently (1).

The underenrollment of minorities in clinical trials is also a significant problem. For example, the Coronary Artery Surgery Study (CASS) was a large multicenter trial that enrolled 24,959 patients, but only 2.3% were black (2). Less than 1% of the CASS sample were black females, and the paucity of data on minority women continues in current studies (2,3), resulting from the lack of specific data on these subgroups, knowledge of the effectiveness of CAD treatment has been predicated on what is effective in primarily white middle-aged and middle-class males. White males had the highest rate of mortality decline (2.9%/year) from coronary heart disease from 1990 to 1994, whereas black women had the lowest decline rate (1.6%/year; 4).

Another challenge is that testing treatment effectiveness must take into account potential physiological and pathophysiological gender differences in the cardiovascular system. Despite anatomic similarities, evidence exists of significant gender differences in cardiovascular structure and function, although these changes may only be apparent in aging or in the adaptation to a stimulus, such as pressure overload (5). Recent studies in a rat model have demonstrated significant gender differences in cardiac output under basal conditions and in response to inotropes (6). Women have smaller coronary arteries and more diffuse stenoses than men (on whom most techniques have been developed), and these characteristics have been cited as reasons for less procedural success, lower symptom relief, and higher procedural mortality for women undergoing revascularization (7,8). Higher rates of hypertrophic left ventricles (LV) in women have also possibly contributed to women's inability to tolerate procedural complications, such as hypovolemic episodes and abrupt closure (8–10).

CAD also differs by prevalence, manifestation, progression, and associated morbidity, along with other host factors among gender and racial groups that can affect treatment effectiveness. Women are typically a decade older than men when CAD develops and, at the time of revascularization, have lower cardiovascular disease (CVD) severity, but similar or greater angina severity, more unstable angina, more heart failure, more frequent coexisting illnesses, higher emergency surgery rates, greater disability, worse socioeconomic status, and smaller body size (7,11–15). However, black women have higher rates of premature CAD than white women (16–18) and have been significantly younger than white women at the time of revascularization (19,20). Black women also have higher rates of certain coexisting illnesses than white women (19,20).

Finally, inequities in access and referral to revascularization by gender, race, and socioeconomic status have been found in studies, which, in turn, affect our ability to determine treatment effectiveness for these groups (21). Ethnic minorities in the United States constitute a large majority of the uninsured or underinsured; therefore, lack of access to cardiac services may greatly contribute to adverse outcomes (22).

The challenge for this chapter is to present evidence for the effectiveness of revascularization by gender and race, considering the multiple issues that are relevant given the paucity of data in these subgroups. Evidence regarding access and referral to revascularization is briefly reviewed in order to place the evidence for revascularization's effectiveness in context.

ACCESS AND REFERRAL

In 1991, two separate large-scale studies reported significant differences in how women and men with CAD were treated (23,24). Women were found to have less aggressive treatment with fewer diagnostic and therapeutic procedures in comparison to men. Since then, differences in access and referral to cardiovascular procedures have been found in many studies that compare women to men and minority patients (primarily black and few Hispanic) to white patients. Revascularization referral is dependent on referral to cardiac catheterization, and evidence shows that undergoing coronary angiography is affected by race and gender considerations, although financial and organizational factors may also play a role in racial differences in treatment (25–29).

Multiple studies have evaluated referral and access to angiography and subsequent revascularization by gender and race, where findings vary given that samples and methods are heterogeneous and potentially confounding variables may or may not be controlled. Generally, findings related to differences in access and referral by gender are inconsistent, possibly reflecting changes in practice since 1991, and inclusion of high-risk samples are already diagnosed with CAD, acute myocardial infarction (AMI), or other coexisting illnesses. Gender differences in cardiac procedures (higher rates for men than women) were found to narrow markedly after diagnosis of a chronic illness (end-stage renal disease [ESRD]), assurance of health insurance, and entry into a comprehensive care system for ESRD and dialysis management. Notably, nearly all of the narrowing of gender disparity occurred in the first year after ESRD development, potentially reflecting unmet clinical needs in women or the overuse of procedures in men at baseline (26).

Results for racial differences in procedure use were more likely to reflect a consistent difference by race and ethnicity. Although most studies evaluated black and white differences, Hispanic patients were also less likely to be referred for angiography or revascularization (25,27,30). In other studies, race differences lessened or disappeared when other factors, such as the type of hospital (with or without revascularization capabilities), insurance status, and extent of CAD, were controlled (31,32).

Sheifer et al. (33) critically reviewed the data on differences in invasive cardiac procedures (angiography, angioplasty, and CABG) by race and gender. Adjusted odds ratios (ORs) for black patients undergoing cardiac procedures when compared to white patients ranged from 0.43 to 0.94, and for women vs men, odds ratios ranged from 0.16 to 0.98. They concluded that CAD management varied significantly across race and sex, and such disparities have clinical implications. No published material after 1997 was reviewed in that article, and some (but not all) recent studies report less racial and gender disparity once adjustment is made for clinical and organizational factors (31,32). However, a more recent review acknowledged that evidence for disparities in referral for revascularization for blacks, Hispanics, and Asians is inconsistent, but persists regardless of data source (i.e., administrative databases, clinical databases, and survey data through May 2000; 34).

However, most of these study types address race or gender, and few have examined their race and gender interaction (25,30,35). Yet, data from the National Hospital Discharge Survey (NHDS) for patients discharged with AMI in 1988–1990 demonstrated that black women were the least likely to undergo cardiac catheterization, angioplasty, and coronary bypass surgery, whereas white men were the most likely. The analysis was adjusted for age, hospital size and type, region, in-hospital mortality, health insurance type, and hospital transfer rates. The odds ratio for black women to undergo CABG was 0.26 (95% confidence interval [CI], 0.11–0.61) when compared to white men *(36)*. A study using Medicare Part A claims data for a random beneficiaries sample in 1991–1992 from five states found no significant disparity by race among women for revascularization appropriateness according to the RAND Institution criteria *(37)*.

Physicians' decisions for cardiac catheterization referral were assessed in 1996–1997 using videotaped scripted interviews of actors portraying patients that represented eight combinations of race, gender, and age. The effects of differing clinical presentation, socioeconomic status, and insurance were negated by using identical scripts for each of three chest pain types. Information on cardiovascular risk, as well as the results of the electrocardiogram and a subsequent Thallium exercise stress test were also provided. More than 700 physicians participated, and the race and gender interaction was significant as black women were the only patients less likely to be referred for cardiac catheterization than white men *(29)*. This study has been criticized for the manner in which findings were presented and subsequently publicized in the general media *(38)*. However, because differences in access and referral to catheterization and revascularization by gender and race continue to be seen, well-designed studies and ongoing health care disparity discussions are needed.

EFFECTIVENESS: OUTCOMES AFTER CABG

Effectiveness is evaluated by reviewing the outcomes literature for CABG. Outcomes to be reviewed include mortality, morbidity, resource utilization, recovery, symptom relief, functional status, and quality-of-life measures. Additionally, race and gender factors will be outlined from the existing CABG literature.

CABG: Mortality

Improved survival is a well-accepted outcome post-CABG for patients with significant CAD (three-vessel, left-main equivalent, and/or reduced ejection fraction ([EF]; *39,40*). In evaluating CABG effectiveness in women and minorities, the same survival benefit should be evident, and mortality can be compared to the white male mortality who are the predominant subjects and reference group in CABG studies.

In CASS, women had an operative mortality (OM) of 4.61% when compared to 1.97% for men *(41)*. The gender difference in OM was most prevalent in the age group of 40–59 years, with OM being similar in patients age 60 and older. In subsequent analysis, CASS investigators and others concluded that when adjustment was made for differences in both the patient's size (smaller physical size was associated with greater mortality) and basic clinical and angiographic variables, gender contributed no predictive information *(8,42)*.

Other investigators have also concluded that female gender is not an independent predictor of mortality in either younger (age 40–65 years, $n = 1464$) or older patients (≥ 75 years, $n = 663$; *43–45*), or in patients overall *(46,47)*. Female gender was not found to be an independent predictor for early postoperative mortality after adjustment for other risk variables in 4823 patients (19.3% female) undergoing CABG in 1989–1998 *(48)*.

However, other studies have documented that for women with higher OM, mortality persists even with adjustment for clinical and physical size variables among CABG patients, including the elderly *(13,49,50)*. The Society of Thoracic Surgeons (STS) National Database was used to evaluate more than 300,000 patients having isolated CABG from 1994 to 1996. Women and men were compared to determine differences in clinical characteristics, and risk stratification was performed to compare OM of subpopulations having similar risk. To fully account for the impact of all risk factors, the STS risk model was used to place patients into similar-risk groups. OM analysis showed a higher OM for women than men in all but the very highest-risk categories (when operative risk approached 30%, no gender difference was found). Effect of body size was evaluated by dividing patients into 10 groups with the same body surface area (BSA). The OM difference was accentuated at higher BSA, and there was no mortality difference by gender for those patients in the smallest BSA groups (BSA < 1.805 m^2). The investigators concluded that there is mounting evidence to support the existence of gender-specific responses to CVD and treatment, and that gender is an independent risk factor for mortality, except when operative risk exceeds 30% *(12)*.

Increased mortality risk in females was evaluated using a risk score from a published logistic risk model in three large CABG patient databases (combined n = 63,116). Female gender was associated with a 58% greater mortality vs men, but after adjustment for differences in risk factor prevalence and BSA, women had a 14% greater mortality than men (OR 1.14, $p = 0.026$). Accounting for BSA essentially eliminates the gender effect, but there is still debate regarding whether gender is a surrogate for BSA or whether gender and BSA represent different underlying mechanisms *(51)*.

Long-term mortality findings post-CABG by gender are different from the findings for OM. After OM adjustment, 5- and 6-year survival for males and females was essentially the same in CASS *(41,52)*. Female gender has also been found to be protective for late survival (60 months) after adjustment for other risk variables *(48)*. In a study of CABG patients less than age 65 (n = 1047) and those 65 and older (n = 953), female gender was associated with higher 5-year mortality in the younger group, but not the older. Men in the older group had a higher risk of death within 5 years than did older women *(53)*. In a small sample (n = 195) of the oldest-old (age 80–91), female gender was not associated with long-term mortality risk *(43)*.

CABG: Morbidity

Female gender may be associated with some increase in complications following CABG as well. In an analysis of 20,614 patients undergoing CABG, female gender was an independent predictor of low-output syndrome (requirement for inotropes or intra-aortic balloon pump [IABP] support to maintain a cardiac index ≥ 2 L/min) among all patients and those with EF of 20–40%, but not in patients with EF less than 20% *(50)*. Female gender was a weak independent predictor for the prespecified composite endpoint of death, perioperative myocardial infarction (MI), IABP use, or stroke in a study of 932 women and 3891 men undergoing isolated CABG from 1989 to 1998 *(48)*.

Conversely, Geraci et al. *(54)* did not find female gender to be associated with a higher risk of adverse events (serious postoperative complications) post-CABG in a study of 2213 Medicare patients. Similarly, in an analysis of 1743 consecutive patients (30% women) undergoing isolated CABG from 1994 to 1997, female gender was not an independent predictor of postoperative complications, but the higher incidence of female complications was associated with their higher rate of comorbid conditions

(46). Ferraris and Ferraris *(55)* found that congestive heart failure (CHF), hypertension, previous stroke, and the combined variable of age/red blood cell volume (indicative of smaller body size and anemia) were independent predictors of serious postoperative morbidity. They concluded that variables reflecting chronic health status and older age seem to be more predictive of increased morbidity.

Although there seems to be some evidence that female gender has some intrinsic association with increased operative mortality and morbidity in patients undergoing CABG, adjusting for other risk factors decreases and, in some studies, erases the greater mortality and morbidity risk of women when compared to men.

CABG: Resource Utilization

Female gender has been found to be associated with longer length of stay following CABG, including longer intubation duration and longer intensive care unit (ICU) stay *(46,56–59)*. Because there is a trend toward shorter postoperative length of stay (PLOS; median 4 days; *60*), a length of stay longer than average may be an obvious marker of a more complicated high-risk patient. Lahey et al. *(61)* found higher 30-day readmission rates for patients discharged at 7 days (33%) and 8 days (36%) than for those discharged on or before day 6 (16.2%). A recent abstract also reported that the cardiac surgery cost was also 1.2 times higher in women than men (mean difference $3997, $p < 0.02$) after adjusting for preoperative risk factors and age. Women's duration of mechanical ventilation and postoperative length of stay were longer than men's, although mortality was comparable *(62)*.

Women have higher rehospitalization rates post-CABG than men in many studies. Among Medicare beneficiaries, women had higher age-adjusted rates than men for all rehospitalizations ($p < 0.001$) and for related event rehospitalizations ($p < 0.001$) during 1-year follow-up *(63)*. Deaton et al. *(64)* found a 41% rate of unplanned rehospitalization 3 months post-CABG in women vs a 22% rate for men, and another study *(61)* reported that 53% of re-admitted patients were women vs 33% of the patients ($p < 0.001$) who were not re-admitted. Cardiovascular re-admission 60 days post-CABG discharge was positively associated with female gender *(65)*. In contrast, Ai et al. *(66)* did not find female gender to be associated with higher rates of rehospitalization 1 year after CABG in 151 patients.

CABG: Recovery, Symptom Relief, and Functional Status

Women and men also differ in their recovery experiences following CABG as well as in the extent of symptom relief and functional status improvement. Some investigators have documented that women have worse functional status prior to CABG than men, and that this is maintained or even increased throughout recovery *(64,67)*. Slower attainment of physical functioning after CABG was reported in women when compared to men (measured by the Short Form [SF]-36), although the study was limited by a very small sample *(68)*. Female gender was found to be an independent predictor of worse functional status (measured by the Duke Activity Status Index) preoperatively and at 1 year in a study of 199 patients age 65 and older *(69)*. In another study, women's self-rated health was significantly worse than men's at 1-year post-CABG *(66)*.

Artinian and Duggan *(70)* described 6-week recovery in 132 men and 47 women after CABG. Women had more comorbid conditions, cardiovascular risk factors and urgent or emergent surgery, and lower education and income. However, women and men did not differ by preoperative functional status or health perception. Women reported greater ambulation dysfunction, home management dysfunction, more symptoms, worse depression scores, and poorer physical health perceptions at 1-, 3-, and 6-week postsurgery than men, although both genders improved over time. The decrease in reported symptoms was greater in men over time than in women. The investigators concluded that women appeared to have a slower physical recovery than men during the first 6-week postsurgery follow-up.

These findings may be put into context when preoperative male and female differences at the time of CABG are taken into account. Importantly, one study found that women's functional and health status 6 months following CABG was not worse than men's once adjustment was made for women's older age, greater comorbid illnesses, CVD severity, and significant psychosocial variables (71).

Additionally, in some studies, women actually have greater gains in functional recovery than men do, yet continuing to have worse functional status scores than men. Women had worse preoperative functional status, lower life satisfaction, and poorer social support than men (undergoing CABG and valve surgery), but social support was only worse for women at 3 months (72). Women were significantly less likely than men to return to their normal activities at 3 months, but women demonstrated more improvement in functional status than men (72). Rankin (58) compared women's recovery (n = 24) and men's (n = 93) during the first 3 months post-CABG. Preoperatively, women were more functionally compromised than men, with longer ICU stays and higher in-hospital mortality at 6 weeks. However, no gender differences were found for measures of biophysical, sexual, recreational, or return-to-work variables at 1 or 3 months.

Women may also have an advantage in psychological recovery, despite that women have higher depression incidence than men pre-CABG and at the time of postsurgical discharge (73). Women reported significantly less mood disturbance (anxiety, anger, and depression measured by the Profile of Mood States) than men at 1 and 3 months post-CABG in one study (58). Similarly, Sokol et al. (74) found that psychological changes after CABG were not worse in women when compared to men, and that women experienced improvement in emotional well-being 6 and 12 months post-CABG, whereas men did not. The number of noncardiac chronic conditions (rather than gender) has been found to be the strongest predictor of depression (66).

Many studies of long-term symptom relief following CABG have demonstrated that women report more angina postsurgery than men (48,53). Female gender was an independent predictor of recurrent angina in the first and subsequent postoperative years in the CASS Registry (75).

CABG: RACE AND GENDER

Race was evaluated in CASS to determine the therapy's effect on survival in blacks when compared to whites. Overall, 5-year survival was worse for black men, but among women, only black women age 50–54 had lower survival than same-age white women. In multivariate analysis, the black race was associated with worse survival in the medical group, but not the surgical group (3).

Preoperative characteristics and in-hospital outcomes were compared in 336 black women with an equal number of randomly selected age-matched white women who had CABG from 1995 to 1999. In the total sample of women prior to age matching, white women were significantly older than black women (61.2 ± 11 years vs 66 ± 11 years, $p < 0.0001$). Black females in comparison to white had higher rates of diabetes, hypertension, renal insufficiency, obesity, and clustering of risk factors, whereas white women tended to have more emergency surgery. Mortality and morbidity did not differ by race, although black women tended to have more prolonged mechanical ventilation, and white women had more atrial fibrillation. PLOS was significantly longer for black women (67).

The influence of gender was investigated in a large cohort of black patients who underwent coronary angiography for suspected CAD, were hospitalized for AMI, or had CABG (780 men and 939 women) in 1983–1989. Women and men undergoing CABG (n = 159; 71 women) did not differ by age, comorbid conditions, or CAD extent. Mean EF was higher in women (62 ± 15) than men (55 ± 15, $p < 0.01$). Women undergoing CABG had better 30-day and 48-month survival than men, but the difference was not significant (76).

EFFECTIVENESS: OUTCOMES AFTER PCI

PCI outcomes include mortality, morbidity, resource utilization, procedural success, recovery, symptom relief, functional status, and quality-of-life measures. Additionally, race and gender interaction is outlined from the existing PCI literature.

PCI: Mortality

As reported in the review by Philippides and Jacobs (7), acute mortality was higher in women undergoing PCI than men in multiple studies in the 1980s and early 1990s. For example, women's PCI-related mortality in the National Heart, Lung, and Blood Institute Percutaneous Transluminal Coronary Angioplasty (NHLBI PTCA) registry 1977–1981 was six times that of men (1.7% vs 0.3%), and multivariate analysis found that female gender was the only predictor of mortality. In subsequent years of the registry (1985–1986), women continued to have a higher procedural mortality rate (2.6% vs 0.3%). In fact, Kelsey and colleagues adjusted for baseline differences and found female gender to impart an independent 4.5-fold increased risk of in-hospital mortality following PCI (77).

Greater procedural mortality for women in comparison to men was reported for PCI performed from 1980 to 1990, with in-hospital mortality being higher for women at every decade of age. Multivariate predictors of in-hospital death were female gender, older age, multivessel disease, and reduced LVEF (78). Bell et al. (79) found that women's in-hospital mortality post-PCI was higher from 1988 to 1990 than from 1979 to 1987 (5.4% vs 2.9%, p = 0.04) and was significantly higher than male mortality (3.1%, p = 0.01) in 1988–1990. Female gender was a weak, but significant, independent predictor of in-hospital death (OR 1.51, 95% CI: 1.00–2.29), and the association was decreased slightly when BSA was added to the multivariate model.

Although reports of gender differences in long-term outcome post-PCI are limited, female gender is not a consistent predictor of higher mortality. At 16-month follow-up, men had higher cumulative mortality (2.2% vs 0.3%, p < 0.05) than women in 1397 patients from the NHLBI PTCA registry in 1977–1981. In this analysis, male gender was an independent predictor of late mortality (80). In other analyses, cumulative mortality (follow-up ranging from 34 months to 7 years) did not differ between men and women *(78,81,82)*. Other investigators contend that female sex is an independent predictor of improved 5-year survival following PCI and CABG after controlling for women's higher risk profile *(83)*.

In a comparison of 1001 women and 3263 men receiving coronary artery stents from 1992 to 1998, women were older and had more hypertension, diabetes, and hypercholesterolemia, but presented with higher EF, less current smoking, multivessel disease, previous MI, and CABG than men. Periprocedural and postprocedural therapy did not differ by gender. Thirty-day outcomes were worse for women who had a higher risk of death, nonfatal MI, or any event (e.g., revascularization) than men. Excess female risk declined over the subsequent months so that 1-year outcomes were similar between women and men. The major risk factor for death at 1 year for women was diabetes; for men, it was older age *(84)*.

Following PCI, outcomes for women and men were evaluated using the large observational National Cardiovascular Network (NCN) registry database ($n = 109,708$ PCI patients in 1994–1997, 33% women). Excess in-hospital mortality for women overall and in device subgroups (balloon-only, stent, and atherectomy) disappeared after adjustment for age, comorbid illness, disease severity, and BSA. The study confirmed BSA's importance when considering mortality risk, in that patients of equivalent size, regardless of gender, had equivalent mortality rates. Another important finding was that in those unstable or severely ill patients with higher predicted PCI mortality risk, women faced a lower relative risk of dying when compared with men *(85)*.

PCI: Morbidity

Reports differ as to whether complication rates are higher for women than men post-PCI. In-hospital reportable outcomes for men and women are similar with comparable rates of Q-wave MI, emergency CABG, and abrupt vessel closure, although women experienced higher CHF rates and pulmonary edema *(79,83,86)*. Vascular (arteriovenous fistula and need for blood transfusion) and renal complications have been found to be more prevalent in women *(87,88)*. In a current data review concerning restenosis following PTCA, however, Califf et al. *(89)*, concluded that female gender is not associated with increased restenosis risk and, in fact, noted that some studies have indicated restenosis was more common in males.

Findings on complications differed by gender in an analysis of PCI outcomes from 1994 to 1997 from the NCN registry. Even after adjustment for age, comorbid illness, disease severity, and BSA, female gender was associated with an increased risk of stroke (OR 1.36; 95% CI 1.1–1.7), Q wave MI (OR 1.25; 95% CI 1.1–1.4), and vascular complications (OR 1.48; 95% CI 1.3–1.7). Overall complication rates were very low for both women and men. Additionally, women more often required a repeat revascularization procedure (repeat PCI or bypass surgery) prior to hospital discharge (OR 1.09 [1.03, 1.16]; *85*).

PCI: Procedural Success

Early PCI procedural success (≥20% reduction in luminal diameter narrowing) and clinical success (procedural success plus the absence of death, MI, and emergent CABG) were lower in women when compared to men. Data from the 1977–1981 NHLBI PTCA registry found procedural success to be 60% in women vs 66% in men, and clinical success was 57% in women vs 62% in men *(80)*. Subsequent reports from the 1985–1986 NHLBI PTCA registry found that success rates had improved for both genders and there were no male and female differences (77). Possible explanations regarding early gender differences in PCI outcomes may be the use of 3-mm balloons, which were oversized for women and the fact that many early analyses did not adjust for baseline differences (i.e., older age and comorbidities) for women vs men. Later investigators reported similar procedural and clinical success rates for women and men (78,79,86). However, in an early report of the use of directional coronary atherectomy and stents, procedural success was lower in women (90).

More recent reports of coronary artery stenting (1992–1998) indicated similar procedural success in 1001 women and 3263 men. Lesion and vessel characteristics differed only in that women had more left-anterior descending lesions, shorter lesion length, smaller vessel size, and fewer restenotic lesions than men. Final minimal lumen diameter was less in women, but most procedural characteristics were similar between genders. Procedural success was achieved in 98% of both women and men (84).

PCI: Recovery, Symptom Relief, and Functional Status

Few data exist regarding quality of life and functional status, specifically for women undergoing PCI. Krumholz et al. (91) examined health-related quality of life after elective PCI for 103 consecutive patients; however, only a small percentage was female (24%). Nonetheless, physical functioning, vitality, and social functioning scores improved as well as improvement in CCSC class, whereas no significant change occurred in general health perceptions.

Predictors of physical component subscale (PCS) score on the SF-36 6 months after PCI were baseline (preoperative) PCS, comorbidity index, baseline mental component subscale (MCS) score, prior CABG, age, and thrombolysis. Only when the cut-off for inclusion of variables was relaxed to $p < 0.15$ did female gender enter as an independent predictor of lower PCS at 6 months (92).

Female patients in the Randomized Intervention Treatment of Angina trial (RITA-2) had significantly worse physical functioning baseline ratings and vitality by the SF-36 than males. The baseline scores were the strongest predictor of 1-year scores, indicating consistency over time in patient self-assessment of quality of life (93). Other investigators have reported greater difficulties initiating sleep and worse quality of life post-PCI in females when compared with age-matched males (94).

PCI: RACE AND GENDER

Similar to the findings in patients undergoing surgical revascularization, women undergoing PCI are different from men undergoing the procedure. Data have consistently indicated that women were older and had more hypertension, diabetes, unstable angina, class IV angina, and heart failure (7,78,79) at the time of procedure. In contrast, women had better LV systolic function, were less likely to be smokers, and have had a previous MI or CABG vs men (83,84). Women have also been found to have smaller coronary arteries and more diffuse stenoses (77,95). Consistent with women's higher CHF rates and preserved LV systolic function, women have also been found to have more LV hypertrophy (9,10).

Comparisons of black and white women in the NHLBI 1985–1986 PTCA registry found that white women were older, but had less unstable angina, diabetes, hypertension, and current smoking than black women. A small number of black women ($n = 38$) and black men ($n = 38$), over half of whom came from one institution, limited the conclusions that could be drawn and the generalizability of the findings in this registry. The number of black patients was less than expected, again indicating that potential referral and access bias limits our ability to confirm conclusions about revascularization in minority patients. Generally, black patients were younger, more often female, had more unstable angina, current smoking, and hypertension. Black patients had a higher multivessel disease incidence, but there was no difference in the number of lesions attempted or the number of vessels treated. Black and white patients also did not differ by lesion location, morphology, geometry, or calcium presence, but stenosis pre- and post-PTCA was higher in black patients. Procedural success and complications were similar except for a higher rate of branch occlusion in blacks. Clinical success and outcomes were similar except that black patients had higher residual vessel disease, consistent with the higher incidence of multivessel disease prior to PTCA. Long-term (5-year) outcomes were similar as well, except for a trend for fewer black patients to report no angina *(96)*.

A small number of black patients ($n = 200$, 51% female) were compared to 4079 white patients undergoing PCI in the NACI registry. Black patients were younger, more likely to be female, and had higher rates of other concomitant disease, hypertension, diabetes, CHF, and a higher body mass index (BMI) than white patients. Black patients were less likely to undergo urgent or emergent procedures, but there were no differences in use of new devices or number of vessels treated. Procedural success and in-hospital outcomes did not differ by race. Sex analysis by race demonstrated a lower rate of hospital MI in black men in comparison to black women. One-year follow-up demonstrated no differences by race, but again showed gender differences among blacks. The composite endpoint of death, QMI, or any revascularization, occurred in 38.4% of black men and 28.7% of black women (*p* value not given). Black men were less likely to report improved angina when compared to black women (63% vs 77%). Kaplan-Meier plots from discharge to 1 year revealed greater event-free survival for black women vs black men, but no sex difference among white patients. Black males had a relative risk of 4.06 (95% CI 1.48–11.13) for death/Q wave MI/CABG when compared to black females. White women and black women were not compared *(97)*.

CONCLUSIONS

Coronary revascularization is effective for women, including minority women. Initially, higher in-hospital mortality and morbidity rates for women largely (although not completely) disappear when women's high-risk profiles are controlled in the analysis. Additionally, it is important to remember that although women and minorities may have somewhat higher relative risk than men and whites, absolute risk differences are small. Gender and race are relatively weak risk predictors, and other patient characteristics (age, heart disease severity, coexisting conditions) are important factors to consider when making patient-specific risk estimates or treatment recommendations.

Long-term female outcomes after revascularization are equal to and sometimes better than male outcomes. Black and white women have similar outcomes and survival and do not exhibit the disparity that is seen in black and white men. Women's outcomes have improved over time, which may reflect a "learning curve" for providers as they gain experience in dealing with older women who have multiple coexisting conditions, smaller coronary anatomy, and physiological therapy responses that may be different from men. Therapies developed specifically for women with CAD are needed, rather than relying on the indiscriminate application of therapies developed on the prevailing male model. Early diagnosis in women is imperative, particularly in black women who develop heart disease earlier than white women. Because many women will be older and "sicker" at the time of revascularization, particular attention needs to be paid to improving women's recovery and quality of life after surgery and PCI.

Patients should not be denied revascularization on the basis of gender, race, or ethnicity. CABG and PCI are effective therapies for women, men, minorities, and whites. Nonetheless, continuing research is necessary on the access and referral to revascularization, along with interventions to improve outcomes for women, minorities, and indeed, all patients.

REFERENCES

1. Harris DJ, Douglas PS. Enrollment of women in cardiovascular clinical trials funded by the National Heart, Lung and Blood Institute. New Engl J Med 2000;343:475–480.
2. Curry CL, Crawford-Green, C. Coronary artery disease in blacks: Past perspectives and current overview. In: Brest AN, Saunders E (eds.) Cardiovascular Disease in Blacks. F.A. Davis, Philadelphia, PA: 1991, pp. 197–204.
3. Maynard C, Fisher LD, Passamani ER. Survival of black persons compared with white persons in the Coronary Artery Surgery Study (CASS). Am J Cardiol 1987;60:513–518.
4. Rosamond WD, Chambles LE, Folsom AR, et al. Trends in the incidence of myocardial infarction and in mortality due to coronary heart disease, 1987 to 1994. N Engl J Med 1998;339:861–867.
5. Hayward CS, Kelly RP, Collins P. The roles of gender, the menopause and hormone replacement on cardiovascular function. Cardiovasc Res 2000;46:28–49.
6. Schwertz D, Vizgirda V, Solaro RJ, et al. Sexual dimorphism in rat left atrial function and response to adrenergic stimulation. Mol Cell Biochem 1999;200:143–153.
7. Phillipides GJ, Jacobs GK. Coronary angioplasty and surgical revascularization: Emerging concepts. Cardiology 1995;86:324–338.
8. Fisher LD, Kennedy JW, Davis KB, et al. and the participating CASS Clinics. Association of sex, physical size, and operative mortality after coronary artery bypass in the Coronary Artery Surgery Study (CASS). J Thorac Cardiovasc Surg 1982;84:334–341.
9. Mendes LA, Davidoff RR, Ryan TJ, Jacobs AK. Congestive heart failure and left ventricular ejection fraction: The gender paradox. J Am Coll Cardiol 1994:6A.
10. Greenberg MA, Mueller HS. Why the excess mortality in women after PTCA? Circulation 1993;87:1030–1032.
11. Czajkowski SM, Terrin M, Lindquist R, et al., for the POST CABG Biobehavioral Study Investigators. Comparison of preoperative characteristics of men and women undergoing coronary artery bypass grafting (The Post Coronary Artery Bypass Graft [CABG] Biobehavioral Study. Am J Cardiol 1997;79:1017–1024.
12. Edwards FH, Carey JS, Grover FL, et al. Impact of gender on coronary bypass operative mortality. Ann Thorac Surg 1998;66:125–131.
13. Hannan EL, Bernard HR, Kilburn HC, O'Donnell JF. Gender differences in mortality rates for coronary artery bypass surgery. Am Heart J 1992;123:866–872.
14. Weintraub WS, Wenger NK, Jones EL, et al. Changing clinical characteristics of coronary surgery patients: Differences between men and women. Circulation 1993;88:79–86.
15. Wenger NK. Coronary heart disease in women: Clinical syndromes, prognosis, and diagnostic testing. In Heart Disease in Women.
16. Garfinkel L. Cigarette smoking and coronary heart disease in blacks: Comparison to whties in a prospective study. Am Heart J 1984;108:802–807.

17. Gerhard GT, Sexton G, Malinow MR, et al. Premenopausal black women have more risk factors for coronary heart disease than white women. Am J Cardiol 1998;82:1040–1045.
18. Keil JE, Loadholt CB, Weinrich MC, et al. Incidence of coronary heart disease in blacks in Charleston, South Carolina. Am Heart J 1984;108:779–786.
19. Warner CD, Arrington K, Weintraub WS, et al. Do Race and Gender Impact Outcomes After Coronary Artery Bypass Graft Surgery? Proceedings of the Southern Nursing Research Society, Eleventh Annual conference, Norfolk, VA, April 1997.
20. Deaton C. Preoperative characteristics and outcomes: differences between black and white women undergoing coronary bypass surgery. Circulation 2000;102(Suppl II):II-511.
21. Philbin EF, McCullough PA, DiSalvo TG, et al. Socioeconomic status is an important determinant of the use of invasive procedures after acute myocardial infarction in New York state. Circulation 2000;102(Suppl III):III-107–III-115.
22. Lewis CE, Raczynski JM, Oberman A, Cutter GR. Risk factors and the natural history of coronary heart disease in blacks. In: Brest AN, Saunders E (eds.). Cardiovascular Disease in Blacks. F.A. Davis, Philadelphia, PA: 1991, pp. 29–43.
23. Ayanian JZ, Epstein AM. Differences in the use of procedures between women and men hospitalized for coronary heart disease. N Engl J Med 1991;325:221–225.
24. Steingart RM, Packer M, Hamm P, et al., for the Survival and Ventricular Enlargement Investigators. Sex differences in the management of coronary artery disease. N Engl J Med 1991;325:226–230.
25. Carlisle DM, Leake BD, Shapiro MF. Racial and ethnic disparities in the use of cardiovascular procedures: Association with type of health insurance. Am J Pub Health 1997;87:263–267.
26. Daumit GL, Hermann JA, Powe NR. Relation of gender and health insurance to cardiovascular procedure use in persons with progression to chronic renal disease. Med Care 2000;38:354–365.
27. Hannan EL, van Ryn M, Burke J, et al. Access to coronary artery bypass surgery by race/ethnicity and gender among patients who are appropriate for surgery. Med Care 1999;37:68–77.
28. Leape LL, Hilborne LH, Bell R, et al. Underuse of cardiac procedures: Do women, ethnic minorities, and the uninsured fail to receive needed revascularization? Ann Intern Med 1999;130:183–192.
29. Schulman KA, Berlin JA, Harless W, et al. The effect of race and sex on physicians' recommendations for cardiac catheterization. New Engl J Med 1999;340:618–626.
30. Ford E, Newman J, Deosaransingh K. Racial and ethnic differences in the use of cardiovascular procedures: Findings from the California Cooperative Cardiovascular Project. Am J Public Health 2000;90:1128–1134.
31. Peniston RL, Lu DY, Papademetriou V, Fletcher RD. Severity of coronary artery disease in black and white male veterans and likelihood of revascularization. Am Heart J 2000;139:840–847.
32. Peterson ED, Lansky AJ, Anstrom KJ, et al. for the National Cardiovascular Network. Evolving trends in interventional device use and outcomes: Results from the National Cardiovascular Network database. Am Heart J 2000;139:198–207.
33. Sheifer SE, Escarce JJ, Schulman KA. Race and sex differences in the management of coronary artery disease. Am Heart J 2000;139:848–857.
34. Kressin NR, Petersen LA. Racial differences in the use of invasive cardiovascular procedures: Review of the literature and prescription for future research. Ann Intern Med 2001;135:352–366.
35. Peterson ED, Shaw LK, DeLong ER, et al. Racial variation in the use of coronary revascularization procedures: Are the differences real? Do they matter? New Engl J Med 1997;336:480–486.
36. Giles WH, Anda RF, Casper ML, et al. Race and sex differences in rates of invasive cardiac procedures in US hospitals: Data from the National Hospital Discharge Survey. Arch Intern Med 1995;155:318–324.
37. Schneider EC, Leape LL, Weissman JS, et al. Racial differences in cardiac revascularization rates: Does "overuse" explain higher rates among white patients? Ann Intern Med 2001;135:328–337.
38. Schwartz, LM Woloshin S, Welch HG. Misunderstandingsabout the effects of race and sex on physicians'referrals for cardiac catheterization. N Engl J Med 1999;341:279–283.
39. Anderson RP. Will the real CASS stand up? A review and perspective on the Coronary Artery Surgery Study. J Thorac Cardiovasc Surg 1986;91:698–709.
40. Chaitman BR, Davis KB, Kaiser GC, et al. and participating CASS Hospitals. The role of coronary bypass surgery for "left main equivalent" coronary disease: The Coronary Artery Surgery Study Registry. Circulation 1986;74(Suppl III): III-17–III-25.
41. Myers WO, Davis K, Foster ED, et al. Surgical survival in the Coronary Artery Surgery Study (CASS) Registry. Ann Thorac Surg 1985;40:245–259.

42. Grover FL, Hammermeister KE, Burchfiel C, and Cardiac Surgeons of the Department of Veterans Affairs. Initial report of the Veterans Administration preoperative risk assessment study for cardiac surgery. Ann Thorac Surg 1990;50:12–28.

43. Freeman WK, Schaff HV, O'Brien PC, et al. Cardiac surgery in the octogenarian: Perioperative outcome and clinical follow-up. J Am Coll Cardiol 1991;18:29–35.

44. Khan SS, Kupfer JM, Matloff JM, et al. Interaction of age and predictive risk factors in predicting operative mortality for coronary bypass surgery. Circulation 1992;86(Suppl II): II-186–II-90.

45. Kirsch M, Guesnier L, LeBesnerais P, et al. Cardiac operations in octogenarians: Perioperative risk factors for death and impaired autonomy. Ann Thorac Surg 1998;66:60–67.

46. Aldea GS, Gaudiani JM, Shapira OM, et al. Effect of gender on postoperative outcomes and hospital stays after coronary artery bypass grafting. Ann Thorac Surg 1999;67:1097–1103.

47. Khan SS, Nessim S, Gray R, et al. Increased mortality of women in coronary artery bypass surgery: Evidence for referral bias. Ann Intern Med 1990;112:561–567.

48. Abramov D, Tamariz MG, Sever JY, et al. The influence of gender on the outcome of coronary artery bypass surgery. Ann Thorac Surg 2000;70:800–805.

49. Curtis JJ, Walls JT, Boley TM, et al. Coronary revascularization in the elderly: Determinants of operative mortality. Ann Thorac Surg 1994;58:1069–1072.

50. Yau TM, Fedak PWM, Weisel RD, et al. Predictors of operative risk for coronary bypass operations in patients with left ventricular dysfunction. J Thorac Cardiovasc Surg 1999;118:1006–1013.

51. Buell HE, DeLong ER, Peterson ED, et al. Examining increased CABG mortality risk in females. J Am Coll Cardiol 1999;33:566A.

52. Eaker ED, Kronmal R, Kennedy JW, Davis K. Comparison of the long-term postsurgical survival of women and men in the Coronary Artery Surgery Study (CASS). Am Heart J 1989;117:71–81.

53. Herlitz J, Brandrup-Wognsen G, Karlson BW, et al. Mortality, risk indicators for death, mode of death and symptoms of angina pectoris during 5 years after coronary artery bypass grafting in men and women. J Intern Med 2000;247:500–506.

54. Geraci JM, Rosen AK, Ash AS, et al. Predicting the occurrence of adverse events after coronary artery bypass surgery. Ann Intern Med 1993;118:18–24.

55. Ferraris VA, Ferraris SP. Risk factors for postoperative morbidity. J Thorac Cardiovasc Surg 1996;111:731–741.

56. Butterworth J, James R, Prielipp R, et al. Female gender associates with increased duration of intubation and length of stay after coronary surgery. CABG Clinical Benchmarking Database Participants. Anesthesiology 2000;92:414–424.

57. Paone G, Higgins RSD, Havstad SL, Silverman NA. Does age limit the effectiveness of clinical pathways after coronary artery bypass graft surgery? Circulation 1998;98:II-41–II-45.

58. Rankin SH. Differences in recovery from cardiac surgery: A profile of male and female patients. Heart Lung 1990;19:481–485.

59. Weintraub WS, Jones EL, Craver JM, et al. Determinants of prolonged length of hospital stay after coronary bypass surgery. Circulation 1989;80:276–284.

60. Warner, C Deaton, Weintraub WS, et al. Factors associated with postoperative lengths of stay after coronary artery bypass graft surgery 1981 through 1995. J Am Coll Cardiol 1997(Suppl A);29:289A (abstract).

61. Lahey SJ, Campos CT, Jennings B, et al. Hospital readmission after cardiac surgery: Does "fast track" cardiac surgery result in cost saving or cost shifting? Circulation 1998;98:II-35–II-40.

62. Fontes ML, Lin Z-Q, Matthew JP, et al. Is the cost of cardiac surgery influenced by gender? Anesthesiology 1998;89:A269.

63. Lubitz JD, Gornick ME, Mentnech RM, Loop FD. Rehospitalization after coronary revascularization among Medicare beneficiaries. Am J Cardiol 1993;72:26–30.

64. Deaton C, Weintraub WS, Ramsay J, et al. Patient health status, hospital length of stay, and readmission after coronary artery bypass surgery. J Cardiovasc Nurs 1998;12:62–71.

65. Cowper PA, Peterson ED, DeLong ER, et al. for the Ischemic Heart Disease Patient Outcomes Research Team Investigators. Impact of early discharge after coronary artery bypass graft surgery on rates of hospital readmission and death. J Am Coll Cardiol 1997;30:908–913.

66. Ai AL, Peterson C, Dunkle RE, et al. How gender affects psychological adjustment one year after coronary artery bypass graft surgery. Women Health 1997;26:45–65.

67. Deaton C. Preoperative characteristics and outcomes: differences between black and white women undergoing coronary bypass surgery. Circulation 2000;102(Suppl II):II-511.

68. Barnason S, Zimmerman L, Anderson A, et al. Functional status outcomes of patients with a coronary artery bypass graft over time. Heart Lung 2000;29:33–46.
69. Jaeger AA, Hlatky MA, Paul SM, Gortner SR. Functional capacity after cardiac surgery in elderly patients. J Am Coll Cardiol 1994;24:104–108.
70. Artinian NT, Duggan CH. Sex differences in patient recovery patterns after coronary artery bypass surgery. Heart Lung 1995;24:483–494.
71. Ayanian JZ, Guadagnoli E, Cleary PD. Physical and psychosocial functioning of women and men after coronary artery bypass surgery. JAMA 1995;274:1767–1770.
72. King KM. Gender and short-term recovery from cardiac surgery. Nursing Res 2000;49:29–36.
73. Burker EJ, Blumenthal JA, Feldman M, et al. Depression in male and female patients undergoing cardiac surgery. Brit J Clin Psychol 1995;34:119–128.
74. Sokol RA, Folks DG, Herrick RW, Freeman AM. Psychiatric outcome in men and women after coronary bypass surgery. Psychosomatics 1987;28:11–16.
75. Cameron AA, Davis KB, Rogers WJ. Recurrence of angina after coronary artery bypass surgery: predictors and prognosis (CASS Registry). J Am Coll Cardiol 1995;26:895–899.
76. Liao Y, Cooper RS, Ghali JK, Szocka A. Survival rates with coronary artery disease for black women compared with black men. JAMA 1992;268:1867–1871.
77. Kelsey SF, James M, Holubkov AL, et al. Results of percutaneous transluminal coronary angioplasty in women: 1985–1986 National Heart, Lung and Blood Institute's Coronary Angioplasty Registry. Circulation 1993;87:720–727.
78. Weintraub WS, Wenger NK, Delafontaine P, et al. PTCA in women compared to men: Is there a difference in risk? Circulation 1992;86(Suppl I):I-253.
79. Bell MR, Holmes DR, Berger PB, et al. The changing in-hospital mortality of women undergoing percutaneous transluminal coronary angioplasty. JAMA 1993;269:2091–2095.
80. Cowley MJ, Mullin SM, Kelsey SF, et al. Sex differences in early and long-term results of coronary angioplasty in the NHLBI PTCA Registry. Circulation 1985;71:90–97.
81. Phillipides G, Jacobs AK, Kelsey SF, et al. and Registry Investigators. Late outcome of PTCA in women vs men: A report from the NHLBI PTCA Registry. Circulation 1992;86(Suppl I):I-254.
82. Welty FK, Mittleman MA, Healy RW, et al. Similar results of percutaneous transluminal coronary angioplasty for women and men with postmyocardial infarction ischemia. J Am Coll Cardiol 1994;23:35–39.
83. Jacobs AK, Kelsey SF, Brooks MM, et al. Better outcome for women compared with men undergoing coronary revascularization: A report from the Bypass Angioplasty Revascularization Investigation (BARI). Circulation 1998;98:1279–1285.
84. Mehilli J, Kastrati A, Dirschinger J, et al. Differences in prognostic factors and outcomes between women and men undergoing coronary artery stenting. JAMA 2000;284:1799–1805.
85. Peterson ED, Lansky AJ, Kramer J, et al. National Cardiovascular Network Clinical Investigators. Effect of gender on the outcomes of contemporary percutaneous coronary intervention. Am J Cardiol 2001;88:359–364.
86. Moran BP, Laramee LA, Gordon JE, Davies RF. Does gender influence short term outcome of coronary angioplasty? Circulation 1992;86(Suppl I):I-253.
87. Agrawal SK, Hearn JA, Cannon AD, et al. Vascular complications following coronary artery stenting – implications for females and elderly. Circulation 1992;86(Suppl I):I-254.
88. Steen MK, Jacobs AK, Freney D, et al. Gender related differences in complications during coronary angiography. Circulation 1992;86(Suppl I):I-254.
89. Califf RM, Fortin DF, Frid DJ, et al. Restenosis after coronary angioplasty: An overview. J Am Coll Cardiol 1991;17:2B–13B.
90. Fishman RF, Friedrich SP, Gordon PC, et al. Acute and long-term results of new coronary interventions in women and the elderly. Circulation 1992;86(Suppl I):I-253.
91. Krumholz HM, McHorney CA, Clark L, et al. Changes in health after elective percutaneous coronary revascularization: A comparison of generic and specific measures. Med Care 1996;34:754–759.
92. Nash IS, Curtis LH, Rubin H. Predictors of patient-reported physical and mental health 6 months after percutaneous coronary revascularization. Am Heart J 1999;138:422–429.
93. Pocock SJ, Henderson RA, Clayton T, et al. for the RITA-2 Trial Participants. Quality of life after coronary angioplasty or continued medical treatment for angina: Three-year follow-up in the RITA-2 Trial. J Am Coll Cardiol 2000;35:907–914.
94. Edell-Gustafsson UM, Hetta JE. Fragmented sleep and tiredness in males and females one year after percutaneous transluminal coronary angioplasty (PTCA). J Adv Nurs 2001;34:203–211.

95. Dodge JT, Brown BG, Bolson EL, Dodge HT. Lumen diameter of normal human coronary arteries: Influence of age, sex, anatomic variation and left ventricular hypertrophy or dilation. Circulation 1992;86:232–246.
96. Scott NA, Kelsey SF, Detre K, et al. and the NHLBI PTCA Registry Investigators. Percutaneous transluminal coronary angioplasty in African-American patients (The National Heart, Lung and Blood Institute 1985–1986 Percutaneous Transluminal Coronary Angioplasty Registry). Am J Cardiol 1994;73:1141–1146.
97. Marks DS, Mensah GA, Kennard ED, et al. Race, baseline characteristics, and clinical outcomes after coronary intervention: The new approaches in coronary interventions (NACI) registry. Am Heart J 2000;140:162–169.

19 Electrophysiology
Treatment Considerations in Women

Michael S. Bailey, MD
and Anne B. Curtis, MD

CONTENTS

INTRODUCTION

Only in the last decade have physicians truly recognized that heart disease may present and behave differently in women when compared to men. In addition, there are sensitivity and specificity differences in diagnostic tests for coronary heart disease (CHD). This recognition of gender differences, critical to heart disease diagnosis and management, extends to electrophysiology as well. Significant differences in the natural history of arrhythmias in women are being discovered, leading to a new understanding of gender differences and more importantly, inspiring research into the basic mechanisms of that difference. Currently, the major thrust is to determine reproductive hormones' influence on normal and abnormal cardiac conduction. Estrogen, particularly estradiol, has many effects on conduction tissue. Testosterone may influence basic conduction properties as well. Reproductive hormones play a significant role in modulating the presentation and behavior of numerous arrhythmia types. The following discussion centers on the most important aspects of clinical electrophysiology in women with CHD, namely atrial fibrillation (AF), long QT syndrome, and sudden cardiac death, preceded by a review of the basic differences in heart rate (HR) and repolarization between the sexes.

From: *Contemporary Cardiology: Coronary Disease in Women: Evidence-Based Diagnosis and Treatment*
Edited by: L. J. Shaw and R. F. Redberg © Humana Press Inc., Totowa, NJ

BASIC ELECTROPHYSIOLOGY: SIMILARITIES
AND DIFFERENCES BETWEEN THE SEXES

The most basic electrophysiological parameter is HR. Men typically have a slightly slower HR (longer sinus cycle length) than women. Debate arises over the possibility of an intrinsic difference between men and women regarding sinus cycle length. After autonomic blockade, Jose and Collison found that women had a higher intrinsic HR than men *(1)*, which suggests that autonomic tone does not have a significant impact on HR disparity between men and women. Burke et al. also showed that men have a slower intrinsic HR than women with autonomic blockade *(2)*. Additionally, they compared HRs in men and women undergoing maximal exercise. Interestingly, covariance analysis identified maximal exercise capacity as the only significant predictor of HR. Thus, a greater capacity for higher exertion levels in men appears to underlie the gender HR difference.

HR also appears to vary depending on what phase of the female reproductive cycle the measurement is taken *(3)*. During the high estrogen state, HR is relatively faster than at low estrogen state. Fluctuations in circulating blood volume and metabolic rate may underlie these changes.

Another basic electrophysiological parameter is the QT interval. In 1920, Bazett identified a length difference in the QT interval between women and men *(4)* and also defined how the QT interval changes with HR fluctuations. Since Bazett's work, several methods have been described to correct the QT interval for HR *(5)*. A 10–20-ms difference exists between the shorter adult male-corrected QT interval and the longer adult female-corrected QT interval. Moreover, the QT interval undergoes circadian variation, where the most QT variability occurs during sleep, and the maximal QT interval is found shortly after awakening before it declines to daytime levels *(6)*.

To explain the 10–20-ms difference in corrected QT intervals, prepubertal QT intervals should be examined. The QT interval is basically the same for boys and girls until puberty. The QT male interval shortens with the growth spurt associated with puberty, a time of increased male hormone production *(7;* Fig. 1), and remains shorter until about age 50. Recent data from Biggodia et al. compares repolarization differences in normal women and men, castrated men, and women with virilization syndromes, revealing information that corroborates an androgen effect on the QT interval *(8)*. Electrocardiograms (ECGs) from castrated men, specifically the QT interval and T-wave morphology, closely resembled that of normal females. Interestingly, the castrated men's QT intervals and T waves returned to near-precastration levels with testosterone administration. Another interesting facet of this study involved virilized females. The QT interval and T-wave morphology closely reflected that of normal men. This study validated its findings with clear differences between the groups' plasma androgen assays and the inclusion of normal male and female controls.

Autonomic blockade has been carried out in women and men while the QT interval was measured *(9)*. The QT interval difference between men and women was preserved. The same female group was studied at menses, during the follicular phase, and during the luteal phase, with and without autonomic blockade. During autonomic blockade, the QT interval was longest in the follicular phase and shortest in the luteal phase. This difference was not present without autonomic blockade and does not explain the QT interval disparity between men and women.

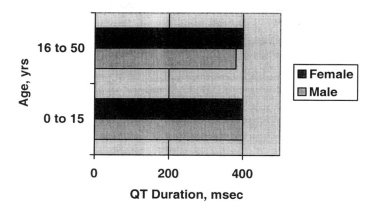

Fig. 1. Age-related differences in QT duration in males and females. Prepubertal males and females have similar QT durations. The male QT interval shortens at puberty (by 20 ms) and remains shorter throughout the reproductive years.

Other QT interval facets affected by gender are the QT-relative risk (RR) relationship, T-wave morphology, and QT dispersion. The QT-RR relationship is different between men and women. In women, the QT interval shortens more rapidly as cycle length shortens and approaches the QT interval for men at higher HRs (10–12). Thus, gender differences in QT interval disappear as HR increases (Fig. 2). In postmenopausal women who were given estrogen replacement therapy (ERT), the QT-RR relationship became similar to that of premenopausal women (13). The QT-RR regression slope increased by 93% with the addition of ERT. No variability change of the RR or QT interval was noted in the ERT state when compared to the postmenopausal state.

T-wave morphology in women differs from that in men. The area under the T wave is less in women, and the upsloping and downsloping limbs are more horizontal than in men (8,14). This difference may be a significant contributor to the increased QT interval length in women, as the overall T-wave duration is shorter. As shown by Biggodia, T-wave morphology is modifiable through testosterone administration in men who were previously in a low-testosterone state. This finding suggests that the shape of the QT and T-wave morphology are more influenced by androgens than estrogens (8).

QT dispersion is defined as the difference between the longest and shortest QTc intervals on a single 12-lead ECG tracing. The normal value will not exceed 60 ms, with values greater than 100 ms believed to confer additional arrhythmia risk (5). QT dispersion has been noted to be greater in men than in women. It has been postulated that a higher degree of QT dispersion may lead to increased arrhythmic events. Controversy exists in the literature regarding the validity of this arrhythmia predictor. Zabel et al. demonstrated in post-myocardial infarction (MI) patients that the presence of "significant" QT dispersion did not confer a worse prognosis over those without significant QT dispersion (15). Day found that patients with congenital long QT syndrome had greater QT dispersion than those with drug-associated (sotalol) long QT syndrome (16).

QT dispersion persists after autonomic blockade, although the degree of QT dispersion is less, suggesting that the autonomic nervous system does not account for the gender-based differences (9). QT dispersion is reduced in estrogen-deficient women

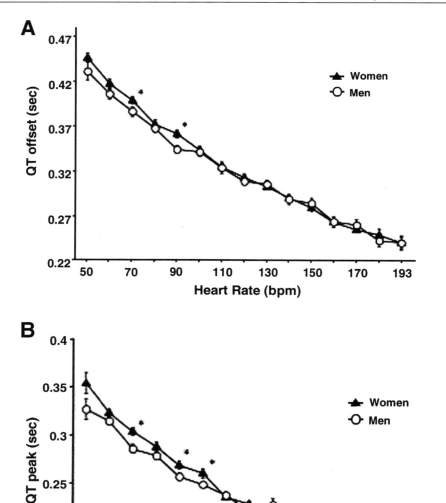

Fig. 2. As heart rate (HR) increases, the QT interval difference between the genders decrease. The QT peak and QT offset are measured from the beginning of the QRS to the T-wave peak and at the repolarization endpoint, respectively. **(A).** HR-independent analysis of gender effects on the QT offset interval. Data are shown as mean ± 1 SE. Women have a longer QT interval than men (up to 100 beats/min for QT offset), with significant differences found at 70 and 90 beats/min HR bins. $p < 0.05$. **(B).** HR-independent analysis of gender effects on the QT peak interval. Data are shown as mean ± 1 SE. Women have a longer QT interval than men [up to 110 beats/min for QT peak], with significant differences found at 70, 90, and 100 beats/min HR bins. $p < 0.05$. (Adapted from ref. *12.*)

Table 1
Population-Attributable Risk of the Risk Factors Associated With AF

Variables	Men	Women
Cigarette smoking	2	8
Diabetes	4	4
Electrocardiographic LV hypertrophy	2	1
Hypertension	14	14
MI	5	1
CHF	10	12
Valve disease	5	18

AF, atrial fibrillation; MI, myocardial infarction; CHF, congestive heart failure. (Adapted from ref. 19.)

when ERT is supplied (17). This may be a possible explanation for the difference in risk of sudden cardiac death in pre- vs postmenopausal women, but a consensus does not exist to confirm this as a bona-fide mechanism for sudden cardiac death in women.

In summary, the estrogen impact on normal and abnormal cardiac conduction is still not fully established. Estrogen is certainly active in different aspects of cardiac conduction, such as in the QT-RR relationship, T-wave morphology, and QT dispersion, but it does not explain the disparity between men and women. Indeed, androgens may have more influence on this disparity than female hormones, and the QT interval difference begins during greatly increased androgen production. These differences likely account for at least some variation in the presentation of cardiac arrhythmias in men and women.

ATRIAL FIBRILLATION

The most common sustained arrhythmia in either sex is AF. AF prevalence begins to rise after age 40, with a marked increase in the general population above age 65. Evaluation of epidemiological data reveals a higher AF prevalence in men than in women at all ages. As age increases, the gap in prevalence between gender widens, with men above age 75 twice as likely to be affected. However, because of their longer life expectancy, the absolute number of women with AF is larger than the number of men with this arrhythmia. Overall, women appear to account for 53% of all patients with AF (18).

The Framingham Heart Study recruited numerous men and women and followed them for 30 years, yielding important epidemiological data regarding AF. Men with AF were more likely to have coronary artery disease (CAD) and a history of MI, with five times the risk of women of developing AF with prior coronary disease. Men also were at five times greater risk than women to develop AF after coronary artery bypass surgery (CABG) (Coronary Artery Surgery Study [CASS] Registry). Women were more likely to have congestive heart failure (CHF) and valvular heart disease than men with AF (Table 1; 19,20).

Some data suggests that lower AF incidence in women results from estrogen status. Tse et al. found significant differences in the shortening of the atrial effective refractory period with rapid pacing in men and women (21). Although premenopausal women had the shortest atrial effective refractory periods during sinus rhythm, they had less of a decline in atrial effective refractory period with rapid atrial pacing and elevated atrial pressure compared to postmenopausal women and age-matched men. The attenuated shortening of the atrial effective refractory period observed under these conditions in premenopausal women suggests that estrogen may exert a protective effect against AF in premenopausal women. The effect seen is not because of age, as there were no age-related differences in atrial effective refractory periods observed in men.

There appear to be differences between men and women in the rate and duration of paroxysmal AF, as reported by Hnatkova et al. *(23)*. In a male and female population with paroxysmal AF, women had statistically higher HRs at AF onset (123 ± 35 vs 115 ± 20 beats/min) and during the episode (120 ± 25 vs 112 ± 22 beat/min). They also tended to have longer episodes (83.8 vs 46.9 min, mean, p = ns). The study demographics were well-matched in all categories, but the mean age was somewhat higher in women when compared to men (65.5 ± 12.4 years vs 58.5 ± 12.6 years, p = ns). As the conduction system ages, mean HR decreases, likely from age-accrued defects in the conduction system. However, even though the women were older, the mean HR during AF was higher in women than men. The authors proposed autonomic differences between men and women as a possible explanation *(22)*. The faster HRs and longer AF duration in women may necessitate the more frequent use of antiarrhythmic drugs for quality of life.

In the Canadian Registry of Atrial Fibrillation (CARAF), it was found that the age of AF presentation in women tended to be older than in men. Women also had higher HRs during AF than men. Interestingly, women were half as likely to receive warfarin than men. In this study, women were also 3.35 times more likely to sustain a major bleed from warfarin than men. Apparently, the major factor in these serious bleeds was poor control of the international normalized ratio (INR; *23*).

When cardioversion of paroxysmal AF or atrial flutter is successful, women are less likely to maintain sinus rhythm. In a study of 124 consecutive patients, Suttorp et al. investigated the risk factors for recurrence of paroxysmal AF or atrial flutter. Subjects with reduced left ventricular (LV) function were excluded, and antiarrhythmic medications were not utilized. The endpoint was the first recurrence of the arrhythmia. Significant risk factors for recurrence included CAD, history of paroxysms of AF or atrial flutter, pulmonary disease and valvular heart disease. In addition, there was a higher risk of recurrence in women, with a relative risk of 2.3 *(24)*.

Women may be more at risk for embolic stroke than men with AF, but they also tend to derive more of a benefit from anticoagulation usage than men *(25)*. Women are also at higher risk for death because of AF, even when matched for comorbid cardiac conditions. Additionally, women are at higher risk for proarrhythmia than men with the use of QT-prolonging antiarrhythmic medications *(26)*.

LONG QT SYNDROME

A female predominance exists in congenital long QT syndrome, with a 70% female-to-male split *(27)*. In addition to the prevalence disparity, females make up more than 60% of symptomatic family members in the International Long QT Syndrome (LQTS) registry *(28)*. Males are more likely to be younger and to have higher event rates before age 15 than females. After age 15, the trend is reversed, with females comprising the

Table 2
Observed vs Expected Incidence of Torsades de Pointes (TdP) Among Women Given
QT-Prolonging Agnets

Drug	No[a]	Median Age. Y	Observed female prevalence		Expected female prevalence	
			%	95% CIC[b]	%	p
Quinidine	108	64	60	50–70	43[c]	<.00
Procainamide hydrochloride	39	66	49	32–66	38[c]	.21
Disopyramide	49	66	86	72–94	63[c]	<.00
Amiodarone	28	64	68	47–85	32[c]	<.00
Sotalol hydrochloride	21	65	76	52–92	50[d]	<.04
Bepridil hydrochoride	27	73	74	53–89	50[d]	<.02
Prenylamine	23	71	78	56–89	50[d]	<.02
Two drugs	19	66	89	63–99	NA	NA

[a] Total number of patients adds up 314 (rather than 332) because two aggregate studies (30,31) totaling 18 patients included cases of exposure to more than one drug, making it impossible to calculate female prevalence for specific drugs.

[b] CI indicates confidence interval.

[c] Based on data provided though a large national pharmaceutical marketing research database produced by IN American, Plymouth Meeting, PA with specific reference to outpatient use of antiarrythmic drugs in 1986 original reported by Hine et al. (36) and supplemented by written communication (Richard A. Fehing, IMS America, January 1992).

[d] For sotalol, bepridil, and prenylamine, where extensive data were not available to estimate expected female prevalence, a conservative estimate of 50% was used. (An even lower prevalence is actually expected, because the drugs are mainly used to treat male predominant conditions.)

NA, not applicable.

These data represent pooled information from literature sources from 1964 to 1992 reporting TdP in patients undergoing clinical trials and from various case reports. (Adapted from ref. 30.)

majority of the affected population and as well as the most symptomatic. In LQT2 and LQT3, the event rate is similar when comparing males and females, regardless of age.

It is unclear the reason for the gender difference in congenital long QT syndrome. Perhaps the underlying difference in the QT interval, with the QT interval being 10–20 ms shorter in males, protects against the potentially fatal syndrome. The difference becomes obvious after puberty, as females suffer most of the symptomatic episodes attributed to congenital long QT syndrome in older patients. Also apparent is the fact that the potassium channel defect associated with certain long QT syndrome phenotypes does not affect the naturally shorter QT interval in men. Lehman et al. provided interesting data showing that the shorter male QT interval is preserved with or without the chromosome defect in LQT1 or LQT2 (29). Both of these genetic defects affect the potassium channel, causing prolonged myocardium repolarization.

Sudden death because of torsades de pointes from QT-prolonging drugs is more common in females than males. Makkar et al. reported an overabundance of torsades de pointes in women who receive prescriptions for QT-prolonging agents (Table 2; 30). In that study, 70% of torsades de pointes occurred in women that receive cardiovascular drugs, although they received only 44% of prescribed drugs. Marker et al. also reviewed other data, all of which revealed a more than 50% predominance of torsades de pointes in women who take cardioactive medications.

Benton et al. administered a single placebo or quinidine dose, a class IA antiarrhythmic agent, to 12 women and 12 men *(31)*. Each group crossed over to the other arm after the first administration. Using Bazett's QT correction, these two groups were compared. Quinidine caused greater QT prolongation in women than men at equivalent serum concentrations. The QT interval change was 44% greater in women than men, a highly significant result ($p < 0.001$).

There are intriguing new data from Rodriguez regarding changes in the risk of drug-induced torsades de pointes during the menstrual cycle. In a cohort study, men and women receiving ibutilide, a class III antiarrhythmic agent, were compared regarding the risk of torsades de pointes. Low-dose ibutilide was administered to women on three separate occasions, at different menstrual cycle phases, as verified by hormonal analysis. Maximum QT prolongation with ibutilide occurred during menses (63 ms over baseline). A 59-ms QTc prolongation occurred during the ovulatory phase, and a 53-ms prolongation occurred during the luteal phase. Men exhibited a 46-ms prolongation of QTc in response to ibutilide. Progesterone and progesterone-to-estradiol ratio inversely correlated with ibutilide-induced QT prolongation *(32)*.

No data exist that define a time during the menstrual cycle when a woman is most at risk for torsades de pointes in response to QT-prolonging agents. However, given the previous Rodriguez observations above, it might be reasonable to postulate that the greatest risk of torsades de pointes in premenstrual women would coincide with the menses. Thus, hospitalization for the initiation of QT-prolonging agents might best be scheduled during the menses.

For women with CHD who require treatment with antiarrhythmic drugs, hospitalization for initiation of therapy with telemetry monitoring is usually advisable. In such patients, therapy with the class IC antiarrhythmic drugs flecainide and propafenone is generally contraindicated because of the findings from the Cardiac Arrhythmia Suppression Trial (CAST; *33*). This is unfortunate, as an advantage of these two drugs is that they do not prolong the QT interval, they do not cause torsades de pointes, and they can safely be started in the out-patient setting for supraventricular tachycardia in patients without structural heart disease. The class IA antiarrhythmic drugs (quinidine, procainamide, and disopyramide) as well as the class III antiarrhythmic drugs (sotalol, ibutilide, and amiodarone) can all cause torsades de pointes. Therapy should be initiated in the hospital for most women with coronary disease, particularly if the indication for treatment is ventricular arrhythmias. The only exception is amiodarone; it is the least likely drug mentioned to cause torsades de pointes. For that reason and because of its unique pharmacokinetics (need for loading doses and long time to steady state), amiodarone can be initiated as an out-patient for most patients for the treatment of supraventricular tachycardia or symptomatic ventricular ectopy.

SUDDEN CARDIAC DEATH

Sudden cardiac death occurs within 1 hour of the onset of symptoms after other possible modes of death have been ruled out. Approximately 300,000 people per year are victims of sudden cardiac death in the United States. The problem of sudden cardiac death in women of all age groups is generally not as prevalent as in men. Women enjoy a prevalence of sudden cardiac death less than half that of their male counterparts. There appears to be a 10–20-year lag in the sudden cardiac death incidence in women when matched for standard male risk factors (34). In men and women, the incidence of sudden cardiac death increases with age.

In a breakdown of risk factors and associations of sudden cardiac death, women are at lower risk for individual variables, such as CAD, LV hypertrophy, and CHF when compared with men. Interestingly, a significant predictor of sudden cardiac death is childlessness, with an odds ratio of 6.7 when compared to women who bore children. Reflecting our inability to adequately screen women for significant CAD, only 37% of women who suffer sudden cardiac death have a preceding diagnosis of overt CAD. In contrast, 56% of men had a CAD diagnosis prior to sudden cardiac death. In patients who have survived a cardiac arrest, CAD is the most significant predictor of mortality in women, whereas impaired LV function is most important in men (35).

In women with CAD and decreased LV function, standard screening for the risk of sudden cardiac death may be less effective than in men. Electrophysiological studies may be less predictive in women than in men as suggested by the Multicenter Unsustained Tachycardia Trial (MUSTT; 36). The rate of inducibility of sustained ventricular tachycardia was found in this population to be lower in women (34% men vs 21% women $p = 0.001$). Additionally, the Framingham Study revealed that the presence of premature ventricular contractions with concomitant CAD did not increase the risk of sudden cardiac death in women as it did in men (33).

Treatment to reduce the risk of sudden cardiac death remains effective in both sexes, as beta blockade is effective in each gender post-MI (37). Implantable defibrillators are also equally effective in men and women, with less frequent device firings in women than their male counterparts in follow-up (38,39).

CONCLUSIONS

There are significant differences in the manifestations of AF and sudden cardiac death in women with CHD in comparison to men. With AF, a greater number of intense symptoms may necessitate therapy with antiarrhythmic drugs more often, yet drug-induced torsades de pointes is a higher risk in women. The older age of most women with AF may make anticoagulation with warfarin more difficult. With sudden cardiac death, most women have no prior evidence of coronary disease, making risk stratification and primary prevention difficult. However, recognition of these gender differences is the first step in designing strategies to manage these arrhythmias more effectively in women.

REFERENCES

1. Jose A, Collison D. The normal range and determinants of the intrinsic heart rate in man. Cardiovasc Res 1970;4:160–167.
2. Burke JH, Goldberger JJ, Ehlert FA, et al. Gender differences in heart rate before and after autonomic blockade: evidence against an intrinsic gender effect. Am J Med 1996;100:537–543.
3. Moran VH, Leathard HL, Coley J. Cardiovascular functioning during the menstrual cycle. Clin Physiol 2000;20:496–504.
4. Bazett H. An analysis of the time-relations of electrocardiograms. Heart 1920;7:353–370.

5. Bednar M, Harrigan E, Anziano R, et al. The QT interval. Prog Cardiovasc Dis 2001;43(5 Suppl 1):1–45.
6. Molnar J, Zhang F, Weiss J, et al. Diurnal pattern of QTc interval: How long is prolonged? J Am Coll Cardiol 1996;27:76–83.
7. Rautaharju PM, Zhou SH, Wong S, et al. Sex differences in the evolution of the electrocardiographic QT interval with age. Can J Cardiol 1992;8:690–695.
8. Biggodia H, Maciel J, Capalozza N, et al. Sex differences on the electrocardiographic pattern of cardiac repolarization: Possible role of testosterone. Am Heart J 2000;140:678–683.
9. Burke JH, Ehlert FA, Kruse JT, et al. Gender-specific differences in the QT interval and the effect of autonomic tone and menstrual cycle in healthy adults. Am J Cardiol 1997;79:178–181.
10. Klingfield P, Lax K, Okin P. QT interval heart rate relation during exercise in normal men and women: Definition by linear regression analysis. J Am Coll Cardiol 1996;28:1547–1555.
11. Stramba-Badiale M, Locati E, Martinelli A, et al. Gender and the relationship between ventricular repolarization and cardiac cycle length during 24-hour Holter monitor recordings. Eur Heart J 1997;18:1000–1006.
12. Mayuga KA, Parker M, Sukthanker ND, et al. Effects of age and gender on the QT response to exercise. Am J Cardiol 2001;87:163–167.
13. Vrtovek B, Starc V, Meden-Vrtovek H. The effect of estrogen replacement therapy on ventricular repolarization dynamics in healthy post-menopausal women. J Electrocardiol 2001;34:277–283.
14. Yang H, Elko P, Fromm BS, et al. Maximal ascending and descending slopes of the T wave in men and women. J Electrocardiol 2001;34:183.
15. Zabel M, Klingenheben T, Franz MR, Hohnloser SH. Assessment of QT dispersion for prediction of mortality or arrhythmic events after myocardial infarction: results of a prospective, long-term follow-up study. Circulation 1998;97:2543–2550.
16. Day CP, McComb JM, Campbell RW. QT dispersion: an indication of arrhythmia risk in patients with long QT intervals. Br Heart J 1990;63:342–344.
17. Yildirir A, Aybar F, Kabakci MG, et al. Hormone replacement therapy shortens QT dispersion in healthy postmenopausal women. Ann noninvasive Electocardiol 2001;6:193–197.
18. Feinberg WM, Blackshear J, Laupacis A, et al. Prevalence, age distribution and gender of patients with atrial fibrillation. Arch Intern Med 1995;155:469–473.
19. Benjamin EJ, Levy D, Vaziri SM, et al. Independent risk factors for atrial fibrillation in a population-based cohort: The Framingham Study. JAMA 1994;27:840–844.
20. Benjamin EJ, Wolf PA, D'Agostino RB, et al. Impact of atrial fibrillation on the risk of death: The Framingham Heart Study. Circulation 1998;98:946–952.
21. Tse HF, Oral H, Pelosi F, et al. Effect of gender on atrial electrophysiologic changes induced by rapid atrial pacing and elevation of atrial pressure. J Cardiovasc Electrophysiol 2001;12:986–989.
22. Hnatkova K, Waktare J, Murgatroyd F, et al. Age and gender influences on rate and duration of paroxysmal atrial fibrillation. Pacing Clin Electrophysiol 1998;21:2455–2458.
23. Humphries K, Kerr C, Connolly S, et al. New-onset atrial fibrillation: sex differences in presentation, treatment, and outcome. Circulation 2001;103:2365–2370.
24. Suttorp M, Kingma J, Koomen E, et al. Recurrence of paroxysmal atrial fibrillation or flutter after successful cardioversion in patients with normal left ventricular function. Am J Cardiol 1993;71:710–713.
25. Michelena H, Ezekowitz M. Atrial fibrillation: are there gender differences. J Gend Specif Med 2000;3:44–49.
26. Rodriguez LM, deChillou C, Schlapfer J, et al. Age at onset and gender of patients with different types of supraventricular tachycardias. Am J Cardiol 1992;70:1213–1215.
27. Albert C, McGovern B, Newell J, Ruskin J. Sex differences in cardiac arrest survivors. Circulation 1996;93:1170–1176.
28. Moss A, Schwartz P, Crampton R, et al. The long QT syndrome. Prospective longitudinal study of 328 families. Circulation 1991;84:1136–1144.
29. Lehmann MH, Timothy KW, Frankovich D, et al. Age-gender influence on the rate-corrected QT interval and the QT-heart rate relation in families with genotypically characterized long QT syndrome. J Am Coll Cardiol 1997;29:93–99.
30. Makkar RR, Fromm BS, Steinman RT, et al. Female gender as a risk factor for torsades de pointes associated with cardiovascular drugs. JAMA 1993;270:2590–2597.
31. Benton RE, Sale M, Flockhart DA, Woosley RL. Greater quinidine-induced QTc interval prolongation in women. Clin Pharmacol Ther 2000;67:413–418.

32. Rodriguez I, Kilborn MV, Liux K, et al. Drug induced QT prolongation in women during the menstrual cycle. JAMA 2001;285:1322–1326.
33. The Cardiac Arrhythmia Suppression Trial (CAST) Investigators. Preliminary report: effect of encainide and flecainide on mortality in a randomized trial of arrhythmia suppression after myocardial infarction. N Engl J Med 1989;321:406–12.
34. Kannel WB, Wilson P, D'Agostino R, Cobb J. Sudden coronary death in women. Am Heart J 1998;136:205–212.
35. Albert CM, McGovern BA, Newell JB, Ruskin JN. Sex differences in cardiac arrest survivors. Circulation 1996;93:1170–1176.
36. Buxton AE, Hafley GE, Lehmann MH, et al. Prediction of sustained ventricular tachycardia inducible by programmed stimulation in patients with coronary artery disease: Utility of clinical variables. Circulation 1999;99:1843–1850.
37. Olsson G, Wikstrand J, Warnold I, et al. Metoprolol-induced reduction in postinfarction mortality: Pooled results from five double-blind randomized trials. Eur Heart J 1992;13:28–32.
38. Kudenchuk PJ, Bardy GH, Poole JE, et al. Malignant sustained ventricular tachyarrhythmias in women: Characteristics and outcome of treatment with an implantable cardioverter defibrillator. J Cardiovasc Electrophysiol 1997;8:2–10.
39. Engelstein ED, Friedman PL, Yao Q, et al. Gender differences in patients with life-threatening ventricular arrhythmias: Impact on treatment and survival in the antiarrhythmics versus implantable defibrillators (AVID) trial. Circulation 1997;96:I–720.

20 Exercise Training and Cardiac Rehabilitation for Women

Elisa Yuen Man Chiu, RN, MS,
Maria Vivina T. Regis, RN, MS,
and Erika Sivarajan Froelicher, RN, PhD, FAAN

CONTENTS

INTRODUCTION

This chapter presents the role of physical activity in the risk reduction of cardiovascular disease (CVD). The unique aspects of exercise training and exercise modalities as they pertain to women are discussed. Exercise interventions regarding prescription and progression are recommended and reviewed. Education, counseling, and behavioral issues about cardiac rehabilitation in women are also included. Sections regarding special populations, such as women with different cardiac diagnoses, focuses on myocardial infarction (MI), coronary artery bypass graft (CABG), and heart transplants, as well as issues that involve elderly women. Finally, strategies to improve exercise compliance and cardiac rehabilitation recommendations for women follow.

From: *Contemporary Cardiology: Coronary Disease in Women: Evidence-Based Diagnosis and Treatment*
Edited by: L. J. Shaw and R. F. Redberg © Humana Press Inc., Totowa, NJ

CORONARY HEART DISEASE IN WOMEN

Lifestyle modification, education, treatments, and medications have begun to control risk factors involved in coronary heart disease (CHD) and have helped to reduce the mortality rates resulting from CVD. Some of these risk factors cannot be changed, such as gender, age, and genetics. But there are many interventions for modifiable risk factor reduction that can be prescribed to decrease CHD risk. Physical inactivity is a very modifiable risk factor that needs to be addressed, especially because of its increasing prevalence today and the availability of the exercise training sciences.

PHYSICAL ACTIVITY

Physical activity is "bodily movement produced by skeletal muscles that requires energy expenditure and produces overall health benefits" *(1)*. "Exercise, a type of physical activity, is defined as a planned, structured, and repetitive bodily movement done to improve or maintain one or more components of physical fitness" *(1)*. Although the meanings of these terms differ, physical activity and exercise are often used interchangeably in the literature and research regarding physical fitness, as well as are in this chapter.

Today, it is undisputed that physical activity has beneficial effects in the prevention of CVDs *(2,3,4)* and is now recognized by the American Heart Association (AHA) as an independent risk factor for CHD *(5)*. In a quantitative meta-analysis *(6)*, it was estimated that there was a doubling of CHD risk among inactive persons when compared with their active peers. Studies evaluating occupational physical activity showed that inactivity was associated with a 90% increase risk of CHD death *(6)*. Physical inactivity plays a major contributing role in many chronic diseases, such as obesity, diabetes mellitus, stroke, as well as CHD. Convincing epidemiological studies have shown that an inverse relationship exists between physical activity and CHD incidence *(7)*. Also shown is a dose-response relationship between the amount of physical activity performed and all-cause mortality and cardiovascular mortality *(8–10)*. Those who remain sedentary have the highest risk of all-cause and cardiovascular mortality. Therefore, the greatest potential for overall reduced mortality is in those who are sedentary and become moderately active *(8)*. In other words, those who are most unfit (or at least fit) can reap the greatest gains.

An abundance of scientific evidence provides consistent evidence that light-to-moderate adult physical activity reduces the risk for all-cause mortality and CVD in both men and women *(11)*. Research also indicates that physical activity and fitness reduces morbidity and mortality for at least six chronic conditions: CHD, hypertension, obesity, diabetes, osteoporosis, and mental health disorders *(12)*. Physical activity can also have many other cardioprotective benefits and seems to be an independent protective factor for CHD mortality and premature total mortality *(7)*. Regular physical activity increases exercise capacity and plays a major role in the primary and secondary prevention of CVDs *(8)*. It can positively modify several coronary risk factors, such as improving lipid and carbohydrate metabolism, lowering elevated blood pressure, reducing body fat, and reducing elevated blood glucose levels *(4)*. Several studies have shown that regular, constant, and long-term exercise training reduces low-density lipoprotein (LDL), increases high-density lipoprotein (HDL) fractions, and facilitates the storage of glucose in liver cells, even in the absence of insulin *(2)*. The benefits of regular exercise can be seen in the body's increased ability to use oxygen to derive energy. Exercise training increases maximum ventilatory oxygen uptake by increasing both cardiac output and the ability of the muscles to extract oxygen from the blood *(8)*. Short-term and long-term exercise training has also proven to be beneficial in improving various indexes of psychological functioning. Cross-sectional studies revealed that active persons, when compared with sedentary individuals, are more likely able to perform cognitive functioning activities, have reduced cardiovascular responses to stress, and report fewer depression symptoms *(8,13)*.

PHYSICAL ACTIVITY IN WOMEN

In past studies, physical activity was proven to be beneficial in CHD reduction; this main benefit was initially demonstrated primarily in men. Exercise has proven beneficial for many conditions, ranging from osteoporosis, depression, and particularly CHD *(14)*. Later studies show that these benefits are also conferred on women. More research studies have shown that physical activity also plays a major role in CHD prevention and reduction in women. Most epidemiological studies in women have shown that a comparable 50% risk reduction is also present among active women in comparison to sedentary women *(15)*. As more women die of CHD today, the AHA recommends a shift in the health paradigm to emphasize healthy lifestyles in women to help prevent the development of risk factors for CHD *(15,16)*. Among the many lifestyle modifications that were recommended, physical activity was emphasized as a major factor in reducing CHD risk *(16)*.

Large national surveys have shown that women, especially minority women, are less likely to be physically active than men. In a recent minority study, women were among the least active subgroup in US society compared with their white counterparts *(17)*. A large body of research has established that regular physical activity in postmenopausal women reduces the risk of premature death and disability in CHD *(17)*. Physical inactivity is a highly prevalent and independent risk factor in women. Moderate amounts of leisure time activity can reduce the risk of MI by half in women *(7)*. Despite these benefits, fewer women (particularly elderly and minority women) are referred for exercise rehabilitation after a coronary event when compared to men *(18)*. Exercise and physical training is not emphasized in women nearly as much as it is in men, which is especially true for referral to cardiac rehabilitation programs. Sedentary lifestyle rates increase with age, and these rates for women exceed those of men *(19)*. See Chapter 7 for a more detailed discussion of this topic.

SIGNIFICANCE OF PROBLEM

Physical inactivity in the United States is now widespread. The evidence of sedentary lifestyle is increasing at an alarming rate in the United States. It has been estimated that 250,000 deaths per year in the United States are attributable to lack of regular physical activity *(20)*. Approximately 60% of US adults are not regularly active, and 25% are completely inactive *(11)*. National surveillance programs have documented that one in four adults (more women than men) currently has a sedentary lifestyle with no leisure time activity *(1)*. CHD is the leading cause of mortality in the United States and the predominant risk factor that is associated with a sedentary lifestyle *(12)*.

Despite this evidence, the majority of Americans in the United States remain effectively sedentary. According to the National Institutes of Health (NIH) Consensus Statement in 1991, 54% of adults reported little or no regular leisure physical activity *(1)*. In 1996, the Surgeon General's Report estimated that approximately one in four adult Americans is completely sedentary *(22)*. AHA's 2001 Heart and Stroke Statistical Update shows that in 1996, approx 28% of Americans age 18 and older had no leisure-time physical activity in the previous 30 days *(21)*. The relative risk (RR) of CHD associated with physical activity and exercise ranges from 1.5 to 2.4, a risk increase comparable to that for high blood cholesterol, high blood pressure, or cigarette smoking *(21)*. These associations are statistically significant and represent the magnitude and severity of the problem.

The AHA also shows that physical inactivity is more prevalent in women than in men, among African Americans and Hispanics than whites, among older than younger adults, and among the less affluent than the more affluent *(21)*. In 1996, the Surgeon General produced the strongest policy statement the US government had made to date with a publication regarding physical activity and health. It is abundantly clear that Americans can substantially benefit and improve their health and quality of life by including physical activity in their daily lives *(22)*, being the first time that numerous governmental health agencies arrived at a consistent statement.

UNDERSTANDING PHYSICAL ACTIVITY IN WOMEN

The benefits of physical activity have become more recognized by health professionals, leading to an increased need for interventions that can help to promote this healthy behavior. The overwhelming statistics of Americans leading sedentary lifestyles warrants practitioners to continue their efforts in counseling patients about the efficacy of physical activity in relation to reducing CHD risk and mortality in women. The statistics also warrant the need for further research on the physical activity recommendations, especially in women. Much of the available research on physical activity has traditionally been performed on middle-aged men. During the past 10–15 years, further research has yielded a sufficient amount of new information about CHD in women and the role of physical activity.

Clinical trials and motivational theories show that there is strong support for the efficacy of physical activity and its relationship to CHD in women. Physical activity is important in the treating patients with known CHD, those with developing risk factors, and also in its secondary prevention. Intervention strategies have been reviewed and successfully implemented among health care providers for women in many randomized clinical trials, such as those performed by Dunn and associates *(23,24)*. and Pereira and associates *(25)*. These studies showed a statistically significant increase in physical activity in the women engaged in a successful intervention of lifestyle vs structured and walking intervention, respectively. Cross-sectional and longitudinal studies, such as those conducted by Manson et al. *(26)*, Kokkinos et al. *(4)*, and Folsom et al. *(27)* have shown that physical activity reduces CHD risk and mortality equally in women as well as men. Many of these studies show that physical activity is also beneficial to an individual's overall well-being and cardiovascular health.

A REVIEW OF LITERATURE ON PHYSICAL ACTIVITY

A review of the literature reveals that many research studies have been conducted on the efficacy of physical activity to CHD in women. Results lend support that physical activity reduces CHD risk and cardiovascular mortality. There is considerable evidence in cross-sectional studies that yield information about physical activity in women. These results vary from the physical activity patterns in women to the beneficial evidence showing increased physical activity in women. One study published by Bernstein, Morabia, and Sloutskis *(28)* sought to identify the prevalence of "sedentarism" and the activities performed by active people that could serve as effective preventive goals. The study stated that leading a sedentary lifestyle is an independent risk factor in CHD. The sedentarism rate in a population-based sample of 919 men and women, age 35–74 years, was 79.5% in men and 87.2% in women *(28)*. The study concluded that given the large number of sedentary individuals, it is essential that physical activity levels be increased in all age groups.

Physical inactivity has also been analyzed among different subpopulations of women. In another cross-sectional study, the objectives were to describe the patterns of physical activity among minority women. The results yielded that African Americans and Native Americans/Alaskan Natives reported the lowest "no leisure-time activity" when compared to white women *(17)*. The probability of being active during leisure time also tended to increase with increased educational level. Women who lived in rural areas were 33% more likely to be completely inactive during their leisure time than women living in urban areas *(17)*. Increased occupational activity was highest among women who were college graduates *(17)*. Although the study did not differentiate between educational level and area of residence, until such studies are done, it is unclear whether rural residence or low educational achievement has the strongest influence on low physical activity in rural populations of women. These results are particularly helpful in identifying high-risk populations and designing intervention strategies for behavior modification.

The literature review of physical activity and women has also yielded information about the many beneficial properties of increased physical activity. Increased physical fitness has been associated with a decrease in CHD risk factors for women. Triglyceride, LDL cholesterol levels, ratio of total cholesterol to HDL cholesterol, glucose levels, and resting systolic and diastolic blood pressures all have an inverse relationship with exercise time *(4)*. All of these CHD risk factors were significantly lowered as exercise time increased in a 522 women *(4)*. The study showed that an increased treadmill time correlated with an increase in HDL cholesterol levels *(4)*. Treadmill time was also associated with a decrease in LDL cholesterol and triglyceride levels *(4)*. This substantiates that increased exercise will raise HDL and lower LDL cholesterol levels, both predictors of decreased coronary risk. The results concluded that increased exercise time has an independent and strong association with CHD risk in women.

An important aspect of physical activity is that simply avoiding a sedentary lifestyle is not enough to reap all the physical activity benefits. The intensity, duration, and frequency of physical activity in women must also be taken into consideration. A study conducted as part of the German Cardiovascular Prevention Study, using a sample of 6039 women, revealed that energy spent on low-intensity activities at a constant energy level was significantly associated with beneficial health conditions, such as a decrease in triglycerides, diastolic blood pressure, and body mass index (BMI) *(29)*. Energy spent on moderately intense activities was significantly associated with an increase in HDL cholesterol, decrease in HDL/total cholesterol ratio, triglycerides, and BMI in women *(29)*. The strongest relationship with coronary risk factors was seen in the high-intensity activities, which correlates with many studies to date that have documented a dose-response relationship to CHD risk factors and physical activity. Duration of exercise training had a significant positive association with systolic blood pressure and peak expiratory flow in women *(29)*. Exercise frequency was also significantly positively associated with HDL cholesterol, HDL/total cholesterol ratio, triglycerides, heart rate, and BMI in women *(29)*. Overall, exercise frequency had the strongest association with reducing coronary risk factors when compared with intensity and duration. The importance of this study is seen in its correlation between the frequency dimensions and physical activity outcomes. It also substantiates the 1995 federal guideline recommendations that every adult should accumulate 30 minutes or more of moderate physical activity on most, preferably all, days of the week *(15,30)*.

EXERCISE TESTING/MEASURES OF PHYSICAL FITNESS IN WOMEN

Exercise testing is a useful diagnostic tool in providing information about a woman's cardiovascular health status in a dynamic state, and when used with a thorough history and physical examination, increases the likelihood of diagnosing CAD in women. There are, however, special considerations when using exercise testing to evaluate women patients. See Chapter 7 for a more detailed discussion of exercise testing as a diagnostic tool and Chapters 12 and 13 for a discussion of the modalities of exercise testing and special considerations for women.

PHYSICAL ACTIVITY PROGRAMS/INTERVENTIONS RECOMMENDED FOR WOMEN TODAY

The Surgeon General's Report on Physical Activity and Health calls for all Americans to engage in a physically active lifestyle *(22)*. According to the Surgeon General's Report, "significant health benefits can be obtained by including a moderate amount of physical activity (i.e., 30 minutes brisk walking or raking leaves, 15 minutes running) on most, if not all, days of the week; through a modest increase in daily activity, most Americans can improve their health and quality of life" *(22)*. Furthermore, evidence shows that physical activity increases in previously sedentary or unfit individuals resulted in subsequent gains through mortality reduction and increase in longevity *(9)*. Current physical activity recommendations from a consensus statement of national health agencies and organizations (i.e., AHA, American College of Cardiology [ACC], CDC, American College of Sports Medicine [ACSM], and Agency for Health Care Policy and Research [AHCPR]) indicate that lower levels of physical activity also provide health benefits *(31)*. This requires a change in the myth, "no pain–no gain." It is also noted that numerous health benefits are associated with regular participation in intermittent moderately intense physical activity (i.e., short bouts instead of long bouts of exercise; VO_{2max} 50%; *31*).

Physical Activity Benefits Older Women

Strength training is defined as training with resistance against which a muscle generates force. This resistance is progressively increased over time, thus resulting in an increase in muscle size *(32)*. Regularly performed strength training exercise results in positive changes in older women, such as improved insulin action, bone density, energy metabolism, and functional status. Strength training results in increased levels of spontaneous activity in the elderly, both the healthy free-living and very frail elderly women *(33)*.

Postural stability and the role of exercise remain unclear *(32)*. Postural instability is usually measured by frequency of falling, and it is assumed that the desire to improve postural stability through exercise will lead to reduction in falls among older women. However, there is no general agreement by investigators on an optimal measure of postural stability. *(32)*. Also, ACSM noted that the multifaceted nature of most intervention programs being effective in preventing falls makes it difficult to identify specific mechanisms by which postural stability is improved *(32)*. Even so, sufficient evidence supports the recommendation of a broad-based exercise program that encompasses balance training, resistive exercise, walking, and weight transfer, which should all be included as part of a multifaceted intervention to decrease the risk of falling *(32)*. According to ACSM, the program's optimal frequency and intensity remains to be clearly identified *(32)*.

Osteoporosis is more common in women than among men for three main reasons: (1) women have lower peak bone mass than men; (2) women lose bone mass at an accelerated rate postmenopause when estrogen levels decline; (3) and women have a longer life span than men *(22)*. Scientific evidence exists that physical activity reduces osteoporosis *(22,34)*. Data from studies *(22,35–39)* support bone loss retardation in postmenopausal women through physical activity. It is also suggested that the rate of bone loss in premenopausal women with normal hormone levels is reduced *(22,39–43)*. Still, there is a need to further understand the different effects of endurance and resistance exercises on bone mineral density and the role and impact of physical activity with the use of estrogen replacement therapy *(34)*.

ACSM recommends that exercise (e.g., walking, aerobic dance, and stretching) should be included in a general exercise program for older women to improve flexibility *(32)*. The exact dose-response relationship remains to be determined, along with an understanding of the benefits of daily living activities that accrue from increased flexibility.

SPECIAL CLINICAL POPULATIONS

Women With Cardiac Conditions

The current Clinical Practice Guideline on Cardiac Rehabilitation *(44)* recommends that participation in cardiac rehabilitation (CR) exercise training for women with cardiac conditions (i.e. MI, CHD, coronary artery bypass surgery [CABG], percutaneous transluminal coronary angiogram [PTCA]) is safe. Based on the guideline, total morbidity rates and mortality from cardiovascular complications following participation in CR exercise training are very low. The scientific evidence on the safety of CR exercise related to morbidity risk was drawn from the results of 15 randomized controlled trials (RCTs), 14 non-RCTs, and 13 observational reports *(44)*. Similarly, the results of 17 RCTs, 8 non-RCTs, 6 observational investigations, and 2 survey questionnaires provided scientific evidence of the association of CR exercise training with mortality *(44)*.

Risk stratification is essential, although not the only factor to consider when ensuring patient safety during exercise *(31)*. It pertains to symptoms and risk factor screening and evaluation suggestive of CHD, so that decisions about the level of medical clearance, the need for exercise testing before starting an exercise program, and the supervision level for both the exercise testing and program should be made judiciously

Table 1
Clinical Indications and Contraindications for In-Patient and Out-Patient CR

Indications
- Medically stable postmyocardial infarction
- Stable angina
- Coronary artery bypass graft surgery
- Percutaneous transluminal coronary angioplasty
- Compensated congestive heart failure
- Cardiomyopathy
- Heart or other organ transplantation
- Other cardiac surgery, including valvular and pacemaker insertion (e.g., implantable cardioverter defibrillator)
- Peripheral vascular disease
- High-risk cardiovascular disease ineligible for surgical intervention
- Sudden cardiac death syndrome
- End-stage renal disease
- At risk for coronary artery disease, with diagnoses of diabetes mellitus, hyperlipidemia, hypertension, etc.
- Other patients who may benefit from structured exercise and/or patient education (based on physician referral and consensus of the rehabilitation team)

Contraindications
- Unstable angina
- Resting systolic blood pressure of >200 mmHg or resting diastolic blood pressure of >110 mmHg should be evaluated on a case-by-case basis
- Orthostatic blood pressure drop of >20 mmHg with symptoms
- Critical aortic stenosis (peak systolic pressure gradient of > 50 mmHg with an aortic valve orifice area of <0.75 cm^2 in an average size adult)
- Acute systemic illness or fever
- Uncontrolled atrial or ventricular arrhythmias
- Uncontrolled sinus tachycardia (>120 beats/min)
- Uncompensated CHF
- 3° AV block (without pacemaker)
- Active pericarditis or myocarditis
- Recent embolism
- Thrombophlebitis
- Resting ST-segment displacement (>2 mm)
- Uncontrolled diabetes (resting blood glucose of >400 mg/dL)
- Severe orthopedic conditions that would prohibit exercise
- Other metabolic conditions, such as acute thyroiditis, hypokalemia or hyperkalemia, hypovolemia, etc.

Source: ref. *31.*

(31). Risk stratification also ensures that patients, both men and women, follow the exercise regimen suitable to their needs with the level of electrocardiogram (ECG) monitoring, clinical supervision, and length of exercise program specific to each individual.

Clinical indications and contraindications for in-patient and out-patient cardiac rehabilitation are presented in Table 1 *(31)*. However, sound clinical judgment is neces-

Table 2
Recommended Exercise Activity for Cardiac Patients (Both Genders)

Intensity
  RPE < 13 (6–20 scale)
  Post-MI: HR < 120 beats/min or HR_{rest} + 20 beats/min (arbitrary upper limit)
  Postsurgery: HR_{rest} + 30 beats/min (arbitrary upper limit)
  To tolerance if asymptomatic
Duration
  Intermittent bouts lasting 3–5 minutes
  Rest periods
    At patient's discretion
    Lasting 1–2 minutes
    Shorter than exercise bout duration
  Total duration of up to 20 minutes
Frequency
  Early mobilization: three to four times per day (days 1–3)
  Later mobilization: two times per day (beginning on day 4)
Progression
  Initially increase duration to 10–15 minutes of exercise, then increase intensity

Source: ref. *31.* RPE, rating of perceived exertion; HR, heart rate.

sary to consider exceptions to the conditions listed. The recommended exercise activity for cardiac patients (for both genders) by ACSM are detailed in Table 2 *(31).*

Elderly Women With Cardiac Conditions

Elderly women patients with cardiac conditions have a low rate of entry into exercise training programs and high dropout rates. They are less likely than men to be referred to CR. Although elderly women have similar clinical profiles, their acute and chronic exercise adaptations can be achieved similarly to elderly men with cardiac disease. Of eligible women, 15% in comparison to 20–25% entry rate for men, were referred into CR after hospital discharge *(33).* Referral differences may reflect the attitude of referring physicians, patients' families, and participants themselves.

Initial evaluation provides information for establishing goals in exercise training programs. There should be a careful and complete patient evaluation before a training regimen is advised, including all the medical indications, as well as the woman's preferences and convenience in carrying out the exercise regimen. Exercise testing and prescription methods must be flexible and modifiable for many elderly women patients with cardiac conditions, especially if they have one or more chronic diseases that can affect both responses to exercise testing and exercise prescription. Modifying testing procedures allows for more appropriate functional capacity measurement and cardiovascular exertion response. Modifying exercise prescriptions permits elderly women patients with cardiac conditions that vary in the range of functional limitations to begin an exercise program at a level suitable and beneficial to them *(33).* The previous recommendations are the goals to strive for based on the individual woman's deconditioning level; a level far below this is often used initially, and once tolerance and acceptance of that level has been demonstrated, the prescription is gradually increased to a higher level.

General recommendations for early short-term exercise in elderly women patients with cardiac conditions are as follows: (a) intensity—50–80% peak oxygen uptake at most recent exercise test that corresponds to 60–85% peak HR at same test; (b) frequency—participation in a formal training program 3 days per week, home exercise (walking or cycle ergometry) 3–5 days a week; (c) duration—shorter bouts with similar prescribed duration per session. Each session includes 10 minutes of warm-up and stretching exercises, 20–40 minutes of aerobic exercise that are broken up into shorter periods, allowing 1–2-minute intervals for rest when appropriate, and 10 minutes of cool-down and flexibility exercises; (d) mode—including both arm and leg exercises using treadmill walking, leg exercises, and arm exercises to strengthen or improve endurance in upper body and lower limbs *(33)*.

Women With Heart Failure

Exercise training can be safe and beneficial to women with heart failure. CR exercise training in patients with heart failure provides improvement in functional capacity and quality of life *(44)*. Peripheral muscle adaptation is suggested to explain the improvement in exercise tolerance in this group of patients.

The screening and evaluation for exercise training of patients with heart failure are systematic processes that include previous data obtained about the disease process and the symptoms present, knowledge of the patient's current history and physical examination, review of pharmacological agents and comorbid status, laboratory data, and most importantly, exercise testing *(45)*. Patients with heart failure who are chosen for participation in an exercise program should be medically stable and without absolute contraindications, such as obstruction to left-ventricular outflow, decompensated congestive heart failure (CHF), or life-threatening dysrrhythmias *(31)*. Additionally, ACSM recommends that HF patients should have an exercise capacity of greater than 3 metabolic equivalents (METs) to be considered for exercise training *(31)*. Certainly, ECG and blood pressure monitoring are helpful, and supervision is indicated to monitor for signs and symptoms suggestive of worsening clinical condition (i.e., increased shortness of breath on exertion, fatigue, arrhythmias, and sudden weight gain). Continuous ECG monitoring from 6 to 12 sessions are generally enough except when the patient's clinical status is unstable *(46)*.

ACSM recommends the following exercise prescription for patients with heart failure (31). Initially, exercise sessions should be brief (i.e., 10–20 minutes) with intervals of 2–6 minutes separated by 1–2-minute rest periods. Progression is prolonged as the patient's exercise tolerance improves. A recent investigation by Meyer and group (31) demonstrated that interval exercise training—applying short bouts of intense muscular loading—in subjects with chronic heart failure yielded good clinical results and improved rehabilitation outcomes. The exercise intensity (utilizing a THR range) corresponds to 40–75% maximal oxygen uptake that is based on symptom-limited exercise protocol (treadmill or cycle ergometer) 3–7 days per week. Activities like walking, stationary cycling, and upper extremity exercises are recommended that can be coupled with resistance training. A minimum of 10–15 minutes for both warm-up and cool-down periods is warranted. Isometric exercises are to be avoided. Rating of perceived exertion (RPE) of 11–14 on the scale of 6–20 are helpful guides.

Exercise testing prior to entering exercise training is strongly recommended for elderly women with heart failure. For a more complete discussion of the topic of elderly women with heart failure and heart failure in general, see Chapter 5.

Women Patients Who Have Received Heart Transplants

The rehabilitation team must rely on clinical judgment and the perceived exertion level to guide therapy. Ideally, transplant candidates should initiate exercise, both aerobic and resistive training, as soon as they undergo evaluation (if possible) to prevent deconditioning and to remain at optimum function before surgery.

After the transplant, exercise usually consists mainly of passive and active range of motion, accompanied by incentive spirometry to facilitate optimum pulmonary ventilation. Sitting in a chair follows soon where leg raising and hip girdle exercises become useful as preparation to transfer weight from sitting to standing. Once able to stand, ambulation initially follows in the patient's private room that progresses to the ward. Patients who continue to have arrhythmias should be on a telemetry monitor. Intensity continues to be assessed by RPE using the Borg scale. Prior to discharge, if no rejection occurs, the patient may be able to exercise on a stationary bicycle ergometer and/or treadmill. It is preferable to perform a predischarge cardiopulmonary exercise test to better define an exercise prescription for an out-patient program *(47)*.

Exercise prescription includes all the essentials of intensity, duration, frequency, and progression. The RPE at anaerobic threshold is a useful indicator of intensity, because the HR usually used to guide exercise response, is not a useful guide for the patient after a heart transplantation *(47)*. Warm-up and cool-down are essential with a 20-minute minimum at prescribed intensity. Longer warm-up and cool-down periods are indicated because of longer recovery from and physiological responses to exercise *(31)*. Exercises should be performed in a monitored setting three times a week for 6–8 weeks. A walking program is recommended for alternate days. An extension of this timetable is often necessary to take into account early episodes of rejection or infection, which may preclude exercise for several days at a time *(47)*. According to Piña *(47)*, results of the exercise regimen will significantly depend on the individual's motivation.

CARDIAC REHABILITATION NEEDS FOR WOMEN

There is a scarcity of research focused on women in CR. Research that supports CR's beneficial effects is based almost entirely on men under the age of 70 *(48)*. A survey constructed from a literature review and advice from key informants examined factors that affect a women's decision to engage in CR. The study included 129 attendees and 61 referred nonattendees who were asked to complete the questionnaire. The findings showed that physician recommendation was considered most important, followed by encouragement by family members, in the women's choice for CR involvement. For women who attended CR programs (CRPs), encouragement from their adult children was significantly more influential in their decision to attend CR than it was for men *(49)*. The meta-analysis documenting CR benefits on mortality included 4554 subjects in 22 trials *(50)*. However, women comprised approx 3% of the randomized subjects. There are few data on the beneficial effects of rehabilitation efforts in women *(51)*. Because most data about CR have been obtained from men and applied to women, current CRPs might not meet women's unique needs. However, research is now forthcoming, which demonstrates that CR is beneficial for women *(44,52–54)*. Numerous studies report that although women may have lower baseline exercise function, when they participate in exercise CR, they experience benefits similar to men in their ability to improve their exercise performance *(52,53)*.

Attention to health behaviors was also a significantly more powerful motivator for women than for men. For people who did not choose to attend CRP, their reasons included concomitant illness, transportation problems, and inconvenient timing of program offerings—the three most often identified barriers to participation for both men and women. Yet, for women, concomitant illness was a much greater contributor to nonattendance than it was for men. Their decision to participate involved several factors, some of which are different and much more important for women in comparison to men. Physician recommendations continued to be the single most important factor in motivating both men and women to attend a CRP. The authors concluded that increased physician endorsement would likely encourage higher CRP participation rates. Furthermore, they suggest that women should be encouraged to discuss CRP advantages and benefits with their adult children, as they appear to be very influential in the female patients' decision to enroll. As women nonattendees are more concerned than men about the effects of concomitant illness, reassurance should be provided about the rehabilitation staff's ability to customize exercise and incorporate the needs and limitations of persons with other health conditions *(48)*.

Education, Counseling, and Behavioral Interventions in CR

In any discussion of CR education, counseling, and behavioral interventions, it is important to define the terms. According to the CR clinical practice guidelines, *education* is defined as a systematic instruction; *counseling* is defined as providing advice, support, and consultation; and *behavioral intervention* is defined as the systematic instruction in techniques to modify health-related behaviors *(44)*. In an effort to further and continue CR improvements, education must always be considered and included. However, education alone is insufficient to affect behaviors that result in risk-factor reduction. Therefore, a combined approach of education, counseling, and behavioral interventions in CR should encompass efforts to address the following issues: smoking cessation, lowering lipid levels, decreasing excess body weight, reducing blood pressure, and promoting physical activity and stress reduction for those at risk. Several reports in the CR literature have focused on education, counseling, and behavioral interventions to reduce some of the CHD risks.

A decline in cigarette smoking can provide many cardiovascular benefits. A multifactorial rehabilitation study, which included exercise training and education, yielded results that showed a significantly lower percent of participants (post-CABG) were smoking in the intervention group 12% vs 15% when compared to the control group at the end of the 12-month follow-up *(44)*. In another RCT that involved participants post-MI, intervention strategies included informational mailing supplements, concurrent pharmacological intervention, and nurse-managed home-based care. Results showed that smoking cessation rates were 70% in the intervention patients when compared to 53% in the control group *(44)*. These studies show that education, counseling, and behavioral interventions are beneficial in smoking cessation programs.

Intensive educational counseling can also be used to improve dietary fat and cholesterol intake. Education about nutrition, with or without pharmacological lipid-lowering therapy, can prove to be very beneficial and is a recommended CR component. Several studies with low-level exercise training intervention and dietary counseling have shown significant levels of decreased total cholesterol, LDL cholesterol, and triglyceride levels in the intervention group when compared with the control group *(44)*. Intensive nutritional counseling has also been performed in noncardiac rehabilitation settings. These results lend further support for the dietary intervention's efficacy to lower lipid levels. Achievement of lipid-lowering may also require pharmacological therapy in certain patients.

Education alone, in many studies, has not proven favorable in the achievement and maintenance of weight loss and/or hypertension management (44). Therefore, a multifactorial cardiovascular risk-reduction intervention must be used and should be included in any comprehensive CRP. Although education is an essential component, other efforts must also be introduced in order to address the issues of body weight reduction and hypertension. Education, combined with other intervention strategies, may prove very helpful. Nutritional counseling and behavioral interventions of exercise can achieve modest and sustained weight loss. Lifestyle modifications, including weight reduction, physical activity, dietary sodium moderation, and pharmacological therapy, can be effective in the management of hypertension. These strategies should be considered in a multifactorial CRP, which emphasizes education, counseling, and behavioral interventions.

Scientific evidence also shows that education, counseling, and psychosocial interventions, either alone or as part of a multifaceted CRP, improve an individual's psychological well-being and thus, these interventions are recommended to complement the psychosocial benefits of rehabilitative exercise training (44,55). These interventions also improve a patient's quality of life (56).

Research shows that recovery from an acute cardiac event (e.g., MI, HF or a surgical procedure (e.g. CABG, cardiac transplantation) is accompanied by depression, anxiety, and change in self-esteem and self-image (56,57). Dracup (57) posits that emotional distress, particularly depression, presents itself more after hospitalization than during the hospital stay. More importantly, in population-based studies, women have been reported to have higher depression rates than men (56). In the study of patients following MI (58), women had higher rates of moderate-to-severe depression during hospitalization and after the first year of illness than men. One of the roles of CRP education, counseling, and behavioral interventions is to facilitate and enhance the patient's social support system.

The Clinical Practice Guideline on CR by the US Department of Health and Human Services (44) and the Best Practice Guidelines for CR and Secondary Prevention by the Heart Research Center (55) modeled after the US federal guidelines used the meta-analytic approach to review studies that involved different interventions to describe the effects of education, counseling, and behavioral strategies on the psychosocial well-being of cardiac patients. Both concluded that clinical and observational studies support the effectiveness of these CR elements in improving psychosocial outcomes. Research studies found that interventions, such as stress management, behavior modification training, and relaxation therapy, are effective in reducing levels of self-reported emotional stress (44,55). However, limitations in the studies that were reviewed, were noted (44,55). First, varying interventions demonstrated improvements in psychological well-being, making it difficult to pinpoint which particular interventions were more effective than others. Second, effective interventions were delivered by health care personnels with varied expertise. However, it was noted, that the better designed studies that utilized more expert providers demonstrated greater benefit (44). Interventions also differed in their duration, frequency, and intensity. There was also a lack of uniformity in the outcome measures and measurement tools used across studies, thus making their results difficult to compare. Consequently, further investigation is needed as to the intervention types that would most benefit specific patient subsets, particularly women (55).

Referral To and Compliance With CRP

Literature pertaining to CR has frequently included the discussion of compliance and/or adherence. These terms, which are very similar in meaning, are often used interchangeably in the literature. For the purposes of this chapter, *compliance* is used to refer to the behavior response to treatment.

Statistics for physical inactivity prevalence in women and the beneficial effects of physical activity have been well-documented in research studies thus far. What might be important to discuss next is the exercise pattern in women following completion of a CRP; this leads to women's adherence to exercise programs. Long-term exercise maintenance studies after acute cardiac events have been conducted almost exclusively in men, and these results cannot be generalized to women (59). Results from a prospective cohort study showed that 30% of women exercise only five times or fewer during the 3 months after CRP completion (59). Only 27.5% of women exercised three or more times per week post-CRP (59). Although 83% of the women were enrolled in the study and continued to exercise during the first month post-CR, one-third had stopped completely after the first month (59). Finally, during the last week of the study (12 weeks after CR completion), only half of women continued to exercise (59).

Understanding women's patterns and compliance to exercise is a key step toward increasing their recommended activity levels. Women have just as much to gain as men by participating in exercise programs. Despite this fact, women are 10–25% less likely to begin a CRP than men, and they have higher dropout rates (59). Women's compliance to exercise programs and CR participation is very low. Study findings have clearly demonstrated that most women do less exercise than current recommendations (59). Research has also shown that sedentary lifestyles increase with age, and the rates for elderly women exceed those of elderly men (19).

The subject of compliance is central to CRPs. Despite documented CR benefits (44), a basic problem that persists in CRP is the lack of patient participation and compliance with the prescribed regimen. Compliance is a behavioral response to illness, "involving perception, decision making, and resultant action" (60). Compliance includes the patient's adherence to a prescribed CRP along with the continued independent follow-up for months and years after the program is completed. Because the benefits of regular physical activity and exercise (and other lifestyle changes) are realized only when patients comply over long periods of time, possibly even for the rest of their lives, it is not surprising that some suggest that noncompliance needs to be treated like a chronic health problem.

Several theories have been proposed for the study of CRP compliance, including the relationship between wellness motivation, social support, health locus of control, health value orientation, and self-efficacy (61,62). No significant correlation was found between wellness motivation and spousal support. However, Fleury (62) did find that patients who valued their families had the highest correlations with wellness motivation. Internal locus of control reportedly has the highest correlation with wellness motivation. The belief in provider control also has a positive correlation. Additionally, a future-oriented health value was found to be positively correlated with wellness motivation, as were activities that resulted in external recognition and individual development in this sample of mostly men *(62)*. In addition to this, the self-efficacy theory has been applied to compliance research *(50,52,60,63)*. Self-efficacy is the belief that one can successfully perform a certain activity. A recent study reported that self-efficacy and exercise behavior measures were highly correlated *(50)*. Self-efficacy scores were also highly correlated with long-term compliance after the formal CRP was completed. Yet, only 14% of subjects in the study were women. The research suggests that because women begin at a lower baseline, CRPs may have greater effects for women than men *(53)*.

Do we know why women drop out at high rates? Despite the growing evidence of beneficial effects for women who participate in CRPs, women are often perceived as being less motivated to attend CR and unwilling to participate in vigorous exercises *(49)*. But it is unclear if the underrepresentation of women is related to motivation or logistical constraints (e.g., transportation). It appears that although 40% of coronary events occur in women, men make up a disproportional number of rehabilitation patients. Obviously, women are not enrolling in CRPs in proportion to the expected ratio based on coronary events *(52)*. Considering men who have had CABG, nearly all men participated in formal CRPs, whereas few women participated *(64)*. Evidence in support of this notion is also available from the work in geriatric groups. Physicians reportedly recommend CRPs more emphatically for elderly men than for elderly women *(54)*. Interestingly, physician referral is one of the strongest predictors of CRP participation *(54)*.

Large national surveys show that women are less likely to be physically active than men *(17)*. According to one cross-sectional study, some of the reasons why people failed to exercise were convenience, motivation, and also a prevalent misconception that only vigorous continuous exercise would provide health benefits *(28)*. Recent studies also show that women are less likely than men to receive counseling after an acute MI *(65)*. Studies reveal that compliance with medications, long-term preventive regimens, and doctors appointments are approx 50%, with the lowest compliance rates being for lifestyle regimens, such as exercise programs, weight control, and smoking cessation. Generally, compliance with cardiac exercise programs is low, with about half of patients dropping out before completion of the program. The literature review further supports this, with reported exercise compliance rates varying between 44 and 65% at best. Reasons cited by patients who drop out of their CRP include medical, logistical, personal, financial, and work conflicts. Numerous factors contribute to noncompliance in CR, but are not limited to lack of self-motivation, lack of spousal support, angina, blue collar occupations, and external locus of control *(61,66)*. Depression, anxiety, and low self-esteem are other factors that affect CRP participation and adherence. The literature suggests that the more risk factors a given individual has to modify, the greater the chance of noncompliance. One factor cited frequently in the literature as being an important predictor of noncompliance is lack of spousal support *(67)*. In addition, older women are less likely to participate in a CRP than are older men *(65)*. A study done on gender differences in CR revealed that women were less aerobically fit than men at baseline measurements *(65)*. Several compliance studies to CR also revealed that women have a 10–30% higher dropout rate than men *(65)*. These statistics are significant, being relevant to the highly inadequate counseling and support for women in CRPs and exercise programs.

Moore et al. *(59)* studied women after they had completed CR in order to learn how well their exercise patterns continued to be carried out over time. They found that 30% of the women exercised five times per week or less during the 3-month period after completion of CR post-CABG. Another 27.5% exercised three or more times per week. The women exercised an average of 5.2 sessions within their target HR during the entire study period. Exercise maintenance dropped consistently during the course of the 3-month follow-up. Although 83% of the participating women started exercising during the first month, after 1 month, one-third of the women had stopped exercising. During the study's last week, only half of the women were still exercising. Moore et al. *(59)* concluded that women exercised well below the recommended guidelines after an acute cardiac event.

Moore's approaches to CR are based on middle-aged men and may not be useful in explaining female participation *(68,69)*. She conducted focus groups to learn about the attitudes and experiences of women toward CR participation. Her results indicate that prior to participation in CR, women did not knew what to expect from a CRP. Once they had participated, the features the women said they liked most were "feeling safe during exercise because of monitoring, peer group support during rehabilitation, and pleasant and encouraging staff" *(68)*. Women desire more social interaction during CR exercise sessions, emotional support from staff members about their cardiac recovery dimensions, and exercise options other than cycle or treadmill. Moore concluded that several CRP design and operational features are perceived by many women as not meeting their needs *(68)*. Although her findings were limited by the sample size (*n* = 11), findings from this study provide valuable insights into women's CR perceptions.

Another report by Moore *(69)* evaluated women and men's preferences for CRP features. Moore's study aimed to identify and compare women and men's preferences for specific CRP features. She used a descriptive design to study 33 men and 32 women who participated in a CRP by asking them to complete a questionnaire, where they were asked to identify both the importance of each of 17 CR features and the extent to which they had experienced each of the features. The results indicate that convenience factors (e.g., driving time, transportation, noninterference with other life activities, and ease of learning the exercise) were well-met preferences by men and women. Men's and women's preferences were not well met for being able to choose their own exercise. Men indicated that the ability to set their own goals was their greatest unmet preference. Women's preferences for no pain or fatigue while exercising were significantly less well met than in men. Moore suggests that a CRP that is responsive to patients' preferences should emphasize joint goal setting with participants and progress discussion, offer encouragement from health professionals, and provide a range of exercise choices *(69)*. Attention to women's concerns about pain and fatigue while exercising should also be addressed.

Additional research and theories have continued to address the issue of CR compliance. Ginzel suggests that one reason for the lower attendance and compliance in women is the older average age of women with CVD *(61)*. But the literature is conflicting, in this regard. One study done in Ireland reported that men in their 70s were twice as likely as women of the same age to attend CR *(49)*. Although others have reported no gender differences in compliance rates, as age increased compliance decreased in women *(70)*. Older women are often physiologically ineligible for CR or unable to drive to the CRP. In contrast, other studies found that as age increased, compliance rates increased (71,72). Similarly, it has been reported that younger women and women smokers are less likely to be compliant than older women or nonsmokers (53). Only 19% of women under the age of 50 completed the program. Riegel and Gocka (73) reported that both men and women had improved psychological adjustments within 4 months post-MI. The specific improvement areas differed by gender. Returning to work was comparable in men and women despite the differences in functional class. Women were more likely than men to ask for social support post-MI. However, the study was seriously flawed by a misunderstanding of the principles in matching and overmatching men to women on the very aspects for which effect estimates were planned, which make these results suspect.

Some of the factors thought to contribute to the high dropout rates from CRPs or exercise and activity recommendations vary for women and men. Various factors, particularly in women, need to be analyzed so that interventions can be developed and implemented. Possible reasons include cost (limited or no insurance reimbursement), inconvenience of program hours or facility location, schedule conflicts with work and family commitments, concurrent illnesses, exercise-related symptomatology, or a combination of these factors (65). For many women, the time of their heart conditions coincides with adult children's return to the home, and thus, women are care providers and unable to care for themselves. Similarly, women are the caregivers for elderly parents, sick siblings, or disabled family members. Health professionals must realize that women are faced with several obstacles unique to their gender that may hinder their participation in exercise programs. Another factor that should also be considered is that most exercise programs are designed to accommodate men, and activities are geared toward exercise activities favored by men because men have been the predominant recipients of CRPs (65). However, because greater numbers of women are taking an interest in CRPs, such programs need to be re-evaluated for their suitability and interest to the women patients. These issues are relevant and need to be addressed in order to begin developing intervention strategies to increase physical activity and exercise in women.

Limited research shows that women have unique psychological and physical needs that are different from those of men during their recovery process. Moore (68) points out that despite a growing number of studies on gender differences that point to CRP problems, the progress in making such programs more "friendly" to women is slow. Because programs do not address the general needs of women, as well as women from minority groups in particular, compliance with CR and women's recovery is hindered. As the women in the population age, consequently CVD incidence in women increases, there is an urgent need for research on the special needs of women in CR. Only by improving our knowledge about what is relevant to CR in women can we intervene effectively to improve participation.

Women who have sustained a major cardiac event are in need of CR. CRPs assist women in the recovery from the cardiac event and teach them the knowledge, skills, and new behaviors to minimize any future risk of a cardiac event. Additionally, women can also be taught to reduce CVD risk in other family members, such as their children, by adopting healthy lifestyles through physical activity and healthy eating. Comprehensive programs, such as the one described by Sivarajan (74,75) and Wenger et al. (44), that include education, counseling, and behavioral intervention, are useful in providing the information and opportunities for problem solving. The program by Sivarajan (74–76) also provides group counseling, where women have the opportunity to discuss their concerns about recovery and issues related to managing their multiple roles. Education and counseling programs have shown improvements in psychosocial outcomes *(44,77)*.

SUMMARY AND CONCLUSION

Women have much to gain from regular physical activity. The prevalence and significance of physical inactivity is of a magnitude minimized up to this point. The implications of how physical activity affects women's health, particularly cardiovascular health, are generously provided in a variety of scientific studies. Continuing studies have shown that women are more sedentary than men, and that this increases with age. National surveys on gender differences reflect that women were less likely to be enrolled in CRP than men, and that women have higher dropout rates *(31)*. Physical inactivity also increases with minority populations and with lower income or education levels *(6,30)*.

It has been clearly shown in several studies that persons with moderate to high levels of physical activity experience lower mortality and have improved cardiovascular health *(22)*. Most studies of women suggest that there is a 50% CVD risk reduction among active women when compared with sedentary women *(78)*. The AHA has shifted its health care paradigm to emphasize healthy lifestyles for women to help prevent the development of risk factors for CHD *(16)*. One aspects in implementing this healthy lifestyle is increasing physical activity. Women also tend to live longer then men and often live alone. Regular physical activity that includes coordination and flexibility can help women live independently, benefiting society as well.

The ACSM recommends that every US adult should accumulate 30 minutes or more of moderately intense activity on most (preferably all) days of the week *(15,30)*. Adopting and maintaining a physically active lifestyle can be influenced by various factors; those that particularly pertain to women have been identified. Health care professionals must use this information to continue to promote a healthy physically active lifestyle for women. Various intervention strategies may need to be employed for high-risk populations, such as the elderly, minorities, and those with lower income or education. At the same time, effective intervention strategies should be implemented and restructured at the individual, community, social, and environmental level to ensure a better chance of increasing the adoption of this healthy behavior in women. One important aspect to remember is that CHD risk reduction must be done comprehensively in women. Preventive measures, such as teaching self-breast exams and the need for regular mammograms, annual pap smears, diabetes, lipid, and cancer screening, should also be emphasized.

IMPLICATIONS FOR PRACTICE

Increasing Physical Activity in Women Today

Health care professionals play an essential role in efforts to decrease the sedentary lifestyle so prevalent among US women today. Initiation of physical activity as primary and secondary prevention strategies should be implemented on a regular basis. In patient-visit settings, physicians and their staff should discuss physical activity and provide exercise prescriptions for patients *(79)*. Prescribed exercise programs should include recreational sports such as running, dancing, and swimming, as well as selected types of resistance exercise to provide a variety of choices for women to increase their activity levels. Intensity, duration, and frequency should also be discussed and modified individually in all types of physical activity programs. The specific role of walking, the most common form of exercise among women, should be fully elucidated to increase activity levels in this population *(26)*. Many factors are associated with adopting and maintaining a physically active lifestyle, such as socioeconomic status, cultural influences, age, and health status. Understanding these factors is necessary to see how these variables influence the adoption of a physically active lifestyle at the individual level. Intervention strategies for encouraging individuals from different backgrounds to adopt and comply to be physically active need to be developed and tested further. Specifics for such intervention strategies can be found in the recent book *Cardiac Rehabilitation: A Practical Approach in the 21st Century (56)* and in the guidelines of the American Association of Cardiovascular and Pulmonary Rehabilitation Program Guidelines that are updated regularly and in the ACSM Manuals *(31)*.

Innovative programs are already being implemented; these should be looked at as excellent examples of how physical activity programs can positively affect women's health. The AHA has developed a website program, titled *Choose to Move,* which instructs women on how to incorporate physical activity into their daily routine through creative and practical ways *(81)*. *Choose to Move* has also expanded to provide guidance with self-management of risk factors. In particular, women who are computer savvy can benefit highly from this program, which uses the internet to provide information and keep an exercise log. This 12-week program shows women how to set realistic health goals, manage their weight, and build a support system. Participants receive informational brochures, a program handbook, and incentive gifts for continued completion of the program.

The National Heart, Lung, and Blood Institute (NHLBI) of the National Health Institute (NIH) has also contributed to efforts in maintaining a healthy lifestyle in women. It has revised its *Healthy Heart Handbook for Women*, which has 100 pages of the latest information on preventing cardiovascular disease like CHD, myocardial infarction, and hypertension *(82)*. This handbook helps women develop a personal action plan to reduce the major risk factors of heart disease. Health care professionals should keep updated regarding the latest research advances and prevention strategies in order to help women be responsible for their overall health and well-being; this includes increasing their levels of physical activity in order to reduce their risk of coronary heart disease. Finally, a new Surgeon General's Report released in Spring 2001 focuses on smoking in women *(83)*.

Increasing Participation in Cardiac Rehabilitation

Current theories on human health behavior suggest that the patient's preferences for specific aspects of health regimen are an important influence on their decision to initiate and continue use of the regimen. Despite low rates of participation in cardiac rehabilitation, especially among women, little research has been done to determine patients' preferences for features of cardiac rehabilitation programs. Moore's study *(68)* suggests that women do not wish to experience pain or tiring while exercising. Therefore, in order for CRPs to be more responsive to patients' preferences, the staff should emphasize joint goal-setting and discussion of progress, offer encouragement to women, and provide a range of exercise choices. It is essential that women's concerns about pain and fatigue while exercising be addressed *(53,84,85)*. Furthermore, women exhibit more shortness of breath, less activity, and more chronic illness during recovery. Because women withdraw from CRPs for medical reasons, and are more likely to have angina while participating in a CRP, they need reassurance that their concerns will be attended to and accommodations will be made for an individualized program (53, 64, 84). Focus groups revealed that the features most liked by women included the positive encouragement they received from professional staff. The women also desired more opportunities to interact with other participants during the sessions. These findings further support the need for concurrent education and counseling sessions, along with the exercise program, with lots of opportunity for women to exchange ideas and share feelings. Such models have existed since the early 1970s but unfortunately too few CRPs have adopted these for incorporation into their exercise program offerings *(76,85)*. Additionally, women in CRPs need a wider range of exercise choices; the *Choose to Move* program and other community programs are likely available although some may need modification according to the findings shown here. Additionally, women may also prefer to use dance as a mode of delivery of exercise.

The methods used by Moore et al. *(68)* could serve as a prototype to be used by other programs in evaluating the extent to which women's preferences exist and to what degree their expectations are being met. This could aid in the development of health care services that can be truly meaningful for patients. In particular, because CRPs are often the first step in long-term lifestyle changes following a cardiac event, it is crucial to have patient input when it comes to program design. Features that are important to women and that match their expectations will result in increased compliance, increased patient satisfaction, and increased overall participation in CRPs. Most importantly, convenience factors such as when the program is offered, transportation, traffic patterns, and resources need to be assessed in each community-based program. More choices also make it easier for working women to attend, promoting higher enrollment *(6,80)*.

RECOMMENDATIONS FOR FUTURE RESEARCH

Despite existing scientific evidence regarding the efficacy and health benefits of physical activity, much more research is needed and must continue to be done. Intervention strategies about how health clinicians can help to increase physical activity in women needs to be emphasized. There is still relatively little empirical data regarding factors that interfere with healthy physical activity in women *(6)*. There is also still a lack of information on how to increase practical ways for women to incorporate physical activity into their daily lives, programs to promote women's cardiovascular health, and what kind of physical activities women are mostly interested in. Factors that affect special populations of women, like minorities and elderly women, still need further understanding. The importance of health care professionals and their influence on encouraging physical activity in women also play an important role in this problem. We must research and create more ways to intervene.

Most of the studies on exercise tolerance, determinants, and barriers have been conducted in men, or results have not been separated by gender *(6)*. Existing data on gender differences need to be interpreted with caution *(6)*. Many studies use self-reported measures to estimate physical activity in women. Some of these self-reported measures, like housework, child and elder care, and walking during non-leisure time, may not be valid because of assessments that may be counted or not counted for women's *(6)*. More randomized clinical trials need to be conducted that provide clear evidence as to the efficacy of physical activity and the strategies that are most effective in promoting this behavior in women. One of the most important aspects of intervention is that it should be individualized with features that help heal women physically, as well as emotionally.

REFERENCES

1. National Institutes of Health. NIH Consensus Statement: Physical activity and cardiovascular health. NIH Consensus Statement 1995;13:1–33.
2. Bernadet P. Benefits of physical activity in the prevention of cardiovascular diseases. J Cardiovasc Pharmacol 1995;25 (Suppl 1):S3–S8.
3. Powell KE, Thompson PD, Caspersen CJ, Kendrick JS. Physical activity and the incidence of coronary heart disease. Ann Rev Pub Health 1987;8:253–287.
4. Kokkinos PF, Holland JC, Pittaras AE, et al. Cardiorespiratory fitness and coronary heart disease risk factor association in women. J Am Coll Cardiol 1995;26:358–364.
5. Fletcher GF, Blair SN, Blumenthal J, et al. Benefits and recommendations for physical activity programs for all Americans. A statement for health professionals by the Committee on Exercise and Cardiac Rehabilitation of the Council on Clinical Cardiology, American Heart Association. Circulation 1992;86:340–344.
6. Leon A. Physical Activity and Cardiovascular Health. Human Kinetics, Inc., Champaigne, IL: 1997.
7. Haapanen N, Miilunpalo S, Vuori I, et al. Characteristics of leisure time physical activity associated with decreased risk of premature all-cause and cardiovascular disease mortality in middle-aged men. Am J Epidemiol 1996;143:870–880.
8. Fletcher GF, Blair SN, Blumenthal J, et al. Statement on exercise: Benefits and recommendations for physical activity programs for all Americans. Circulation 1996;94:857–862.
9. Blair SN, Kampert JB, Kohl HW III, et al. Influences of cardiorespiratory fitness and other precursors on cardiovascular disease and all-cause mortality in men and women. J Am Med Assoc 1995;276:205–210.
10. Blair SN, Kohl HW III, Barlow CE, et al. Changes in physical fitness and all-cause mortality: A prospective study of healthy and unhealthy men. J Am Med Assoc 1995;273:1093–1098.
11. Froelicher ES, Oka RK, Fletcher GF. Evidence Based Cardiology. BMJ Books, London: 1998.
12. United States Department of Public Health. Counseling to promote physical activity: guide to clinical preventive services: report to the U. S. Preventive Services Task Force. Office of Public Health Sci 1989;128:611–624.
13. Lobstein DD, Mosbacher BJ, Ismail AH. Depression as a powerful discriminator between physically active and sedentary middle-aged men. J Psychosom Res 1983;27:69–76.
14. Sherman SE, D'Agostino RB, Silbershatz H, Kannel WB. Comparison of past versus recent physical activity in the prevention of premature death and coronary artery disease. Am Heart J 1999;138:900–907.
15. Mosca L, Manson JE, Sutherland SE, et al. Cardiovascular disease in women: A statement for healthcare professionals from the American Heart Association. Circulation 1997;96:2468–2482.
16. Rose VL. American Heart Association releases scientific statement on cardiovascular disease in women. Am Fam Physician 1998;57:2873–2876.
17. Brownson RC, Eyler AA, King AC, et al. Patterns and correlates of physical activity among U. S. women 40 years and older. Am J Public Health 2000;90:264–271.
18. Wenger NK. Coronary heart disease: An older woman's major health risk. British Med J 1997;315:1085–1091.
19. Christmas C, Anderson RA. Exercise and older patients: Guidelines for the clinician. J Am Geriat Soc 2000;48:318–324.

20. Newton KM, Sivarajan Froelicher ES. Coronary heart disease risk factors. In: Woods SL, Froelicher ES, Motzer SU (ed.). Cardiac Nursing. Lippincott, Philadelphia, PA: 2000, pp. 745–747.
21. American Heart Association. 2001 Heart and Stroke Statistical Update. American Heart Association, Dallas, TX: 2000.
22. US Department of Health and Human Services. Physical Activity and Health: A Report of the Surgeon General. US Department of Health and Human Services, Centers for Disease Control and Prevention, National Center for Chronic Disease Prevention and Health Promotion; Atlanta, GA: 1996.
23. Dunn AL, Marcus BH, Kampert JB, et al. Comparison of lifestyle and structured interventions to increase physical activity and cardiorespiratory fitness. Am J Prevent Med 1999;15:413–430.
24. Dunn AL, Marcus BH, Kampert JB, et al. Comparison of lifestyle and structured interventions to increase physical activity and cardiorespiratory fitness: A randomized trial. J Am Med Asso 1999;281:327–334.
25. Pereira MA, Kriska AM, Day RD, et al. A randomized walking trial in postmenopausal women. Arch Intern Med 1998;158:1695–1701.
26. Manson JE, Hu FB, Rich-Edwards JW, et al. A prospective study of walking as compared with vigorous exercise in the prevention of coronary heart disease in women. N Engl J Med 1999;341:650–658.
27. Folsom AR, Arnett DK, Hutchinson RG, et al. Physical activity and incidence of coronary heart disease in middle-aged women and men. Med Sci Sports Exerc 1997;29:901–909.
28. Bernstein MS, Morabia A, Sloutskis D. Definition and prevalence of sedentarism in an urban population. Am J Pub Health 1999;89:862–868.
29. Mensink GBM, Heerstrass DW, Neppelenbroek SE, et al. Intensity, duration, and frequency of physical activity and coronary risk factors. Med Sci Sports Exerc 1997;29:1192–1198.
30. Pate RR, Pratt M, Blair SN, et al. Physical activity and public health: A recommendation from the Centers for Disease Control and Prevention and the American College of Sports Medicine. J Am Med Assoc 1995;273:402–407.
31. American College of Sports Medicine. ACSM's Guidelines for Exercise Testing and Prescription, 6th Ed. Lippincott Williams & Wilkins, Baltimore, MD: 2000.
32. American College of Sports and Medicine. ACSM's Guidelines for Exercise Testing and Prescription, 5th Ed. Lippincott Williams & Wilkins, Philadelphia, PA: 1998.
33. Williams MA. Exercise Testing and Training in the Elderly Cardiac Patient. Human Kinetics Publisher, Champaign, IL: 1994.
34. National Institute of Health. Counseling to promote physical activity. Guide to Clinical Preventive Services, 2nd Ed.; 1996. Available at http://text.nlm.nih.gov/cps/www/cps.61.html: Accessed April 2001.
35. Smith EL, Gilligan C, McAdam M, et al. Deterring bone loss by exercise intervention in premenopausal and postmenopausal women. Calcif Tissue Int 1989;44:312–321.
36. Dalsky GP, Stocke KS, Ehsani AA, et al. Weight-bearing exercise training and lumbar bone mineral content in postmenopausal women. Ann Intern Med 1988;108:824–828.
37. Bloomfield SA, Williams NI, Lamb DR, et al. Non-weightbearing exercise may increase lumbar spine bone mineral density in healthy postmenopausal women. Am J Phys Med Rehabil 1993;72:204–209.
38. Chow R, Harrison JE, Notarius C. Effect of two randomized exercise programs on bone mass of healthy postmenopausal women. Brit Med J 1987;295:1441–1444.
39. Harris SS, Caspersen CJ, et al. Physical activity counseling for healthy adults as a primary preventive intervention in the clinical setting. J Am Med Assoc 1989;261:3590–3598.
40. Jacobson PC, Beaver W, Grubb SA. Bone density in women: college athletes and older athletic women. J Orthop Res 1984;2:8–32.
41. Chow RK, Harrison JE, et al. Physical fitness effect on bone mass in postmenopausal women. Arch Phys Med Rehabil 1986;67:231–234.
42. Marcus R, Drinkwater B, et al. Osteoporosis and exercise in women. Med Sci Sports Exer 1992;24:S301–S307.
43. Snow-Harter C, Bouxsein ML, Lewis BT, et al. Effects of resistance and endurance exercise on bone mineral status of young women: a randomized exercise intervention trial. J Bone Miner Res 1992;7:761–769.
44. Wenger NK, Froelicher ES, Smith LK, et al. Cardiac Rehabilitation: Clinical Practice Guideline, No. 17. AHCPR Publication No. 96-0672. US DHHS, Public Health Service, Agency for Health Care Policy and Research, and the National Heart, Lung, and Blood Institute; Rockville, MD: 1995.

45. Fletcher GF, Fernandez V. Screening and evaluation of patients for exercise testing. In: Balady GJ, Pina IL (ed.). Exercise and Heart Failure. Futura Publishing Company, Inc., Armonk, NY: 1997, pp. 311–320.
46. Fletcher BJ, Dunbar S. Training methods and monitoring of the heart failure patients. In: Balady GJ, Pina IL (ed.). Exercise and Heart Failure. Futura Publishing Company, Inc., Armonk, NY: 1997, pp. 321–328.
47. Piña IL. Training methods in monitoring of cardiac transplant patients. In: Balady GJ, Pina IL, editors. Exercise and Heart Failure. Futura Publishing Company, Inc., Armonk, NY: 1997, pp. 329–332.
48. Lieberman L, Meana M, Stewart D. Cardiac rehabilitation: gender differences in factors influencing participation. J Womens Health 1998;7:717–723.
49. McGee HM, Horgan JH. Cardiac rehabilitation programs: Are women less likely to attend? Br Med J 1992;305:283–284.
50. Vidmar PM, Rubinson L. The relationship between self-efficacy and exercise compliance in cardiac rehabilitation. J Cardio Rehabil 1994;14:246–254.
51. Murdaugh C. Coronary artery disease in women. J Cardiovasc Nurs 1990;4:35–50.
52. Schuster PM, Waldron J. Gender differences in cardiac rehabilitation patients. Rehab Nurse 1991;16:248–253.
53. Cannistra LB, Balady GJ, O'Malley CJ, et al. Comparison of the clinical trials, profile, and outcome of women and men in cardiac rehabilitation. Am J Cardiol 1992;68:1274–1279.
54. Ades PA, Waldmann ML, Polk DM, Coslesky JT. Referral patterns and exercise response in rehabilitation of female coronary patients aged >62 years. Am J Cardiol 1992;69:1422–1425.
55. Goble AJ, Worcester MUC. Best Practice Guidelines for Cardiac Rehabilitation and Secondary Prevention. Department of Human Services Victoria, Victoria, Australia: 1999.
56. Taylor CB, Cameron RP. Psychosocial risk factors: assessment and intervention for depression. In: Wenger NK, Smith LK, Sivarajan Froelicher E, McCall Commoss P (eds.). Cardiac Rehabilitation: A Guide to Practice in the 21st Century. Marcel Dekker, New York: 1999, pp. 263–277.
57. Dracup K. Cardiac rehabilitation: the role of social support in recovery and compliance. In: Shumaker SA, Czajkowski SM (ed.). Social Support and Cardiovascular Disease. Plenum Press, New York: 1994, pp. 333–353.
58. Freedland KE, Carney RM, Lustman PJ, et al. Major depression in coronary artery disease patients with versus without a prior history of depression. Psychosom Med 1992;54:416–421.
59. Moore SM, Ruland CM, Pashkow FJ, Blackburn GG. Women's patterns of exercise following cardiac rehabilitation. Nurs Res 1998;47:318–323.
60. Lemanski KM. The use of self-efficacy in cardiac rehabilitation. Prog Cardiovasc Nurs 1990;5:114–117.
61. Ginzel AR. Women's compliance with cardiac rehabilitation programs. Prog Cardiovasc Nurs 1996;11:30–35.
62. Fleury JD. The application of motivational theory to cardiovascular risk reduction. Image 1992;24:229–239.
63. Bandura A. Self-efficacy. Toward a unifying theory of behavior change. Psychol Rev 1977;84:191–215.
64. Hawthorn MH. Gender differences in recovery after coronary artery surgery. Image J Nurs Sch 1991;16:1026–1034.
65. Franklin BA, Bonzheim K, Berg T, Bonzheim F. Hospital and home-based cardiac rehabilitation outpatient programs, chapter 15. Heart Disease and Rehabilitation. 3rd ed. Pollock M, Schmidt D (eds.). Human Kinetics, Champaign, IL: 1995.
66. Comoss PM. Nursing strategies to improve compliance with life-style changes in a cardiac rehabilitation population. J Cardiovasc Nurse 1988;2:23–36.
67. Hilbert GA. Spouse support and myocardial infarction patient compliance. Nursing Res 1985;34:217–220.
68. Moore SM. Women's views of cardiac rehabilitation programs. J Cardiopulm Rehabil 1996;16:123–168.
69. Moore SM, Kramer FM. Women and men's preferences for cardiac rehabilitation program features. J Cardiopulm Rehabil 1996;16:163–168.
70. Conn VS, Taylor SG, Abele PB. Myocardial infarction survivors: age and gender differences in physical health, psychosocial state and regimen adherence. J Adv Nurs 1991;16:1026–1034.
71. Oldridge NB, Ragowski B, Gottlieb M. Use of outpatient cardiac rehabilitation services: factors associated with attendance. J Cardiopul Rehabil 1992;12:25–31.

72. Burke LE. Adherence to heart healthy lifestyle – what makes a difference? In: Wenger NK, Smith LK, Froelicher ES, Comoss PM (eds.). Cardiac Rehabilitation, A Guide to Practice in the 21st Century. Marcel Dekker, Inc, New York, NY: 1999, pp. 385–393.

73. Riegel B, Gocka I. Gender differences in adjustment to acute myocardial infarction. Heart Lung 1995;24:457–466.

74. Sivarajan ES, Newton KM. Exercise, education, and counseling for patients with coronary artery disease. Clin Sports Med 1984;3:349–369.

75. Sivarajan ES, Newton KM. Symposium on cardiac rehabilitation: exercise, education and counseling for patients with coronary artery disease. Clin Sports Med 1984;3:349–369.

76. Sivarajan ES, Newton KM, Almes MJ, et al. Limited effects of out-patient teaching and counseling after myocardial infarction: a controlled study. Heart Lung 1983;12:65–73.

77. Ott CR, Sivarajan ES, Newton KM, et al. A randomized study of early cardiac rehabilitation: the sickness impact profile as an assessment tool. Heart Lung 1983;12:162–170.

78. American Heart Association. Silent Epidemic: The Truth about Women and Heart Disease, American Heart Association, Dallas, TX: 1992.

79. Berra K, Froelicher ES. Exercise testing. In: Woods SL, Froelicher ES, Halpenny CJ, Motzer SU (eds.). Cardiac Nursing, 3rd ed. Lippincott, Philadelphia, PA: 1995, pp. 387–406.

80. Sivarajan ES, Halpenny CJ. Exercise testing. Am J Nurs 1979;79:2164.

81. American Heart Association. (March 22, 2001). Choose to move. Available: http://www.women.americanheart.org

82. National Heart, Lung, and Blood Institute & National Institutes of Health. (March 22, 2001). Healthy Heart Handbook for Women. Available: http://www.nhlbi.nih.gov

83. U.S. Department of Health and Human Services. (2001). Women and Smoking: A Report of the Surgeon General. Rockville, MD: U.S. Department of Health and Human Service, Office of the Surgeon General.

84. Ward A, Morgan WP. Adherence patterns of healthy men and women enrolled in an adult exercise program. J Cardiopulmonary Rehabilitation 1984;4:143-152.

85. Sivarajan ES, Bruce RA, Lindskog BD, Almes MJ, Belanger L, Green B. Treadmill test responses to an early exercise program after myocardial infarction: a randomized study. Circulation 1982;65:1420-1428.

21 Menopausal Hormone Therapy
Is There Evidence for Cardiac Protection?

Nanette K. Wenger, MD

CONTENTS

INTRODUCTION

Several converging variables have escalated the interest in menopausal hormone therapy as a unique cardioprotective mechanism for women. These variables include the progressive aging of the population, with women enjoying an increased life expectancy and spending a greater proportion of their lives in the menopausal state; the predominance of clinical coronary events in menopausal women; the excess coronary risk in women with premature menopause or bilateral oophorectomy, which is abolished by estrogen therapy *(1);* and the less favorable outcomes of women than their male counterparts with myocardial infarction (MI) and coronary revascularization procedures, which underscore the need for better preventive strategies *(2).* Furthermore, an array of biologically plausible mechanisms for estrogen-mediated cardioprotection is evident *(3),* and a sizeable compendium of data from observational studies of estrogen use suggests that it might help prevent cardiovascular disease (CVD) in healthy women and curtail illness progression in women with coronary heart disease (CHD). Only recently has information regarding menopausal hormone therapy and cardiovascular

From: *Contemporary Cardiology: Coronary Disease in Women: Evidence-Based Diagnosis and Treatment*
Edited by: L. J. Shaw and R. F. Redberg © Humana Press Inc., Totowa, NJ

outcomes been derived from randomized controlled clinical trials (RCTs). Overwhelmingly conflicted with the traditional assumptions of benefit, this evidence has guided contemporary position papers and scientific statements from professional health organizations. Each of these aspects is examined.

Relatively few women lived past the age of menopause in the early 1900s, whereas today women spend about one-third of their life in menopausal status. The challenge for clinicians is to render these years of health and vitality, rather than a time of disease and disability. CHD is substantially prevalent and highly lethal in menopausal women. Each year, more US women than men die from CHD *(4)*. About one-third of all MIs in the United States occur in women; women have greater mortality from MI than men, even when matched for age, and both with and without the use of coronary thrombolysis. The database of the US Society of Thoracic Surgeons reveals that almost one-third of all coronary artery bypass graft (CABG) surgery procedures are performed in women; female gender independently predicts operative mortality, except in the highest risk category *(5)*.

The greater age dependency for CHD in women than for men has been known since the early years of the Framingham Heart Study. Any initial clinical manifestation of CHD is delayed approx 10 years in women when compared with men, and MI occurs as much as 20 years later *(6)*. However, there is no abrupt increase in CHD incidence or mortality at menopause; rather, the sharp inflection on these curves occurs in the 70s and 80s *(4)*. The etiology of these age–gender differences remains elusive. Does estrogen loss at menopause directly render women vulnerable to CHD? Or can gender differences be attributed to the male–female crossover in coronary risk factor prevalence with aging *(7)*? Whereas hypertension, hypercholesterolemia, and diabetes mellitus predominate in younger and middle-aged men, these characteristics accelerate in middle-aged and older women. For example, after age 50, twice as many women as men develop hypertension, and isolated systolic hypertension predominates in elderly women. Low-density lipoprotein (LDL) cholesterol levels are lower in women than men at middle age; they increase progressively in women after menopause until at least age 80 and exceed levels in men at older age. Total cholesterol levels increase with age in women, particularly in the menopausal years, and continue to increase at least to age 70 (which is where the large data sets end). High-density lipoprotein (HDL) cholesterol levels change little as women age. After age 45, a woman is twice as likely as a man to develop diabetes. Thus, at the age when women begin to develop CHD, they are also more likely to have a higher prevalence of conventional coronary risk factors. Coronary risk factors tend to predominate and cluster in socioeconomically and educationally disadvantaged female populations; these populations have a high prevalence of CHD and increased CHD mortality.

BIOLOGICALLY PLAUSIBLE MECHANISMS FOR ESTROGEN CARDIAC PROTECTION

Lipid and Lipoprotein (Lp) Effects

Although favorable effects of estrogen on lipid subfractions explain only approx 25–50% of the described coronary risk reduction, this aspect has been the most extensively studied *(8,9)*. Estrogen is associated with a 10–15% decrease in LDL cholesterol levels, a comparable increase in HDL cholesterol, and lower levels of Lp(a); estrogen also inhibits LDL oxidation *(10,11)*. Estrogen-receptor polymorphisms have been associated with an augmented response of HDL cholesterol to hormone replacement therapy (HRT). The clinical correlates of these genotypes related to HRT have yet to be determined *(12)*. This same polymorphism (IVS1–401) is also associated with greater reduction in levels of E-selectin, but not an increase in C-reactive protein (CRP; *13*). However, elevation of triglyceride levels is a uniform unfavorable effect of orally administered estrogen. The mechanisms underlying lipid benefit remain uncertain. Possibilities include enhanced stability of the atherosclerotic plaque, improved endothelial function that may limit plaque rupture and vascular thrombosis; and increased bioavailability of nitric oxide, among others.

Variation in lipid effects among studies may reflect the route and type of estrogen administration, estrogen dosage, and/or concomitant progestin administration *(14)*. A metabolic substudy of the Women's HOPE trial in 749 healthy menopausal women, mean age 51, showed favorable changes in lipids, lipoproteins, and hemostatic factors with minimal changes in carbohydrate metabolism. The metabolic profile of 0.45 mg conjugated equine estrogen (CEE) alone or in combination with 1.5 mg medroxyprogesterone acetate (MPA) was similar to 0.625 mg CEE and 2.5 mg MPA *(15)*.

Randomized comparison of the effects of 0.3 mg and 0.65 mg doses of conjugated equine estrogen in menopausal women at risk for CHD showed comparable improvement in lipid profiles and in brachial artery endothelial function *(14a)*. These issues contribute to the continuing debate over the role of estrogen in cardiac protection and accentuate the need for additional studies.

Coagulation Effects

Other potentially atheroprotective effects of estrogen include lowered levels of fibrinogen, plasminogen, and antithrombin III, along with improved fibrinolytic activity as manifest by increased levels of tissue plasminogen activator (tPA) and lowered levels of plasminogen activator inhibitor-1 (PAI-1; *16–19*). However, some study results of hormone effects on hemostatic factors are conflicting; questions remain whether the route of estrogen administration and/or concomitant progestin administration causes variation in coagulation parameters. Despite these favorable coagulation markers, estrogen is associated with an increased occurrence of deep vein thrombosis and pulmonary embolism; the culprit factors have not yet been defined. Potential procoagulant effects include increased levels of protein C and factors VII and X.

Other Metabolic Effects

Estrogen lowers fasting glucose and insulin levels, decreases insulin resistance, and improves body fat distribution *(16)*. Results from the Third National Health and Nutrition Examination Survery (NHANES III) identified that both diabetic and nondiabetic menopausal women who were HRT users had better lipoprotein profiles than never or previous HRT users. Also, diabetic women taking HRT had better glycemic control than never or previous HRT users *(20)*. Another mediator of hormone benefit may be lower levels of homocysteine. However, an unfavorable estrogen effect is increased levels of the inflammatory marker CRP, an independent CHD predictor. Potential mechanisms of risk include vascular inflammation and plaque instability *(19,21,22)*. In a nested case-control study of menopausal women in the Women's Health Initiative (WHI), CRP and interleukin-6 (IL-6) independently predicted vascular events among apparently healthy menopausal women. HRT increased CRP levels, but in this study, the use or nonuse of HRT was less important as a predictor of cardiovascular risk than levels of either CRP or IL-6 *(23)*.

Among healthy menopausal women taking tibolone, transdermal estrogen, and CEE, higher CRP levels were present in women using tibolone and CEE. Glycated hemoglobin was significantly lower in women who received transdermal estrogen and tibolone when compared to women not on HRT, and women on tibolone had significantly higher systolic blood pressures *(24)*.

Another randomized trial compared oral with transdermal estrogen therapy on CRP levels in healthy menopausal women *(24a)*. Oral but not transdermal estrogen increased CRP by a first-pass hepatic effect. Whether CRP elevation with oral estrogen use directly promotes atherosclerosis remains to be ascertained.

Vascular Effects

Estrogen's retardant effect on atherosclerosis may relate to its inhibition of the inflammatory response to atherosclerosis *(25)*. This is manifest as decreased myointimal proliferation; inhibition of platelet adhesion, aggregation, and foam cell formation, as well as decreased expression of adhesion molecules. The correlates of the lower levels of cellular adhesion molecules (E-selectin, intercellular adhesion molecule-1 [ICAM-1], vascular cell adhesion molecule-1 [VCAM-1]) are decreased leukocyte adhesion to, and decreased monocyte infiltration of, the vascular endothelium. Monocyte chemoattractant protein-1 (MCP-1), which stimulates migration of blood monocytes into developing atherosclerotic lesions, is also inhibited by estrogen *(26)*.

Estrogen's modulation of coronary vasoreactivity may explain some of its protective effect. Estrogen promotes endothelium-dependent vascular dilation. This is mediated by an increased bioavailability of nitric oxide and prostacycline, and by lower levels of the potent vasoconstrictor endothelin *(17)*, likely by a decreased vascular response to catecholamines and possibly via an endothelium-independent calcium channel-blocking effect *(27)*. Nitric oxide is an important contributor to vascular benefit *(28)*. Antiatherogenic properties of nitric oxide include vascular dilation promotion, limitation of platelet aggregation and adhesion, decreased vascular smooth muscle cell proliferation and migration, decreased neointimal proliferation, and a decrease in inflammatory cell and platelet adhesion to vascular endothelium. Attenuation of endothelial cell apoptosis *(29)* and augmentation of re-endothelialization are additional estrogen mechanisms that promote vascular benefit.

Furthermore, estrogen may enhance angiogenesis *(30)* with potential favorable effects both on neovascularization and on collateral vessel formation, which has been suggested to improve myocardial perfusion. An autopsy study showed lower coronary calcium plaque content and decreased mean plaque area in estrogen-treated menopausal women *(31)*, suggesting that estrogen may modulate calcium content of atherosclerotic plaques and slow atherosclerotic progression.

Despite this strong biological rationale for cardiovascular benefit, clinical outcome studies are requisite for evidence-based medicine. Data are conflicting as to whether the addition of a progestin attenuates any of these estrogen benefits.

Physiological Consequences of Estrogen Use

Initially in animal models, and subsequently in menopausal women, estrogen has been shown to reverse the paradoxic vasoconstriction response to acetylcholine in atherosclerotic coronary arteries *(32)*. Some studies suggest that this phenomenon may be gender-specific for women *(33)*.

Brachial artery flow-mediated vasodilation studies in 1636 women older than 65 years in the Cardiovascular Health Study showed no difference between hormone users and nonusers. However, in the few women without clinical or subclinical CVD or risk factors, HRT improved flow-mediated vasodilator responses, suggesting a potential favorable estrogen effect prior to CVD development *(34,35)*. Estrogen in combination with a synthetic progestin improved flow-mediated brachial artery dilation and reduced inflammatory markers in hypertensive and/or overweight women, with a response comparable to that seen with estrogen and a natural progesterone *(36)*.

A nonrandomized comparison of menopausal women with elevated resting blood pressures and a positive family history of CHD indicated that the exaggerated hypertensive responses to stress in this population were inhibited with HRT use *(37)*.

Cyclic variation in endothelial function and frequent myocardial ischemia in premenopausal women with variant angina was associated with variation in estrogen levels. Both flow-mediated vasodilation and estradiol levels were lowest from the end of the luteal phase to the beginning of the menstrual phase and highest in the follicular phase *(38)*.

Estrogen has been described to cause false-positive ST segment depression on the stress electrocardiogram (ECG), possibly related to the similar chemical structure of estrogen to digitalis. In the study that compared data from menopausal women not taking HRT, taking estrogen alone, and taking estrogen plus progesterone, the decreased specificity of the stress ECG with estrogen use was countered by the coadministration of progesterone *(39)*.

In menopausal women with CHD who had exercise-induced myocardial ischemia, estrogen administration increased treadmill exercise time and delayed the time to exercise-induced ischemia *(40,41)*. Systemic vasodilator effects are also postulated as a mechanism of benefit. However, many of these studies were performed with supraphysiological estrogen doses, and conflicting data in research reports may relate to different hormone preparations and different administration routes.

Short-term oral estrogen given to healthy menopausal women did not affect myocardial perfusion at rest in response to adenosine or myocardial perfusion reserve, as studied by cardiac positron emission tomography (PET) scanning *(42)*. Estrogen did not increase endothelium-independent vasodilation or directly increase myocardial perfusion, nor was there benefit of short-term HRT on PET scan-measured myocardial blood flow or flow reserve in menopausal women with coronary risk factors or established CHD *(43)*.

In a RCT, 293 menopausal women with unstable angina, mean age 70 years, received estrogen, estrogen plus progestin, or placebo added to standard anti-ischemic therapy. Recurrent ischemia by ambulatory ECG recording and the hospital and 6-month adverse clinical events were similar in the three groups, giving evidence that acute HRT did not reduce ischemia *(44)*.

DATA FROM OBSERVATIONAL STUDIES

Compelling epidemiological evidence of estrogen's cardiovascular benefit has been widely reported. Observational studies and meta-analyses of more than 30 observational studies of oral estrogen use almost uniformly suggested a 35–50% reduction in the risk of coronary events, particularly for women who were current estrogen users.

Comparable benefit was evident in the smaller number of studies of estrogen and progestin use *(45)*. Cardioprotection was described as even more prominent for women with established CHD, showing a 35–80% reduction in recurrent events described among hormone users *(46–48)*.

Information from the Nurses' Health Study statistically favored HRT users when compared with nonusers as having a lower cardiovascular risk, even when progestins were part of the regimen and with lower dose estrogen *(49)*.

A population-based nested case-control study from the United Kingdom in apparently healthy women age 50–74 years showed an absolute risk reduction for MI of 32% among women who used HRT for more than 1 year, without an increased risk during the first year. Oral and transdermal therapy at medium-high doses were thought to have a comparable cardioprotective effect *(50)*.

By contrast, a recent meta-analysis of 22 small randomized hormone trials, in which coronary events were reported as adverse events, showed no cardioprotective effect and an increased odds ratio of 1.4 for hormone users when compared with nonusers, i.e., coronary risk rather than benefit, both with and without the consideration of venous thromboembolism *(51)*. The same authors corroborated these results (i.e., lack of beneficial effect of HRT on cardiovascular risk) in six unpublished clinical studies from Finnish drug-licensing applications *(52)*.

Several pitfalls of observational studies may offer explanations for the conflicting results of epidemiological studies and rigorous clinical outcome information from prospective RCTs, reflecting that observational studies tend to overestimate benefit and underestimate risk. First is the selection bias in that predominantly healthy women, typically those with favorable coronary risk profiles, are those who are prescribed hormones. Common contraindications to estrogen therapy include such medical problems as hypertension, diabetes, MI, stroke, smoking, claudication, and heart failure, i.e., either established CVD or major CVD risk factors. Thus, does the observed benefit reflect a healthy female cohort or favorable estrogen or HRT effects? Additional inherent weaknesses of observational data include a compliance bias, compliance likely being a marker for other health-related behaviors. Women who continue hormone use beyond the duration of menopausal symptoms demonstrate excellent compliance. In several RCTs of nonhormonal cardiovascular therapies, men and women in the placebo groups adherent to placebo had a 40–60% decreased risk of coronary events in comparison to those not adherent to placebo *(53)*. Clearly, compliance appears to be a surrogate for other health-related behaviors that may favorably affect outcomes. Finally, when women discontinue hormone use owing to early adverse effects, they are not captured as users in cross-sectional observational studies.

Observational data based on 10 years of computerized hormone use records in the Group Health Cooperative, a health maintenance organization, examined the risk of recurrent coronary events and HRT use *(54)*. Among women who survived an initial MI, there was no difference in the overall risk of recurrent coronary events between current hormone users and nonusers. An increased risk was suggested during the first 60 days after HRT initiation and reduced risk with current hormone use for more than 1 year.

Other relevant observational data derive from a case-control study in the Group Health Cooperative *(55)*. The prothrombin gene variant 20210G→A was described as a risk factor for incident nonfatal MI in hypertensive women. There was significant interaction between HRT use and this prothrombin variant on MI risk; current HRT users with this prothrombin variant and hypertension had an 11-fold increased nonfatal MI risk. This risk was absent in nonhypertensive women, and there was no interaction of HRT risk with the presence or absence of coagulation Factor V Leiden, either in normotensive or hypertensive women.

Data from the Nurses' Health Study (1976–1996) that involved 2489 menopausal women with previous MI or coronary atherosclerosis, showed an adjusted relative risk with current hormone use of 0.56, with less than 1-year use of 1.06, with 1–1.9-years use of 0.26, and with greater than 2-year use of 0.38; multivariable-adjusted relative risks were 0.65, 1.25, 0.55, and 0.38, respectively. Thus, risk for major recurrent coronary events increased among short-term hormone users, but decreased with long-term use, without differences between estrogen alone or estrogen-progestin use (56).

A retrospective review of menopausal women following percutaneous transluminal coronary angioplasty (PTCA; 57) showed a decline in the combined death or MI outcome among estrogen users, independent of age, cigarette smoking, diabetes mellitus, or the number of diseased coronary arteries. Estrogen did not appear to alter restenosis, as revascularization rates were comparable for estrogen users and nonusers. In contrast, another study of menopausal women showed that estrogen use during elective PTCA was associated with decreased angiographic restenosis and improved survival (48). In a sizeable cohort post-CABG surgery, a small number of women were estrogen users; estrogen users had an improved survival. Only 3% of estrogen users received a concomitant progestin (47).

HRT use and hospital survival after MI was examined in the Third National Registry of Myocardial Infarction (NRMI-3). During 1998–2000, 114,724 women older than 55 years with confirmed MI were included in the NRMI-3 database. Of these, 6.4% (7353 women) were current HRT users. The unadjusted hospital mortality rate post-MI was 7.4% for HRT users vs 16.2% for nonusers, with an odds ratio of 0.41 (CI 0.36–0.43); the adjusted mortality odds ratio was 0.65 (CI 0.59–0.72). The authors describe a significant HRT association with decreased MI mortality in all age strata. This association may relate to a therapeutic HRT effect, reflect selection and adherence bias, or may be a combination of both (58).

In the Coumadin Aspirin Reinfarction Study (CARS), the cohort of menopausal women with recent MI was examined for hormone use status (59). HRT initiation after a recent MI increased the risk of cardiac events when compared with never users or prior/current users. The increased risk largely reflected increased unstable angina during follow-up; death and MI were less frequent in new users than never users. Estrogen-progestin users had fewer cardiac events during follow-up than users of unopposed estrogen. In the NRMI-3 cohort previously described, HRT use did not modify stroke risk in menopausal women with acute MI, either with or without use of thrombolytic therapy (60).

A population-based case-control study at the Group Health Cooperative was designed to assess the HRT association with the risk of incident ischemic and hemorrhagic stroke. After risk-factor adjustment, there was no increase in ischemic or hemorrhagic stroke linked with current estrogen use, with or without a progestin. However, there was a transitory increase in the risk of ischemic and hemorrhagic stroke associated with HRT initiation, a finding that the investigators suggested warrants further evaluation (61).

A case-controlled study of the effects of HRT in menopausal women with diabetes suggested that current HRT use neither increased or decreased the risk of MI in diabetic women both with and without established CHD *(61a)*.

In the observational Cardiovascular Health Study, 62% of women at baseline had never used HRT, 26% were past users, and 12% were current users. Overall, HRT was not associated with the risk of incident congestive heart failure *(61b)*. In this cohort, clinical markers of endogenous estrogen status (body mass index [BMI] and self-reported osteoporosis) suggested a lower risk among menopausal women 65 years and older with presumed lower levels of endogenous estrogen, i.e., those with a lower BMI or with osteoporosis.

As noted, it was well-appreciated that women who used hormone therapy differed from nonhormone users in many aspects, including general health status, health consciousness, coronary risk attributes, and socioeconomic status (SES). Also, higher SES is associated with lower CHD rates. A recent meta-analysis of the observational studies previously cited *(62)* that adjusted for socioeconomical status, education, and major coronary risk factors failed to demonstrate cardiac protection and support hormone use for the primary prevention of coronary disease and CVD. Adjusted analyses showed a relative risk of 1.08. Similarly, a scientific review *(63)* conducted for the US Preventive Services Task Force indicated hormone benefits for the prevention of osteoporotic fracture and colorectal cancer, uncertain prevention of dementia, but illnesses that included coronary disease events, stroke, thromboembolic events, breast cancer with 5 or more years of hormone use, and cholecystitis. Specifically, there was an increased risk of coronary events, hazard ratio (HR) 1.29; an increased stroke risk (RR 1.2); an increased risk of venous thromboembolism (RR 2.14) with the risk highest in the first year; protection against osteoporotic fracture; an increased breast cancer risk that elevated with the duration of use; an increased risk of endometrial cancer; an increased cholecystitis risk (RR 1.8); a decreased risk for colon cancer (RR 0.80); cognitive improvement in women with menopausal symptoms resulting in sleep deprivation; and no definitive information from dementia studies.

HRT RISKS

If a substantial cardioprotective effect was demonstrated for HRT in healthy women and/or in women with established CHD, the magnitude of benefit would likely eclipse HRT risks for many women. Nonetheless, noncoronary HRT risks are highly relevant in clinical decision making *(64)*. Moreover, these risks stand in addition to symptomatic problems of endometrial bleeding and breast pain or tenderness associated with estrogen use.

HRT and Venous Thromboembolic Disease

Although medicine textbooks of a decade ago did not describe venous thromboembolism as a significant adverse consequence of HRT use, recent reports indicate otherwise.

In the Oxford Study, hormone use was associated with a relative risk of 3.5 (CI 1.8–7.0) for venous thromboembolism, and in the Puget Sound Study, a relative risk of 3.6 (CI 1.6–7.8). The Nurses' Health Study, which examined only pulmonary embolism, showed a RR of 2.1 (CI 1.2–3.8) with hormone use. The absolute risk of venous thromboembolism is low in healthy younger menopausal women, but older age and comorbidity increase the absolute risk.

RCT data from the Heart and Estrogen/progestin Replacement Study (HERS) reinforce the substantial increased risk for venous thromboembolism in menopausal women with CHD who use hormone therapy (65). The risk was less in women who used aspirin or statins and greater for women with lower extremity fractures, in-patient surgery, cancer, or hospitalizations.

A nested case-control study in women with documented CHD enrolled in the HERS and the Estrogen Replacement and Atherosclerosis (ERA) trial showed that in women with the factor V Leiden mutation who were treated with HRT, the absolute venous thromboembolism (VTE) incidence was 15.4 per thousand each year when compared with 2.0 in women without the mutation taking placebo. In women with CHD and factor V Leiden, the absolute risk increase associated with HRT use was more than 40-fold greater (8.3/1000/year; 66). Comparable data are reported from the United Kingdom (67).

A recent systematic review and meta-analysis for the US Preventive Services Task Force showed current estrogen use to be associated with a 2.14 increased RR for VTE, with the risk highest in the first year of use. The absolute rate increase is 1.5 VTE events per 10,000 women per year (68). VTE risk must be considered in making HRT recommendations.

Gallbladder Disease

Symptomatic gallbladder disease increased by 30% in HERS women randomized to HRT, 89% of whom required surgery (i.e., a 38% increased relative risk for biliary tract surgery; 69). This translates to one additional gallbladder operation for each of the 69 women receiving HRT for 4 years (70). Statin use decreased the risk for biliary tract surgery. In a retrospective cohort of more than 800,000 women, estrogen users were significantly more likely to undergo cholecystectomy (71).

Urinary Incontinence

Literature reviews concluded that oral estrogen was either of no benefit (72) or was associated with an increased risk of urinary incontinence (73). Among HERS women with urinary incontinence at randomization, HRT was associated with significant worsening of incontinence (74). The clinical community's reluctance to accept these outcomes is unfounded.

Dry Eye Syndrome

In the randomized Women's Health Study, women using HRT, particularly estrogen alone, were at increased risk of dry eye syndrome (75).

HRT and Breast Cancer

Based on a review of the literature, the US Congress Office of Technology Assessment 1995 (76) report cited an RR of breast cancer among hormone users of 1.35 for 10 years or more of hormone use. The 1996 European Position Paper on HRT and the Menopause (77) cited a relative risk of 1.2–1.4 for 8–15 years of hormone use, and the World Health Organization (WHO) Expert Committee 1996 report cited a relative risk of 1.3–1.8 for 10 years or more of hormone use.

Meta-analysis of nonrandomized studies of the breast cancer risk among long-term estrogen users identified comparable risk *(78)*.

It is not believed that hormones cause breast cancer, but rather that hormone-sensitive cancers likely grow more rapidly with hormone use and become readily detected; alternatively, there may be improved surveillance for breast cancer among hormone users. This effect may explain the more favorable outcome for women who develop breast cancer while on hormone therapy than is the case for hormone-naïve women who develop breast cancer. No studies report an increased breast cancer incidence with 5 or less years of hormone use, whereas data are conflicting for 5–10 years of use, and the data previously cited generally reflect more than 10 years of hormone use *(79)*.

Over 3 years, 19–24% of HRT and 8% of ERT users had a significant increase in mammographic density *(80)*. Epidemiological evidence suggests an increased breast cancer risk with greater mammographic density, beyond that ascribed to poorer detection.

HRT and Ovarian Cancer

Based on a study of 44,241 menopausal women, former participants in the Breast Cancer Detection Demonstration Project, evaluation was done for the incidence of ovarian cancer. Estrogen-only replacement therapy, particularly for 10 or more years, was associated with a significantly increased ovarian cancer risk. Short-term estrogen/progestin therapy did not impart an increased risk, but an increased risk was seen in long-term estrogen users and in estrogen users who had switched to estrogen/progestin *(81)*.

DATA FROM RCTS

The Postmenopausal Estrogen/Progestin Interventions (PEPI) Trial

PEPI is an intermediate or surrogate outcomes trial; the hypothesis underlying this study was that women who take estrogen have a lower CHD risk, and that estrogen prevents CHD by its favorable effects on coronary risk factors *(16)*. Thus, PEPI was designed to examine the impact of several hormone regimens when compared with placebo on coronary risk factors, rather than on clinical coronary events. In 28-day cycles, 875 healthy menopausal women were randomly assigned to conjugated equine estrogen 0.625 mg daily or the same estrogen dosage with medroxyprogesterone acetate either on a cyclic or continuous basis or cyclic micronized progestin in comparison to placebo. All hormone regimens significantly improved levels of HDL cholesterol, LDL cholesterol, Lp(a), and fibrinogen, but all significantly raised triglyceride levels. Active treatments had no effect on blood pressure or on 2-hour insulin levels, nor did they have any effect on weight gain. The best improvement in HDL cholesterol levels occurred with unopposed estrogen or estrogen plus micronized progesterone. Importantly, unopposed estrogen in uterine-intact women was associated with a 10% annual occurrence of adenomatous or atypical endometrial hyperplasia, an endometrial cancer precursor, such that unopposed estrogen is no longer considered appropriate for women with an intact uterus, and addition of a progestin is obligatory.

All hormone regimens rapidly increased CRP levels, an inflammatory effect, but decreased soluble E-selectin levels, a potential anti-inflammatory effect *(22)*.

The PEPI investigators concluded that the best PEPI regimen for CHD risk factors in women with a uterus was estrogen and micronized progesterone, and in women after hysterectomy, unopposed estrogen. Whether these effects on coronary risk factors translate into improved clinical cardiovascular outcomes has been studied in several large RCTs.

Postmenopausal Hormone Replacement Against Atherosclerosis (PHOREA)

Another intermediate outcomes trial conducted in Germany examined the effect of 17-β estradiol (with and without gestodine) on subclinical disease progression in 321 healthy menopausal women with increased carotid intima-media thickness (CIMT) at baseline (82). Despite significant favorable effects on LDL cholesterol and fibrinogen levels, there was no hormone therapy benefit on CIMT progression.

Estrogen in the Prevention of Atherosclerosis Trial (EPAT)

In contrast, a favorable effect of 17-β estradiol on CIMT progression was demonstrated in the Estrogen in the Prevention of Atherosclerosis Trial (EPAT; 83). EPAT enrolled 222 healthy menopausal women with LDL levels greater than or equal to 130 mg/dL. All women received dietary counseling and lipid-lowering therapy if the LDL exceeded 160 mg/dl. Hormone therapy slowed CIMT progression, but only in the women who did not receive lipid-lowering medication.

HERS

HERS was a randomized placebo-controlled, double-blind trial designed to examine whether estrogen plus progestin would reduce CHD event risk in menopausal women with established CHD (84). HERS enrolled 2763 such women, all with an intact uterus, and included women up to age 80. All women had documented CHD: MI, CABG surgery, mechanical revascularization, or if only angina was present, at least 50% narrowing of one major coronary artery at angiography.

The women were randomized to one capsule daily containing 0.625 mg conjugated estrogen plus 2.5 mg medroxyprogesterone acetate vs an identical placebo and were followed at 4-month intervals for an average of 4.1 years. The primary outcome was a combination of nonfatal MI and coronary death. Among the secondary cardiovascular outcomes were coronary revascularization, hospitalization for unstable angina or heart failure, resuscitated cardiac arrest, stroke or transient ischemic attack, and peripheral arterial disease. Baseline characteristics of the HERS participants showed their mean age to be 67 years, predominantly white, and an average education of 13 years. Thirteen percent were current smokers, 19% were diabetic, the mean systolic blood pressure was 135 mmHg, and mean diastolic blood pressure was 73 mmHg. At baseline, the mean LDL cholesterol level was 145 mg/dL; this is of concern given the 100 mg/dL-goal for women with documented CHD. Despite approx 46% of HERS women who received statins at baseline, they were not treated to goal levels. Mean HDL cholesterol was 50 mg/dL, and triglyceride level was 168 mg/dL. Fifty-six percent of the women had a body mass index that exceeded 27 kg/m². These women exercised moderately, drank alcohol moderately, and approx 24% had previously used estrogen, although randomization was not permitted for women who had used estrogen within the previous 6 months.

Despite achieving the anticipated changes in lipoprotein levels, a greater decrease in LDL cholesterol in the estrogen/progestin than in the placebo group, and an increase in both HDL cholesterol and triglycerides in the estrogen/progestin group when compared with placebo, there was no statistical difference in the primary outcome of nonfatal MI plus coronary death between the hormone-treated and the placebo groups. In the hormone group, 172 women had a primary outcome event vs 176 women in the placebo group, a relative hazard (RH) of 0.99. There was no difference in either total CHD events, nor in the subsets, CHD death and nonfatal MI. Also, no benefit of hormone use existed in a large number of secondary cardiovascular clinical outcomes. Of concern was a posthoc analysis that showed a significant time trend in CHD events by year since randomization. During the first year, there was a RH of 1.52, a 52% increased occurrence of CHD events in women receiving HRT in comparison to those receiving placebo. For the second year, the results were comparable, and for years 3 and 4–5, there appeared to be a favorable RH trend of 0.87 and 0.67, respectively. The trend to late benefit is uncertain as it reflects both a nonrandomized comparison of survivors and differences from the 1-year excess risk. Although a number of theories have been proposed, the reasons for these results remain controversial (85).

The conclusion of the HERS investigators was that 4.1 years of daily estrogen plus progestin in women with documented CHD did not reduce overall CHD risk. There was a trend to an early increased CHD risk and a later decline. There was also a threefold increased VTE risk and a 38% increased risk for gallbladder disease, primarily operative, with none of these events being fatal.

Important are the conclusions that should not be drawn from the HERS data; there was no study of unopposed estrogen, other estrogen/progestin regimens, or women without CHD; hence, the HERS conclusions and recommendations cannot be applied to these variables.

The recommendations of the HERS investigators were that, for women with documented CHD, this estrogen/progestin regimen should not be started for the secondary prevention of CHD. However, given the favorable pattern of CHD events after several years of therapy, it could be appropriate for women who already receive such hormone therapy to continue use.

Subsequent analysis of the HERS data showed that increased Lp(a) was an independent risk factor for recurrent coronary events. Hormone therapy lowered Lp(a) levels. HRT showed a more favorable effect when compared with placebo in women with initial high Lp(a) than those with low levels (86).

A further analysis of HERS data identified that HRT reduced the incidence of diabetes by 35% in women with established CHD (86a). The authors concluded that this finding provides important insights into the metabolic effects of hormone therapy, but is insufficient to recommend hormone use for the secondary prevention of CHD.

Follow-up with most of the participants has occurred in HERS-II (see below); ongoing laboratory testing of stored serum samples should provide further information regarding HRT benefits and risks.

The Estrogen Replacement and Atherosclerosis (ERA) Trial

ERA was a secondary prevention randomized angiographic trial involving 309 menopausal women whose mean age was 66 years (87). About half had prior MI and comparable number had PTCA. One-fourth were diabetic, and 60% had hypertension.

They were randomized to conjugated equine estrogen 0.625 mg daily vs placebo if they had hysterectomy and conjugated equine estrogen 0.625 mg daily plus medroxyprogesterone acetate 2.5 mg daily if not. Compliance averaged 81% during the mean follow-up of 3.2 years. A coronary angiogram was performed at the initiation of the trial and a follow-up angiogram at termination. The primary outcome was change in the angiographic characteristics of the coronary atherosclerotic lesions. There was no difference in mean minimum luminal diameter between the hormone regimens and placebo, and no difference existed in several secondary outcomes, including the change in percent diameter stenosis, change in minimum luminal diameter, or the number of new lesions. Essentially, there was no difference in regression or progression of the coronary atherosclerotic lesions between the hormone and placebo groups. These results contradict the findings of previous observational studies, which suggested a possible angiographic benefit of hormone therapy (88).

The Papworth HRT Atherosclerosis Survival Enquiry (PHASE)

This randomized secondary prevention clinical trial in the United Kingdom, compared transdermal estrogen alone or with transdermal norethisterone vs placebo in 255 menopausal women with angiographically documented CHD (89). This small trial was terminated early at the interim analysis because of futility and possible harm; after 4-year follow-up, there was no clinical cardiovascular benefit with hormone therapy and a nonsignificant early increase in adverse event rates in the hormone group. The investigators suggested that transdermal HRT should not be initiated for secondary prevention in menopausal women with angiographically proved CHD (89).

The Women's Estrogen for Stroke Trial (WEST)

This randomized double-blind, placebo-controlled trial involved the administration of 1 mg 17-β estradiol daily vs placebo to 664 menopausal women, mean age 71 years, who had had a transient ischemic attack (TIA) or ischemic stroke within 90 days. At a mean follow-up of 2.8 years, estrogen did not decrease the risk of death or recurrence of nonfatal stroke. However, the fatal stroke risk increased with estrogen therapy, and women with nonfatal stroke who took estrogen had slightly worse neurological and functional deficits. The investigators concluded that estradiol should not be prescribed for the secondary prevention of cerebrovascular disease (90). A posthoc analysis suggested that the more severe events occurred in the initial 6 months of hormone therapy.

Heart and Estrogen/progestin Follow-Up Study (HERS II)

To ascertain whether the trend toward a reduced coronary event risk with hormone use in the later years of HERS would persist with additional follow-up and result in overall decrease in the risk of coronary events, the majority of HERS participants (93% of the surviving women) were followed for an additional 2.7 years in an observational study (HERS II). Women in the open-label study were encouraged to remain on their original drug assignment. HERS II results identified that hormone therapy did not reduce the risk of coronary events, overall RH 0.99 (CI 0.84–1.17) even after adjustment for potential confounders and other factors, such as statin use, RH 0.97 (CI 0.82–1.14), nor were the results altered with analysis of women adherent to randomized treatment assignment, RH 0.96 (CI 0.77–1.19; 91). In association with this lack of cardiovascular benefit, the harms included a twofold increase in VTE risk (RH 2.08

overall), predominantly in the initial year (RH 2.66 HERS, 1.40 HERS II); and nearly a 50% increase in the rate of gallbladder disease that required surgery (RH 1.48 overall). Therefore, in older women with established CHD, this estrogen/progestin regimen did not provide cardiovascular benefit and, in fact, caused significant harm. Thus, it should not be used to decrease the risk of cardiovascular events.

The Women's Angiographic Vitamin and Estrogen (WAVE) Trial

Hormone treatment failure for cardiovascular protection was also evident in the Women's Angiographic Vitamin and Estrogen (WAVE) trial, a randomized double-blind trial of 423 menopausal women with at least one 15–75% coronary stenosis at baseline coronary angiography (92). The study involved a 2 × 2-factorial design with women who received 0.625 mg CEE (plus 2.5 mg MPA if they had not had hysterectomy) or matching placebo and vitamin E + C vs placebo. The endpoint was angiographic change at a mean of 2.8 years and intercurrent death or nonfatal MI. Neither HRT nor antioxidant vitamin supplements provided cardiovascular benefits. Rather, a potential for harm was suggested with each treatment. The increased risk associated with HRT was statistically significant ($p = 0.045$).

EStrogen in the Prevention of ReInfarction Trial (ESPRIT)

The ESPRIT trial in the United Kingdom randomly assigned menopausal women aged 50–69 years who had survived an initial myocardial infarction to estradiol compared with placebo therapy (92a). HRT did not reduce the overall risk of subsequent cardiac events, with no difference observed in the frequency of reinfarction or cardiac death at 24 months. Of concern is the low adherence to therapy in the hormone group and the substantial crossover to hormone use in the placebo population.

Hormone Therapy and Unstable Angina

Menopausal women with unstable angina are described to have elevated baseline levels of soluble thrombomodulin, E-selectin, and VCAM-1; these markers of endothelial activation and injury were not affected by a 21-day course of oral CEE or CEE + MPA (92b). Nor did acute hormone therapy added to standard anti-ischemic therapy in menopausal women with unstable angina reduce ambulatory electrocardiographic evidence of myocardial ischemia (92c). Two hundred ninety-three women were randomized to receive intravenous followed by oral estrogen or intravenous estrogen followed by oral CEE and MPA for 21 days compared with placebo.

Secondary Prevention Angiographic Trials in Progress

Ongoing angiographic endpoint trials include the Estrogen and Bypass Graft Atherosclerosis Regression Trial (EAGER) and the Women's Estrogen/progestin and Lipid Lowering Heart Atherosclerosis Trial (WELLHEART).

Women's Health Initiative (WHI)

The overall WHI is the largest study of menopausal women to date, with an enrollment of over 160,000 predominantly healthy women age 50–79 years (93). Within this observational cohort, 27,248 women were participants in a randomized double-blind, placebo-controlled hormone trial. They were randomly assigned to 0.625 mg conjugated equine estrogen plus 2.5 mg medroxyprogesterone acetate daily vs placebo if they had an intact uterus or 0.625 mg conjugated equine estrogen daily vs placebo if they had had a hysterectomy. As in HERS, this regimen was selected as the hormone preparation most commonly used by US women. This trial was designed to reveal hormone therapy's effect in predominantly healthy menopausal women. Further WHI details are available on the National Institutes of Health (NIH) website *(94)*.

In both 2000 and 2001, the Data Safety and Monitoring Board recommended reporting the small increase in MI and stroke to all participants, both in the estrogen and estrogen/progestin groups, when compared with placebo. This unanticipated occurrence involved less than 1% of the women and occurred in addition to the anticipated increase in VTE. Because of the low incidence of adverse events and the potential for a late benefit, the Data Safety and Monitoring Board recommended continuation of the study.

In July 2002, the estrogen/progestin therapy arm of the WHI hormone trial was discontinued prematurely after an average follow-up of 5.2 years because of an increased risk of invasive breast cancer that exceeded the preset trial that stopped boundaries *(95)*, combined with a lack of global risk benefit. The randomized estrogen-only therapy arm vs placebo is continuing. In addition to the 26% increased risk for invasive breast cancer with estrogen/progestin therapy, harms included a 29% increased risk for coronary events, 41% increased stroke risk, and doubled risk for VTE, in contrast to colorectal cancer benefits (37% decrease), hip fracture (33% decrease), and 24% decrease in total fracture. Coronary events, stroke, pulmonary embolism, and invasive breast cancer provided equal contributions to harm. Translated to the care of an individual woman, if 2000 women were treated with this regimen for 5 years, there would be an excess of seven coronary events, eight strokes, eight cases of invasive breast cancer, and eight more pulmonary emboli, in contrast to six less colorectal cancers and five fewer hip fractures. Although the majority of WHI women had no adverse events, the population risk is substantial. Thus, the global risk–benefit profile does not warrant recommendation of this therapy as a widespread preventive intervention on a population basis.

A comparable ongoing primary prevention trial in the United Kingdom is the Women's International Study of Long Duration Oestrogen after Menopause (WISDOM; *96*). Based on 2002 WHI results, WISDOM has been terminated. Britain's Medicines Control Agency has advised that HRT has not been proven to prevent heart disease and may increase risk in women with existing CHD *(97)*.

Subsequent data from the estrogen/progestin arm of WHI addressed health-related quality of life *(97a)*. Based on assessments in all WHI women performed at baseline and at 1 year and assessments in a subgroup of women at 3 years, HRT resulted in no clinically meaningful effects on measures of general health, vitality, mental health, depressive symptoms, or sexual satisfaction. Only among 50- to 54-year-old women with moderate to severe baseline vasomotor symptoms was there an improvement in such symptoms and a small benefit in sleep disturbance; there was no improvement in other health-related quality of life outcomes.

The Women's Health Initiative Memory Study (WHIMS) was an ancillary study of WHI that also reported on the population in the continuous combined estrogen/progestin therapy versus placebo cohort *(97b)*. This study encompassed participants 65 years of age and older and showed a doubled likelihood of developing dementia among hormone-treated women, although the absolute risk of dementia was low. There was no effect of hormone therapy on mild cognitive impairment. In another WHIMS study *(97c)*, again in women 65 years of age and older in the estrogen/progestin vs placebo arm of WHI, global cognitive function was measured by the Modified Mini-Mental State Examination. Hormone-treated women had significantly smaller average increases in total cognition scores, although the differences were not clinically significant. However, more hormone-treated women had statistically significant and clinically important declines in the Mini-Mental State Examination scores.

AMERICAN HEART ASSOCIATION SCIENCE ADVISORY ON HRT AND CVD

In 2001 the American Heart Association (AHA) issued a science advisory for health care professionals addressing HRT and CVD *(98)*. This was based on newly available scientific information and reflected changes in clinical practice guidelines of both the AHA and the National Cholesterol Educational Program (NCEP). Previously, the AHA had recommended hormone therapy as first-line management for lipid lowering in women; the 2001 AHA/American College of Cardiology (ACC) guidelines for preventing MI and death *(99)* now recommend statin therapy, owing to greater lipid lowering in women than occurs with estrogen and documented clinical cardiovascular outcome benefits for women in RCTs of statins for both primary *(100)* and secondary prevention *(101–104)*. HRT decreases levels of LDL cholesterol and increases HDL cholesterol levels, although to a lesser extent than statin therapy. The new guidelines recognize that results of recent RCTs of HRT for secondary prevention showed no cardiovascular benefit and potential early cardiovascular risk, both with oral and transdermal preparations *(84,89)* for healthy women and women with CHD *(84,89,105)*. The same change in recommendations occurred from the Adult Treatment Panel II (ATP II) of the NCEP that had recommended initial hormone therapy for lipid lowering in women to the NCEP ATP-III, which now recommends initial statin use *(106)*.

The following were the AHA 2001 summary recommendations for HRT and CVD.

SECONDARY PREVENTION

1. HRT should not be initiated for secondary CVD prevention.
2. The decision to continue or stop HRT in women with CVD who are undergoing long-term HRT should be based on established noncoronary benefits and risks and patient preference.
3. If a woman develops an acute CVD event or is immobilized while undergoing HRT, it is prudent to consider HRT discontinuance or to consider VTE prophylaxis while she is hospitalized to minimize the VTE risk associated with immobilization. HRT reinstitution should be based on established noncoronary benefits and risks, as well as patient preference.

PRIMARY PREVENTION

1. Firm clinical recommendations for primary prevention await the results of ongoing RCTs.
2. There are insufficient data to suggest that HRT should be initiated for the sole purpose of primary prevention of CVD.
3. Initiation and continuation of HRT should be based on established noncoronary benefits and risks, possible coronary benefits and risk, and patient preference.

Noncardiac benefits include the amelioration of menopausal symptoms and osteoporosis prevention; risks involve VTE, gallbladder disease, and likely breast cancer, the latter with more than 5–10 years of HRT. As noted, the database for primary prevention recommendations was less robust, given the lack of reported primary prevention clinical trials; however, participant notifications from the ongoing WHI raise concern for cardiovascular risks.

The 2002 American Heart Association recommendations *(106a)* cite that women should not start nor continue combined HRT for the prevention of coronary heart disease. This adds recommendations for women who have no evidence of heart disease to recommendations for women with established heart disease and reflects data from the WHI trial reported subsequent to the AHA 2001 recommendations.

A revised coronary prevention statement for women by the AHA is currently being formulated. In the interim, emphasis is appropriate regarding a subset of menopausal women not enrolled in the RCTs previously cited. These are women with moderate-to-severe menopausal symptoms who would be unlikely to volunteer for a study with a 50% likelihood of being randomized to placebo. This population also is unlikely to be studied in comparable trials and remains an important patient component in clinical practice to whom these clinical trial data cannot be reliably applied. For these women, quality-of-life benefits of hormone therapy likely will outweigh the small but definite risks cited previously. Recommendations from the American College of Obstetricians/Gynecologists and the North American Menopause Society include statements that recommend the lowest effective hormone dose for the shortest feasible timespan for such women *(107,108)*.

US PREVENTIVE SERVICES TASK FORCE

A scientific review conducted for the US Preventive Services Task Force *(108a)* identified benefits of hormone therapy as the prevention of osteoporotic fracture and colorectal cancer. Harms included the increased risk of coronary disease, stroke, thromboembolic events, breast cancer (with 5 or more years of hormone use), and cholecystitis. It was an uncertain benefit for the prevention of dementia. The conclusion was that the harms of estrogen/progestin therapy were likely to exceed chronic disease prevention benefits for most women. The US Preventive Services Task Force (USPSTF) recommends against routine estrogen and progestin use for the prevention of chronic conditions in menopausal women. Using hormone therapy to relieve menopause symptoms was not reviewed for these recommendations *(109)*.

BEYOND HORMONES

Most women (62%) believe that cancer is their greatest health problem; less than 10% recognize CHD as their major health threat *(110)*. Many physicians remain unaware of women's vulnerability to CHD *(111)* and fail to adequately counsel women about CHD risk and preventive strategies across the lifespan. Also they have not instituted preventive testing and traditional coronary risk-reduction strategies; therapies such as statins *(112)* and antihypertensive medications, known to protect against CVD, remain underutilized both in healthy women and in women with CHD *(113)*. In HERS, a nonrandomized comparison of statin users and nonusers, identified that statin use was associated with lower rates of cardiovascular events, VTE, and total mortality, further reinforcing the value of statin use in women with CHD *(114)*.

Ample data demonstrate that healthy lifestyle changes, supplemented by medications as necessary to control blood pressure and lipids, result in favorable clinical outcomes for women *(4)* and enhance menopausal health. Rather than focusing on hormone therapy, women and their physicians should direct their attention to lifestyle changes and other pharmacotherapies known to reduce cardiovascular risk. Physicians should encourage both the initiation and maintenance of these therapies *(115)*.

In the 54-month report from the Women's Healthy Lifestyle Project *(116)*, which followed women from perimenopause to postmenopause, a lifestyle program of reduced calorie and fat intake and increased physical activity prevented increases in LDL cholesterol and body weight associated with that transition. The program was effective for hormone users and nonusers.

US FOOD AND DRUG ADMINISTRATION LABELING REQUIREMENTS, 2003

In January 2003 the US Food and Drug Administration (FDA) outlined new labeling requirements for all estrogen and estrogen/progestin products, likely reflecting the lack of clinical trial evidence that other hormone formulations differed significantly in their risk–benefit profiles from those reported above *(116a)*. In the United States, menopausal hormone therapy is approved for the management of menopausal symptoms, the management of symptoms of vulvovaginal atrophy, and the prevention of menopausal osteoporosis. The new labels require the statement that these products are not approved for heart disease prevention and must highlight the increased risk of heart disease, heart attack, stroke, and breast cancer. Prescription of hormone therapy for moderate to severe menopausal symptoms is advised at the lowest effective dose for the shortest possible duration. Topical therapy should be considered for symptoms of vulvovaginal atrophy. Consideration of approved nonestrogen therapy is recommended for the prevention of osteoporosis.

Importantly, the FDA advises women to discuss with their healthcare providers other approaches to reducing heart disease risk factors such as diet, smoking cessation, and blood pressure control. As previously noted, exercise and lipid management should be added to these variables.

SELECTIVE ESTROGEN RECEPTOR MODULATORS (SERMS)

SERMs are nonhormonal agents that bind with high affinity to estrogen receptors and promote specific effects in different tissues. This section addresses the SERM raloxifene, a nonsteroidal benzothiophene derivative, licensed for clinical use in the United States for osteoporosis prevention and treatment. Raloxifene exerts estrogen agonist-like effects on bone and cardiovascular risk factors along with estrogen antagonist-like effects on the breast and uterus, offering the potential to provide cardioprotection without imparting undue noncardiac risks *(117)*. Raloxifene is currently in clinical trial both to evaluate cardioprotective effects and evaluate the prevention of invasive breast cancer.

Cardiovascular Effects of Raloxifene: Preclinical Studies

Preclinical cardiovascular studies of raloxifene suggest that it shares many of the favorable estrogen effects on lipid metabolism and the vascular wall. Raloxifene lowered serum cholesterol levels in an ovariectomized rat model (118) and exerted favorable effects on inflammation and coagulation markers. A raloxifene analog inhibited endothelial VCAM-1 expression, suggesting a potential antiatherogenic effect of raloxifene on the vascular wall. Raloxifene upregulated thrombomodulin in human umbilical vein endothelial cells (119). Increased thrombomodulin expression may reduce thrombotic risk by regulation of protein C.

Raloxifene had a protective effect against LDL oxidation, inhibiting myeloperoxidase activity (120). A raloxifene analog enhanced the endothelium-dependent vasodilation of aortic rings from ovariectomized rats (121). Increased release of nitric oxide (NO) is likely the mechanism that underlies the enhancement of endothelium-dependent vasodilation. An additional vascular protective effect may relate to the acute activation of endothelial nitric oxide synthase (eNOS) by raloxifene in human endothelial cells; this increase in NO production is through a rapid estrogen receptor-mediated mechanism (122). In a study of ovariectomized ewes (123), raloxifene and estrogen produced comparable short-term increases in both coronary and uterine blood flow, at least partially mediated by NO.

Regarding effects on vascular smooth muscle, both estrogen and raloxifene inhibited vascular smooth muscle cell migration without an effect on vascular smooth muscle cell proliferation (124). In animal models of vascular injury and atherosclerosis, both 17-β estradiol and raloxifene inhibited the aortic accumulation of cholesterol in an ovariectomized cholesterol-fed rabbit model (125). By contrast, in an ovariectomized cynomolgus monkey model being fed an atherogenic diet, conjugated equine estrogen reduced coronary artery plaque size, an effect not seen with raloxifene (126). With increased raloxifene doses, both estradiol and raloxifene significantly reduced atherosclerosis progression when compared with placebo in ovariectomized cholesterol-fed rabbits, with the effect only partially explained by lipid lowering (127,128). In an animal vascular injury model, data on raloxifene benefit were conflicting depending on the study (129,130); however, vascular wall changes were at least partially independent of changes in serum cholesterol levels. These changes suggest the potential of raloxifene to favorably limit atherosclerosis development.

In studies of ischemia-reperfusion injury in a canine model, both raloxifene and 17-β estradiol reduced myocardial infarct size in comparison to control animals (131). In a hypertensive rat model, raloxifene improved hypertension-induced endothelial dysfunction by increased NO bioavailability, which decreased blood pressure and decreased vascular damage (132).

Cardiovascular Effects of Raloxifene: Clinical Studies

Raloxifene effects on serum lipids, lipoproteins, and triglycerides derive predominantly from osteoporosis studies in menopausal women. In 601 menopausal women with low and normal bone mineral density, raloxifene lowered total and LDL cholesterol, comparable to changes described with estrogen. Raloxifene did not change HDL cholesterol or triglyceride levels, both of which increase in women who receive estrogen. Importantly, endometrial thickness as ascertained by transvaginal ultrasonography did not increase with raloxifene.

Comparison of raloxifene effects and HRT in 390 healthy menopausal women (133) confirmed that raloxifene decreases LDL levels, fibrinogen, and Lp(a). In contrast to HRT, there was no raloxifene effect on HDL cholesterol and PAI-1, and a lesser effect on HDL_2 and Lp(a), but raloxifene did not raise triglyceride levels.

Raloxifene and CEE were compared with placebo in 56 hysterectomized healthy menopausal women *(134)*. HDL cholesterol increased and PAI-1 decreased with CEE, whereas CRP and triglyceride levels increased with CEE, effects not seen with raloxifene.

Raloxifene significantly reduced homocysteine levels when compared with placebo *(135)* in healthy menopausal women. In a prospective nested case-control study of healthy menopausal women, high-sensitivity CRP (hs-CRP) was the strongest univariate predictor of cardiovascular event risk *(136)*. Although HRT increased CRP levels by 84% *(135)*, raloxifene did not alter CRP levels. The differing effects of HRT and raloxifene on CRP are not explained by different effects on IL-6 or tissue necrosis factor-α (TNF-α; *137)*) and may reflect different effects on the liver.

CEE and raloxifene comparison in healthy menopausal women showed that raloxifene lowered levels of cell adhesion molecules, although less than with CEE, but did not increase inflammation markers as did CEE *(138)*.

The favorable raloxifene effects on some biochemical markers of cardiovascular risk, differing in many ways from those of estrogen, support the need for a randomized trial with clinical cardiovascular outcomes, rather than solely an intermediate outcomes study. The uniform lowering of total and LDL cholesterol, Lp(a), and fibrinogen levels, without effect on triglyceride levels, are potential beneficial effects of raloxifene on cardiovascular risk markers. Data on other coagulation parameters are inconsistent; raloxifene lowers homocysteine levels and does not increase CRP. Limited data suggest improvements in endothelial function.

Brachial artery diameter increased significantly with raloxifene in healthy menopausal women, suggesting an estrogen-like effect on endothelial responses to vasodilator stimuli *(139)*. In another study, raloxifene improved flow-mediated vasodilation, increased plasma NO levels, and lowered plasma endothelin-1 levels *(140)*. Raloxifene and HRT (17β estradiol + norethisterone acetate) comparably improved endothelial function and flow-mediated endothelium-dependent vasodilation *(141)*. Raloxifene also reduced the carotid artery pulsatility index in healthy menopausal women, with the decline comparable to that reported with estrogen therapy *(142)*.

The Multiple Outcomes of Raloxifene Evaluation (MORE) study *(143)* showed that raloxifene improved total and LDL cholesterol and fibrinogen levels, but did not increase either HDL cholesterol or triglyceride levels. Further data from the MORE trial suggested that high endogenous estradiol levels identified women with a high risk of breast cancer, women with potentially the greatest raloxifene benefit *(144)*. Raloxifene did not improve cardiovascular outcomes in the total MORE cohort. However, in the subset of osteoporotic women at increased cardiovascular risk, there was a significant decrease in the risk of cardiovascular events. Four-year data showed no early increase in the cardiovascular event risk with raloxifene. Were the RUTH trial (*see* the following section) not already in progress, these findings would likely have spurred the initiation of a raloxifene trial with cardiovascular outcome endpoints *(145)*.

The safety raloxifene profile assumes enormous importance. There is no evidence of endometrial stimulation and no increased risk of endometrial cancer. Similarly, there are no symptoms of breast pain or tenderness, and there is nearly a 76% reduction in the risk of invasive breast cancer *(146)*. Bone mineral density is preserved, and the risk of vertebral fractures decreased by almost half in an at-risk population *(147)*. The most significant side effect of raloxifene is VTE, a risk comparable to that of estrogen and HRT.

Raloxifene Use for The Heart (RUTH) Trial

RUTH is an ongoing randomized double-blind, placebo-controlled trial designed to evaluate the effect of 60 mg raloxifene daily on the risk of coronary events (coronary death, nonfatal MI, or hospitalized acute coronary syndrome other than MI), and on invasive breast cancer in menopausal women at risk for major coronary events *(148)*. Menopausal women, both those with documented CHD and those at high risk for major coronary events owing to age and/or cardiovascular risk factors, are studied. In 26 countries, 10,101 women age 55 years and older have been randomized with an estimated follow-up of 5–7 years. Several secondary cardiovascular endpoints, as well as hospitalizations, breast cancers, fractures, and VTE events will be evaluated. Baseline characteristics of this population have been described *(149)*.

There are substantial differences between HERS *(84)* and RUTH *(150)*. RUTH is a larger trial that involves an international population. All HERS women had documented CHD, whereas RUTH participants are women with documented CHD and at increased risk of coronary events. In contrast to HERS, a progestin is not needed in RUTH, as raloxifene does not stimulate the endometrium. RUTH involves a larger number of diabetic patients. Concern with HRT elevation of triglyceride levels excluded many diabetic women from HERS, and raloxifene does not increase triglyceride concentrations. Because HERS is a US study, there is higher concomitant use of both cardiovascular drugs and procedures than will be seen in the international RUTH trial.

OTHER HORMONE PREPARATIONS

Little information is available on the cardioprotective effects of other selective estrogen receptor modulators, phytoestrogens, tibolone, and a variety of other hormone preparations not tested or reported in clinical trials for primary or secondary prevention. Data are lacking for safety, for efficacy, and for interactions with other medical therapies.

REFERENCES

1. Colditz GA, Willett WC, Stampfer MJ, et al. Menopause and the risk of coronary heart disease in women. N Engl J Med 1987;316:1105–1110.
2. Wenger, NK. Coronary heart disease in women: an older woman's major health risk. BMJ 1997;315:1085–1090.
3. Mendelsohn ME, Karas RH. The protective effects of estrogen on the cardiovascular system. N Engl J Med 1999;340:1801–1811.
4. American Heart Association. 2002 Heart and Stroke Statistical Update. American Heart Association, Dallas, TX: 2001.
5. Edwards FH, Carey JS, Grover FL, et al. Impact of gender on coronary bypass operative mortality. Ann Thorac Surg 1998;66:125–131.
6. Lerner DJ, Kannel WB. Patterns of coronary heart disease morbidity and mortality in the sexes: a 26-year follow-up of the Framingham population. Am Heart J 1986;111:383–390.
7. Wenger NK. The natural history of coronary artery disease in women: Epidemiology, coronary risk factors, and clinical characteristics. In: Charney P (ed.). Coronary Artery Disease in Women: What All Physicials Need to Know. American College of Physicians/American Society of Internal Medicine, Philadelphia, PA: 1999, pp. 3–35.
8. Espeland MA, Marcovina SM, Miller V, et al for the PEPI Investigators. Effect of postmenopausal hormone therapy on lipoprotein(a) concentration. Circulation 1998;97:979–986.
9. Guetta V, Cannon RO III. Cardiovascular effects of estrogen and lipid-lowering therapies in postmenopausal women. Circulation 1996:93:1928–1937.

10. Hoogerbrugge N, Zillikens MC, Jansen H, et al. Estrogen replacement decreases the level of antibodies against oxidized low-density lipoprotein in postmenopausal women with coronary heart disease. Metabolism 1998;47:675–680.

11. Shwaery GT, Vita JA, Keaney JF, Jr. Antioxidant protection of LDL by physiologic concentrations of estrogens is specific for 17β-estradiol. Atherosclerosis 1998;138:255–262.

12. Herrington DM, Howard TD, Hawkins GA, et al. Estrogen-receptor polymorphisms and effects of estrogen replacement on high-density lipoprotein cholesterol in women with coronary disease. N Engl J Med 2002;346:967–974.

13. Herrington DM, Howard TD, Brosnihan KB, et al. Common estrogen receptor polymorphism augments effects of hormone replacement therapy on E-selectin but not C-reactive protein. Circulation 2002;105:1879–1882.

14. Shulman LP. Effects of progestins in different hormone replacement therapy formulations on estrogen-induced lipid changes in postmenopausal women. Am J Cardiol 2002;89(Suppl):47E-55E.

14a. Mercuro G, Vitale C, Fini M, Zoncu S, Leonardo F, Rosano GMC. Lipid profiles and endothelial function with low-dose hormone replacement therapy in postmenopausal women at risk for coronary artery disease: a randomized trial. International Journal of Cardiology 2003;89:257–265.

15. Lobo RA, Bush T, Carr BR, Pickar JH. Effects of lower doses of conjugated equine estrogens and medroxyprogesterone acetate on plasma lipids and lipoproteins, coagulation factors, and carbohydrate metabolism. Fertil Steril 2001;76:13–24.

16. The Writing Group for the PEPI Trial. Effects of estrogen or estrogen/progestin regimens on heart disease risk factors in postmenopausal women. The Postmenopausal Estrogen/Progestin Interventions (PEPI) Trial. JAMA 1995;273:199–208.

17. Chen F-P, Lee N, Wang C-H, et al. Effects of hormone replacement therapy on cardiovascular risk factors in postmenopausal women. Fertil Steril 1998;69:267–273.

18. Gebara OCE, Mittleman MA, Sutherland P, et al. Association between increased estrogen status and increased fibrinolytic potential in the Framingham Offspring Study. Circulation 1995;91:1952–1958.

19. Cushman M, Meilahn EN, Kuller LH, et al. Hormone replacement therapy (HRT) and markers of hemostasis and inflammation in elderly women. Circulation 1998;97:8A.

20. Crespo CJ, Smit E, Snelling A, et al. Hormone replacement therapy and its relationship to lipid and glucose metabolism in diabetic and nondiabetic postmenopausal women. Results from the Third National Health and Nutrition Examination Survey (NHANES III). Diabetes Care 2002;25:1675–1680.

21. Ridker PM, Hennekens CH, Rifai N, et al. Hormone replacement therapy and increased plasma concentration of C-reactive protein. Circulation 1999;100:713–716.

22. Cushman M, Legault C, Barrett-Connor E, et al. Effect of postmenopausal hormones on inflammation-sensitive proteins: the Postmenopausal Estrogen/Progestin Interventions (PEPI) Study. Circulation 1999;100:717–722.

23. Pradhan AD, Manson JE, Rossouw JE, et al. Inflammatory biomarkers, hormone replacement therapy, and incident coronary heart disease. Prospective analysis from the Women's Health Initiative observational study. JAMA 2002;288:980–987.

24. Prelevic GM, Kwong P, Byrne DJ, et al. A cross-sectional study of the effects of hormone replacement therapy on the cardiovascular disease risk profile in healthy postmenopausal women. Fertil Steril 2002;77:945–951.

24a. Vongpatanasin W, Tuncel M, Wang Z, Arbique D, Mehrad B, Jialal I. Different effects of oral versus transdermal estrogen replacement therapy on C-reactive protein in postmenopausal women. J Am Coll Cardiol 2003;41:1358–1363.

25. Caulin-Glaser T, Farrell WJ, Pfau SE, et al. Modulation of circulating cellular adhesion molecules in postmenopausal women with coronary artery disease. J Am Coll Cardiol 1998;31:1555–1560.

26. Pervin S, Singh R, Rosenfeld ME, Navab M, et al. Estradiol suppresses MCP-1 expression in vivo. Implications for atherosclerosis. Arterioscler Thromb Vasc Biol 1998;18:1575–1582.

27. Collins P, Rosano GMC, Jiang C, et al. Cardiovascular protection by oestrogen–a calcium antagonist effect? Lancet 1993;341:1264–1265.

28. Guetta V, Quyyumi AA, Prasad A, et al. The role of nitric oxide in coronary vascular effects of estrogen in postmenopausal women. Circulation 1997;96:2795–2801.

29. Spyridopoulos I, Sullivan AB, Kearney M, et al. Estrogen-receptor-mediated inhibition of human endothelial cell apoptosis. Estradiol as a survival factor. Circulation 1997;95:1505–1514.

30. Morales DE, McGowan KA, Grant DS, et al. Molecular and cellular cardiology: estrogen promotes angiogenic activity in human umbilical vein endothelial cells in vitro and in a murine model. Circulation 1995;91:755–763.
31. Christian RC, Harrington S, Edwards WD, et al. Estrogen status correlates with the calcium content of coronary atherosclerotic plaques in women. J Clin Endocrinol Metab 2002;87:1062–1067.
32. Reis SE, Gloth ST, Blumenthal RS, et al. Ethinyl estradiol acutely attenuates abnormal coronary vasomotor responses to acetylcholine in postmenopausal women. Circulation 1994;89:52–60.
33. Collins P, Rosano GMC, Sarrel PM, et al. 17β-estradiol attenuates acetylcholine-induced coronary arterial constriction in women but not men with coronary heart disease. Circulation 1995;92:24–30.
34. Herrington DM, Espeland MA, Crouse JR III, et al. Estrogen replacement and brachial artery flow-mediated vasodilation in older women. Arterioscler Thromb Vasc Biol 2001;21:1955–1961.
35. Vita JA, Keaney JF, Jr. Hormone replacement therapy and endothelial function. The exception that proves the rule? Arterioscler Thromb Vasc Biol 2001;21:1867–1869.
36. Koh KK, Ahn JY, Jin DK, et al. Effects of continuous combined hormone replacement therapy on inflammation in hypertensive and/or overweight postmenopausal women. Arterioscler Thromb Vasc Biol 2002;22:1459–1464.
37. McCubbin JA, Helfer SG, Switzer FS, III, Price TM. Blood pressure control and hormone replacement therapy in postmenopausal women at risk for coronary heart disease. Am Heart J 2002;143:711–717.
38. Kawano H, Motoyama T, Ohgushi M, et al. Menstrual cyclic variation of myocardial ischemia in premenopausal women with variant angina. Ann Intern Med 2001;135:977–981.
39. Bokhari S, Bergmann SR. The effect of estrogen compared to estrogen plus progesterone on the exercise electrocardiogram. J Am Coll Cardiol 2002;40:1092–1096.
40. Rosano GMC, Sarrel PM, Poole-Wilson PA, Collins P. Beneficial effect of oestrogen on exercise-induced myocardial ischaemia in women with coronary artery disease. Lancet 1993;342:133–136.
41. Webb CM, Rosano GMC, Collins P. Oestrogen improves exercise-induced myocardial ischaemia in women. Lancet 1998;351:1556–1557.
42. Peterson LR, Eyster D, Dávila-Román VG, et al. Short-term oral estrogen replacement therapy does not augment endothelium-independent myocardial perfusion in postmenopausal women. Am Heart J 2001;142:641–647.
43. Duvernoy CS, Rattenhuber J, Seifert-Klauss V, et al. Myocardial blood flow and flow reserve in response to short-term cyclical hormone replacement therapy in postmenopausal women. J Gend Specif Med 2001;4:21–27.
44. Schulman SP, Thiemann DR, Ouyang P, et al. Effects of acute hormone therapy on recurrent ischemia in postmenopausal women with unstable angina. J Am Coll Cardiol 2002;39:231–237.
45. Barrett-Connor E, Grady D. Hormone replacement therapy, heart disease, and other considerations. Annu Rev Public Health 1998;19:55–72.
46. Newton KM, LaCroix AZ, McKnight B, et al. Estrogen replacement therapy and prognosis after first myocardial infarction. Am J Epidemiol 1997;145:269–277.
47. Sullivan JM, El-Zeky F, Vander Zwaag R, Ramanathan KB. Effect on survival of estrogen replacement therapy after coronary artery bypass grafting. Am J Cardiol 1997;79:847–850.
48. O'Keefe JH Jr, Kim SC, Hall RR, et al. Estrogen replacement therapy after coronary angioplasty in women. J Am Coll Cardiol 1997;29:1–5.
49. Grodstein F, Manson JE, Colditz GA, et al. A prospective, observational study of postmenopausal hormone therapy and primary prevention of cardiovascular disease. Ann Intern Med 2000;133:933–941.
50. Varas-Lorenzo C, García-Rodríguez LA, Perez-Gutthann S, Duque-Oliart A. Hormone replacement therapy and incidence of acute myocardial infarction. A population-based nested case-control study. Circulation 2000;101:2572–2578.
51. Hemminki E, McPherson K. Impact of postmenopausal hormone therapy on cardiovascular events and cancer: pooled data from clinical trials. BMJ 1997;315:149–153.
52. Hemminki E, McPherson K. Value of drug-licensing documents in studying the effect of postmenopausal hormone therapy on cardiovascular disease. Lancet 2000;355:566–569.
53. Petitti DB. Coronary heart disease and estrogen replacement therapy. Can compliance bias explain the results of observational studies? Ann Epidemiol 1994;4:115–118.
54. Heckbert SR, Kaplan RC, Weiss NS, et al. Risk of recurrent coronary events in relation to use and recent initiation of postmenopausal hormone therapy. Arch Intern Med 2001;161:1709–1713.

55. Psaty BM, Smith NL, Lemaitre RN, et al. Hormone replacement therapy, prothrombotic mutations, and the risk of incident nonfatal myocardial infarction in postmenopausal women. JAMA 2001;285:906–913.

56. Grodstein F, Manson JE, Stampfer MJ. Postmenopausal hormone use and secondary prevention of coronary events in the Nurses' Health Study. A prospective, observational study. Ann Intern Med 2001;135:1–8.

57. Abu-Halawa SA, Thompson K, Kirkeeide RL, et al. Estrogen replacement therapy and outcome of coronary balloon angioplasty in postmenopausal women. Am J Cardiol 1998;82:409–413.

58. Shlipak MG, Angeja BG, Go AS, et al. for the National Registry of Myocardial Infarction-3 Investigators. Hormone therapy and in-hospital survival after myocardial infarction in postmenopausal women. Circulation 2001;104:2300–2304.

59. Alexander KP, Newby LK, Hellkamp AS, et al. Initiation of hormone replacement therapy after acute myocardial infarction is associated with more cardiac events during follow-up. J Am Coll Cardiol 2001;38:1–7.

60. Angeja BG, Shlipak MG, Go AS, et al. for the National Registry of Myocardial Infarction 3 Investigators. Hormone therapy and the risk of stroke after acute myocardial infarction in postmenopausal women. J Am Coll Cardiol 2001;38:1297–1301.

61. Lemaitre RN, Heckbert SR, Psaty BM, et al. Hormone replacement therapy and associated risk of stroke in postmenopausal women. Arch Intern Med 2002;162:1954–1960.

61a.Gami AS, Wright RS, Ballman KV, Kopecky SL, Hayes SN. Hormone replacement therapy and risk of acute myocardial infarction in postmenopausal women with diabetes mellitus. Am J Cardiol 2003;91:1275–1277.

61b.Rea TD, Psaty BM, Heckbert SR, et al. Hormone replacement therapy and the risk of incident congestive heart failure: the Cardiovascular Health Study. Journal of Women's Health 2003;12:341–350.

62. Humphrey LL, Chan BK, Sox HC. Postmenopausal hormone replacement therapy and the primary prevention of cardiovascular disease. Ann Intern Med 2002;137:273–284.

63. Nelson HD, Humphrey LL, Nygren P, et al. Postmenopausal hormone replacement therapy. Scientific review. JAMA 2002;288:872–881.

64. McNagny SE, Wenger NK. Menopause and hormone replacement therapy. In: Branch WT (ed). Office Practice of Medicine, 2003, WB Saunders, Philadelphia, PA. pp. 569–580.

65. Grady D, Wenger, NK, Herrington D, et al for the Heart and Estrogen/progestin Replacement Study Research Group. Postmenopausal hormone therapy increases risk for venous thromboembolic disease. The Heart and Estrogen/progestin Replacement Study. Ann Intern Med 2000;132:689–696.

66. Herrington DM, Vittinghoff E, Howard TD, et al. Factor V Leiden, hormone replacement therapy, and risk of venous thromboembolic events in women with coronary disease. Arteriosclero Thromb Vasc Biol 2002;22:1012–1017.

67. Rosendaal FR, Vessey M, Rumley A, et al. Hormonal replacement therapy, prothrombotic mutations and the risk of venous thrombosis. Br J Haematol 2002;116:851–854.

68. Miller J, Chan BKS, Nelson HD. Postmenopausal estrogen replacement and risk for venous thromboembolism: A systematic review and meta-analysis for the U.S. Preventive Services Task Force. Ann Intern Med 2002;136:680–690.

69. Simon JA, Hunninghake DB, Agarwal SK, et al. for the Heart and Estrogen/progestin Replacement Study (HERS) Research Group. Effect of estrogen plus progestin on risk for biliary tract surgery in postmenopausal women with coronary artery disease. The Heart and Estrogen/Progestin Replacement Study. Ann Intern Med 2001;135:493–501.

70. McNagny SE, Wenger NK. Postmenopausal hormone-replacement therapy. N Engl J Med 2002;346:63.

71. Mamdani MM, Tu K, Van Walraven C, et al. Postmenopausal estrogen replacement therapy and increased rates of cholecystectomy and appendectomy, CMAJ 2000;162:1421–1424.

72. Fantl JA, Bump RC, Robinson D, et al. and the Continence Program for Women Research Group. Efficacy of estrogen supplementation in the treatment of urinary incontinence. Obstet Gynecol 1996;88:746–749.

73. Thom DH, Brown JS. Reproductive and hormonal risk factors for urinary incontinence in later life: A review of the clinical and epidemiologic literature. J Am Geriatr Soc 1998;46:1411–1417.

74. Grady D, Brown JS, Vittinghoff E, et al. for the HERS Research Group. Postmenopausal hormones and incontinence: The Heart and Estrogen/progestin Replacement Study. Obstet Gynecol 2001;97:116–120.

75. Schaumberg DA, Buring JE, Sullivan DA, Dana MR. Hormone replacement therapy and dry eye syndrome. JAMA 2001;286:2114–2119.

76. U.S. Congress Office of Technology Assessment. Effectiveness and Costs of Osteoporosis Screening and Hormone Replacement Therapy. OTA-BP-H-160. U.S. Government Printing Office, Washington, DC: 1995.

77. European Menopause Society. European consensus development conference on menopause. Human Reproduction 1996;11:975–979.

78. Clemons M, Goss P. Mechanisms of disease: Estrogen and the risk of breast cancer. N Engl J Med 2001;344:276–285.

79. Collaborative Group on Hormone Factors in Breast Cancer. Breast cancer and hormone replacement therapy: collaborative reanalysis of data from 51 epidemiological studies of 52 705 women with breast cancer and 108 411 women without breast cancer. Lancet 1997;350:1047–1059.

80. Greendale GA, Reboussin BA, Hogan P, et al. for the Postmenopausal Estrogen/Progestin Interventions Trial Investigators. Sympton relief and side effects of postmenopausal hormones: Results from the Postmenopausal Estrogen/Progestin Interventions Trial. Obstet Gynecol 1998;92:982–988.

81. Lacey JV, Jr, Mink PJ, Lubin JH, et al. Menopausal hormone replacement therapy and risk of ovarian cancer. JAMA 2002;288:334–341.

82. Angerer P, Störk S, Kothny W, et al. Effect of oral postmenopausal hormone replacement on progression of atherosclerosis: a randomized, controlled trial. Arterioscler Thromb Vasc Biol 2001;21:262–268.

83. Hodis HN, Mack WJ, Lobo RA, et al. for the Estrogen in the Prevention of Atherosclerosis Trial Research Group. Estrogen in the prevention of atherosclerosis. A randomized, double-blind, placebo-controlled trial. Ann Intern Med 2001;135:939–953.

84. Hulley S, Grady D, Bush T, et al. for the Heart and Estrogen-progestin Replacement Study (HERS) Research Group. Randomized trial of estrogen plus progestin for secondary prevention of coronary heart disease in postmenopausal women. JAMA 1998;280:605–613.

85. Petitti DB. Hormone replacement therapy and heart disease prevention: experimentation trumps observation. JAMA 1998;280:650–652.

86. Shilpak MG, Simon JA, Vittinghoff E, et al. Estrogen and progesting, lipoprotein(a), and the risk of recurrent coronary heart disease events after menopause. JAMA 2000;283:1845–1852.

86a. Kanaya AM, Herrington D, Vittinghoff E, et al. Glycemic effects of postmenopausal hormone therapy: the Heart and Estrogen/progestin Replacement Study: a randomized, double-blind, placebo-controlled trial. Ann Intern Med 2003;138:1–9.

87. Herrington DM, Reboussin DM, Brosnihan KB, et al. Effects of estrogen replacement on the progression of coronary-artery atherosclerosis. N Engl J Med 2000;343:522–529.

88. Sullivan JM. Coronary arteriography in estrogen-treated postmenopausal women. Prog Cardiovasc Dis 1995;38:211–222.

89. Clarke SC, Kelleher J, Lloyd-Jones H, Slack M, Schofield PM. A study of hormone replacement therapy in postmenopausal women with ischaemic heart disease: the Papworth HRT Atherosclerosis Study. BJOG: an International Journal of Obstetrics and Gynaecology 2002;109:1056–1062.

90. Viscoli CM, Brass LM, Kernan WN, et al. A clinical trial of estrogen-replacement therapy after ischemic stroke. N Engl J Med 2001;345:1243–1249.

91. Grady D, Herrington D, Bittner V, et al. for the HERS Research Group. Cardiovascular disease outcomes during 6.8 years of hormone therapy: Heart and Estrogen/progestin Replacement Study follow-up (HERS II). JAMA 2002;288:49–57.

92. Waters DD, Alderman EL, Hsia J, et al. Effects of hormone replacement therapy and antioxidant vitamin supplements on coronary atherosclerosis in postmenopausal women. A randomized controlled trial. JAMA 2002;288:2432–2440.

92a. The ESPRIT Team. Oestrogen therapy for prevention of reinfarction in postmenopausal women: a randomised placebo controlled trial. Lancet 2002;360:2001–2008.

92b. Chou ET, Schulman SP, Thiemann DR, Sohn RH, Bellantoni MF, Rade JJ. Effect of short-term estrogen with and without progesterone therapy on circulating markers of endothelial activation and injury in postmenopausal women with unstable angina pectoris. Am J Cardiol 2003;91:1240–1242.

92c. Schulman SP, Thiemann DR, Ouyang P, et al. Effects of acute hormone therapy on recurrent ischemia in postmenopausal women with unstable angina. J Am Coll Cardiol 2002;39:231–237.

93. Rossouw JE, Finnegan LP, Harlan WR, et al. The evolution of the Women's Health Initiative: Perspective from the NIH. JAMA 1995;50:50–55.

94. http://www.nhlbi.nih.gov/whi/hrt.htm. (Click on "HRT Update-English.") Women's Health Initiative, accessed March 3, 2003.

95. Writing Group for the Women's Health Initiative Investigators. Risks and benefits of estrogen plus progestin in healthy postmenopausal women. Principal results from the Women's Health Initiative randomized controlled trial. JAMA 2002;288:321–333.

96. Vickers MR, Meade TW, Wilkes HC. Hormone replacement therapy and cardiovascular disease: the case for a randomized controlled trial. Ciba Found Symp 1995;191:150–164.

97. MRC stops study of long term use of HRT. London: MRC press release, http://www.mrc.ac.uk/inex/public-interest/public-press_office/public-press_releases_2002/public-23_october_2002.htm. Accessed March, 2003.

97a. Hays J, Ockene JK, Brunner RL, et al. for the Women's Health Initiative Investigators. Effect of estrogen plus progestin on health-related quality of life. N Engl J Med 2003;348:1839–1854.

97b. Shumaker SA, Legault C, Rapp SR, et al for the WHIMS Investigators. Estrogen plus progestin and the incidence of dementia and mild cognitive impairment in postmenopausal women. The Women's Health Initiative Memory Study: a randomized controlled trial. JAMA 2003;289:2651–2662.

97c. Rapp SR, Espeland MA, Shumaker SA, et al for the WHIMS Investigators. Effect of estrogen plus progestin on global cognitive function in postmenopausal women. The Women's Health Initiative Memory Study: a randomized controlled trial. JAMA 2003;289:2663–2672.

98. Mosca L, Collins P, Herrington DM, et al. Hormone replacement therapy and cardiovascular disease. A Statement for Healthcare Professionals from the American Heart Association. Circulation 2001;104:499–503.

99. Smith SC Jr, Blair SN, Bonow RO, et al. AHA/ACC guidelines for preventing heart attack and death in patients with atherosclerotic cardiovascular disease: 2001 update. A Statement for Healthcare Professionals from the American Heart Association and the American College of Cardiology. Circulation 2001;104:1577–1579.

100. Downs JR, Clearfield M, Weis S, et al for the AFCAPS/TexCAPS Research Group. Primary prevention of acute coronary events with lovastatin in men and women with average cholesterol levels: results of AFCAPS/TexCAPS. JAMA 1998;279:1615–1622.

101. The Scandinavian Simvastatin Survival Study Group. Randomised trial of cholesterol lowering in 4444 patients with coronary heart disease: the Scandinavian Simvastatin Survival Study (4S). Lancet 1994;344:1383–1389.

102. Sacks, FM, Pfeffer MA, Moye LA, et al. for the Cholesterol and Recurrent Events Trial Investigators. The effect of pravastatin on coronary events after myocardial infarction in patients with average cholesterol levels. N Engl J Med 1996;335:1001–1009.

103. The Long-Term Intervention with Pravastatin in Ischaemic Disease (LIPID) Study Group. Prevention of cardiovascular events and death with pravastatin in patients with coronary heart disease and a broad range of initial cholesterol levels. N Engl J Med 1998;339:1349–1357.

104. Heart Protection Study Collaborative Group: MRC/BHF Heart Protection Study of cholesterol lowering with simvastatin in 20,536 high-risk individuals: a randomised placebo-controlled trial. Lancet 2002;360:7–22.

105. The Women's Health Initiative Study Group. Design of the Women's Health Initiative Clinical Trial and Observational Study. Controlled Clin Trials 1998;19:61–109.

106. Expert Panel on Detection, Evaluation, and Treatment of High Blood Cholesterol in Adults. Executive Summary of the Third Report of the National Cholesterol Education Program (NCEP) Expert Panel on Detection, Evaluation, and Treatment of High Blood Cholesterol in Adults (Adult Treatment Panel III). JAMA 2001;285:2486–2497.

106a. American Heart Association President Robert Bonow M.D. responds to new findings from the Women's Health Initiative Trial. Available at http://www.americanheart.org/presenter.jhtml?identifier=3003700. Accessed March 3, 2003.

107. Guidelines for Women's Health Care. 2nd ed. American College of Obstetricians and Gynecologists. American College of Obstetricians and Gynecologists, Washington, DC: 2002, pp. 130–133,171–176,314–318.

108. Report from the NAMS Advisory Panel on Postmenopausal Hormone Therapy. The North American Menopause Society. Accessed at www.menopause.org. March 3, 2003.

108a. Nelson HD, Humphrey LL, Nygren P, et al. Postmenopausal hormone replacement therapy. Scientific review. JAMA 2002;288:872–881.

109. U.S. Preventive Services Task Force. Postmenopausal hormone replacement therapy for primary prevention of chronic conditions: Recommendations and rationale. Ann Intern Med 2002;137:834–839.
110. Robertson RM. Women and cardiovascular disease. The risks of misperception and the need for action. Circulation 2001:103:2318–2320.
111. Wenger NK. Coronary heart disease: An older woman's major health risk. BMJ 1997;315:1085–1090.
112. LaRosa JC, He J, Vupputuri S. Effect of statins on risk of coronary disease. A meta-analysis of randomized controlled trials. JAMA 1999;282:2340–2346.
113. Mosca L, Grundy SM, Judelson D, et al. Guide to preventive cardiology for women. AHA/ACC Scientific Statement: Consensus Panel Statement. Circulation 1999;99:2480–2484.
114. Herrington DM, Vittinghoff E, Lin F, et al, for the HERS Study Group. Statin therapy, cardiovascular events, and total mortality in the Heart and Estrogen/progestin Replacement Study (HERS). Circulation 2002;105:2962–2967.
115. Collins P, Wenger NK, Rossouw JE, Paoletti R. Cardiovascular and pulmonary disease. In: Wenger NK, Paoletti R, Lenfant CJM, Pinn VW (eds). International Position Paper on Women's Health and Menopause: A Comprehensive Approach. National Heart, Lung, and Blood Institute, Office of Research on Women's Health, National Institutes of Health, Giovanni Lorenzini Medical Sciencen Foundation, NIH Publication No. 02–3284: 2002, Bethesda, MD, pp. 141–180.
116. Kuller LH, Simkin-Silverman LR, Wing RR, et al. Women's healthy lifestyle project: a randomized clinical trial. Results at 54 months. Circulation 2001;103:32–37.
116a.US Food and Drug Administration. Center for Drug Evaluation and Research. Estrogen and estrogen with progestin therapies for postmenopausal women. Available at 222.fda.gov/cder/drug/infopage/estrogens_progestins/default.htm. Accessed March 3, 2003.
117. Wenger NK. Cardiovascular effects of raloxifene: the potential for cardiovascular protection in women. Diabetes Obes Metab 2002;4:166–176.
118. Black LJ, Sato M, Rowley ER, et al. Raloxifene (LY139481 HCI) prevents bone loss and reduces serum cholesterol without causing uterine hypertrophy in ovariectomized rats. J Clin Invest 1994;93:63–69
119. Richardson MA, Berg DT, Calnek DS, et al. 17β-estradiol, but not raloxifene, decreases thrombomodulin in the antithrombotic protein C pathway. Endocrinology 2000;141:3908–3911.
120. Zuckerman SH, Bryan N. Inhibition of LDL oxidation and myeloperoxidase dependent tyrosyl radical formation by the selective estrogen receptor modulator raloxifene (LY139481 HCL). Atherosclerosis 1996;126:65–75.
121. Rahimian R, Laher I, Dube G, van Breemen C. Estrogen and selective estrogen receptor modulator LY117018 enhance release of nitric oxide in rat aorta. J Pharmacol Exp Therapeut 1997;283:116–122.
122. Simoncini T, Genazzani AR. Raloxifene acutely stimulates nitric oxide release from human endothelial cells via an activation of endothelial nitric oxide synthase. J Clin Endocrinol Metab 2000;85:2966–2969.
123. Zoma WD, Baker RS, Clark KE. Coronary and uterine vascular responses to raloxifene in the sheep. Am J Obstet Gynecol 2000;182:521–528.
124. Wiernicki T, Glasebrook A, Phillips DL, Singh JP. Estrogen and novel tissue selective estrogen receptor modulator raloxifene directly modulate vascular smooth muscle cell functions: Implications in the cardioprotective mechanism of estrogen. Circulation 1996;94(Suppl I):1–278.
125. Bjarnason NH, Haarbo J, Byrjalsen I, et al. Raloxifene inhibits aortic accumulation of cholesterol in ovariectomized, cholesterol-fed rabbits. Circulation 1997;96:1964–1969.
126. Clarkson TB, Anthony MS, Jerome CP. Lack of effect of raloxifene on coronary artery atherosclerosis of postmenopausal monkeys. J Clin Endocrinol Metab 1998;83:721–726.
127. Bjarnason NH, Haarbo J, Byrjalsen I, et al. Raloxifene reduces atherosclerosis: studies of optimized raloxifene doses in ovariectomized, cholesterol-fed rabbits. Clin Endocrinol 2000;52:225–233.
128. Bjarnason NH, Haarbo J, Byrjalsen I, et al. Raloxifene and estrogen reduces progression of advanced atherosclerosis–a study in ovariectomized, cholesterol-fed rabbits. Atherosclerosis 2001;154:97–102.
129. Bakir SE, Chen S-J, Li G, et al. The synthetic estrogen receptor modulator raloxifene hydrochloride is not vasoprotective in the rat carotid injury model. Circulation 1999;100(Suppl I):I–332.
130. Kauffman RF, Bean JS, Fahey KJ, et al. Raloxifene and estrogen inhibit neointimal thickening after balloon injury in the carotid artery of male and ovarectomized female rats. J Cardiovascular Pharmacol 2000;36:459–465.

131. Ogita H, Kitakaze M, Node K, et al. Amelioration of ischemia- and reperfusion-induced myocardial injury by raloxifene: Roles of nitric oxide and the opening of calcium-activated potassium channels. J Am Coll Cardiol 2001;27(Suppl):362A–363A.

132. Wassmann S, Laufs U, Stamenkovic D, et al. Raloxifene improves endothelial dysfunction in hypertension by reduced oxidative stress and enhanced nitric oxide production. Circulation 2002;105:2083–2091.

133. Walsh BW, Kuller LH, Wild RA, et al. Effects of raloxifene on serum lipids and coagulation factors in healthy postmenopausal women. JAMA 1998;279:1445–1451.

134. de Valk-de Roo GW, Stehouwer CDA, Meijer P, et al. Both raloxifene and estrogen reduce major cardiovascular risk factors in healthy postmenopausal women. A 2-year, placebo-controlled study. Arterioscler Thromb Vasc Biol 1999;19:2993–3000.

135. Walsh BW, Paul S, Wild RA, et al. The effects of hormone replacement therapy and raloxifene on C-reactive protein and homocysteine in healthy postmenopausal women: A randomized, controlled trial. J Clin Endocrinol Metab 2000;85:214–218.

136. Ridker PM, Hennekens CH, Buring JE, Rifai N. C-reactive protein and other markers of inflammation in the prediction of cardiovascular disease in women. N Engl J Med 2000;342:836–843.

137. Walsh BW, Cox DA, Sashegyi A, et al. Role of tumor necrosis factor-α and interleukin-6 in the effects of hormone replacement therapy and raloxifene on C-reactive protein in postmenopausal women. Am J Cardiol 2001;88:825–828.

138. Blum A, Schenke WH, Hathaway L, et al. Effects of estrogen and the selective estrogen receptor modulator raloxifene on markers of inflammation in postmenopausal women. Am J Cardiol 2000;86:892–895.

139. Sarrel PM, Nawaz H, Chan W, et al. Raloxifene improves brachial artery and microcirculatory flow-mediated dilation in healthy postmenopausal women. Circulation 2000;102(Suppl):II–107.

140. Saitta A, Morabito N, Frisina N, et al. Cardiovascular effects of raloxifene hydrochloride. Cardiovascular Drug Reviews 2001;19:57–74.

141. Saitta A, Altavilla D, Cucinotta D, et al. Randomized, double-blind, placebo-controlled study on effects of raloxifene and hormone replacement therapy on plasma NO concentrations, endothelin-1 levels, and endothelium-dependent vasodilation in postmenopausal women. Arterioscler Thromb Vasc Biol 2001;21:1512–1519.

142. Setacci C, la Marca A, Agricola E, et al. Effects of the selective estrogen receptor modulator, raloxifene, on carotid artery pulsatility index in postmenopausal women. Am J Obstet Gynecol 2002;186:832–835.

143. Harper KD, Barrett-Connor E, Sashegyi A, et al. The effect of raloxifene on cardiovascular risk in osteoporotic postmenopausal women: 3-year results from the MORE (Multiple Outcomes of Raloxifene Evaluation) Trial. J Am Geriatr Soc 2001;49:S5–S6.

144. Cummings SR, Duong T, Kenyon E, et al., for the Multiple Outcomes of Raloxifene Evaluation (MORE) Trial. Serum estradiol level and risk of breast cancer during treatment with raloxifene. JAMA 2002;287:216–220.

145. Barrett-Connor E, Grady D, Sashegyi A, et al for the MORE Investigators. Raloxifene and cardiovascular events in osteoporotic postmenopausal women. Four-year results from the MORE (Multiple Outcomes of Raloxifene Evaluation) Randomized Trial. JAMA 2002;287:847–857.

146. Cummings SR, Eckert S, Krueger KA, et al. The effect of raloxifene on risk of breast cancer in postmenopausal women. Result from the MORE randomized trial. JAMA 1999;281:2189–2197.

147. Ettinger B, Black DM, Mitlak BH, et al., for the Multiple Outcomes of Raloxifene Evaluation (MORE) Investigators. Reduction of vertebral fracture risk in postmenopausal women with osteoporosis treated with raloxifene: Results from a 3-year randomized clinical trial. JAMA 1999;282:637–645.

148. Mosca L, Barrett-Connor E, Wenger NK, et al. Design and methods of the Raloxifene Use for The Heart (RUTH) study. Am J Cardiol 2001;88:392–395.

149. Wenger NK, Barrett-Connor E, Collins P, et al., for the RUTH Investigators. Baseline characteristics of participants in the Raloxifene Use for The Heart (RUTH) trial. Am J Cardiol 2002;90:1204–1210.

150. Barrett-Connor E, Wenger NK, Grady D, et al. Coronary heart disease in women randomized clinical trials, HERS and RUTH. Maturitas 1998;31:1–7.

IV ECONOMICS AND POLICY ISSUES IN HEALTH CARE RELATED TO WOMEN

22 Gender Bias

*Is It Real and How Does It Affect Diagnosis,
Management, and Outcome?*

Thomas H. Marwick, MD, PhD, FRACP, FACC and Jonathan Chan, MBBS

CONTENTS

INTRODUCTION

Coronary heart disease (CHD) continues to be a dominant cause of mortality in the United States, claiming 500,000 lives of both sexes annually *(1)*. Since the 1980s, the cardiovascular mortality rate in women has remained static, despite the relative decline in cardiovascular mortality in men *(1)*. Several factors may account for this difference in outcome, including differences in risk factor profiles (especially smoking) and the biology of coronary artery disease (CAD; especially older age occurrence in women vs men). Another explanation might be the presence of gender differences in the diagnosis and management of CHD *(2)*, such that coronary disease is underdiagnosed and undertreated in women in comparison to men *(3,4)*.

Partly because of the presence of numerous confounding variables, the assessment of gender-specific differences in CHD management is a complex issue. Two fundamental issues influence the literature on gender and patient outcomes—the limited size of the evidence base and the impact of confounding variables *(5)*. Women are underrepresented in many large therapeutic studies, in part because of the overall lower prevalence of CHD in women, and partly from the exclusion of women of childbearing age and the presence of upper age limits on recruitment *(6)*. The latter affects women disproportionately, as coronary disease in women presents about a decade later than that

From: *Contemporary Cardiology: Coronary Disease in Women: Evidence-Based Diagnosis and Treatment*
Edited by: L. J. Shaw and R. F. Redberg © Humana Press Inc., Totowa, NJ

in men *(7)*. The second concept is that a multitude of gender-related confounding variables, such as age, comorbidity and clinical presentation, may affect decision making and may also have as much impact on outcome as gender-related biological differences. Regression analysis may be utilized to allow independent sex assessment after consideration of other variables.

GENDER BIAS IN DIAGNOSIS OF CORONARY DISEASE

Clinical Presentation

An evaluation of disease probability is the initial step of the diagnostic process and may potentially explain bias in the investigation of coronary disease. Chest pain is usually the main presenting symptom in CAD, and gender differences in the clinical presentation of chest pain may lead to differences in diagnosis and subsequent management, particularly among patients without a previous history of proven CAD *(8)*. Atypical chest pain is more common in women than in men, perhaps because of the higher prevalence of microvascular and vasospastic angina in women and other causes of nonischemic chest pain, such as mitral valve prolapse *(9)*. Angina at rest, during sleep, or stress-provoked are also more common in women *(10)*. Even in patients who present with typical angina, the likelihood of angiographically proven CAD is lower in women *(11)*. In the Coronary Artery Surgery Study (CASS), 62% of women with typical angina had coronary disease when compared with 40% with probable angina and only 4% with nonischemic pain *(12)*. These differences in clinical presentation influence the predictability of positive angiography findings in those who present with chest pain. It is quite possible that lower referral rates to noninvasive and invasive testing may reflect the perception that chest pain is a less reliable symptom in women *(13)*.

Regardless the reason, there seems little doubt that physicians use different criteria for managing chest pain in men and women. In a study of 720 primary care physicians *(14)*, recommendations were made about the management of patients with particular characteristics portrayed by actors. Estimates of the CAD probability were lower for women than men ($64 \pm 19\%$ vs $69 \pm 18\%$, $p < 0.001$), and women were less likely to be referred for cardiac catheterization (odds ratio [OR], 0.60; 95% confidence interval [CI], 0.4–0.9; $p = 0.02$).

Evidence shows that risk factors in women are more prevalent *(15)* and have a greater correlation with CAD when compared to men. Diabetes is a strong predictor of CAD in women *(16,17)*. Intermediate predictors include hypertension *(18,19)*, smoking *(20,21)*, central obesity *(22)*, family history, and presence of peripheral vascular disease. The assessment of CAD pretest probability might be enhanced by the combination of chest pain evaluation with the assessment of cardiovascular risk factors.

Noninvasive Diagnostic Testing

Noninvasive testing is employed in CAD diagnosis and risk stratification to identify those patients who will potentially benefit from further medical therapy or revascularization procedures. There is a general perception among physicians that the diagnostic accuracy of noninvasive testing is less reliable in women than their male counterparts but this is imperfectly supported by evidence simply because women have been underrepresented in published studies of noninvasive testing *(23)*. Accuracy differences in each of the noninvasive testing modalities in men and women likely impact decision making regarding subsequent angiography and may therefore be responsible for gender bias.

EXERCISE ELECTROCARDIOGRAM

The exercise electrocardiogram (ECG) remains the most widely utilized noninvasive testing modality. Although exercise testing guidelines continue to recommend the exercise ECG as an accurate test in women *(24)*, evidence suggests that both the sensitivity and specificity of exercise testing is lower in women when compared to men *(25–30)*. Furthermore, the incremental value of exercise testing to clinical data is of lesser significance in women than men *(31)*.

The perception of lower diagnostic accuracy of exercise testing—as with the clinical presentation—may lead to a gender bias that influences both lower utilization of this test or if the test is performed and positive toward less frequent female referral to angiography. A recent paper from the Rochester Epidemiology Project *(32)* examined a population-based cohort of 2624 exercise tests in Olmsted County residents. The utilization of stress testing was lower in women than men across all age strata, being 1888 per 100,000 in men and 703 for women (rate ratio for men over women 2.7, 95% CI 2.5–2.9). At the time of initial testing women were more symptomatic and had poorer exercise performance than men. The age-adjusted rate ratios for stress test utilization were 2.8 (95% CI 2.5–3.0) and that for CHD mortality was 1.9 (95% CI 1.7–2.2).

The data regarding onward referral to angiography are conflicting. In a study of 840 patients (47% women) with suspected CAD, Shaw and colleagues *(33)* found that 62% of men were referred to subsequent angiography in comparison to only 38% of women (*p* = 0.002). Even after multiple logistic regression analysis, male gender was identified to have an increased likelihood of follow-up testing (relative risk [RR] 1.9; 95% CI 1.6–6.0, *p* = 0.005). The consequence of this referral bias was that at 2-year follow-up, women who had less follow-up and angiography referrals had higher rates of cardiac mortality and nonfatal myocardial infarction (MI). On the other hand, no bias was detected when a group of cardiologists from an academic medical center were asked to predict the probability of any obstructive coronary disease, severe coronary disease, and the survival probability in a cohort of 410 symptomatic outpatients undergoing exercise testing for possible CAD *(34)*. Although the 130 women were referred for cardiac catheterization significantly less often than men (18% vs 27%, *p* = 0.03), this was explained by a lower rate of positive exercise tests and a significantly lower pretest probability of coronary disease in women. Moreover, the cardiologists neither underestimated coronary disease risk, nor the coronary disease probability.

Although the results of exercise ECG testing are unfavorable, numerous steps may be taken to minimize the reliance on ST response alone. Gender-specific criteria that improve the accuracy of treadmill testing in women have been obtained by application of the ST heart rate index. Integration with hemodynamic and functional capacity data improves the predictive power of the exercise ECG in women *(35)*, and the Duke treadmill score appears to be valid for the separation of high- and low-risk groups in both sexes. To the extent that functional impairment (particularly likely in the elderly) may compromise sensitivity, selection for pharmacological stress imaging tests may be a better choice in many patients.

NUCLEAR PERFUSION IMAGING

The higher diagnostic accuracy of stress perfusion imaging over conventional stress electrocardiography in CAD detection in unselected groups has been defined for many years with both thallium and technetium tracers *(36,37)*. However, both sensitivity and specificity of this imaging modality may be compromised in women *(38,39)*. False-positive test results may be because of breast soft-tissue attenuation artifacts, which may mimic anterior and anterolateral perfusion defects *(40)*. False-negatives may arise because of the failure to resolve ischemic zones in the smaller female heart *(41)* and the performance of submaximal exercise *(42,43)*. As noted previously, a low threshold should be applied to the decision to perform pharmacological testing in women because of concern in the possibility of submaximal stress; pharmacological tests have been shown to have equivalent accuracy *(44,45)* in women and men. There is no question that the results of single photon emission tomography (SPECT) are prognostically useful in women *(46,47)*. Moreover, the diagnostic problems are not insoluble—examination of the unprocessed images is an effective means for recognizing artifactual defects as false rather than true positive findings *(48)*. The extent of perfusion defects is related to the likelihood of significant disease and risk *(49)*, and gated imaging has substantially improved specificity *(50)*. Finally, some groups have integrated scanning results with an assessment of disease probability *(51)*.

It is unclear whether the possibility of inaccurate findings might influence subsequent decision making. In a study of 2137 men and 1074 women performed at Cedars-Sinai Medical Center, it was found that more men than women were referred to angiography (11% vs 7%, $p < 0.001$) after exercise dual-isotope SPECT imaging, but after stratification by the amount of malperfused myocardium, the angiography rate was similar *(52)*. Interestingly, these results were almost simultaneously obtained in another study of 1318 women and 2351 men who underwent exercise thallium SPECT at the Cleveland Clinic *(53)*. This study showed that angiography was less frequently performed (6% in women vs 14% in men, $p < 0.001$), but this was for good reason—women had a lower frequency of abnormal thallium results (8% vs 29%, $p < 0.001$). After correction for these other variables in a multiple logistic regression analysis, there was no difference in the referral rate to angiography between men and women (RR 1.00, 95% CI, 0.75–1.34). In conclusion, although referral bias to angiography exists following exercise testing, there is no evidence of its occurrence after nuclear imaging procedures.

STRESS ECHOCARDIOGRAPHY

Stress echocardiography is now a well-established diagnostic test for CAD at many centers and has proven to have at least equivalent accuracy to nuclear stress perfusion imaging *(54)*, with the additional benefit of being quite cost-effective *(55)*. Stress echocardiography also yields high specificity in women *(56–58)*, and the only study that showed a lower specificity demonstrated that specificity was actually 83–86% after correction for verification bias *(59)*. High specificity levels are important from a cost standpoint, as they avoid unnecessary angiography and may be translated into better cost-efficiency than standard exercise testing *(58)*. A meta-analysis of studies from 1966 to 1995 *(60)* showed that exercise echocardiography had a weighted mean sensitivity and specificity of 86% (95% CI 75–96%) and 79% (95% CI 72–86%), more favorable than the exercise ECG—with a 61% sensitivity and specificity (95% CI

54–68%) and 70% (95% CI 64–75%) and exercise thallium imaging—with results of 78% (95% CI 72–83%) and 64% (95% CI 51–77%). Nonetheless, the sensitivity of exercise echocardiography in women may still be compromised by submaximal exercise testing. In this situation, sensitivity can be improved by the adoption of pharmacological stress testing, although the reported sensitivity is less than in unselected populations (61,62). Therefore, it appears that stress echocardiographic techniques avoid the pitfalls of exercise ECG in a similar way (and perhaps even better) than exercise SPECT. However, currently there is insufficient data whether these benefits translate to avoidance of gender differences in angiography referral following stress echocardiography.

ELECTRON BEAM COMPUTED TOMOGRAPHY (EBCT)

This test is presently in use for the detection of subclinical atherosclerosis and the evaluation of symptoms suggestive of CAD (63). Generally, the absence of coronary calcification is considered to be a sensitive marker of the absence of significant CAD, but its presence may be explained by mild subclinical disease. Indeed, one early study showed the results to reflect risk factor status, but only modest accuracy for angiographic stenoses (64). Evidence does suggest that the sensitivity of coronary calcification was less in women than men (65), perhaps related to lower pretest CAD probability. Moreover, perhaps because women present at an older age than men, and the finding of coronary calcification becomes less specific with increasing age, specificity may be as low as 50% (65–67). Although the combination with SPECT may not increase EBCT accuracy (68), a widely applied investigative strategy is that patients with a positive test undergo some other form of functional testing to clarify whether significant stenoses are present. In this situation, the lower specificity in women may impact onward referrals from positive tests. However, there is no current evidence that a positive EBCT result is managed any differently in women vs than men.

Angiography As a Diagnostic Test

The results of coronary angiography have traditionally been considered to be the "gold standard" test for CAD identification. Unfortunately, however, the reduction of coronary flow by stenoses is influenced by vessel location, association with bifurcations, and vessel curvatures and morphology, among other factors (69). Therefore, the use of a single cut-off clearly cannot define coronary disease as the cause of patient symptoms in all situations. Moreover, although the results of angiography form the cornerstone to identify the highest risk levels (and thereby the patients who might be best served by revascularization) (70), these criteria miss other patients at significant risk, and other functional testing may be prognostically at least as powerful (71,72). Finally, coronary angiography may not necessarily be applied appropriately for either diagnostic or prognostic reasons. For all of these reasons, angiography referral may not be a particularly good standard for evaluating the quality of care.

Nonetheless, coronary angiography may be seen as a necessary prelude to revascularization decisions. Therefore, the study of how gender affects the difference in patient referral to angiography and subsequent referral from angiography for further management may help the understanding of the impact of gender bias on CHD treatment. In several studies (Table 1), the performance of angiography is almost universally greater in men than in women, although only the combination of these results with outcomes

Table 1
Relationship of Gender to the Performance of Coronary Angiography in Patients With Chronic CAD

Author (ref.)	Study group	n	Women	Cath rate (M|W)	RR (M|W)	Comments
Tobin (8)	Stress nuclear studies	390	35%	40%|4%	6.3	Other predictors: age, symptoms, MI, stress results
Morise (73)	Abnormal exercise test	1980	44%	21%|24%	—	
Shaw (33)	Abnormal exercise test	840	47%	45%|34%	—	Revascularization more in men, death/MI more in women
Gregor (74)	Chronic CAD (MONICA)	9737	33%	24%|18%		Differences also in exercise testing
Ayanian (75)	Chronic CAD (MA)	49623	43%	28%|16%	1.28	Revascularization more in men; same findings in MI group
Kee (76)	Chronic CAD (MD)	33159	46%	29%|18%	1.15	
	Acute and chronic CAD	24179	37%	7%|3%	2.1	No differences between women across social class
D'Hoore (77)	Acute and chronic CAD	33940	34%	—	1.47	Differences between men and women unrelated to cost
Hachamovitch (52)	Stress nuclear studies	3211	33%	11%|7%		No differences after stratified by amount of abnormal left ventricle
Lauer (53)	Stress nuclear studies	3669	36%	14%|6%	2.4	Not different after adjusting for age and thallium result
Miller (78)	Stress nuclear studies	14499	41%	17%|8%	1.3	Gender weaker correlate of angiography than imaging variables

MONICA, Monitoring Trends and Determinants in Cardiovascular Disease.

data can identify whether these findings imply underuse on women, overuse in men, or both *(8,33,52,53,73–78)*. Presently, 40–50% of women undergoing angiography are reported to have normal coronary arteries *(79)*, so that it is difficult to justify an unfocused application of angiography in more patients.

Summary: Sources of Bias in the Diagnostic Evaluation of CAD

The initial evaluation of the quality of the pain and risk factors remains important in the determination of CAD likelihood in women who present with chest pain *(9)*. Patients at high-pretest clinical risk (e.g., typical angina and multiple risk factors) warrant direct referral to angiography. Those with intermediate or low risk can be referred for risk stratification by noninvasive stress testing. Those with positive stress test results should be referred to angiography and based on the previous evidence, the use of stress imaging approaches may reduce the perception of lower reliability and diagnostic accuracy of exercise ECG testing in women, thereby avoiding underreferral of women for angiography. Female selection for angiography based on positive stress imaging results as opposed to positive conventional stress ECG testing or clinical symptoms may minimize costs of unnecessary investigations. At present, there are still insufficient data to alter the recommendations for angiography in women in comparison to men.

GENDER BIAS IN MANAGEMENT AND OUTCOME OF CHRONIC CAD

Coronary Bypass Surgery

Table 2 displays a summary of the major trials that concerning gender influence on the performance of myocardial revascularization *(33,75,77,79–81)*. These data show that women have a lower frequency of bypass surgery than men. This lower prevalence for intervention may be explained by both the lower frequency of referral to noninvasive stress testing and initial angiography as well as less angiography despite positive stress testing (as discussed previously). Importantly, however, after CAD diagnosis is confirmed, revascularization rates are equal in men and women *(82)*.

The decision to refer to surgery is based on the nature of the symptoms, the perception of the correlation between symptoms and severity of disease, and the operative risks associated with surgery. The long-term survival after bypass graft surgery is similar in men and women *(83,84)*. However, women are reported to have a higher mortality from cardiac surgery than men *(85,86)*, with perioperative mortality in women being reported to be twice that of men *(87)*. Even in more recent data from the Bypass Angioplasty Revascularization Investigators (BARI) trial *(82)*, women have a higher incidence of postoperative complications, including postprocedural MI and pulmonary edema. Additionally, they enjoy less effective angina relief, and increased frequency of graft occlusion *(88)*. Some of these phenomena reflect the older age, instability, and greater comorbidity of many female patients at presentation *(5)*, as well as intervention effects later in the course of disease, the atherogenic milieu and especially the smaller size of grafted vessels in women.

In the context of these differences, surgery avoidance may merely reflect good clinical judgement to avoid surgery in situations where there is a high risk to benefit ratio, rather than true gender bias. Indeed, when all these variables were taken into account, Bickell and colleagues *(81)* examined nearly 6000 patients from Duke University and found no

Table 2
Influence of Gender on the Performance of Revascularization in Chronic Coronary Disease

Author (ref.)	Study group	n	Women	PTCA rate (M|W)	CABG rate (M|W)	PTCA (M|W)	CABG (M|W)	Comments
Kuykendall (80)	Chronic CAD	31657	28%	—	33%|32%	0.92	—	Revasc also predicted by age, race, HT, CHF, rhythm, medical disorders (e.g., COPD)
Bickell (81)	Post angiography	5795	19%	—	46%|44%		1.23 high risk 0.84 (low risk)	Women as likely to undergo revasc when benefit is greatest
Sullivan (79)	Chronic CAD	886	23%	16%|26%	43%|12%	—	—	Revasc also predicted by age, HT, DM, F/H, angiographic severity
Shaw (33)	Abnormal exercise test	840	47%	4.9|2.0 ^	4.9|2.0 ^	—	—	—
Ayanian (75)	Chronic CAD (MA)	49623	43%	16%|7% ^	16%|7% ^	1.31 ^	1.31 ^	Combined revascularization (PTCA and CABG)
	Chronic CAD (MD)	33159	46%	14%|7% ^	14%|7% ^	1.4 ^	1.4 ^	Combined revascularization (PTCA and CABG)
D'Hoore (77)	Acute and chronic CAD	33940	34%	—	—	1.38 ^	1.38 ^	Combined revascularization (PTCA and CABG)

CABG, coronary bypass surgery; PTCA, percutaneous transluminal coronary angioplasty; revasc, revascularization; CHF, congestive heart failure; DM, diabetes mellitus; CAD, coronary artery disease; HT, hypertension; COPD, chronic obstructive pulmonary disease.

gender difference exists between men and women referred to surgery (46% and 44%, respectively). However, among low-risk patients, more men were referred to surgery with an OR of 1.23 (95% CI, 1.05–1.58). Among high-risk patients, the contrary occurred, with more women referred to surgery, OR 0.84 (95% CI, 0.68–1.04). This observation may suggest that men were overtreated, whereas women were referred more appropriately for surgery. Similarly, 74% (95% CI, 71–77%) of 631 patients who met the RAND expert panel criteria for necessary revascularization actually underwent revascularization, irrespective of patient gender, ethnic group, or payer status *(89)*.

In summary, the indications for coronary bypass surgery should be reserved for those patients with symptoms refractory to conventional medical therapy, those with failed or complicated percutaneous angioplasty, and those with left-main CAD or multivessel disease with reduced left ventricular function in both men and women. Factors that influence the risk of the procedure and likelihood of success should also be taken into account—including the age of the patient, the presence of comorbidity, availability of suitable conduits and targets, and the demonstration of inducible ischemia on noninvasive stress testing. Although differential rates of surgical revascularization have been shown, this may reflect the application of these principles and good clinical judgement, rather than gender bias.

Coronary Angioplasty

Women referred to angioplasty present at an older age, with greater comorbidity and more severe unstable symptoms *(90,91)*, which reflect the older presentation of coronary disease in women as well as the difficulties of interpreting symptoms. This may delay diagnostic investigations, as described previously. Not surprisingly, the initial studies that compare the efficacy of angioplasty between genders showed women to have a greater mortality with the procedure than men. In the National Heart, Lung and Blood Institute (NHLBI) report, women who underwent angioplasty had a mortality three times that of men, and on multivariate analysis, female gender was an independent correlate of mortality *(92)*. However, modern technology improvements and the accumulation of experience have led more recent data to suggest that the efficacy of the procedure has improved in women, so that the long-term prognosis after successful coronary angioplasty is excellent and similar to that of men *(93)*. In the BARI trial, the angioplasty success rate was actually higher in women than men (76% vs 71%, *p* < 0.01), and this was achieved at a lower mortality *(82)*.

Several studies have suggested that women are referred to angioplasty rather than bypass surgery. For example, in a study of 22,795 patients at the Mayo Clinic, more women were referred to angioplasty whereas more men underwent bypass surgery *(91)*. However, once again this may be a reflection of good clinical judgement rather than gender bias, because of the higher mortality rates noted in women undergoing surgery, so that angioplasty may be the therapeutic option of lower risk.

GENDER BIAS IN DIAGNOSIS AND MANAGEMENT OF ACUTE CORONARY SYNDROMES

MI

The results of follow-up studies post-MI suggest that men have a better prognosis than women, at least in the short term. In the Framingham Heart Study, 30-day mortality rates were higher in women than in men (28 vs 16%), as were the early reinfarction rates (25% vs 22%; *94*). These differences reflect the older age at presentation of women, greater comorbidity *(95)*, and smaller coronary arteries even after correction for other aspects of body habitus—given the differences in biology between men and women, they do not necessarily indicate undertreatment. Nonetheless, these greater risks highlight the greater need for careful risk stratification in women postinfarction. However, other causes of adverse outcome include factors like later presentation and less rapid infarction recognition *(96–98)*, that reflect differences in awareness and presentation that are amenable to intervention.

Acute infarction should be treated with thrombolytic therapy or primary angioplasty, depending on the availability of resources on a timely basis. Primary angioplasty is specifically indicated in the presence of contraindications to thrombolysis or infarction associated with hemodynamic compromise *(99,100)*. Very little data is available regarding the gender influence in patients after primary angioplasty. Antoniucci et al. *(101)* found the 6-month mortality rate was 12% in 230 women and 7% in 789 men (*p* = 0.03), with nonfatal reinfarction in 3% and 1%, respectively (*p* = 0.01). However, these differences likely reflected the older age of women, as well as a greater diabetes incidence and cardiogenic shock, so that after multivariate analysis, gender did not emerge as a significant variable in relation to 6-month mortality.

Although thrombolysis offers benefit to both men and women *(102)*, this benefit appears to be less marked in women *(95)*. For example, the ISIS-2 trial showed a 45% reduction in mortality in men who received streptokinase plus aspirin, in comparison to only 31% reduction in women *(103)*. Women have been reported to have a lower tendency to be receive thrombolysis than men *(104)*, but given the older age of presentation, greater comorbidity, lower perceived benefit and higher intracranial bleeding rates *(105)* in women, this may not so much represent gender bias than good clinical judgement of the balance of thrombolysis benefits with higher RR.

The current American Heart Association/American College of Cardiology (AHA/ACC) guidelines on the treatment of MI suggest that invasive and noninvasive strategies are equally justifiable. However, whatever strategy is used, early risk stratification is appropriate because the majority of complications occur early in the course. Patients that receive thrombolytic treatment have fewer subsequent events, but despite their lower risk status, appropriately powered studies show that risk stratification is still valuable after thrombolysis. Maximal symptom limited stress testing is preferred over submaximal testing because it offers better assessment of functional capacity and nearly doubles the yield of ischemic responses *(106,107)*, but if the patient is unable to exercise, pharmacological stress imaging studies are a promising alternative *(108,109)*. Whether studies exist that address any gender-based variation in the performance of these investigations is unknown.

Table 3 summarizes studies that have examined gender's role in the referral of patients to coronary angiography following infarction—most have shown that men have a greater tendency to undergo angiography than women *(96,110–118)*. Udvarhelyi and colleagues *(110)* examined 218,000 patients, of whom 28% of men but only 18% of women underwent angiography post-MI, giving an OR of 1.22. In 1994, Kostis and colleagues *(111)* examined more than 42,000 patients and found that frequency of angiography in men was 32% in comparison to 18% in women, with an OR of 1.39 (95% CI, 1.32–1.47). Similarly, in a study performed by Chirboga and col-

Table 3
Relationship Between Gender and Angiography After MI

Author	n	Women	Cath rate (M|W)	RR (M|W)	Other predictors of angiography
Udverheyli (110)	218427	50%	28%|18%	1.22	Age, race, sympt, HT, DM, CHF, COPD
Kostis (111)	42595	24%	32%|18%	1.39	Age, race, HT, DM, CHF, rhythm dis, medical dis (e.g., COPD)
Krumholtz (112)	2473	45%	34|22%	1.01	Age, FC, EF
Chiriboga (113)	4762	39%	12%|8%	1.46	Age, HT, DM, CHF, symptoms
Dellborg (114)	1515	33%	1.9%|0.2%	—	
Maynard (96)	4891	34%	58%|40%	—	
Steingart (115)	2231	17%	27%|15%	1.87	
Kilaru (116)	439	40%	63%|64%	0.97	Age, ACC/AHA class but not gender
Oka (117)	3016	33%	60%|50%	1.50	
Kudenchuk (118)	1097	22%	76%|67%	2.0	Age, symptoms, heart rate, ST elevation, past bypass surgery

CHF, congestive heart failure; DM, diabetes mellitus; EF, ejection fraction; HT, hypertension; COPD, chronic obstructive pulmonary disease; FC, functional capacity.

leagues (113) on 4763 patients with MI, 12% of men and 8% of women were referred to angiography (OR 1.46, 95%CI, 1.18–1.80).

In contrast, Krumholz and colleagues (112) have reported contradicting data that there are no gender differences in the use of angiography post-MI. In this study, which included 2473 patients (45% women), the angiography frequency in men was 34% when compared with 22% in women, giving an OR of 1.01 (95% CI, 0.89–1.33). In a smaller Scottish study with 3.5-year follow-up, the frequency and mortality were similar in both genders, as were the proportions returning to work after 1 year. Moreover, other aspects of care (admission to a monitored bed, inpatient cardiac rehabilitation and risk factor intervention) appeared the same in both groups (119). In a substudy of the Survival and Ventricular Enlargement (SAVE) trial with 1842 men and 389 women, Steingart and colleagues (115) reported that more men than women (27% vs 15%, p < 0.001) were referred to angiography before their index MI, despite greater functional disability from angina in women. However, during index MI, both men and women had equal rates of undergoing angiography. These findings are consistent with the "Yentl syndrome" phenomenon previously discussed, whereby once disease is diagnosed, no difference in management is witnessed. Table 4 emphasizes revascularization frequency after infarction in men and women (96,110–113,115,117,118,120), which shows comparable management by PTCA—gender issues may limit the use of bypass surgery, also discussed previously.

Angiography should be recommended for patients refractory to medical therapy (e.g., those with failed thrombolysis with potential benefit from rescue angioplasty), in patients with a complicated clinical course (e.g. hemodynamic instability), or to those considered to be at high risk (e.g., presentation with heart failure, significant left ven-

Table 4
Influence of Gender on the Performance of Percutaneous Intervention

Author	Study group	n	Women	PTCA rate (M|W)	CABG rate (M|W)	RR of PTCA (M|W)	RR of CABG (M|W)
Udverheyli (110)	Post-MI	218427	50%	21%|22%	32%|27%	0.94	1.15
Krumholtz (112)	Post-MI	?2473	45%	55%|51%	21|16%	0.86	1.54
Chiriboga (113)	Post-MI	?4762	39%	3.4%|1.0%	1.5|1.1	2.48	1.02
Kostis (111)	Post-MI	42595	24%	6.9|3.5	10.4|6.0	—	—
Maynard (96)	Post-MI	4891	34%	22%|14%	11%|8%	—	—
	MI/Post-cath			38%|36%	18%|20%	—	—
Steingart (115)	Post-MI	2231	17%	—	13%|6%	—	1.84
	MI/Post-cath			—	46%|38%	—	NS
Johnstone (120)	Post-MI (LV dysf)	2568	20%	—	30%|24%	—	—
	Post-MI	4215	13%	—	41%|28%	—	—
Oka (117)	Post-MI	3016	33%	—	56%|51%	—	NS
Kudenchuk (118)	Post-MI	1097	22%	33%|29%	15%|11%	NS	NS

LV dys, left ventricular dysfunction.

tricular dysfunction, or where stress testing shows ischemia). There is no evidence base for a systematic selection of men rather than women for angiography, and based on current data, the same indications for angiography apply to both men and women postinfarction. Although some studies show that women are referred to angiography less than men, it is difficult to elucidate whether this is the result of true gender bias or can be justified by clinical characteristics. Overall, women present with higher intervention risks, with greater age and comorbidity, and so their subsequent lower referral rates may reflect good clinical judgement rather than gender bias.

Unstable Angina

Unstable angina is a clinical syndrome characterized by a change in the previously stable pattern of angina, manifest as chest pain at rest, at a lower exertional threshold, or with increased frequency and intensity. The underlying substrate for unstable angina is plaque rupture with subtotal occlusion of a coronary artery by a platelet-rich thrombus overlying a complicated plaque (121). The place of angiography and interventional therapy is currently contested. Standard practice involves the use of intravenous heparin and nitrates, with referral to coronary angiography and intervention if medical treatment fails, and in those considered high risk because of their clinical course, biochemical findings or positive stress testing results (122). Although more recent studies have suggested that an interventional approach is of prognostic benefit (123), an early invasive strategy did not reduce the risk of future events among women when compared to men (124).

In 1991, Ayanian et al. (75) examined the gender differences in the utilization of invasive diagnostic and therapeutic procedures between men and women with CAD. The retrospective study analyzed nearly 83,000 patients hospitalized in Massachusetts and Maryland. After adjustment for age, race, insurance status, and primary and secondary diagnosis, the study concluded that more men (28%) than women (15%) were referred for coronary angiography. Subsequently, men also underwent more revascularization procedures than women. Similar findings have been reported more recently by Roger et al. *(125)*. In a study of 2271 Olmsted County residents who presented with unstable angina, men were more likely than women to undergo noninvasive cardiac tests (RR 1.27; 95%CI 1.14–1.40), as well as invasive cardiac procedures (RR 1.72; 95% CI 1.51–1.97). Women had a worse outcome than men, but after multivariate adjustment, male sex was associated with greater risk of death (RR 1.23; 95% CI 0.99–1.54) and cardiac events (RR 1.21; 95% CI 1.03–1.42).

The cause of this discrepancy is incompletely understood, but it may reflect insecurity to the overdiagnosis of unstable angina in women. This has at least two explanations—women with chronic stable angina show a greater incidence of rest angina, nocturnal angina, and angina provoked by mental stress *(126)*, as well as having a higher prevalence of vasospasm, microvascular disease, or noncardiac chest pains. However, the findings in the Thrombolysis in Myocardial Infarction (TIMI IIIb) study show that at least 25% of women who present with unstable angina have normal coronary arteries when compared with 16% of men *(127)*. Interestingly, there seems to be no gender differences in male and female treatment once CAD diagnosis has been established in women. This phenomenon known as the *Yentl syndrome* seems to suggest that a confirmed diagnosis of heart disease in women alters the physician's attitude in treating women in a manner similar to men *(128)*.

The presence of gender bias in unstable angina is difficult to assess because of differences in the significance of rest angina in men and women. Perhaps the development of inflammatory markers may help in the distinction of rest angina resulting from these features and the more hazardous situation of plaque rupture. However, currently, insufficient data exist to alter the current referral guidelines between gender.

CONCLUSIONS

To date, the evaluation of gender bias in the diagnosis and management of CAD is difficult because women have been underrepresented in many studies. The different clinical presentation, greater comorbidity, greater operative mortality, and less reliable noninvasive testing in women may affect a physician's attitude and approach to CAD management in women. The majority of the existing data indicate that the frequency of diagnostic angiography and subsequent therapeutic intervention is less in women. It is controversial to decide whether this observed difference reflects true gender bias or whether it reflects merely good clinical judgement to reduce risks. Insufficient data exist to justify the different treatment of women and men in acute or chronic CAD. Sound clinical judgement with the incorporation of factors other than gender should be taken into account in the patient selection for invasive intervention.

REFERENCES

1. American Heart Association. 2001 Heart and Stroke Statistical Update. American Heart Association, Dallas, TX: 2000.
2. Chandra NC, Ziegelstein RC, Rogers WJ, et al. Observations of the treatment of women in the United States with myocardial infarction: a report from the National Registry of Myocardial Infarction-I. Arch Intern Med 1998;158:981–988.

3. American Heart Association. Silent epidemic: the truth about women and heart disease. American Heart Association Publication 64-9702. 1995, Dallas, TX, pp. 1–3.

4. Weintraub WS, Kosinski AS, Wenger NK. Is there a bias against performing coronary revascularization in women? Am J Cardiol 1996;78:1154–1160.

5. Fetters JK, Peterson ED, Shaw LJ, et al. Sex-specific differences in coronary artery disease risk factors, evaluation and treatment: Have they been adequately evaluated? Am Heart J 1996;131:796–813.

6. Wenger NK, Speroff L, Packard B. Cardiovascular health and disease in women. N Engl J Med 1993;329:247–256.

7. Lerner DJ, Kannel WB. Patterns of coronary heart disease morbidity and mortality in the sexes: A 26 year follow-up of the Framingham population. Am Heart J 1986;111:383–390.

8. Tobin JN, Wassertheil-Smoller S, Wexler JP, et al. Sex bias in considering coronary bypass surgery. Ann Intern Med 1987;107:19–25.

9. Douglas PS, Ginsburg GS. The evaluation of chest pain in women. N Engl J Med 1996;334:1311–1315.

10. Pepine CJ, Adams J, Marks RG, et al. Characteristics of a contemporary population with angina pectoris. Am J Cardiol 1994;74:226–231.

11. Diamond GA, Forrester JS. Analysis of probability as an aid in the clinical diagnosis of coronary artery disease. N Engl J Med 1979;300:1350–1358.

12. Weiner DA, Ryan TJ, McCabe CH, et al. Exercise stress testing. Correlations among history of angina, ST-segment response and prevalence of coronary-artery disease in the country artery surgery study (CASS). N Engl J Med 1979;301:230–235.

13. Birdwell BG, Herbers JE, Kroenke K. Evaluating chest pain: The patient's presentation style alters the physician's diagnostic approach. Arch Intern Med 1993;153:1991–1995.

14. Schulman KA, Berlin JA, Harless W, et al. The effect of race and sex on physicians' recommendations for cardiac catheterization. N Engl J Med 1999;340:618–626.

15. Frishman WH, Gomberg-Maitland M, Hirsch H, et al. Differences between male and female patients with regard to baseline demographics and clinical outcomes in the Asymptomatic Cardiac Ischemia Pilot (ACIP) Trial. Clin Cardiol 1998;21:184–190.

16. Barrett-Connor EL, Cohn BA, Wingard DL, Edelstein SL. Why is diabetes mellitus a stronger risk factor for fatal ischemic heart disease in women than in men? The Rancho Bernardo Study. JAMA 1991;265:627–631.

17. Manson JE, Colditz GA, Stampfer MJ, et al. A prospective study of maturity-onset diabetes mellitus and risk of coronary heart disease and stroke in women. Arch Intern Med 1991;151:1141–1147.

18. Stokes J, III, Kannel WB, Wolf PA, et al. Blood pressure as a risk factor for cardiovascular disease. The Framingham Study—30 years of follow-up. Hypertension 1989;13(5 Suppl):I13–I18.

19. Keil JE, Sutherland SE, Knapp RG, et al. Mortality rates and risk factors for coronary disease in black as compared with white men and women. N Engl J Med 1993;329:73–78.

20. Prescott E, Hippe M, Schnohr P, et al. Smoking and risk of myocardial infarction in women and men: longitudinal population study. BMJ 1998;316:1043–1047.

21. Hansen EF, Andersen LT, Von Eyben FE. Cigarette smoking and age at first acute myocardial infarction, and influence and extent of smoking. Am J Cardiol 1993;71:1439–1442.

22. Kaplan NM. The deadly quartet. Upper-body obesity, glucose intolerance, hypertriglyceridemia, and hypertension. Arch Intern Med 1989;149:1514–1520.

23. Johnson LL. Sex specific issues relating to nuclear cardiology. J Nucl Cardiol 1995;2:339–348.

24. Gibbons RJ, Balady GJ, Beasley JW, et al. ACC/AHA Guidelines for Exercise Testing. A report of the American College of Cardiology/American Heart Association Task Force on Practice Guidelines (Committee on Exercise Testing). J Am Coll Cardiol 1997;30:260–311.

25. Hlatky MA, Pryor DB, Harrell FE, et al. Factors affecting sensitivity and specificity of exercise electrocardiography: Multivariable analysis. Am J Med 1984;77:64–71.

26. Linhart JW, Laws JG, Satinsky JD. Maximum treadmill exercise electrocardiography in female patients. Circulation 1974;50:1173–1178.

27. Sketch MH, Mohiuddin SM, Lynch JD, et al. Significant sex differences in the correlation of electrocardiographic exercise testing and coronary arteriograms. Am J Cardiol 1975;36:169–173.

28. Barolsky SM, Gilbert CA, Faruqui A, et al. Differences in electrocardiographic response to exercise of women and men: A non-Bayesian factor. Circulation 1979;60:1021–1027.

29. Hung J, Chaitman BR, Lam J, et al. Noninvasive diagnostic test choices for the evaluation of coronary artery disease in women: a multivariate comparison of cardiac fluoroscopy, exercise electrocardiography and exercise thallium myocardial perfusion scintigraphy. J Am Coll Cardiol 1984;4:8–16.

30. Guiteras P, Chaitman BR, Waters DD, et al. Diagnostic accuracy of exercise ECG lead systems in clinical subsets of women. Circulation 1982;65:1465–1474.

31. Goldman L, Cook EF, Mitchell N, et al. Incremental value of the exercise test for diagnosing the presence or absence of coronary disease. Circulation 1982;66:945–953.

32. Roger VL, Jacobsen SJ, Pellikka PA, et al. Gender differences in use of stress testing and coronary heart disease mortality: a population-based study in Olmsted County, Minnesota. J Am Coll Cardiol 1998;32:345–352.

33. Shaw LJ, Miller DD, Romeis JC, et al. Gender differences in the noninvasive evaluation and management of patients with suspected coronary artery disease. Ann Intern Med 1994;120:559–566.

34. Mark DB, Shaw LK, DeLong ER, et al. Absence of sex bias in the referral of patients for cardiac catheterization. N Engl J Med 1994;330:1101–1106.

35. Shaw LJ, Peterson ED, Shaw LK, et al. Use of a prognostic treadmill score in identifying diagnostic coronary disease subgroups. Circulation 1998;98:1622–1630.

36. Anonymous. Thallium scintigraphy for diagnosis and risk assessment of coronary artery disease. Lancet 1991;338:786–788.

37. Berman DS, Kiat H, Van Train K, et al. Technetium 99m sestamibi in the assessment of chronic coronary artery disease. Sem Nucl Med 1991;21:190–212.

38. Friedman TD, Greene AC, Iskandrian AS, et al. Exercise thallium-201 myocardial scintigraphy in women: correlation with coronary arteriography. Am J Cardiol 1982;49:1632–1637.

39. Chae SC, Heo J, Iskandrian AS, et al. Identification of extensive coronary artery disease in women by exercise single-photon emission computed tomographic (SPECT) thallium imaging. J Am Coll Cardiol 1993;21:1305–1311.

40. Stolzenberg J, Kaminsky J. Overlying breast as cause of false-positive thallium scans. Clin Nucl Med 1978;3:229.

41. Hansen CL, Crabbe D, Rubin S. Lower diagnostic accuracy of thallium-201 SPECT myocardial perfusion imaging in women: An effect of smaller chamber size. J Am Coll Cardiol 1996;28:1214–1219.

42. Verzijlbergen JF, Vermeersch PH, Laarman GJ, Ascoop CA. Inadequate exercise leads to suboptimal imaging. Thallium-201 myocardial perfusion imaging after dipyridamole combined with low-level exercise unmasks ischemia in symptomatic patients with non- diagnostic thallium-201 scans who exercise submaximally. J Nucl Med 1991;32:2071–2078.

43. Iskandrian AS, Heo J, Kong B, Lyons E. Effect of exercise level on the ability of thallium-201 tomographic imaging in detecting coronary artery disease: analysis of 461 patients [see comments]. J Am Coll Cardiol 1989;14:1477–1486.

44. Kong BA, Shaw L, Miller DD, Chaitman BR. Comparison of accuracy for detecting coronary artery disease and side-effect profile of dipyridamole thallium-201 myocardial perfusion imaging in women versus men. Am J Cardiol 1992;70:168–173.

45. Amanullah AM, Berman DS, Hachamovitch R, et al. Identification of severe or extensive coronary artery disease in women by adenosine technetium-99m sestamibi SPECT. Am J Cardiol 1997;80:132–137.

46. Marwick TH, Shaw LJ, Lauer MS, et al. The noninvasive prediction of cardiac mortality in men and women with known or suspected coronary artery disease. Economics of Noninvasive Diagnosis (END) Study Group. Am J Med 1999;106:172–178.

47. Hendel RC, Chen MH, L'Italien GJ, et al. Sex differences in perioperative and long-term cardiac event- free survival in vascular surgery patients. An analysis of clinical and scintigraphic variables. Circulation 1995;91:1044–1051.

48. DePuey EG, III. How to detect and avoid myocardial perfusion SPECT artifacts. J Nucl Med 1994;35:699–702.

49. Shaw LJ, Iskandrian AE, Hachamovitch R, et al. Evidence-based risk assessment in noninvasive imaging. J Nucl Med 2001;42:1424–1436.

50. Taillefer R, DePuey EG, Udelson JE, et al. Comparative diagnostic accuracy of Tl-201 and Tc-99m sestamibi SPECT imaging (perfusion and ECG-gated SPECT) in detecting coronary artery disease in women. J Am Coll Cardiol 1997;29:69–77.

51. Melin JA, Wijns W, Vanbutsele RJ, et al. Alternative diagnostic strategies for coronary artery disease in women: demonstration of the usefulness and efficiency of probability analysis. Circulation 1985;71:535–542.

52. Hachamovitch R, Berman DS, Kiat H, et al. Gender-related differences in clinical management after exercise nuclear testing. J Am Coll Cardiol 1995;26:1457–1464.

53. Lauer MS, Pashkow FJ, Snader CE, et al. Gender and referral for coronary angiography after treadmill thallium testing. Am J Cardiol 1996;78:278–283.

54. Fleischmann KE, Hunink MG, Kuntz KM, Douglas PS. Exercise echocardiography or exercise SPECT imaging? A meta-analysis of diagnostic test performance. JAMA 1998;280:913–920.

55. Kuntz KM, Fleischmann KE, Hunink MG, Douglas PS. Cost-effectiveness of diagnostic strategies for patients with chest pain. Ann Intern Med 99;130:709–718.

56. Masini M, Picano E, Lattanzi F, et al. High dose dipyridamole-echocardiography test in women: correlation with exercise-electrocardiography test and coronary arteriography. J Am Coll Cardiol 1988;12:682–685.

57. Williams MJ, Marwick TH, O'Gorman D, Foale RA. Comparison of exercise echocardiography with an exercise score to diagnose coronary artery disease in women. Am J Cardiol 1994;74:435–438.

58. Marwick TH, Anderson T, Williams MJ, et al. Exercise echocardiography is an accurate and cost-efficient technique for the detection of coronary artery disease in women. J Am Coll Cardiol 1995;26:335–341.

59. Roger VL, Pellikka PA, Bell MR, et al. Sex and test verification bias. Impact on the diagnostic value of exercise echocardiography. Circulation 1997;95:405–410.

60. Kwok Y, Kim C, Grady D, et al. Meta-analysis of exercise testing to detect coronary artery disease in women. Am J Cardiol 1999;83:660–666.

61. Secknus M-A, Marwick TH. Influence of gender on physiologic response and accuracy of dobutamine echocardiography. Am J Cardiol 1997;80:721–724.

62. Lewis JF, Lin L, McGorray S, et al. Dobutamine stress echocardiography in women with chest pain. Pilot phase data from the National Heart, Lung and Blood Institute Women's Ischemia Syndrome Evaluation (WISE). J Am Coll Cardiol 1999;33:1462–1468.

63. Fiorino AS. Electron-beam computed tomography, coronary artery calcium, and evaluation of patients with coronary artery disease. Ann Intern Med 1998;128:839–847.

64. Wong ND, Vo A, Abrahamson D, et al. Detection of coronary artery calcium by ultrafast computed tomography and its relation to clinical evidence of coronary artery disease. Am J Cardiol 1994;73:223–227.

65. Devries S, Wolfkiel C, Fusman B, et al. Influence of age and gender on the presence of coronary calcium detected by ultrafast computed tomography. J Am Coll Cardiol 1995;25:76–82.

66. Rumberger JA, Sheedy PF, III, Breen JF, Schwartz RS. Coronary calcium, as determined by electron beam computed tomography, and coronary disease on arteriogram. Effect of patient's sex on diagnosis. Circulation 1995;91:1363–1367.

67. Detrano R, Hsiai T, Wang S, et al. Prognostic value of coronary calcification and angiographic stenoses in patients undergoing coronary angiography. J Am Coll Cardiol 1996;27:285–290.

68. Aoyagi K, Inoue T, Yamauchi Y, et al. Does myocardial thallium-201 SPECT combined with electron beam computed tomography improve the detectability of coronary artery disease?—comparative study of diagnostic accuracy. Ann Nucl Med 1998;12:197–204.

69. Gould KL. Percent coronary stenosis: battered gold standard, pernicious relic or clinical practicality? J Am Coll Cardiol 1988;11:886–888.

70. Gibson RS, Watson DD, Craddock GB, et al. Prediction of cardiac events after uncomplicated myocardial infarction: A prospective study comparing predischarge exercise thallium-201 scintigraphy and coronary angiography. Circulation 1983;68:321–336.

71. Alderman EL, Fisher LD, Litwin P, et al. Results of coronary artery surgery in patients with poor left ventricular function (CASS). Circulation 1983;68:785–795.

72. Caracciolo EA, Davis KB, Sopko G, et al. Comparison of surgical and medical group survival in patients with left main equivalent coronary artery disease. Long-term CASS experience. Circulation 1995;91:2335–2344.

73. Morise AP, Singh P, Duval R. Correlation of reported exercise test results with recommendations for coronary angiography in men and women with suspected coronary artery disease. Am J Cardiol 1995;75:180–187.

74. Gregor RD, Bata IR, Eastwood BJ, et al. Gender differences in the presentation, treatment, and short-term mortality of acute chest pain. Clin Invest Med 1994;17:551–562.

75. Ayanian JZ, Epstein AM. Differences in the use of procedures between women and men hospitalized for coronary heart disease. N Engl J Med 1991;325:221–225.

76. Kee F, Gaffney B, Currie S, O'Reilly D. Access to coronary catheterisation: fair shares for all? BMJ 1993;307:1305–1307.

77. D'Hoore W, Sicotte C, Tilquin C. Sex bias in the management of coronary artery disease in Quebec. Am J Public Health 1994;84:1013–1015.
78. Miller TD, Roger VL, Hodge DO, et al. Gender differences and temporal trends in clinical characteristics, stress test results and use of invasive procedures in patients undergoing evaluation for coronary artery disease. J Am Coll Cardiol 2001;38:690–697.
79. Sullivan AK, Holdright DR, Wright CA, et al. Chest pain in women: clinical, investigative, and prognostic features. BMJ 1994;308:883–886.
80. Kuykendall DH, Johnson ML. Administrative databases, case-mix adjustments and hospital resource use: the appropriateness of controlling patient characteristics. J Clin Epidemiol 1995;48:423–430.
81. Bickell NA, Pieper KS, Lee KL, et al. Referral patterns for coronary artery disease treatment: gender bias or good clinical judgment? Ann Intern Med 1992;116:791–797.
82. Jacobs AK, Kelsey SF, Brooks MM, et al. Better outcome for women compared with men undergoing coronary revascularization: a report from the bypass angioplasty revascularization investigation (BARI). Circulation 1998;98:1279–1285.
83. Laskey WK. Gender differences in the management of coronary artery disease: bias or good clinical judgement? Ann Intern Med 1992;116:869–871.
84. Eaker ED, Kronmal R, Kennedy JW, Davis K. Comparison of the long-term, postsurgical survival of women and men in the Coronary Artery Surgery Study (CASS). Am Heart J 1989;117:71–81.
85. Loop FD, Golding LR, MacMillan JP, et al. Coronary artery surgery in women compared with men: analyses of risks and long-term results. J Am Coll Cardiol 1983;1:383–390.
86. Hannan EL, Bernard HR, Kilburn HC, Jr., O'Donnell JF. Gender differences in mortality rates for coronary artery bypass surgery. Am Heart J 1992;123:866–872.
87. Marwick TH, Case C, Vasey C, et al. Prediction of mortality by exercise echocardiography : a strategy for combination with the duke treadmill score. Circulation 2001;103:2566–2571.
88. Douglas JS, Jr., King SB, III, Jones EL, et al. Reduced efficacy of coronary bypass surgery in women. Circulation 1981;64:II11–II16.
89. Leape LL, Hilborne LH, Bell R, et al. Underuse of cardiac procedures: do women, ethnic minorities, and the uninsured fail to receive needed revascularization? Ann Intern Med 1999;130:183–192.
90. Chaitman BR, Bourassa MG, Davis K, et al. Angiographic prevalence of high-risk coronary artery disease in patient subsets (CASS). Circulation 1981;64:360–367.
91. Bell MR, Berger PB, Holmes DR, Jr., et al. Referral for coronary artery revascularization procedures after diagnostic coronary angiography: evidence for gender bias? J Am Coll Cardiol 1995;25:1650–1655.
92. Kent KM, Rosing DR, Ewels CJ, et al. Prognosis of asymptomatic or mildly symptomatic patients with coronary artery disease. Am J Cardiol 1982;49:1823–1831.
93. Bell MR, Grill DE, Garratt KN, et al. Long-term outcome of women compared with men after successful coronary angioplasty. Circulation 1995;91:2876–2881.
94. Kannel WB, Sorlie P, McNamara PM. Prognosis after initial myocardial infarction: the Framingham study. Am J Cardiol 1979;44:53–59.
95. Lincoff AM, Califf RM, Ellis SG, et al. Thrombolytic therapy for women with myocardial infarction: is there a gender gap? Thrombolysis and Angioplasty in Myocardial Infarction Study Group. J Am Coll Cardiol 1993;22:1780–1787.
96. Maynard C, Litwin PE, Martin JS, Weaver WD. Gender differences in the treatment and outcome of acute myocardial infarction. Results from the Myocardial Infarction Triage and Intervention Registry. Arch Intern Med 1992;152:972–976.
97. Weaver WD, White HD, Wilcox RG, et al. Comparisons of characteristics and outcomes among women and men with acute myocardial infarction treated with thrombolytic therapy. GUSTO-I investigators. JAMA 1996;275:777–782.
98. Fiebach NH, Viscoli CM, Horwitz RI. Differences between women and men in survival after myocardial infarction. Biology or methodology? JAMA 1990;263:1092–1096.
99. Ryan TJ, Anderson JL, Antman EM, et al. ACC/AHA Guidelines for the management of patients with acute myocardial infarction. A report of the American College of Cardiology/American Heart Association Task Force on Practice Guidelines (Committee on Management of Acute Myocardial Infarction). J Am Coll Cardiol 1996;28:1328–1428.
100. Aroney C, Boyden AN, Jelinek MV, et al. Current guidelines for the management of unstable angina: a new diagnostic and management paradigm. Intern Med J 2001;31:104–111.

101. Antoniucci D, Valenti R, Moschi G, et al. Sex-based differences in clinical and angiographic outcomes after primary angioplasty or stenting for acute myocardial infarction. Am J Cardiol 2001;87:289–293.

102. Indications for fibrinolytic therapy in suspected acute myocardial infarction: collaborative overview of early mortality and major morbidity results from all randomised trials of more than 1000 patients. Fibrinolytic Therapy Trialists' (FTT) Collaborative Group. Lancet 1994;343:311–322.

103. Randomised trial of intravenous streptokinase, oral aspirin, both, or neither among 17,187 cases of suspected acute myocardial infarction: ISIS-2. ISIS-2 (Second International Study of Infarct Survival) Collaborative Group. Lancet 1988;2:349–360.

104. Maynard C, Althouse R, Cerqueira M, et al. Underutilization of thrombolytic therapy in eligible women with acute myocardial infarction. Am J Cardiol 1991;68:529–530.

105. GISSI-2: a factorial randomised trial of alteplase versus streptokinase and heparin versus no heparin among 12,490 patients with acute myocardial infarction. Gruppo Italiano per lo Studio della Sopravvivenza nell'Infarto Miocardico. Lancet 1990;336:65–71.

106. Juneau M, Colles P, Theroux P, et al. Symptom-limited versus low level exercise testing before hospital discharge after myocardial infarction. J Am Coll Cardiol 1992;20:927–933.

107. Senaratne MP, Hsu LA, Rossall RE, Kappagoda CT. Exercise testing after myocardial infarction: relative values of the low level predischarge and the postdischarge exercise test. J Am Coll Cardiol 1988;12:1416–1422.

108. Carlos ME, Smart SC, Wynsen JC, Sagar KB. Dobutamine stress echocardiography for risk stratification after myocardial infarction. Circulation 1997;95:1402–1410.

109. Leppo J, O'Brien J, Rothlendler J, et al. Dipyridamole thallium-201 scintigraphy in the prediction of future cardiac events after acute myocardial infarction. N Engl J Med 1984;310:1014–1018.

110. Udvarhelyi IS, Gatsonis C, Epstein AM, et al. Acute myocardial infarction in the Medicare population. Process of care and clinical outcomes. JAMA 1992;268:2530–2536.

111. Kostis JB, Wilson AC, O'Dowd K, et al. Sex differences in the management and long-term outcome of acute myocardial infarction. A statewide study. MIDAS Study Group. Myocardial Infarction Data Acquisition System. Circulation 1994;90:1715–1730.

112. Krumholz HM, Douglas PS, Lauer MS, Pasternak RC. Selection of patients for coronary angiography and coronary revascularization early after myocardial infarction: is there evidence for a gender bias? Ann Intern Med 1992;116:785–790.

113. Chiriboga DE, Yarzebski J, Goldberg RJ, et al. A community-wide perspective of gender differences and temporal trends in the use of diagnostic and revascularization procedures for acute myocardial infarction. Am J Cardiol 1993;71:268–273.

114. Dellborg M, Swedberg K. Acute myocardial infarction: difference in the treatment between men and women. Qual Assur Health Care 1993;5:261–265.

115. Steingart RM, Packer M, Hamm P, et al. Sex differences in the management of coronary artery disease. Survival and Ventricular Enlargement Investigators. N Engl J Med 1991;325:226–230.

116. Kilaru PK, Kelly RF, Calvin JE, Parrillo JE. Utilization of coronary angiography and revascularization after acute myocardial infarction in men and women risk stratified by the American College of Cardiology/American Heart Association guidelines. J Am Coll Cardiol 2000;35:974–979.

117. Oka RK, Fortmann SP, Varady AN. Differences in treatment of acute myocardial infarction by sex, age, and other factors (the Stanford Five-City Project). Am J Cardiol 1996;78:861–865.

118. Kudenchuk PJ, Maynard C, Martin JS, et al. Comparison of presentation, treatment, and outcome of acute myocardial infarction in men versus women (the Myocardial Infarction Triage and Intervention Registry). Am J Cardiol 1996;78:9–14.

119. Bannerman A, Hamilton K, Isles C, et al. Myocardial infarction in men and women under 65 years of age: no evidence of gender bias. Scott Med J 2001;46:73–78.

120. Johnstone D, Limacher M, Rousseau M, et al. Clinical characteristics of patients in studies of left ventricular dysfunction (SOLVD). Am J Cardiol 1992;70:894–900.

121. Fuster V, Badimon L, Badimon JJ, Chesebro JH. The pathogenesis of coronary artery disease and the acute coronary syndromes (1). N Engl J Med 1992;326:242–250.

122. Braunwald E, Mark DB, Jones RH, et al. Unstable angina: Diagnosis and treatment. US Dept of Health and Human Services, Rockville, MD: 1994.

123. Invasive compared with non-invasive treatment in unstable coronary- artery disease: FRISC II prospective randomised multicentre study. FRagmin and Fast Revascularisation during InStability in Coronary artery disease Investigators. Lancet 1999;354:708–715.

124. Lagerqvist B, Safstrom K, Stahle E, et al. Is early invasive treatment of unstable coronary artery disease equally effective for both women and men? FRISC II Study Group Investigators. J Am Coll Cardiol 2001;38:41–48.

125. Roger VL, Farkouh ME, Weston SA, et al. Sex differences in evaluation and outcome of unstable angina. JAMA 2000;283:646–652.

126. Pepine CJ, Abrams J, Marks RG, et al. Characteristics of a contemporary population with angina pectoris. TIDES Investigators. Am J Cardiol 1994;74:226–231.

127. Hochman JS, McCabe CH, Stone PH, et al. Outcome and profile of women and men presenting with acute coronary syndromes: a report from TIMI IIIB. TIMI Investigators. Thrombolysis in Myocardial Infarction. J Am Coll Cardiol 1997;30:141–148.

128. Healy B. The Yentl syndrome. N Engl J Med 1991;325:274–276.

23   The Role of Women's Health Centers in Improving Access and Process of Care

Susan Kendig, RNC, MSN, WHCNP and
D. Douglas Miller, MD, CM, MBA, FACC, FRCP(c)

Contents

INTRODUCTION

The origins of the broadly based interest in women's health issues can be traced to three main causes:

1. The emergence of women into more prominent societal, professional, and public service roles.
2. Significant advances in the scientific fields of reproductive medicine, endocrine physiology and pharmacology, and diagnostic technology.

From: *Contemporary Cardiology: Coronary Disease in Women: Evidence-Based Diagnosis and Treatment*
Edited by: L. J. Shaw and R. F. Redberg © Humana Press Inc., Totowa, NJ

3. The recognition by public and private health care payers that women's health is big business.

The health care industry has recognized that women are a major interest group in family health care decision making *(1)*. It is estimated that 70–80% of health care is delivered to or controlled by women, making them a formidable market force with significant influence on health care utilization and profitability *(2)*. Yet often, women's health care needs were not adequately addressed by traditional health care systems based on a male model of care, with resulting negative impact on their outcomes *(3)*.

The biomedical and health care communities have responded to these major trends in US heath care in several ways. Curriculum reform intended to improve physician training through the integration of gender-specific information has been implemented in several specialties. Indeed, women's health, once thought of in terms of obstetrics/gynecology (OB/GYN) practice, has earned a place as a subspecialty or clinical focus of internal medicine, family practice, and other specialties. Conversely, 4-year OB/GYN residencies are now required to provide 6-month primary care *(4)*. An increasing number of women are entering medicine and the biomedical research professional workforce, thus influencing attention to women's issues.

The impact of women's power as consumers has not been lost on the business community. The altruism and business interests of large pharmaceutical firms with significant financial interest in women as consumers of their products has fostered the development of large media campaigns that target gender-focused conditions affecting mortality, morbidity, and quality of life.

The paucity of gender-focused research was addressed through increased research funding at the basic translational and outcomes levels to augment evidence in women's health. Similarly, public health efforts by governmental and nongovernmental organizations (NGOs) to benchmark and improve access and delivery systems for women's health care, nationally and internationally has contributed to the development of women's centers. By establishing diverse women's health care advocates drawn from the public, private, and professional sectors with focused interests and expertise on one or more of these areas, it is hoped that these activities will lead to improved health among all women.

What began in the latter part of the last century as a "movement" has evolved into an evidence-based standard of practice, with established benchmarks for services, quality, accreditation and outcomes. The field of women's health is complicated by the facts that:

1. Scientific advances are a rapidly moving target with which providers, payers, and patients (consumers) must constantly struggle to keep pace.
2. Women, as a subset of the US population and the global population, are a highly heterogeneous target group, whose health risks and needs vary widely by age, socioeconomics, geography, genetics, and interest level.
3. Competitive market forces and contradictory evidence of risk and benefit, fueled by pop-cultural and media-marketing influences, create confusion among expert and ingénue consumers alike as to the best practices in a wide range of fundamental and niche areas.
4. Successes (screening mammography) and failures (hormone replacement therapy [HRT] for secondary coronary event prevention) may not be evenly or equally reported. "Sex sells," and gender-based scientific reports may garner greater interest and lower peer scrutiny in the lay and medical presses. Unrecognized biases and overt fraud may degrade this literature, along with other subjects.

WHAT'S DRIVING WOMEN'S CARDIOVASCULAR HEALTH CARE?

Because women control the majority of health care decisions, they have a direct impact on the traditional provider's revenue stream. Additionally, women are leaders in a consumer dynamic that is changing health care. It is estimated that 42% of women utilize complementary therapies, and approx 52% utilize the Internet (2). These market forces, in combination with women's increasingly busy lives, are indications that health care providers must consider adapting in meeting the increased consumer demand for accessibility or lose their business to other sources of care and information.

In planning women's health services, consideration must be given to demographics and market trends. For instance, 21% of women report feeling "super-stressed" vs 15% of men; the average woman sleeps 20% less than her grandmother did; and, 70% of health care visits by women can be traced to stress-related causes (2). The ethnic makeup of the female population is projected to change from a predominantly (71%) white demographic today to a 47% minority population by 2050. The aging of this population from primarily childbearing age to menopausal and postmenopausal demographic, combined with increased ethnic diversity among women, has many implications for providers. Ethnic and cultural influences, as well as gender influences, will become a more prominent component of health care in terms of incidence of disease, treatment responses, and competence in working with a diverse population. The emphasis on reproductive health, long the dominant force in women's health, will be replaced with a focus on gender-specific specialty programs, postmenopausal services, and wellness and lifestyle preservation (2).

PROMOTING HEALTH AND WELLNESS IN WOMEN

The emerging care model for women extends well beyond the obstetrical experience, addressing the life continuum from adolescence through maturity. The model that women want, and that fits best with their emerging leadership in the consumer market, is one that embraces a wellness philosophy that is directed in partnership by the woman and her health care provider.

Access to basic primary care services is key to women's cardiovascular health. In 2001, The National Women's Law Center published a national and state-by-state report card regarding women's health in an attempt to assess women's overall health status. According to the report, women's accessibility to health services is severely compromised by inadequate health insurance coverage. Nearly one in ten persons lives in a "medically underserved area," with limited access to primary care, and only one state has adequate policies that affect reimbursement for prescription medications. In terms of cardiovascular health, no state has met the national goals for increasing physical activity, reducing overweight status, and improving diet; and, no state has met the goal for reducing the percentage of women with hypertension. Minnesota, the state with the best ranking for women and heart disease, where 65.4 per 100,000 women died of coronary heart disease (CHD) when compared to Mississippi, where 141.2 per 100,000 died (5). Beyond lost lives, CHD takes a huge economic toll, with an estimated cost of $326.6 billion in 2000 in health-related outlays and lost productivity (6).

CARDIOVASCULAR HEALTH AS A WOMEN'S HEALTH ISSUE

Currently, three major trends influence women's health care. Increasing evidence of the health and financial advantages of prevention has resulted in payers' and providers' focus on health promotion and education. Managed care systems have emerged and continue to evolve as primary insurers within the goal of cost control. The emphasis on outcome-focused care has increased funding for female-focused health research *(7)*. The study of chronic conditions affecting women is another factor that influences women's health programs. For the first time, the causes of mortality and morbidity among postmenopausal women (age 50–79) are under investigation. The National Institutes for Health's (NIH) Research Agenda is a primary factor of this trend, through their emphasis on disease prevention, health promotion, and directives to include women in clinical trials. The NIH established the Women's Health Initiative (WHI) in 1991. This 15-year initiative is one of the largest US prevention studies of its kind, with $628 million projected funding.

Epidemiological studies and randomized clinical trials provide evidence that CHD is largely preventable. Health promotion and wellness behaviors have been directly associated with positive cardiac health. Stamper et al. *(8)* applied data from the Nurse's Health Study over a 14-year period to assess the effect of a combination of lifestyle practices on the risk of CHD and stroke. Among women, this study found that adherence to lifestyle guidelines involving diet, exercise, and smoking abstinence was associated with a risk of CHD more than 80% lower than in the rest of the population. The single most important factor was smoking, with a relative risk of 5.48 for those smoking 1–14 cigarettes per day vs nonsmokers.

Although heart disease is recognized by the health care profession as the leading cause of death for postmenopausal women, disease severity and potential is not well understood by the general public. Mosca et al. *(9)* concluded that most women do not perceive heart disease as a substantial health concern and report that they are not well-informed about their risk. Of the 1000 respondents in this study, 61% rated cancer as the greatest health problem for women vs 8% who cited heart disease or stroke. Generally, cancer was the disease that caused the greatest worry to the most women (30%), followed by breast cancer (28%), heart disease (22%), and heart attack (20%). Although over 70–90% of women believe they discuss heart disease and prevention with their health care provider, less than 30% reported doing so *(9,10)*. Significantly, a majority of women reported that they were not well-informed about heart disease prevention. Of those who did have information, magazines were identified as the major source of information (43%), followed by television (24%), and health care providers (18%).

This information underscores the importance of incorporating cardiovascular health promotion into women's health encounters. Likewise, evidence of gender differences regarding cardiac disease onset, intervention, and management must be considered across all practice settings. Cardiovascular disease (CVD) is more lethal and less aggressively treated in women than in men *(11)*. Intragender differences, such as higher risk of stroke, hypercholesterolemis, diabetes, and obesity among minority women also affect CVD risk. Gender and ethnic differences in factors, such as the implications of lipid levels, onset of disease, and presenting symptoms, further support the integration of cardiovascular health into women's health center programs.

Designing meaningful primary care services that women want and need requires a combination of replicating successful evidence-based health and wellness programming with market research. Most surveys regarding ideal women's health programs identify convenience, a wholistic approach to care, and amenities as components that are important to women. Although many programs offer female practitioners as an additional marketing advantage, research shows that provider gender is not a primary concern for women. Only 17% actually select a provider based on gender (12). The female majority indicate that attention to their concerns and provider empathy are more important attributes than gender.

TECHNOLOGICAL ADVANCES

A variety of technological advances have also influenced the progress of women's health care and have influenced the development of women's health specialty centers. Examples of such advances are as follows:

1. Therapeutic
   a. Isolation and characterization of the estrogen receptor
      - Target for antagonist and agonists (R_x)—natural, synthetic, and mimetic
      - Tissue distribution of receptors in health and disease—tumor growth-modulating effects (direct or indirect)
   b. Pharmacological modulation of the female reproductive cycle
      - Menstrual cycle
      - Birth control
      - Secondary effects (i.e., immunological)
      - Ovarian failure (drugs, surgical techniques, egg harvesting, artificial insemination, and so forth)
   c. Dose-response variability
      - Efficacy of R_x (different dosing)
      - Safety of R_x (biodistribution)
      - Teratogenicity (thalidomide)
      - Toxicity (end-organ differences, cytotoxicity profiles, and so forth)
   c. OTC market
      - Direct marketing to patient
      - Common illnesses
      - Local pharmacy
2. Devices and techniques
   a. Surgical approaches
      - Anatomy differences
      - Left internal mammary artery (LIMA), coronary artery bypass grafting (CABG)
   b. Implantable devices
      - Sizing constraints (stents)
   c. Trends
      - Ultrasound/noninvasive
      - Minimally invasive (laparoscopic)
   d. Percutaneous
      - Delivery systems (vascular, other)
   e. Prosthetics
      - Cosmetic and reconstruction

- Materials testing
- Breast-augmentation surgery

3. Diagnostics
   a. Home testing
      - Privacy issues (reproductive), convenience
   b. Screening approaches
      - High-risk populations (mandated)
      - General recommendations
      - Standardized/credentialed, facilities/regs (pap smears, mammography, and so forth)
      - Payer recognition of cost efficiency
   c. Noninvasive imaging
      - Ultrasound ($\pm$ contrast agents)
      - Nuclear medicine/radiotracers/software
      - Attenuation, hardware
      - Echocardiogram (ECG) gating, resolution of single photon emission tomography (SPECT)/photon emission tomography (PET), and so on.
      - Computed tomography (CT; mammography)
      - Digital data
      - Mammoscintigraphy (Tc^{99m} cardiolite)
   d. Information technology (IT)
      - Web-based (Web MD, Mayo, and so on)
      - Tele-medicine (telepathology, pap)
      - Consumer driven (general inquiry, comparison shopping, and so forth)

Although technology has significantly improved women's health outcomes and life expectancy, it has also created service delivery challenges because of increased demand for services and lack of reimbursement resources. These technological advances and benefits of screening tests, such as pap smears and mammograms, have been instrumental in transitioning women's health care from episodic, system-based medical visits to regular, routine, prevention-focused care.

DESIGNING AN EFFECTIVE WOMEN'S CARDIOVASCULAR HEALTH PROGRAM

Effective delivery of women's cardiovascular services requires that health care systems and/or practices have a strong organization commitment to improving women's health outcomes. The founders must be prepared to invest the resources necessary to deliver top-quality, convenient services in an environment that women value. From the outset, it is extremely important to capture patient outcomes data that can be used to benchmark quality and performance to parent organizations, payers, national data repositories, and government watchdogs. Underresourced or virtual women's health care delivery programs that do not significantly consider quality, fail to document their positive results, or lack commitment to task, are generally ineffective and destined to fail in the future.

It must be recognized early in the planning process that such commitment requires significant investment, and financial returns will not be immediate. A careful capital-budgeting process must also be in place to assure that the providers are equipped with the best in modern health care technology, and practice facilities are state-of-the-art.

However, chasing every new diagnostic and therapeutic advance can lead to bleeding edge, not leading edge performance. Every effort should be made to assemble a team of highly trained and experienced providers, who are each individually committed to their own specialized tasks within the broader mission of the women's health care practice. The growing number of credentialed graduate medical and nursing education programs in women's health are a rich source of well-trained and expertly mentored health care professionals.

Although advanced training and modern technology are important, around-the-clock health care provider availability and high-practice site ambiance are frequently cited as key attributes by women health care consumers. As with any business, practice location is a critical element to provide convenient public services. Operating hours must take into consideration the business hours of working women, the school-day schedules of students, and the desirability of offering limited services on holidays. Administrative and support staff who present the practice to patients and families on a daily basis are often the greatest attribute of any women's health care practice.

It is also important that insurers, press, and local health officials come to recognize the importance of cardiovascular health to their women constituents, which requires a continual education process. The women's health message is now being consistently delivered by nonprofit organizations with the mission of promoting good health at both the regional and national levels, such as the American Heart Association (AHA). Development is the major source of funding or the educational efforts and public awareness campaigns of the organizations. Although corporate donors, foundations, and endowments are critical contributors, the practice must also participate in such programs and be generous with its in kind and actual giving activities.

Those forming a women's cardiovascular program should therefore initiate effective business planning, raise public awareness on the subject, participate in philanthropy, and keep pace with emerging technology. Successful and progressive practices in the area of cardiovascular women's health care have usually mastered all of these facets of new practice development.

A LIFESPAN APPROACH TO CARDIOVASCULAR HEALTH

Cardiovascular health is just one component of women's health. Because of its significance to women's health, it is important to consider the mechanisms to incorporate cardiovascular health into all stages of the health care continuum. Risk assessment, health promotion education, and appropriate and timely referral is essential in maintaining optimal cardiac health, yet may be challenging to operationalize in practice. Table 1 summarizes the range of services that can be featured, separated by age.

PRIMARY PREVENTION

The health care setting is one venue for primary prevention activities. Ideally, health promotion interventions in the primary care setting complement those in place through public health initiatives and other community venues. At a minimum, health promotion education and support for lifestyle change should be incorporated into the primary care visit. Risk reduction information in primary care encounters should include:

Table 1
Services to Consider in Women's Health Programs

Adolescent Services:
- Assessment of risk taking behaviors (motor vehicle behavior—seat belt use, helmet use, unsafe sexual practices, and risk of STDs, HIV, pregnancy, and ATOD use)
- Exposure to violence—intimate partner violence and violent home/school/work environment
- Depression and suicide risk. (Suicide is third leading cause of death)
- Nutrition—screening for disordered eating (anorexia, bulimia, and overeating)
- Routine health screenings—immunizations, growth, iron status, scoliosis, and so forth.
- Cardiovascular health—blood pressure, cholesterol, and obesity interventions

Young/Early Adult Services:
- Preconception health
- Interconceptional counseling
- Well woman exams, including screenings for STDs, cervical cancer, breast exams, and risk factors associated with the development of chronic disease conditions
- Infertility assessment
- PMS, perimenstrual symptoms, and dysmennorrhea
- Mental health screening, including depression, anxiety, stress, and ATOD use
- Exposure to interpersonal violence

Midlife and Postmenopausal Services:
- Physical/psychological changes associated with perimenopause/menopause
- Knowledge deficits related to physiological changes
- Identification of risk factors associated with CVD
- Mental health screening, including depression, anxiety, stress, and ATOD use
- Exposure to interpersonal violence
- Mammography
- Bone densitometry/osteoporosis screening and interventions
- HRT

Other Services: Self-Advocacy Activities Across Populations
- Special events, including educational programs, resource libraries, and newsletters
- Evidence-based information related to complementary therapies
- Cosmetic surgery
- Services for populations with special needs (i.e., culturally competent programs for minority and immigrant women, women with disabilities, and so on)

- Smoking prevention/cessation. An estimated 60,000 women die each year from smoking-related heart disease *(13)*. Tobacco use impacts women's health throughout the lifespan. Elementary school-age initiators of cigarette smoking are least likely to attempt to quit or successfully quit and are most likely to smoke as adults *(14)*.
- Increase physical activity. More than 50% of women are inactive. Sedentary lifestyle has been linked to a 1.5–2.5 fold increased risk of CVD *(10,13)*. Yet, reported areas for physical activity is generally higher among men than women, with lack of time, feeling tired, and lack of motivation being the most commonly cited barriers to exercise *(15)*. Inactivity begins early, as activity levels drop sharply during adolescence. Despite the proven benefits of physical activity, only New Jersey requires students in grades 9–12 to take 4 years of physical education *(5)*.
- Weight reduction. Obesity significantly affects cardiovascular health. Data from the Nurses' Health Study indicates that women who gain more than 20 pounds after age 18

increase their risk of coronary disease by 30% *(16)*. Approximately 11% of children are overweight, and an additional 14% are at risk for being overweight *(17)*. Disease risk increases as body mass index (BMI) exceeds 25, however, even a 5–10-pound weight loss can be cardioprotective *(16,18)*.

Interventions that targeting modifiable risk factors should be designed to meet the needs of women at each developmental stage. Addressing nonmodifiable risk factors, from the standpoint of individual risk, can serve as a motivator *(19)*.

Women utilize a variety of health care providers to obtain reproductive and nonreproductive health care. According to the Commonwealth Fund Survey of Women's Health, 33% of women reported seeing both a family practitioner or internist and an OB/GYN; 16% saw only an OB/GYN, 39% saw only a family practitioner or internist, 3% saw only other specialists, and 10% had no regular physician *(20)*. Therefore, it is important for health care providers in these specialties to be cognizant of cardiovascular risk factors, lifestyle modifications, current recommendations, and interventions pertinent to women.

Currently, there are three models of primary care women's health centers: (1) hospital owned/operated centers in community hospitals and academic centers; (2) independent-for-profit centers founded by physicians, advanced practice nurses, or entrepreneurs, and marketed to privately insured women; and (3) community-based nonprofit centers. Six case studies of primary care women's health centers in the United States found the centers usually functioning at full capacity, require little marketing to attract patients, and have high patient satisfaction. One study comparing three women's primary care centers with three internal medicine practices found that women accessing care at the centers received more clinical preventive services, more preventive counseling, and reported higher satisfaction levels than women attending traditional internal medicine practices *(4)*. Health care providers may be challenged to consider more integrated models of care that address women's total health needs in order to be competitive in the women's health market.

BUILDING THE TEAM—AN INTERDISCIPLINARY MODEL OF CARE

Interdisciplinary integrative models of care consider the whole person in relation to health and utilize a team approach to health care. This model requires health care providers to work on a team where "individual members understand cognitive maps of other members and try to modify their perspective in light of the other's perspective" *(21)*. This differs from a unidisciplinary model in which providers function individually and from a multidisciplinary model where "individuals representing different professions work together as a team" *(21)*. The interdisciplinary team works interdependently with each other to provide care, contrary to unidisciplinary and multidisciplinary teams where members remain highly autonomous. Interdisciplinary collaboration requires providers to interact with each other toward patient-centered outcomes. Providers in interdisciplinary practices have an intimate understanding of one another's disciplines.

Unidisciplinary models of care have been the most common in medical care. Multidisciplinary models have often been employed to provide care to clients with complex medical problems or with at-risk populations for poor outcomes. Interdisciplinary teams are the most time-intensive to form, but have significant potential to affect patient outcomes and differentiating practice.

An integrative model forms the basis of a comprehensive framework for women's health assessment and health maintenance across the lifespan *(22)*. It requires the provider to view the woman as a whole person on a continuum of health at a given point in the lifespan. At a minimum, the integrated team of women's health experts consists of physicians and/or advanced practice nurses, nurses, behavioral health experts, lifestyle change consultants, and nutritionists. Access to specialists in various services that affect women's health, such as cardiology, endocrinology, gerontology, bone health, and other services are essential to the team. The integrated approach accomplishes the following outcomes in addressing CVD prevention.

- Incorporates biological, psychosocial, environmental, and professional sciences into a "whole person" understanding of health.
- Incorporates linkages between prenatal, childhood and adult health throughout the lifespan that includes health promotion, disease prevention, and disease management *(22)*.
- Addresses a full range of issues that impact health throughout the continuum.

THE ROLE OF ADVANCED PRACTICE NURSES AND PHYSICIAN ASSISTANTS IN IMPROVING PATIENT AND FINANCIAL OUTCOMES

Advanced practice nurses (APNs) and physician assistants (PAs) have been shown to effectively expand practice capacity and profitability while enhancing patient outcomes. The term *APN* encompasses nurse practitioners in all specialties, clinical nurse specialists, and certified nurse midwives. Typically, APNs are educated within their specialty at the Masters level, have completed extensive didactic coursework and precepted practicum experiences beyond that of the registered nurse, achieved national certification in their specialty, and meet state Board of Nursing requirements for practice. Considerable clinical literature supports the claim that primary care nurse practitioners (NPs) can satisfy the medical needs of 50–90% of the ambulatory patient population. According to the Office of Technology Assessment Report *(23)*, NPs can deliver as much as 80% of primary health care for adults and 90% of pediatric care. A randomized study of 1316 patients to either NPs or physicians found no significant differences in patient health status or health service utilization. Additional studies support the effectiveness of APNs and PAs in providing appropriate health care, selecting prescriptions appropriate to the diagnosis, and positively affecting patient outcomes *(24–26)*. Naylor et al. *(27)* also found that hospitalized elders who received comprehensive discharge planning and home follow-up by APNs had fewer hospital readmissions, increased readmission time, and fewer hospital days per patient. Patients in collaborative APN/MD practices receive more comprehensive care than care provided by either discipline alone. The practice that offers the most comprehensive services will be the most competitive *(28)*. Clearly, utilization of advanced practice providers can benefit patient outcomes at all levels of care.

APNs have also been shown to positively impact practice financial outcomes. One study conducted in a large health maintenance organization (HMO) setting found that adding a NP to the practice could double the typical panel of patients seen by the physician *(29)*. In an American College of Obstetrics and Gynecology survey of OB-GYN practices, respondents who employed an advanced practice professional were more likely than their counterparts to report revenue in the upper one-third of revenue producers *(30)*.

Rules governing advanced practice providers' scope of practice are typically defined by the Board of Nursing for APNs and the medical licensing board for PAs in the state of practice. Generally, services provided by APNs are independently reimbursable by third-party payers. In the Balanced Budget Act of 1997, direct reimbursement of NPs was defined. According to the Medicare rules, NPs may bill in their own name and are reimbursed at 85% of the physician rate or 80% of the fee schedule, whichever is greater. However, the NP may be reimbursed at 100% of the physician fee schedule if the service is billed as "incident to" physician services. Several rules govern "incident to" claims, the most significant being that the physician must be in the office suite when the services are performed. Physician practices that employ NPs and other advanced practice providers must have a clear understanding of the Medicare rules when billing for services to prevent audits and loss of income *(31,32)*.

FINDING AND UTILIZING COMMUNITY RESOURCES TO SUPPORT HEALTH

Health and human service providers who work with women emphasize issues affecting individuals. The next intervention stage at the community level focuses on building programs and services that promote and support women's health. Understanding women's resources within a community and building mechanisms for appropriate referral and access can enhance health care practices and leverage provider time. Often, women enter primary care services for routine care, such as female exams, family planning, and screenings. Access to the primary care provider offers the opportunity for a comprehensive analysis of physical, emotional, environmental, and sociocultural factors affecting women's health, with concomitant health care guidance and referral to community resources. Because community resources vary widely between communities, it is essential to be familiar with resources in the practice area. Examples of community resources that may be important to support cardiovascular health include:

- Recreation resources—fitness centers, YM/WCA programs, community walking trails, and mall walking programs.
- Nutrition resources—dieticians and local Weight Watcher programs.
- Behavioral Health Resources—private providers, hotlines, help centers, and chemical-dependent treatment centers.
- Interpersonal violence programs—women's shelters and hotline numbers.

However, awareness of community resources is not enough. Access to community resources may be intimidating and requires time and effort on the part of the client. Women involved in caring for children, aging parents, work, volunteer commitments, and school may not have the time or financial resources to make frequent telephone calls, know the economical intricacies of their situation, or have the flexibility in their schedule to make repeated attempts to explore resources. Therefore, it is important for women's health centers to establish links with community resources that enhance and complement their services and meet their client's needs. Basic information regarding any referral should be made available to the client to facilitate a positive entry into recommended resources. Before referring a woman to a new resource, it is important for the health care provider to become familiar with the resource. A file of basic information about referral resources can easily be updated and shared with patients. Minimum information in the office referral file should include: referral name, address and phone number, contact person, required source of referral, eligibility requirements (i.e., financial need, nutritional status, and so on), fees, services provided, appointment policy, and items to take to the appointment (i.e., physician consult form, proof of address, and so forth).

MARKETING THE PROGRAM

Women's health programs, including those featuring cardiovascular services, exist in an increasingly competitive environment. It is difficult to differentiate the services provided in one practice from those offered by another. Effective branding of a practice can be enhanced through naming, ad placements, and novel offerings. However, the best practices are fundamentally characterized by their quality and by an established track record of excellence in health delivery. These attributes lend credibility to the practice in the viewpoint of patients, press, and the general public. With quality and credibility come the professional accolades and public recognitions that can be rightfully claimed as a mark of quality. It takes tremendous effort to sustain a position of prominence.

Routine marketing tactics rely on the accurate identification of what the consumer wants and the subsequent promotion of services that satisfy these needs. Focus groups and outside consultants can be helpful at the early stages of a marketing campaign, serving as an interface between the desires of the potential patient population and the vested interests of the practice group. In the creative phase, the best ideas and aspirations of both groups can be brought into play. Eventually, the marketing experts refine a product that can be brought before the public in a variety of deliverables, including targeted mailings, print ads, radio and TV spots, and so on—creating awareness. The budget is often the only constraint as to the level of marketing coverage that can be provided.

Practices have effectively combined the announcement of the services and a measure of philanthropy by sponsoring public radio and TV programs or by placing their providers before the public as "experts" in media health information areas. Being affiliated with the organization of prominent not-for-profit-sponsored events, such as the network of regional AHA Heart Balls in February Heart Month, can be an effective means to gain exposure. Involvement of practice members on the boards of such organizations of a practice is to plan or participate in public education and continuing medical education programs that feature subjects of interest to the patients and their referring physicians. In addition to promoting the clinical services offered by the practice, value-added activities, such as nutritional support, exercise training, and lifestyle modification advice, can be noted to add substance. Case-based teaching using real-life success stories is highly effective with both patients and physicians.

One recent development that has brought prominence to some practices is the offer of new medical advances through clinical trails within the practice (33). Practices that participate in phase 3 and 4 clinical research studies are frequently perceived as being "cutting edge," and are viewed as more advanced than their competitors. The infrastructure required for safe and compliant clinical trails operations is significant, with

Institutional Review Board, data management, and clinical research coordinator capabilities being essential. Although the research infrastructure can be expensive, the direct return on investment from sponsor grants and contracts, as well as the intangible perceived quality benefits bestowed on the practice, frequently make this a good investment.

The final element of highly effective marketing, which accrues measurable financial and reputation benefits, is constant concept review and marketing program renewal. Although it is attractive to stick with a winner, who can rebut the value of a marketing slogan that pervades the consciousness of pop culture, most major health systems and nearly all practices cannot aspire to achieve this level of market penetration. As such, quality must remain a constant, but the introduction of fresh faces and offerings to pique public interest can be invaluable, even in the health care arena. In addition, the capacity to link the practice to health habits, not just disease management, can prove useful.

CASE STUDIES IN PRIMARY PREVENTION

Health care providers can participate in primary prevention activities at the individual, family, and community level. Many health care providers are collaborating with communities to bring cardiovascular health messages to patients in a variety of venues, as well as using innovative staff-led models of patient education within the office setting. The following are two examples of such primary prevention initiatives.

- One small Midwestern community on the outskirts of a large urban area noted an increase in the number of children with obesity, diabetes, lung disease, and poor nutrition habits. Dr. Dolores Gunn, a family practice physician, in collaboration with the community school district and the Institute for Research and Education in Family Medicine, (St. Louis, MO) developed an innovative school health program. Offered weekly to children in primary and secondary grades in lower income and at-risk neighborhoods, the program focuses on preventative health education and the development of healthy lifestyles. Educational classes, seminars, and demonstrations in exercise and low cholesterol nutrition have been implemented, along with aggressive campaigns that target substance abuse prevention. The overall goal is to improve the quality-of-health education and prevention messages in the community and foster a healthier generation of adults.
- In 2000, the Association of Women's Health, Obstetric, and Neonatal Nurses (AWHONN) in collaboration with the American Nurses Foundation launched the Cardiovascular Health for Women Initiative. The program is designed to educate nurses and women about CVD within the context of a health promotion and disease prevention framework. A panel of women's health experts, including physicians and APNs, researchers, national consumer advocates, AHA representatives, and professors in health policy worked in partnership with organizational staff to develop an evidence-based guideline and tool kit to support the implementation of cardiovascular primary prevention activities to target women in clinical and community settings.

CONCLUSIONS

In final analysis, we must consider the various motives and motivations of the stakeholders in what has become a major life sciences industrial segment. These include: profit, professional advancement, public notoriety and acclaim, pure altruism, reaction to personal loss, and so on.

If we can conclude anything from this complex evolutionary process, we must agree that the women's health "project" is a work in progress. As we emerge from the era of potential gender bias against women into the neocontemporary phase of gender equity in the women's health field, it is appropriate to critically consider whether this is cause for celebration or a starting point for the next phase of progress.

At the risk of being politically incorrect, one could rightfully posit that this recent phase of playing health care "catch up" should be naturally followed by an era of over-reaching goals, and biomedical advances that would place women's health at the forefront of *all* health and biomedical activities. The benefits of this novel realignment of the health sciences world should not be prejudged as being bias to men or negative toward society. On a global population basis, there is at least a 51:49 chance that a paradigm of women's health superiority would represent a fundamental advance for mankind, leading to benefits for all.

The next logical step down from the specific identifiers of homosapiens to the geopolitical ideal of "citizens of the world," is being left as male or female from a pluripotential stem cell at the moment of creation. This sentinel event, and the resulting hormonal sequelae that define our gender biology and disease pathophysiology, are what largely determine our individual health risks and medical futures.

REFERENCES

1. Travis CB, Gressley DL, Phillippi RH. Medical decision making, gender, and coronary heart disease. J Womens Health 1993;2:269–279.
2. Tiber Group. Women's health: A Practical Application of on the Road to Consolidation III: The New Market Makers Tiber Group, Chicago, IL: 2000.
3. Wenger NK, Speroff L, Packard B. Coronary heart disease in women: An overview (myths, misperceptions, and missed opportunities). Cardiovascular Rev Reports 1993;14:24–41.30.
4. Weisman CS. Changing definitions of women's health: Implications for health care and policy. Matern Child Health J 1997;1:179–189.
5. National Women's Law Center, FOCUS on Health and Leadership for Women at the Center for Clinical Epidemiology and Biostatistics—University of Pennsylvania School of Medicine and the Lewin Group. Making the grade on women's health: A national and state-by-state report card. National Women's Law Center, Washington, DC: 2000.
6. Forum for State Health Policy Leadership. Women's health: Mandates, state offices help close some of the gaps. State Health Notes 2000;21:1,6.
7. Kendig S, Kiel, D. Promoting health and wellness in women. Health & Sciences Television Network, A Division of PRIMEDIA Healthcare, Carrollton, TX: 1999.
8. Stampfer MJ, Hu FB, Manson JE, et al. Primary prevention of coronary heart disease in women through diet and lifestyle. N Engl J Med 2000;343:16–22.
9. Mosca L, Jones WK, King KB, et al. Awareness, perception, and knowledge of heart disease risk and prevention among women in the United States. Arch Family Med 2000;9:506–551.
10. Women and heart disease: A study of women's awareness and attitudes towards heart disease and stroke. Prepared for the American Heart Association. Yankelovich Partners, Norwalk, CT: 1997.
11. Shaw L, Miller D, Romeis J, et al. Patterns in coronary heart disease—Morbidity and mortality in the sexes: A 26-year follow up of the Framingham population. Ann Intern Med 1994;111:383.
12. Roper Starch Worldwide. Presented at Enhancing patient interaction in a changing medical environment. California Permenente Medical Group, CA: 1997.
13. American Heart Association. Take charge: A woman's guide to fighting heart disease. American Heart Association, Dallas, TX: 1997.
14. Ershler J, Leventhal H, Fleming R, Glynn K. The quitting experience for smokers in sixth through twelfth grades. Addic Behav 1989;14:365–378.
15. Brownson RC, Baker EA, Houseman RA, et al. Environmental and policy determinants of physical activity in the United States. Am J Pub Health 2001;91:1995–2003.

16. Manson JE, Colditz GA, Stampfer MJ, et al. A prospective study of obesity and coronary heart disease. N Engl J Med 1990;322:882.

17. Troiano RP, Flegle KM. Overweight children and adolescents: Description, epidemiology, and demographics. Pediatrics 1998;101:497–504.

18. Meisler JG, St. Jeor S. Summary and recommendations from the American Health Foundation's Expert Panel on Healthy Weight. Am J Clin Nutr 1996;63(Suppl 1):474S.

19. Giardina EV. Call to action: Cardiovascular disease in women. J Womens Health 1998;7:37–43.

20. Weisman CS. Women's use of health care. In Falik, MM & Collins, KS (Eds) Women's health: The Commonwealth Fund Survey. Johns Hopkins University Press, Baltimore, MD: 1996.

21. Sheer B. Reaching collaboration through empowerment: A developmental process. J Obstet Gynecol Neonatal Nurs 1996;25:513–517.

22. Walker LO, Tinkle MG. Toward integrated science of women's health. J Obstet Gynecol Neonatal Nurs 1996;25:379–382.

23. Office of Technology Assessment. Nurse practitioners, physician assistants, and certified nurse midwives: A policy analysis. Government Printing Office (Health Technology Case Study 37, OTA-HCS-37), Washington, DC: 1986.

24. Diamond F. Nurse Practitioners inch onto the field. Managed Care 2000; (http://www.managed-caremag.com), retreived Sept. 28, 2000.

25. Rudy EB, Davidson LJ, Daly B, et al. Care activities and outcomes of patients cared for by acute care nurse practitioners, physician assistants, and resident physicians: a comparison. Am J Crit Care 1998:267–281.

26. Brown SA, Grimes DA. A meta-analysis of nurse practitioners and nurse midwives in primary care. Nurs Res 1995;44:332–339.

27. Naylor MD, Brooten D, Campbell R, et al. Comprehensive discharge planning and home follow-up of hospitalized elders: A randomized clinical trial. JAMA 1999;281:613–620.

28. Mundinger MO. Advanced Practice Nursing—Good medicine for physicians? N Engl J Med 1994;330:211–214.

29. Hummel J, Pirzada S. Estimating the cost of using non-physician providers in primary care teams in an HMO: Where would the savings begin? HMO Practice 1994;8:161–164.

30. ACOG. Practice Expenses for OB-GYNs. Economic Impact Nov. 3, 2000.

31. Buppert C. HEDIS for the primary care provider: Getting an "A" on the managed care report card. Nurse Pract 1999;24:84–99.

32. Gosfield AG. The ins and outs of "incident to" reimbursement. Family Practice Management (http://www.aafp.org/fpm/20011100/23thei.html). Nov-Dec, 2001.

33. Merkatz RB, Temple R, Sobel S, et al. Women in clinical trials of new drugs, a change in food and drug administration policy. N Engl J Med 1993;329:292–296.

24 Obstetrician/Gynecologists, Primary Care, and Cardiovascular Disease

William W. Hurd, MD, Sheela Barhan, MD, and Robert E. Rogers, MD

CONTENTS

INTRODUCTION

Obstetrics and gynecology (OB/GYN) is a distinctive field of medicine that combines the most basic aspects of office preventive medicine and the unique medical-surgical specialties of obstetrics and gynecology. The obvious common denominator in these disparate areas is the health care of women. With the evolution of managed care over the last decade, fitting the multifaceted field of OB/GYN into the standard "either primary care or specialty care" paradigm has been difficult for both the specialty itself and the health care industry.

The fact that a majority of women reported a preference for seeing an obstetrician/gynecologist for their routine gynecological care, despite having a primary care physician (PCP), may be a reflection of the unique and strong bond often found between the patient and her physician in the field *(1)*. The substantial contribution of the preventive medicine specialty is obvious because of the preventive procedures popularized by the obstetrician/gynecologist (i.e., the annual examination, pap smears, and mammograms) are among the most commonly measured indicators of health care quality used today *(2)*. Problems are also inherent in the combination of primary care with a surgical specialty, clearly illustrated by that fact that most common surgical procedures

From: *Contemporary Cardiology: Coronary Disease in Women: Evidence-Based Diagnosis and Treatment*
Edited by: L. J. Shaw and R. F. Redberg © Humana Press Inc., Totowa, NJ

performed primarily by obstetrician/gynecologists (i.e., hysterectomy and cesarean section) now account for one-third of all surgical procedures in this country today *(3)*. The close scrutiny of these procedures by the health care industry addresses both their importance to health maintenance for women and to the unique role of the obstetrician/gynecologist as both primary care "gatekeeper" and surgeon.

A primary question for both the specialty and our managed care system is "just where does obstetrician/gynecologist fit in?" Many obstetrician/gynecologists and their patients insist that we offer both primary care and specialty care *(4)*. Traditional primary care specialties (e.g., family practice, internal medicine, and pediatrics) are not convinced that surgical specialists can simultaneously be PCPs. Many practicing obstetrician/gynecologists agree with this contention, and traditional Obstetrics and Gynecology Residency training has not included much information on the diagnosis and treatment of nongynecological problems. In response, postgraduate education in obstetrics and gynecology has made a major shift toward primary care to address these objections. However, before these questions can be answered and training can be appropriately readjusted, a more basic question of "what is a primary care physician?" must be answered.

This chapter examines the ways in which obstetrician/gynecologists serve as PCPs, along with their special role in preventive and long-term care of women at risk for cardiovascular disease (CVD). A critical evaluation of the specialty's successes and limitations evokes several areas where the primary care roles of obstetrician-gynecologists should be more clearly defined.

DEFINITION OF PRIMARY CARE

Many physicians are referred to as PCPs, but the term *primary care* is difficult to precisely define. Primary care has been defined from an institutional perspective as "the provision of integrated, accessible, health care services by clinicians that are accountable for addressing a large majority of personal health care needs, developing a sustained partnership with patients, and practicing within the context of family and community" *(5)*. This definition addresses important psychosocial aspects, but is somewhat vague as to the types of health care services that are provided.

The US Public Health Service has defined primary care from a research perspective as "care that is first contact, comprehensive, longitudinal, and person-centered care (rather than disease- or problem-specific), and that maximizes health and well-being by providing preventive, curative, rehabilitative care for the most common medical problems" *(6)*. Again, the psychological aspects of the patient-provider relationship are alluded to. Additionally, all types of health care (preventive, curative, and rehabilitative) are incorporated. Although both of these definitions touch on important aspects of primary care, their global nature makes it difficult to determine what type of practitioners would be included.

Controversies that concern which specialists should be considered PCPs are long-standing. Most authors agree that specialists in the fields of family practice, internal medicine, and pediatrics should be considered PCPs *(7,8)*. These markedly different specialties are similar because they all are heavily weighted toward preventive care, provide relatively limited amounts of tertiary care, and are nonsurgical in nature. In sharp contrast, obstetrician/gynecologists are surgical specialists who provide tertiary care.

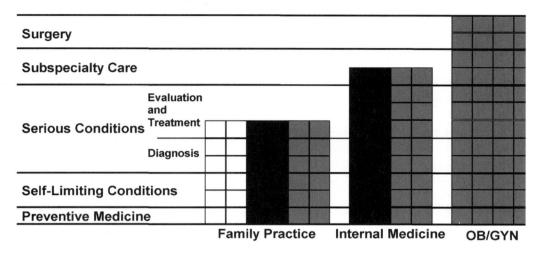

Fig. 1. Practice profiles of PCPs based on their training and patient populations for family practice, internal medicine, and obstetrics and gynecology (OB/GYN). Each block is equivalent to 1 month of postgraduate training. Clear blocks, children; black blocks, adult males; gray blocks, adult females.

It is this very different mode of practice that explains why the controversy remains as to whether obstetrician-gynecologists are PCPs. Even when systematical analysis results in the placement of obstetrician/gynecologists in the "primary care quadrant," there is hesitancy in designating obstetrician/gynecologists as PCPs *(9)*. Nevertheless, it is clear that many women consider their obstetrician-gynecologists to be their PCPs *(10)*. Fresh insights into this conundrum may be obtained when various specialists are analyzed from the perspective of a patient-oriented primary care definition.

The Committee on the Future of Primary Care of the Institute of Medicine has defined primary care as "the provision of integrated, accessible health care services by clinicians who are accountable for addressing a large majority of personal health care needs" *(11)*. However, few knowledgeable patients expect their PCP to know all things about all medical conditions (e.g., "Dr. Welby"). Patients want a PCP who possesses the combination of knowledge and judgment required to keep them healthy without unnecessary tests or treatments. From this perspective, we have recently published a patient-oriented definition of PCP *(12)*. From the patients' perspective, PCPs may be defined as trusted physicians who (1) perform all preventive care necessary to safeguard health; (2) diagnose and treat self-limiting conditions; (3) diagnose serious conditions; and either (4) treat serious conditions for which they have expertise or (5) refer the patient to the best available expert for treatment of serious conditions. The strength of this functional definition is that it delineates the various health care tiers routinely provided by all PCPs (Fig. 1).

HEALTH CARE TIERS

Preventive Medicine

The first health care tier is preventive medicine, which includes cancer screening, immunization, and health counseling. Cancer screening includes pelvic and breast examinations, both by physical examination and specific screening tests, along with cervical cytology (pap smears) and mammograms. In an aging population, screening for other common diseases (e.g., osteoporosis, diabetes, hypothyroidism, hypercholesterolemia, and CVD) brings about increased importance.

CVD is especially important because it remains the single leading cause of morbidity and mortality in the United States, accounting for almost 1 million annual deaths *(13)*. Fortunately, identifying and altering several risk factors has been shown to reduce CVD risk *(14)*. Certainly, the most obvious of these risk factors is cigarette smoking. If obstetrician/gynecologists are to be effective PCPs, identifying smokers and helping them implement smoking cessation strategies are extremely important.

Several common health risks for CVD relate to physical activity and diet. Our common sedentary lifestyles and high-calorie, high-fat, and low-fiber diets, appear to increase the risk of CVD, both directly and indirectly, as a result of obesity, hypercholesterolemia, and type 2 diabetes mellitus. Screening for these secondary risk factors and patient counseling on changes in diet and physical activity remain the cornerstone of effective preventive therapy for CVD.

Self-Limiting Conditions

The next health care tier is the diagnosis and treatment of self-limiting conditions. The patient has two primary purposes for making the effort necessary to see a physician for the most common symptoms: (1) to make sure that the symptoms do not indicate a serious disease and (2) to relieve the discomfort caused by the symptoms as quickly as possible. Patients depend on a PCP to get them in quickly for an appointment, to effectively rule out serious disease, and treat any self-limiting condition with the safest and most effective therapy. Health maintenance organizations (HMOs) are also there to make sure that both diagnosis and care are cost-effective.

The treatment of self-limiting conditions warrants special attention. Although most physicians can diagnose most self-limiting conditions with a reasonable degree of confidence, it is perhaps the crucial indication of an effective PCP to be able to treat these conditions appropriately. When a patient is diagnosed as having a viral upper respiratory tract infection and otitis media, it is less than ideal to refer them to another PCP or an urgent care facility. To be considered a PCP, appropriate knowledge in this area is requisite.

Serious Conditions

DIAGNOSIS OF SERIOUS CONDITIONS

The final health care tier is the management of serious conditions, which can be further subdivided into diagnosis and evaluation/treatment. The patient is often unable to distinguish symptoms of self-limiting conditions from those of serious conditions. Obviously, it is critical that the PCP is able to tell the difference. Unfortunately, all experienced clinicians are aware that it is often difficult to recognize a serious illness early in its course.

It is clear from the previous discussion that to be cost-effective, PCPs must have exceptional diagnostic abilities. Cautious utilization of expensive diagnostic tests may save money for many self-limiting illnesses *(15)*. However, treatment of serious chronic conditions by PCPs may save money at the expense of decreased quality of life in some cases *(16)*. A more serious concern is that underutilization of certain diagnostic tests that could result in late diagnosis and increased cost for the treatment of serious illness, although this possibility has not been well-studied. On the other end of the spectrum, it has been well-documented that overutilization of diagnostic and treatment modalities (particularly surgical) dramatically increases the health care cost without measurably increasing patient health *(17)*. The importance of excellent diagnostic ability among PCPs cannot be overemphasized.

Several common serious diseases are well-established as modifiable risk factors for CVD, which include hypertension, hypercholesterolemia, and diabetes mellitus. The obstetrician/gynecologist is in an ideal position to diagnose these conditions during the annual examination that many women undergo at the time of pap smear. Blood pressure measurement is a routine part of both obstetric and gynecological physical examinations; thus, obstetrician/gynecologists routinely detect new onset hypertension in both pregnant and nonpregnant patients *(18)*. Similarly, screening for hypercholesterolemia has long been a standard part of health maintenance routinely practiced by obstetrician/gynecologists *(19)*.

Obstetrician-gynecologists are aware of the importance of screening for diabetes mellitus (DM). Because of its serious implications, DM is almost universally screened for during early pregnancy *(20)*. Likewise, obstetrician-gynecologists are aware of the importance of postpartum follow-up of patients with gestational diabetes to detect type 2 diabetes mellitus. More than half of obstetrician-gynecologists screen for diabetes in nonpregnant patients with a positive family history.

MANAGEMENT AND TREATMENT OF SERIOUS ILLNESSES

Once a serious illness is diagnosed, the PCPs must either treat the condition or refer the patient to an appropriate expert. Thorough evaluation and treatment of serious illnesses, contrary to diagnosis, are not obligatory in primary care. Treatment ability varies dramatically among specialties and practitioners. Suboptimal treatment of a serious condition by a less experienced and confident provider could be detrimental. In contrast, expert evidence-based treatment can be advantageous from both a health and a cost perspective *(21)*. Patients prefer to believe that their trusted PCPs know when to treat and when to refer.

The ability of the obstetrician/gynecologist to treat chronic serious conditions that put patients at risk for CVD may be increasing with the modern emphasis of primary care training. Treatment of mild hypertension is certainly within the realm of expertise of many obstetrician/gynecologists *(18)*. However, the actual percentage of obstetrician/gynecologists who primarily manage uncomplicated hypertension is uncertain. The effect of hypoestrogenemia and hormone replacement therapy (HRT) on serum lipid levels has been of great interest to PCP caring for postmenopausal women. The treatment of hypercholesterolemia is usually relatively simple; however, the number of obstetrician/gynecologists who primarily manage hypercholesterolemia in their patients remains uncertain. Conversely, at least one-third of obstetrician/gynecologists feel comfortable managing type 1 and type 2 DM, perhaps because management of gestational DM is a standard part of most obstetric practices *(20)*.

REQUIREMENTS FOR EXPERTISE

The ability to provide either effective primary care or appropriate treatment for life-threatening illnesses is not limited to certain specialists. Rather, these abilities depend on three requirements: (1) appropriate training, (2) continued interest in the area of care, and (3) continued experience based on an appropriate number of cases.

Training

The first requirement, an appropriate level of training, includes both residency training and appropriate continuing medical education (CME). It is not enough to be adequately trained during residency in primary care for the treatment of a serious disease or high-risk procedure, because training often becomes outdated with emerging lightning advances being made in clinical medicine. The dangers associated with out-of-date treatments are well-recognized by most state medical boards, which require documentation of a minimum CME amount for continued licensure.

The problem is particularly significant in very comprehensive practices, where the broad aspects of specialty care may be difficult to keep up with. Although most state licensure requires CME credit throughout the year, it is uncommon for these credits to be directed toward the practice needs of individual physicians. It remains the responsibility of individual PCPs to ensure that they remain current in the modern management of conditions that they elect to diagnose or treat. Also, it remains the specialists' responsibility to provide primary care so that they remain current in the modern screening and diagnostic methods for conditions outside their realm of expertise.

Interest

The second requirement necessary for physicians to provide primary care or treat a serious medical condition is a special interest in that particular process. Only the individual physician's interest will assure that appropriate continuing self-education is carried out. An excellent example of the need for CME is the evaluation of abnormal pap smears. For many years, pap smears were classified as grade I–V. A change occurred in 1989 with the Bethesda system, adding terms such as "Cervical Intraepithelial Neoplasia (CIN) I-III." The classification system was revised in 1991. Although the techniques for obtaining an adequate pap smear have remained relatively constant over time, appropriate interpretation and management have dramatically changed. A keen interest in the field and targeted CME is required to avoid practicing out-of-date medicine.

Experience

The final requirement is continued experience based on an appropriate number of cases. In other words, the requirement for a screening test must be common enough in the patient population treated by the PCP to maintain expertise. CME alone is not enough to maintain skills, especially for complex illnesses and disease processes where the treatment is highly technical. Surgical examples are the most obvious. It is clear that surgeons who perform a particular procedure on a weekly basis are much more likely to be technically excellent than surgeons who perform the same procedure on an annual basis. It is important for PCPs to be able to judge whether or not their current skills and knowledge are either first-rate or "rusty."

With this in mind, it makes sense that some PCPs can appropriately evaluate and treat common serious conditions if they fulfill the previous criteria. Certainly, colonoscopy and obstetrical care fit in this category for many family practitioners. Some have even extended their expertise to include cesarean section and other surgical techniques *(22)*. Similarly, obstetrician/gynecologists can appropriately and effectively provide primary care and treat chronic medical conditions, such as hypertension and DM, with the appropriate training, interest, and continued experience *(18)*.

PCP PROFILES

Profiles may be created for different primary specialties using this three-tiered definition of primary care; these profiles should be based on training and practice populations (Fig. 1). Profiles should consider the relative time available during residency for training in the various areas. The relative amount of CME required to stay updated in the various aspects of care would be expected to be roughly proportional as well. Although somewhat imprecise, these theoretical profiles can serve as a basis to compare and contrast the various primary care specialties.

Family Practice

The ideal model for a PCP in many ways is the family practitioner. Although much primary care was performed in the past by general practitioners with a limited amount of postgraduate education, the complexity of modern health maintenance, diagnostic modalities, and treatments has made this approach impractical. Experience and CME alone are rarely sufficient to make up for the lack of formal postgraduate training in the modern age of medicine.

Family practitioners undergo 3 years of postgraduate training that focuses on techniques for health maintenance, diagnosis, and treatment of self-limiting illnesses, as well as the diagnosis of serious conditions that span from pediatrics to geriatrics for both men and women (Fig. 1). The result is a broad-based area of expertise. Postgraduate education time constraints necessitate a limited amount of training in the in-depth evaluation and treatment of serious conditions. Many family practitioners develop limited areas of specialty expertise during or subsequent to their residency, which often include diagnostic procedures (e.g., colonoscopy and colposcopy) and surgical procedures (e.g., cesarean section).

Internal Medicine

Internists are a group of specialists that commonly function as PCPs. Their profile is somewhat more narrow than family practice, because they infrequently take care of children. This results in a greater proportion of time during both their 3-year postgraduate training and subsequent practice devoted to evaluation and treatment of serious adult illnesses, including hypertension, heart disease, and diabetes. Evolution of the specialty toward primary care has required increased emphasis on preventive care and diagnosis of a broader sphere of conditions, particularly in the gynecology area.

Many internists are comfortable providing primary gynecological care. Although they routinely diagnose self-limiting gynecological conditions, their ability to thoroughly evaluate and treat these conditions is often less than family practitioners and markedly less than gynecologists. For example, it is unlikely that a woman with perimenopausal uterine bleeding would be evaluated with an endometrial biopsy in many internists' offices. Conversely, this condition might be routinely evaluated with a biopsy in a family practitioner's office and with a biopsy and vaginal ultrasound in a gynecologist's office. This difference in diagnostic sophistication is most likely a reflection of both the level of training in residency and experience in managing this common condition and is likely to decrease as training in primary care becomes more standardized across specialties.

Obstetrician/Gynecologists

Obstetrician/gynecologists, like internists, perform primary care on a relatively narrow range of patients when compared to family practitioners. By definition, the practice is limited to women and occasionally female children. An important difference is that the postgraduate training is 4 years in length in comparison to 3 years for family practice and internal medicine.

The most striking aspect of the profile results from the fact that, contrary to the other PCPs, the obstetrician/gynecologist is a surgical specialty. In addition to preventive medicine of women, the specialty combines the procedure-dependent area of obstetrics with the surgical specialty of gynecology. Surprisingly, the most common major surgical procedures done in the United States are cesarean section and hysterectomy *(3)*.

CVD AND THE OBSTETRICIAN/GYNECOLOGIST

Health Maintenance

Effective patient screening for health risk factors remains the cornerstone of primary care that delineates this field from other medical activity. Several of the most ubiquitous health risk factors involve lifestyles. Smoking has been said to be the most important preventable independent risk factor for CVD *(23)*. Although multiple medical and psychological approaches to smoking cessation have been developed, interventions by busy physicians have been shown to significantly increase their patients' cessation rates *(24)*. It is an important role of all PCPs to ask about tobacco use, provide advice on smoking cessation, determine a smoker's readiness to take action, and offer assistance in cessation and follow-up. Interestingly, physicians do not alienate smokers by showing their concern, even in those smokers not interested in quitting *(25)*.

Other lifestyles that increase the risk of CVD are poor dietary habits, a lack of physical activity, and the often-associated obesity *(13)*. The problem appears to be increasing in our populations, and presently more than 25% of all women in the United States are considered to be obese (body mass index [BMI] $\geq$ 30 kg/m^2) *(26)*. Because improvements in diet, activity, and body weight have all been shown to independently and collectively reduce CVD risk, the role of the PCP in identifying and addressing these problems cannot be overstated. Unfortunately, safe and effective methods for helping patients make long-term changes in these areas are still at issue.

Equally important for the PCP in the prevention strategy is the early diagnosis of serious chronic medical conditions that increase the risk of CVD, including diabetes, hypercholesterolemia, and hypertension *(13)*. These three serious conditions share a subtle nature that requires careful screening for early detection. Diabetes appears to be increasing in frequency in this country, possibly as a result of increasing obesity. Type 2 diabetes may now affect more than 7% of US adults *(13)*, in contrast to hypercholesterolemia, which may actually be decreasing in the United States, likely resulting from decreased dietary intake of saturated fat and cholesterol, despite the increased obesity prevalence *(27)*. Hypertension continues to be a widespread condition in the United States, affecting more than 20% of adult females *(28)*. Surprisingly, it has been estimated that nearly half of the patients with hypertension in the United States are not treated, and another quarter are not well-controlled *(13)*. Because the obstetrician/gynecologist remains the physician most often seen by women in this country, effective screening to diagnose these conditions, and referral for appropriate evaluation, treatment, and follow-up, is our critical responsibility in CVD *(29)*.

Hypoestrogenemia, associated with the postmenopausal period, is another common chronic condition that increases the risk of CVD. There is Ample evidence exists that indicates bilateral oophorectomy in premenopausal women increases the risk of CVD unless exogenous hormones are given *(30)*. However, it is less certain that natural menopause alone is a risk factor for CVD. The Framingham Heart Study indicated that natural menopause was associated with a fourfold increase in the 10-year incidence of coronary heart disease (CHD) when compared with premenopausal women, but no adjustment was made for age or cigarette smoking *(31)*. The Nurses' Health Study adjusted for age in 5-year categories and found that the rate of CHD was significantly elevated in postmenopausal women, with an relative risk (RR) of 1.7 (95% CI, 1.1–2.8), but adjustment for cigarette smoking diminished the relative risk to 1.0 (95% confidence interval [CI], 0.8–1.3; *30)*. The role of hypoestrogenemia in the increased CVD incidence postmenopause will certainly be more accurately defined by further studies.

Hypoestrogenemia diagnosis is a relatively simple matter in most women. The earliest signs are often vasomotor "hot flashes" that may signal dropping estrogen levels months to years before the subsequent hypoestrogenemia becomes a significant health issue. A good clinical indication is that cessation of menses (menopause) is the best clinical indicator that hypoestrogenemia has reached a point where medical concerns, such as increased bone loss and an increased CVD risk, become a concern *(32)*. Signs of chronic estrogen deficiency include vaginal atrophy and the somewhat subtle signs of vertebral compression fractures, which include height decline and an exaggerated curvature of the thoracic spine.

Treatment

Treatment of these chronic serious diseases by PCPs is related to both the provider's belief as to the risk of the condition to the patient's health and the provider's expertise. It is well-accepted that the treatment of both hypertension and hypercholesterolemia can reduce the risk of CVD. Both internal medicine specialists and family practitioners view treatment of these conditions as part of their primary roles in health prevention. Although most obstetrician/gynecologists may be comfortable in diagnosing these conditions, few believe that they are appropriately trained to chronically treat them. For this reason, a referral by obstetrician/gynecologists to another specialist for the long-term treatment of these conditions is common. Interestingly, many academicians and clinicians believe that, with improved training, first-line treatment of these conditions can be effectively carried out by the practicing obstetrician/gynecologists, although long-term studies of this belief do not yet exist *(18,32)*.

With hypoestrogenemia, it appears to be exactly the opposite: there is significant disagreement as to whether HRT is effective in decreasing the risk of CVD, but obstetrician/gynecologists are well-trained to treat this condition *(32)*. The vast majority of clinical studies have consistently showed a 40–50% reduction in CVD risk with use of HRT *(33)*. It has been estimated that 25–30% of the observed protective effects can be accounted for by lipid-dependent mechanisms (e.g., increases in high-density lipoprotein [HDL] cholesterol and decreases in low-density lipoprotein [LDL] cholesterol). The remaining 70–75% can be accounted for by lipid-independent mechanisms related to the estrogen's ability to modify the function of the endothelium and vascular smooth muscle (e.g., increased vascular dilation and decreased coronary artery uptake of LDL; *34*).

Additionally, multiple studies have supported HRT's beneficial effect on lipoprotein profiles. For example, a 3-year randomized double-blind trial showed that estrogen alone or in combination with progestins increased HDL cholesterol and decreased LDL cholesterol *(35)*. A randomized double-blind study of newer HRT preparations suggests that this beneficial lipoprotein profile is maintained and perhaps enhanced in terms of triglyceride levels *(36)*.

However, it remains uncertain as to whether HRT can decrease the risk of CVD in postmenopausal women with known CHD *(37,38)*. The Heart and Estrogen/Progestin Replacement Study (HERS) suggested that HRT might not prevent secondary coronary events (i.e., myocardial infarction [MI] or CHD death) in postmenopausal women with CHD in the first 3 years of use and might actually increase the risk of venous thromboembolism during the first year of use *(37)*. However, by years 4 and 5, the rate of CHD events was lower in the HRT group, suggesting that HRT might not prevent the early thrombosis-related CHD events, but may decrease the risk of later occurring CHD events related to atherosclerotic disease. Hopefully, The Women's Health Initiative (WHI) a 12-year prospective randomized, controlled study of 164,500 postmenopausal women scheduled for completion in 2010) will help answer many of the questions concerning the risks and benefits of CHD therapies for women.

DIAGNOSIS OF CVD

CHD diagnosis presents a greater challenge in women when compared with men both because of the gender differences in the clinical presentation of ischemic heart disease and the diminished accuracy of diagnostic tools. Follow-up reports from the Framingham study indicate that women develop chest pain more often than men, but are less likely to progress to MI *(31)*. Chest pain remains the most common initial CHD manifestation in women, and nearly 90% of women with MI (similar to that of men) will have chest pain as a feature of initial clinical presentation *(39)*. However, women with MI appear to be significantly more likely than men to present with atypical symptoms of angina, such as upper abdominal pain, dyspnea, nausea, and fatigue. For this reason, any woman at risk of CVD with chest pain or atypical symptoms of angina should be carefully evaluated for CHD. Because of the unique challenges presented for the definitive diagnosis and evaluation of CHD in women, the choice and interpretation of an array of noninvasive diagnostic procedures for CHD should be deferred to a specialist expert in this diagnosis.

OBSTETRICIAN/GYNECOLOGISTS AS PCPS

Several obstetrician/gynecologists serve as PCPs for many of their patients. The majority of obstetrician/gynecologists have an interest in an ongoing relationship with their patients. One of the primary reasons that many medical students choose obstetrics and gynecology for further study is that it is unique among the surgical specialties because of their continuing relationships with their patients, rather than seeing patients only when they have been referred for surgery.

Unfortunately, in past years, obstetrician/gynecologists have not received a significant amount of primary care training during their residencies. However, an attempt has been made over the last decade to rectify this situation *(40)*. As the profession strives to realign its residency programs, an ongoing debate has developed as to whether surgical training is suffering as a result, and whether the primary care taught during residency is of use to obstetrician/gynecologists in practice *(41)*.

AREAS FOR IMPROVEMENT IN EDUCATION

Although obstetrician/gynecologists often provide primary care for many of their patients, insufficiencies in their training remain that must be addressed. The challenge will be to assure that not only are obstetrician/gynecologists appropriately trained during their residencies, but also ensure that they have a continuing medical education and clinical experience to maintain and update their knowledge.

Health Maintenance

If obstetrician/gynecologists are to fulfill the role of PCPs, they must be adequately trained and strive to remain updated on contemporary recommendations for health maintenance and health screening. Obstetrician/gynecologists who perform pap smears and mammograms on every postmenopausal patient, but fail to provide other health maintenance services (e.g., check cholesterol or provide routine immunizations), are not providing their patients with complete primary care.

Diagnosis and Treatment of Serious Nongynecological Conditions

Every obstetrician/gynecologist who provides primary care must be willing and able to diagnose serious nongynecological conditions. Failure to recognize the symptoms of serious medical conditions, such as cardiac ischemia, could have tragic results for patients. Residency training and CME must be provided in this area if we are to provide appropriate primary care.

It has yet to be determined the best role for the obstetrician/gynecologist in the evaluation and treatment of common chronic conditions, including those that increase the patient's risk of CVD, and CVD itself. Although all obstetrician/gynecologists should be able to screen for these conditions, not all of them will be qualified to evaluate and treat them. Just as many family practitioners and internists refer women with postmenopausal bleeding to obstetrician/gynecologists, many obstetrician/gynecologists will continue to refer women with diabetes, hypertension or CVD to other PCPs and specialists with the training and interest necessary to take care of the patient with the most current techniques. Few would argue that PCPs must avoid treating serious conditions outside of their realm of expertise if they wish to maintain their patients' trust.

CONCLUSION

PCPs must be skilled in providing care for their patients at many levels. Because of the complexities involved in achieving and maintaining expertise in any area of medicine, the most important characteristic of PCPs, as with all physicians, is personal integrity. Patients must feel confident that PCPs care first and foremost for the patient, rather than for the disease. Patients expect their physicians to be up-to-date relative to current diagnostic and treatment modalities. Patients also trust PCPs to know their limitations and make the best referrals at the appropriate time. To adequately serve patients' trust as PCPs, obstetrician/gynecologists must strive to improve their capability to provide comprehensive preventive care, diagnosis, and treatment of self-limited conditions as well as recognize serious nongynecologic conditions. Because CVD remains the leading cause of death for women in America, obstetrician/gynecologists must be prepared to provide prevention, diagnosis, and perhaps treatment of this condition *(42)*.

REFERENCES

1. Schmittdiel J, Selby JV, Grumbach K, Quesenberry CP Jr. Women's provider preferences for basic gynecology care in a large health maintenance organization. J Womens Health 1999;8:825–833.
2. Ruffin M, Gorenflo DW, Woodman B. Predictors of screening for breast, cervical, colorectal, and prostatic cancer among community-based primary care practices. J Am Board Fam Pract 2000;13:1–10.
3. Graves EJ, Kozak LJ. Detailed diagnosis and procedures, National Hospital Discharge Survey, 1996. Vital Health Stat 1998;138:1–155.
4. Herman CJ, Hoffman RM, Altobelli KK. Variation in recommendations for cancer screening among primary care physicians in New Mexico. J Community Health 1999;24:253–267.
5. Donaldson M, Yordy K, Vanselow N. Primary care: America's health in a new era. Institute of Medicine, National Academy Press, Washington, DC: 1996.
6. USPHS Agency for Health Care Policy and Research. Primary care and health care reform (PA-93-063). NIH guide 22(10), Bethesda, MD, 1993.
7. Scherger JE, Rucker L, Morrison EH, et al. The primary care specialties working together: a model of success in an academic environment. Acad Med 2000;75:693–698.
8. Irigoyen MM, Kurth RJ, Schmidt HJ. Learning primary care in medical school: does specialty or geographic location of the teaching site make a difference? Am J Med 1999;106:561–564.
9. Franks P, Clancy CM. Nutting PA. Defining primary care. Empirical analysis of the National Ambulatory Medical Care Survey. Med Care 1997;35:655–668.
10. Brown CV. Primary care for women: the role of the obstetrician-gynecologist. Clin Obstet Gynecol 1999;42:306–313.
11. Institute of Medicine Committee on the Future of Primary Care. Primary care: America's health in a new era. The Institute, Washington, DC: 1996.
12. Hurd WW, Barhan S, Rogers RE. Obstetrician gynecologist as primary care provider. Am J Managed Care 2001;7:SP71–SP77.
13. Cooper R, Cutler J, Desvigne-Nickens P, et al. Trends and disparities in coronary heart disease, stroke, and other cardiovascular diseases in the United States: findings of the national conference on cardiovascular disease prevention. Circulation 2000;102:3137–3147.
14. Stampfer MJ, Hu FB, Manson JE, et al. Primary prevention of coronary heart disease in women through diet and lifestyle. N Eng J Med 2000;343:16–22.
15. Heudebert GR, Centor RM, Klapow JC, et al. What is heartburn worth? A cost-utility analysis of management strategies. J Gen Intern Med 2000;15:175–182.
16. Lave J, Frank RG, Schulberg HC, Kamlet MS. Cost-effectiveness of treatments for major depression in primary care practice. Arch Gen Psychiatry 1998;55:645–651.
17. Ofman JJ, Rabeneck L. The effectiveness of endoscopy in the management of dyspepsia: a qualitative systematic review. Am J Med 1999;106:335–346.
18. Nolan TE. Evaluation and treatment of uncomplicated hypertension. Clin Obstet Gynecol 1995;38:156–165.
19. Grimes DA. Prevention of cardiovascular disease in women: role of the obstetrician-gynecologist. Am J Obstet Gynecol 1988;158:1662–1668.
20. Gabbe S, Hill L, Schmidt L, Schulkin J. Management of diabetes by obstetrician-gynecologists. Obstet Gynecol 1998;91:643–647.
21. Eccles M, Freemantle N, Mason J. North of England evidence based development project: guideline for angiotensin converting enzyme inhibitors in primary care management of adults with symptomatic heart failure. BMJ 1998;316:1369–1375.

22. Anonymous. Joint position paper on training for rural family practitioners in advanced maternity skills and cesarean section. College of Family Physicians of Canada, Society of Rural Physicians of Canada, Society of Obstetricians and Gynaecologists of Canada. Can Fam Physician 1999;45:2416–2422, 2426–2432.

23. Toobert DJ, Strycker LA, Glasgow RE. Lifestyle change in women with coronary heart disease: what do we know? J Womens Health 1998;7:685–699.

24. Lancaster T, Stead L, Silagy C, Sowden A. Effectiveness of interventions to help people stop smoking: findings from the Cochrane Library. BMJ 2000;321:355–358.

25. Solberg LI, Boyle RG, Davidson G, et al. Patient satisfaction and discussion of smoking cessation during clinical visits. Mayo Clin Proc 2001;76:138–143.

26. Clinical Guidelines and Identification, Evaluation, and Treatment of Overweight, and Obesity in Adults: The Evidence Report. National Institutes of Health: National Heart, Lung, and Blood Institute in cooperation with the National Institute of Diabetes and Digestive and Kidney Diseases, NIH Publication no. 98-4083, Bethesda, MD: 1998.

27. Cleeman JI, Lenfant C. The National Cholesterol Education Program: progress and prospects. JAMA 1998;280:2099–2104.

28. The Sixth Report of the Joint National Committee on Prevention, Detection, Evaluation, and Treatment of High Blood Pressure. National Institutes of Health: National Heart, Lung, and Blood Institute, National High Blood Pressure Education Program, NIH Publication no. 98-4080, Bethesda, MD: 1997.

29. Brett KM, Burt CW. Utilization of ambulatory medical care by women: United States, 1997–98. Vital Health Stat 2001;13:1–46.

30. Colditz GA, Willett WC, Stampfer MJ, et al. Menopause and risk of coronary heart disease in women. N Engl J Med 1987;316:1105–1110.

31. Lerner DJ, Kannel WB. Patterns of coronary heart disease morbidity and mortality in the sexes: a 26-year follow-up of the Framingham population. Am Heart J 1986;111:383–390.

32. Hurd WW, Amesse LS, Randolph JF Jr. Chapter 29: Menopause. In: Berek JS (ed.). Novak's Gynecology, 13th ed. Baltimore, MD: Williams and Wilkins, 2002.

33. Wagner JD. Rationale for hormone replacement therapy in atherosclerosis prevention. J Reprod Med 2000;45(Suppl 3):245–258.

34. Clarkson TB, Anthony MS. Effects on the cardiovascular system: basic aspects. In: Lindsay R, Dempster DW, Jordan VC (eds.). Estrogens and Antiestrogens. Lippincott-Raven, Philadelphia, PA: 1997, p. 89–118.

35. The Writing Group for the PEPI Trial. Effects of estrogen or estrogen/progestin regimens on heart disease risk factors in postmenopausal women: the Postmenopausal Estrogen/Progestin Interventions (PEPI) Trial. JAMA 1995;273:199–208.

36. Lobo RA, Zacur HZ, Caubel P, Lane R. A novel intermittent regimen of norgestimate to preserve the beneficial effects of 17[beta]-estradiol on lipid and lipoprotein profiles. Am J Obstet Gynecol 2000;182:41–49.

37. Hulley S, Grady D, Bush T, et al. Randomized trial of estrogen plus progestin for secondary prevention of coronary heart disease in postmenopausal women. JAMA 1998;280:605–613.

38. Herrington DM, Reboussin DM, Brosnihan KB, et al. Effects of estrogen replacement on the progression of coronary-artery atherosclerosis. N Engl J Med 2000;343:522–529.

39. Kudenchuk P, Maynard C, Martin J, et al. Comparison of presentation, treatment, and outcome of acute myocardial infarction in men versus women (the Myocardial Infarction Triage and Intervention Registry). Am J Cardiol 1996;78:9–14.

40. Laube DW, Ling FW. Primary care in obstetrics and gynecology resident education: a baseline survey of residents' perceptions and experiences. Obstet Gynecol 1999;94:632–636.

41. Morrison JC, Cowan BD, Hampton HL, et al. Medical practices of past graduates from one obstetric/gynecologic training program. South Med J 1998;91:227–230.

42. American Heart Association. 1997 Heart and Stroke Facts: Statistical Update. American Heart Association, Dallas, TX: 1996.

25   Health Technology Assessment in the Era of Managed Care
Issues in Women's Health Care

Laura Sampietro-Colom, MD, MPH,
Shawna Jackson, MS, Erin Williams, BSN, RN,
and Frank J. Papatheofanis, MD, MPH, PhD

CONTENTS

INTRODUCTION

As a result of an aging population and emerging new health technologies, health care providers throughout the world have begun to search for ways to reduce and stabilize the cost of health care while maintaining or improving its quality. Many changes have been implemented based on a growing emphasis on evidence-based decision making and medical practices.

Evidence-based approaches to health care include health policies and clinical practices that are motivated by the conclusions drawn from systematically collected and analyzed data. The health care field experienced a widespread integration of the evidence-based paradigm into its decision-making processes both nationally and internationally during the 1980s and 1990s. However, the concordance between evidence-based health recommendations and formally stated health policy remains incomplete *(1,2)*.

In the late 1960s, the term *technology assessment* was coined by policymakers in the United States who defined it as policy research to provide a balanced analysis and perspective of a new technology for decision makers *(3)*. Subsequently, the Office of Technology Assessment (OTA) was introduced in the early 1970s, with the objective to

From: *Contemporary Cardiology: Coronary Disease in Women: Evidence-Based Diagnosis and Treatment*
Edited by: L. J. Shaw and R. F. Redberg © Humana Press Inc., Totowa, NJ

research and assess new health technologies for the purpose of informing decision makers at the government policy level (4). Since then, health technology assessment (HTA) has spurred much interest and has been used in various ways in health care organizations throughout the world.

This chapter focuses on how the evidence-based paradigm has affected change through HTA development and integration in the increasingly managed health care environment, emphasizing the United States. The association of heath technology and cardiovascular disease (CVD) in women is also addressed.

EVIDENCE-BASED HEALTH CARE IN THE UNITED STATES

Health insurance coverage policies often determine the rate at which a new health technology is diffused into clinical practice (5–7). Private payers (e.g., Blue Cross–Blue Shield) and government-funded health care programs (e.g., Medicaid and Medicare) must balance the need and drive for the discovery and development of more effective treatment and prevention programs within a necessarily defined, and often constrained, budget. Consequently, both public and private health care providers have a vested interest in the search for health technologies that will provide quality care for patients and also keep rising health care costs at a minimum (5).

With the rapid advent of new health technologies, illustrated by the many innovative pharmaceuticals that have been developed in the past few years, health care costs (including employee and employer premiums) have risen in the United States. Many patients are unwilling to pay for treatments unless insurance companies will provide reimbursement. As a result, how the payers, both public and private, determine which new technologies will be reimbursed and at what rate remains the primary importance to pharmaceutical and medical device manufacturer's commercialization plans (5).

Many public and private health care payers have instituted policies that require HTA and economic analyses to determine whether or not the recently approved technology will be reimbursed by their coverage policy (Table 1) . Most coverage policies state that the services the patient receives must be both reasonable and necessary for the treatment or diagnosis of a current health condition. However, the US Food and Drug Administration (FDA) approves new health technologies by evaluating their safety and effectiveness, not their necessity (5). As a result, a new pharmaceutical drug that received FDA approval for the treatment of a specific disease may not be placed as a high priority on health plan-covered benefits' lists because of its cost and/or lack of evidence when compared to other accepted treatments. Additionally, unless there are sufficient conclusive data to support a new technology's effectiveness (data beyond clinical trials required by the FDA), it may not be approved for reimbursement by payers, or it may be placed under strict reimbursement limitations pending more data acquisition, as in the case of electron beam computed tomography (EBCT) and genetic screening technologies during the last decade (6,7). Accordingly, the medical device and pharmaceutical industries have begun to generate and use HTAs to predict the likelihood of FDA approval and favorable reimbursement policy.

HTAS

Currently, health professionals and health care organizations worldwide have yet to come to a consensus as to how the term *health technology assessment* should be

Table 1
Health Care Organizational Use of HTA

Organization/country	HTA objective(s)
Blue Cross–Blue Sheild Association TEC/ United States	To determine whether or not the new technology improves health outcomes, such as length of life, quality of life, and functional ability, it must meet the following five criteria: 1. The technology must have final approval from the appropriate governmental regulatory bodies. 2. The scientific evidence must permit conclusions concerning the effect of the technology on health outcomes. 3. The technology must improve the net health outcome (i.e., the health benefits must be greater than the adverse events). 4. The technology must be as beneficial as established alternatives. 5. The improvement must be attainable outside the investigational setting.
Department of Health's Research and Development program–National Institute for Clinical Excellence (NICE)/United Kingdom	The objective of the HTA program is to assess the cost, effectiveness, and impact of new and some established health technologies through efficient high-quality research in order to manage and provide care within the National Health Service (NHS). Each assessment seeks to answer four questions (27): 1. Does the technology work? 2. For whom does the technology work? 3. What is the cost of the technology? 4. How does the technology being evaluated compare with the alternatives?
Danish Center for Evaluation and Health Technology Assessment (DACEHTA)/ Denmark	Established in April 2001. Its aim is to carry out HTAs to (28): 1. Integrate HTA principles into the decision-making policies and procedures at all levels of public health services 2. Improve the quality and standards of public health services 3. Improve the value of the money that is spent by the public health services
Canadian Coordinating Office of Health Technology Assessment (CCOHTA)/ Canada	The Canadian Coordinating Office of Health Technology Assessment (CCOHTA) defines HTA as the process of evaluating medical technologies (devices, equipment, procedures and drugs) and their use through the systematic collection and critically evaluated and synthesized available research data. Factors such as efficacy, safety, effectiveness, quality of life, patient use as well as economic, ethical, and social implications are all considered, when appropriate, within the assessments (29).

Table 2
US Preventive Services Task Force Grading for Strength of Recommendations

A. There is good evidence to support the recommendation that the condition be specifically considered in a periodic health examination.
B. There is fair evidence to support the recommendation that the condition be specifically considered in a periodic health examination.
C. There is insufficient evidence to recommend for or against the inclusion of the condition In a periodic health examination, but recommendations may be made on other grounds.
D. There is fair evidence to support the recommendation that the condition be excluded from consideration in a periodic health examination.
E. There is good evidence to support the recommendation that the condition be excluded from consideration in a periodic health examination.

Source: ref. *45.*

defined *(8).* In the early 1980s, the US National Center for Health Care Technology defined it as "the careful evaluation of a medical technology for evidence of its safety, efficacy, cost, cost-effectiveness and ethical and legal implications, both in absolute terms and in comparison with other competing technologies" *(9).* The International Network of Agencies for Health Technology Assessment (INAHTA) defines health care technology as anything that is used for the prevention, rehabilitation, or treatment of a health condition. These parameters include vaccines, pharmaceuticals, medical devices, medical and surgical procedures, and the systems within which health is protected and maintained. The INAHTA defines HTAs as multidisciplinary analyses of the medical, social, ethical, and/or economic implications of technology development, diffusion, and/or use to support policy changes in health care *(10).* INAHTA's broad definition of HTA is inclusive of the major health organizations different views on what an HTA is and how it should be used (Table 1). Today, most institutions involved in producing HTAs agree that the main purpose of this research is to improve decision making regarding the use and diffusion of health technology *(8,11).*

Ideally, a health technology must be proven safe, efficacious, and effective before it becomes widely available in the clinical field. HTA uses the best scientific evidence from clinical trials to assess the short-term safety and efficacy of any health technology. However, if this evidence is not available, HTA also uses observational studies to determine the technology's effects. As observational studies could be affected by factors that may confound the relationship between a health technology and a health effect, their inclusion is guided by the significance of their quality, and their results are considered with caution in any assessment recommendation. For that reason, when analyzing evidence, HTA uses a quality checklist to establish a hierarchy of the evidence assessed, which leads to grade recommendations *(12–14).* Effectiveness is usually assessed through observational studies; however, megatrials or randomization of settings, rather than patients, are being advocated as techniques to address the effectiveness of a health technology *(15)* (Tables 2 and 3).

Patient preferences is a novel area of study in HTA. However, knowledge of patient preferences is very important when assessing health technologies, particularly for those associated with benefits as well as risks. Preferences may also affect its effectiveness (e.g., unaccepted drugs lead to low compliance, and low compliance may preclude the

Table 3
US Preventive Services Task Force Grading for Quality of Evidence

I: Evidence obtained from at least one properly conducted RCT.
I-1: Evidence obtained from well-designed controlled trials without randomization.
II-2: Evidence obtained from well-designed cohort or case-control analytic studies, preferably from more than one center or research group.
II-3: Evidence obtained from multiple time series with or without the intervention. Dramatic results in uncontrolled experiments (such as the results of the introduction of penicillin treatment in the 1940s) could also be regarded as this type of evidence.
IIII: Opinions of respected authorities, based on clinical experience; descriptive studies and case reports; or reports of expert committees.

Source: ref. 45.

Table 4
HTA Economics Questions Asked by NICE*

What are the added costs over what we do at present?
Are there savings?
Where and when do costs and savings fall?
Where are the margins (where we consider the added benefit no longer commensurate with the added cost)?
How do the benefits of using resources in this way compare with other ways of using the same amount of resource?
Is there some other, perhaps unrelated, area of activity in which we should now disengage?

* NICE, National Institute for Clinical Excellence.

achievement of expected benefits). Health technologies also have to demonstrate their superiority or additional value against other available competition for the same clinical purpose. Moreover, these technologies should ideally prove to be more cost-effective. The results of this study give a more comprehensive view of the value of a health technology in a specific health care context (Table 4).

US AGENCY FOR HEALTH CARE POLICY AND RESEARCH

In 1995, the US Congress voted to eliminate the OTA, which left the United States without a federal organization charged with the task to evaluate new health technologies. In December 1999, the US Department of Health and Human Services formed the Agency for Health Research and Quality (AHRQ), formerly known as the Agency for Health Care Policy and Research (AHCPR), as one of its Public Health Service agencies. The AHRQ's mission is "to support research designed to improve the outcomes and quality of health care, reduce its costs, address patient safety and medical errors, and broaden access to effective services. The research sponsored, conducted, and disseminated by AHRQ provides information that helps people make better decisions about health care" *(16).* One of the nine components of AHRQ is the Center for Practice and Technology Assessment (CPTA). CPTA coordinates the evidence-based practice program of AHRQ and is accountable for the research on the assessment of new and established medical technologies, including conducting and performing assessments to assist other agencies in making quality changes in their current health care policies. The CPTA reports have historically been requested by Center for Medicare and Medicaid Services (CMS) and the Civilian Health and Medical Program for the Uniformed Services to update policymakers with the current "best-practices" and data to support coverage policy decisions *(17)*.

CPTA has 12 evidence-based practice centers throughout the United States and Canada, which include both public organizations and private companies. Each center develops evidence reports and technology assessments on assigned topics of special interest to Medicare and Medicaid populations, with a high burden of disease, and/or treatments or diagnostic procedures that have high costs. Among these reports are rigorous reviews of scientific literature and, when appropriate, economical analyses and meta-analyses *(17)*. Technology assessments and evidence reports have also been used recently at a national level of influence by several professional societies, such as the American College of Physicians–American Society for Internal Medicine, the American College of Cardiology/American Heart Association (ACC/AHA), the American Urological Association *(5)* and the American Society of Anesthesiologists *(18)*, to develop evidence-based clinical practice guidelines.

In 1999, Health Care Finance Administration (HCFA), now CMS, established the Medicare Coverage Advisory Committee (MCAC). MCAC was charged with improving the decision-making process by which health technologies became a part of Medicare services. The executive committee decided to evaluate evidence for a technology in a two-step process. First, the investigating panel determined whether or not the available evidence was sufficient to draw conclusions applicable to Medicare patients. Second, the panel evaluated and compared the technology's effectiveness to that of current treatments in a structured review of the literature. Once both steps were completed and the findings presented to the MCAC executive committee, public recommendations were made as to whether or not the evidence was conclusive in the effectiveness of the new technology *(5)*. This process is fairly new and continues to evolve.

HTA'S ROLE IN WOMEN'S HEALTH CARE

In the United States, one of the most significant HTA contributions to the improvement of women's health care is in the development and adoption of mammography as a tool for breast cancer detection. The following section examines the development and diffusion of breast cancer screening technology, a case study exemplifying HTA impact on improving female health outcomes. The fundamental HTA questions that pertain to breast cancer screening and health outcomes discussed next are: Is there evidence that early detection is beneficial; and, do persons identified with early-stage disease through screening have better health outcomes than those who present clinically without screening? *(19)* (Tables 5–7).

WOMEN, HEALTH TECHNOLOGY, AND CVD

Fueled by a heightened awareness that women have unique health care issues and experiences, a growing effort exists to develop strategies for improved care and quality of life for women. Within the last decade, HTAs have played an integral role in the

Table 5
Clinical Advantages and Disadvantages of Mammography

Advantages	Disadvantages
Noninvasive, simple procedure Widely available	Production of consistent, high-quality images may be technically difficult
Routine screening can result in 25–35% reduction in breast cancer mortality among women ages 50–70 *(3)*	Cannot detect all breast lesions Results are difficult to interpret in women with dense breast tissue, leading to higher rates of false-negative and false-positive results Optimal screening intervals not well-defined
Generally considered safe	Radiation tolerance may be patient-specific

Source: ref. 46.

Table 6
Objectives of the Breast Cancer Surveillance Consortium (BCSC) in 1994

1. Enhance the understanding of breast cancer screening practices in the United States through assessment of accuracy, cost, and quality of screening programs and the relation of these programs to changes in breast cancer mortality or other short-term outcomes, such as diagnosis stage or survival.
2. Foster collaborative research among consortium participants to examine such issues as regional and health care system differences in the provision of screening services and subsequent diagnostic evaluations.
3. Provide a foundation for the conduct of clinical and basic science research that can improve the understanding of breast cancer etiology and prognosis. The intent is to collect a core set of pathological data on established prognostic indicators and to provide the capability to examine the prognostic potential of other, more investigational indicators *(13)*.

Source: ref. 47.

development and standardization of guidelines for the screening and treatment of diseases prevalent among women.

HTA in women's health care has primarily focused on those clinical conditions that affect women solely or predominantly, such as breast cancer *(20)*, ultrasound prenatal screening *(21)*, in vitro fertilization *(22)*, and hormone replacement therapy (HRT) for osteoporosis *(23)*, among others. For those clinical conditions that affect both women and men (e.g., CVDs), HTA has barely distinguished between genders in its analysis. Therefore, until now, HTA availability in CVD with exclusive focus in women is generally lacking. One of the potential explanations may be the gender research bias in the past *(24)*, although improvements have been made during the end of the last century.

The principles followed by any HTA, as mentioned previously, can also be applied to the technology assessment addressed to CVD in women. An overview is provided here of HTA principles using examples of technology addressing CVD in women. Notably, they are not based on a systematic literature review, but instead exemplify the thoughts underlying an HTA process.

HRT has been widely prescribed to postmenopausal women during the last decades and has been proven in clinical trials to be safe and efficacious in the treatment of vaso-

Table 7
US Preventive Services Task Force 1996 Guidelines for Clinical Preventive Services Grading
of Strength of Recommendations for Clinical Interventions for Breast Cancer Screening

Grade	Ages of women (years)	Clinical intervention
C	70+	Insufficient evidence regarding clinical benefit of mammography or CBE. Recommendation for mammography may be made on basis of high burden of suffering and lack of evidence of differences in test characteristics in age group vs those age 50–69
A	50–69	Screening for breast cancer every 1–2 years with mammography alone or mammography and annual clinical breast examination (CBE)
C	50–69	There is insufficient evidence to recommend annual CBE
C	40–49	There is conflicting evidence of fair to good quality for women age 40–49 regarding the clinical benefit from mammography with or without CBE, and insufficient evidence regarding benefit from CBE alone; recommendations for or against routine mammography or CBE cannot be made based on current evidence.
C	All	Insufficient evidence to recommend for or against teaching breast self-examination in periodic health examination

Source: ref. *45.*

motor symptoms (hot flashes and night sweats), vaginal dryness, and urethritis after menopause *(25)*. HRT has also demonstrated, through randomized controlled trials (RCT), to slow down the loss of bone mass or reverse it postmenopause *(23)*. During the past two decades, a significant amount of large-scale observational studies have suggested that women taking estrogen (opposed or unopposed to progesterone) have one-third of the risk for coronary heart disease (CHD) when compared to those women estrogen-free *(26)*. The veracity of this effect is very important for women because coronary disease is the leading cause of mortality in women, with incidence after menopause equal to that of men *(25)*. In the past, the evidence from these observational studies has led to several scientific associations recommending the HRT use in all postmenopausal women, especially for those at CHD risk (i.e., to recommend the estrogen use for CVD's primary or secondary prevention; *27*).

From an HTA perspective, the benefits attributed to any health technology should be valued against any other available in the market, addressing the same clinical purpose. Low-dose aspirin therapy has been shown to have a significant benefit in the primary prevention of myocardial infarction (MI; *28–30*). In 1989, the Physicians's Health Study demonstrated that low-dose aspirin reduced MI risk *(28)*. More recently, the combination of information (using the general variance-based method) from four randomized trials (one trial included 47% women), including 51,000 subjects and 2284 important vascular events, showed a significant reduction of 32% (95% confidence interval [CI]: 21–41%) for nonfatal MI and 13% (95% CI: 5–19%) for any important vascular events in those patients assigned to aspirin *(29)*. Additionally, a case-control study nested in a cohort of 164,769 postmenopausal women (50–74 years of age, followed from 1991 to 1995), showed that the relative risk of MI associated with the current aspirin use for more than 1 month duration was 0.56 (95% CI: 0.26–1.21), and nonfatal MI was 0.28 (95% CI: 0.08–0.91; *30*). For secondary prevention, low-dose aspirin has also shown its safety and effectiveness *(31)*.

With this knowledge, what then should a physician recommend to women regarding taking aspirin or hormones to prevent CVD? To answer this question, a RCT that compares HRT efficacy with aspirin in primary and secondary CVD prevention in women is needed. Until now, there has been no such study. Additionally, to comprehensively analyze the added value of one health technology against the other, the impact of each option's costs and benefits should be considered. When comparing the cost and effect of both aspirin and HRT, although aspirin may appear to be a potentially cheaper option, a statement regarding the better cost-effectiveness of aspirin related to HRT cannot be performed. To our knowledge, there is a lack of cost-effectiveness studies that compare these two HT options either for primary or secondary prevention.

As mentioned previously, HTA uses the best available scientific evidence in its analysis. Therefore, because observational studies can be subject to bias, their results should be taken into account with caution until high-quality scientific evidence becomes available, such as an RCT. HRT in postmenopausal women for secondary CVD prevention has been recently questioned through RCT *(32,33)*. The Heart Estrogen/Progestine Replacement Study (HERS) did not show a significant reduction of coronary events in postmenopausal women who took HRT *(32)*. The HERS study randomized 2763 postmenopausal women to estrogen and placebo. After 4.1-year followup, the incidence of cardiac events was almost identical in the two groups. The results from this study were supported by the Estrogen Replacement and Atherosclerosis (ERA) randomized trial of 309 postmenopausal women who underwent coronary angiography and showed no effect in the progression of coronary atherosclerosis with established disease as assessed by quantitative coronary angiography *(33)*. Limitations have been associated with these studies *(34)*. Nevertheless, in light of this new evidence, the AHA has stated its recommendation of not prescribing HRT for CVD secondary prevention and is awaiting ongoing RCT results in primary prevention *(35)*. This case shows the importance of considering evidence by its quality when assessing a health technology as HTA does.

HRT has also been associated with several adverse effects, such as an increased risk of venous tromboembolism, gallbladder disease, endometrial cancer (when estrogen is given without progesterone), and likely to an increase of breast cancer *(25,26)*. As a result of the risk and benefits associated with HRT, several guidelines have recommended taking into account women's preferences when prescribing this therapy *(27,36)*. A before-and-after study that used a decision aid for women who considered HRT following menopause shows the presence of different treatment preferences when the same information about benefits and risks is given to a group of women *(37)*.

In general, women's values have not been incorporated into health care decisions, which is certainly true in the area of CVD, where few studies have addressed preferences in women's health care *(38)*. Assessing female preferences is important, as previous research has shown that men and women value risk differently. For example, white men perceive risks to be much smaller and more acceptable than women *(39)*. Moreover, considering patient preferences for specific intervention aspects may influence a patient's decision to initiate or continue the use of health care services. Men and women may also differ in their preferences for cardiovascular-related improvement programs (e.g., cardiac rehabilitation program features; *[40]*). Generally, women give more importance to "not getting tired while exercising" than men ($t = 2.42$, $p = 0.02$).

No clinically justified variations in the diagnosis and treatment of ischemic heart disease between men and women have been well-documented in the literature during the past decade *(41,42)*. Despite the abundant scientific evidence produced, differences still remain *(43,44)*. However, non-HTA institutions worldwide have formally assessed this lack of access for women to scientifically proven diagnostic and therapeutic technologies for CVD. To our knowledge, there is no governmental strategy that addresses this inequity. An HTA document on gender differences in access to CVD diagnostic and therapeutic interventions is recommended in order to solve this issue.

CONCLUSION

The role and measure of HTA continues to evolve in the United States, European Union, and elsewhere. HTA as a contribution in the identification of appropriate diagnostic and therapeutic options for women's health also continues to gain valuable momentum. Many examples can be explored that illustrate HTA impact in decision making regarding technologies relevant to health care in women. Methodologies for conducting HTA must begin to account for gender-specific health outcomes to become more effective tools for decision makers. Such methodologies must extend beyond currently practiced approaches that essentially go no further than outline demographic differences in study results or clinical outcomes, eliminating gender as a required subset analysis. HTA results must be based on technology assessment criteria that captures specific female responses to health interventions. In that way, the gender-based understanding of efficacy can be explored without the intricacies associated with general population studies. HTA will assume a more important and vital role in women's health care as institutions, such as managed care and other health service models, wax and wane as optimal choices for health care delivery. Having a constant benchmark methodology and decision-making technique like HTA will stabilize the evaluation of new technology, despite the health service model of the epoch, and guarantee the adoption and diffusion of the most useful health care technologies.

REFERENCES

1. Niessen LW, Grijseels EWM, Rutten FFH. The evidence-based approach in health policy and health care delivery. Soc Sci Med 2000;51:859–869.
2. Murray CJ. Toward an analytical approach to health sector reform. Health Policy 1995;32:93–109.
3. Hettman F. Society and the Assessment of Technology. Organization for Economic Opportunity and Development; Paris, France: 1973.
4. Institute of Medicine. Assessing Medical Technologies. National Academic Press; Washington, DC: 1985.
5. Garber AM. Evidence-based coverage policy: Insurers can borrow from research into medical effectiveness to help them allocate medical resources wisely. Health Affairs 2001;20:63–80.
6. Shaw LJ, Redberg RF. From clinical trials to public health policy: The path from imaging to screening. A Symposium: First International SAI Meeting. Am J Cardiol 2001;88:62E–65E.
7. Schoonmaker MM, Bernhardt BA, Holtzman NA. Factors influencing health insurers' decisions to cover new genetic technologies. Intl J Technol Assess Health Care 2000;16:178–189.
8. Lange M, Jørgensen T, Kristensen FB, Stilven S. The concept of Health Technology Assessment: Views of applications to funding of HTA projects. Intl J Technol Assess Health Care 2000;16:1201–1224.
9. Perry S. Technology assessment in health care: The US perspective. Health Policy 1988;9:17–24.

10. International Network of Agencies for Health Technology Assessment (INAHTA). Available at: http://www.inahta.org/. Accessed October 5, 2001.

11. Drummond M, Weatherly H. Implementing the findings of Health Technology Assessments: If the CAT got out of the bag, can the TAIL wag the dog? Intl J Technol Assess Health Care 2000;16:1–12.

12. http://www.shef.ac.uk/~~scharr/ir/units/systrev/hierarchy.htm, HTA; February, 2002.

13. http://cebm.jr2.ox.ac.uk/docs/levels.html, HTA; February, 2002

14. http://www.cche.net/usersguides/economic.asp, HTA; February, 2002

15. Meadows A, ed. Tools for evaluating health technologies. Five background papers. Office of Technology Assessment. Congress of the United States, Washington, DC 1995.

16. AHRQ Profile: Quality Research for Quality Healthcare. AHRQ Publication No. 00-P005, March 2001. Agency for Healthcare Research and Quality, Rockville, MD. Available at: http://www.ahrq.gov/about/profile.htm. Accessed October 5, 2001.

17. Center for Practice and Technology: Assessment Mission and Programs. AHRQ Publication no. 00-Po65, August 2001. Agency for Healthcare Research and Quality, Rockville, MD. Available at: http://www.ahrq.gov/about/cptafact.htm. Accessed October 5, 2001.

18. Connis RT, Nickinovich DG, Caplan RA, Arens JF. The development of evidence-based clinical practice guidelines: Integrating medical science and practice. Int J Technol Assess Health Care 2000;16:1003–1012.

19. Oortwijn W, Banta HD, Cranovsky R. Introduction: Mass screening, Health Technology Assessment, and health policy in some European countries. Intl J Technol Assess Health Care 2001;17:269–274.

20. Borràs JM (coordinator). Breast cancer screening in Catalonia: cost-effectiveness, health care impact and cost of the treatment of breast cancer. Catalan Agency for Health Technology Assessment & Catalan. Institute of Oncology, Barcelona: 1996.

21. Aymerich M, Almazán C, Jovell AJ. Assessment of obstetric ultrasonography for the control of normal pregnancies in primary care. Catalan Agency for Health Technology Assessment, Barcelona: 1997.

22. Dahlquist G, Alton Lundberg V, Bergh T, et al. Children born from in vitro fertilization (IVF). SBU 2000 (report no. 147): p. 102.

23. Hailey D, Sampietro-Colom L, Marshall D, et al. The effectiveness of bone density measurement and associated treatments for prevention of fractures. An international collaborative review. Internt J Health Technol Assess Health Care 1998;14:237–254.

24. Sherman SS. Gender, health and responsible research. Clin Geriat Med 1993;9:261–269.

25. Barret-Connor E, Stuenkel CA. Hormone replacement therapy (HRT): risk and benefits. Int J Epidemiol 2001;30:423–426.

26. Barret-Connor E, Grady D. Hormone replacement therapy, heart disease, and other considerations. Annu Rev Public Health 1998;19:55–72.

27. American College of Physicians. Guidelines for counseling postmenopausal women about preventive hormone replacement therapy. Ann Intern Med 1992;117:1038–1041.

28. Steering Committee of the Physician's Health Study Group: final report on the aspirin component of the ongoing Physician's Health Study. N Engl J Med 1989;321:129.

29. Hebert PR, Hennekens CH. An overview of the 4 randomized trials of aspirin therapy in the primary prevention of cardiovascular disease. Arch Intern Med 2000;160:3123–3127.

30. Garcia Rodriguez LA, Varas C, Patrono C. Differential effects of aspirin and non-aspirin nonsteroidal antiinflammatory drugs in the primary prevention of myocardial infarction in postmenopausal women. Epidemiology 2000;11:382–387.

31. Anonymous. Collaborative overview of randomised trials of antiplatelet therapy. I: Prevention of death, myocardial infarction, and stroke by prolonged antiplatelet therapy in various categories of patients. Antiplatelet Trialists' Collaboration. BMJ 1994;308:81–106.

32. Hulley S, Grady D, Bush T, et al. Randomized trial of estrogen plus progestins for secondary prevention of coronary heart disease in postmenopausal women. JAMA 1998;280:605–613.

33. Herrington DM, Reboussin DM, Brosnihan B, et al. Effects of estogen replacement therapy on the progression of coronary-artery atherosclerosis. N Engl J Med 2000;343:522–529.

34. Nabel EG. Coronary heart disease in women. An ounce of prevention. N Engl J Med 2000;343:572–574.

35. American Heart Association. Hormone replacement therapy and cardiovascular disease: a statement for healthcare professionals from the American Heart Association. Circulation 2001;104:499–503.

36. Society of Obstetricians and Gynaecologists of Canada, Canadadian Menopause Consensus Conference. Journal of the Society of Obstetricians and Gynecologists of Canada 1994;16:4–40.

37. O'Connor AM, Tugwell P, Wells GA, et al. A decision aid for women considering hormone replacement therapy after menopause: decision support framework and evaluation. Patient Educ Counsel 1998;33:267–279.
38. Sampietro-Colom L, Phillips V, Blair A. Eliciting women's preferences in health care. A review of the literature (Submitted for publication).
39. Flynn J, Slovic P, Mertz C K. Gender, race and perception of enviromental health risks. Risk Analysis 1994;14:1101–1108.
40. Moore SM, Kramer F M. Women's and men's preferences for cardiac rehabilitation program features. J Cardiopulmonary Rehabil 1996;16:163–168.
41. Shaw LJ, Miller D, Romeis JC, et al. Gender differences in the nonivasive evaluation and management of patients with suspected coronary artery disease. Ann Intern Med 1994;120:559–566.
42. Clarke KW, Gray D, Keating NA, Hampton JR. Do women with acute myocardial infarction receive the same treatment as men?. BMJ 1994;309:563–566.
43. Rathore S, Chen J, Wang Y, et al. Sex differences in cardiac catherization: the role of physician gender. JAMA 2001;286:2849–2856.
44. Hippisley-Cox J, Pringle M, Crown N, et al. Sex inequalities in ischaemic heart disease in general practice: cross sectional survey. BMJ 2001;322:832.
45. US Preventative Services Task Force. Guide to Preclinical Preventative Services: Appendix A Task Force Ratings. 2nd ed., 1996; Available at http://hstat.nlm.nih.gov/ftrs/ directbrowse.pl?dbName=cps&href=APPA&t=1002299264. Accessed October 5, 2001.
46. American College of Radiology and Radiological Society of North America. Mammography. Available at http://www.radiologyinfo.org/content/mammogram.htm. Accessed October 5, 2001.
47. Jepson R, Clegg A, Forbes C, et al. The determinants of screening uptake and interventions for increasing uptake: A systematic review. Health Technol Assess 2000;4:1–148. Available at: http://www.hta.nhsweb.nhs.uk/fullmono/mon414short.pdf. Accessed October 4, 2001.

26 Issues in the Analysis of Cost-Effectiveness in the Diagnosis and Treatment of Coronary Artery Disease in Women

Adam Atherly, PhD and Steven D. Culler, PhD

INTRODUCTION

In 1997, 30% of total health care expenditures ($326.6 billion) in the United States were directly or indirectly related to cardiovascular disease (CVD) *(1)*. Given the enormous financial burden placed on society by CVD, there is an increasing interest in evaluating the efficiency with which the dollars are spent. Cost-effectiveness analysis (CEA) is a methodology designed for such evaluations.

The purpose of this chapter is to explore the implications of cost-effectiveness for the treatment of coronary artery disease (CAD) in women. It begins by discussing the key issues in CEA that impact the analysis of subgroups (including women). Then, the chapter provides an example of the implications of subgroups analysis by using published data to create gender-specific cost-effectiveness ratios for coronary stents. Finally, the chapter concludes by discussing the implications of the previous sections.

COST-EFFECTIVENESS ANALYSIS

CEA's purpose is to provide a measurement of the gain in health per dollar spent on an intervention. In the modern era, proliferation of new treatments and technologies has led to a decline in mortality rates for some conditions (particularly in CAD), increases in life expectancy and improved quality of life. However, new treatments and technology have also led to spiraling health care costs and both explicit and implicit

From: *Contemporary Cardiology: Coronary Disease in Women: Evidence-Based Diagnosis and Treatment*
Edited by: L. J. Shaw and R. F. Redberg © Humana Press Inc., Totowa, NJ

rationing of care as the care payers struggle to accommodate new innovations into health care budgets. As a result, payers and policymakers are increasingly questioning the actual contributions of expensive technological and pharmaceutical advances to the health of the population. CEA is a tool that is well-suited to provide guidance to the "bang for a buck" provided by different interventions.

CEA explicitly measures the trade-off between "cost" and "effectiveness." CEA compares a monetary measure of the treatment or intervention cost (e.g., dollars, pounds) to a effectiveness measure (e.g., life years saved) in the form of a ratio. By convention, the cost-effectiveness ratio puts effectiveness in the numerator and cost in the denominator (e.g., a new drug cost $5000 per life year saved or a new surgery cost $10,000 per life year saved; 2). Because cost-effectiveness ratios are inherently relative, absolute conclusions regarding the cost-effectiveness of a treatment can rarely be drawn (3). Instead, after calculating cost-effectiveness ratios, comparisons can be made across different treatments for the same condition or even across different conditions.

The use of CEA can be theoretically justified both on the grounds of efficiency and equity (4). From an efficiency perspective, selecting the treatments with the greatest cost-effectiveness will ensure the dollars spent on health care yield the greatest benefit for society. Also, concentrating health care resources on those with the greatest benefit will produce an equitable spending distribution. However, a complicating factor is a heterogeneous treatment response based on observable characteristics. If, for example, the treatment's effectiveness varies depending on age, sex, or race, then maximal efficiency and equity can be achieved by calculating separate cost-effectiveness ratios for the subgroups (5). Conducting a subgroup analysis has implications throughout the analysis, and decisions about the framework for the analysis will contribute to the end result.

CEA typically takes the societal perspective (6). When studies adopt the societal perspective, all economic resources consumed in an intervention are included, rather than the costs of medical care to a particular individual or organization. Although studies that adopt the societal approach may not answer key questions asked by particular stakeholders, studies using the societal approach will provide accurate intervention evaluations from the perspective of overall welfare. Studies using other perspectives may omit significant costs that are paid by other organizations, thus, providing an incomplete perspective of the overall impact of a program or intervention. For example, for a particular health plan, it may be cost-effective to not pay for hypertension treatments because most members will unenroll before untoward health effects are realized. However, high-cost adverse health events associated with untreated hypertension will lead to increased costs for other payers and should be included in the total cost calculation.

Taking the societal perspective is particularly important when examining subgroups (e.g., women). If a study examined the cost-effectiveness from the payer perspective, such as an employer, the lower labor force participation rates among women could lead to an undervaluing of treatments that are particularly effective for women. The use of a uniform societal perspective ensures balance in the evaluation of costs and benefits.

Measuring Costs

The denominator of the cost-effectiveness ratio measures the marginal intervention cost. Health care interventions always have costs even in the absence of market prices. If a consumed resource has an alternate use, then an economic cost was incurred. Economic and accounting costs are not synonymous. Some costs that appear in a financial report are not considered economic costs, whereas some economic costs do not appear in financial reports.

Costs included should be marginal costs, which only include costs that would not have occurred if the treatment had not been given. CEA should include all economic costs associated with an intervention, including both direct and indirect medical costs. Direct medical costs include all costs directly attributable to the intervention. Examples would include the cost of medical supplies, physician charges, costs associated with hospitalizations, and the value of the patient time required for treatment and travel. Indirect medical costs are costs that are associated with the patient care, but that cannot be directly attributed to a particular patient or intervention. Examples include costs associated with maintaining a hospital, such as heating, laundry, and janitorial services.

In some situations, treatment cost may vary significantly across subgroups. For example, older men tend to have shorter hospitalizations than older women because men tend to die earlier. That is, an elderly man is more likely to be discharged home after a hospitalization because he will have his wife available to care for him. However, an elderly woman—with the exact same medical condition—may be discharged to a skilled nursing facility because her husband has died and, therefore, cannot provide care at home. There are two important implications of this difference: first, although nonmarket care provided to the man from his wife should be included in the cost of care, often it is not. This will make the cost of care for the man artificially lower than the cost of care for the woman. Second, even if the appropriate societal cost of nursing care for the man is calculated and included, the value of economic alternatives for an elderly woman (which provides her imputed wage) are likely to be lower than for the nursing home employees, again yielding a lower cost estimate for the man.

Notably, the difference in cost calculated in the latter case is correct. In truth, the societal cost of providing care for the man *is* lower than for the similar woman. This is a result of the shorter life expectancy rates for men, the limited economical alternatives for elderly women, and the social contract in many societies that requires women to provide nursing care for their husbands, but not necessarily vice versa. These realities are biased to both sexes, but the result is that men are discharged more quickly from hospitals, requiring less formal nursing support and consequently using fewer health care resources.

Income transfers (e.g., payments to individuals in exchange for participating in a trial) are not economic costs. Transfers merely move dollars from one individual to another; from the societal perspective, one individual has gained and another has lost, and there is no net change in societal welfare.

Measuring Benefits

The numerator of the cost-effectiveness ratio measures the benefits associated with the intervention or treatment. There are numerous possible endpoints that could be selected for evaluation; most clinically meaningful endpoints could be used to measure the benefit of a treatment. The clinical endpoint most commonly used is mortality. Mortality rates can be used to calculate the life expectancy for both those who receive an intervention and those who do not. The two life expectancies can then be compared, and the marginal effectiveness can be calculated.

In CAD, mortality is often used as the effectiveness measure. Mortality has several advantages as an outcome measure. First, its definition is widely agreed on and, second, its importance of mortality as an outcome is obvious to all observers. Finally, mortality is relatively straightforward and inexpensive to measure.

The use of mortality rates has important implications for comparisons of the effectiveness of CAD interventions for men and women. Because women have a longer life expectancy than men at all ages, treatments without gender-specific morality effects administered to men and women at the same age will be more effective in women than men. However, women tend to experience CAD later in life than men, which, for treatments without gender-specific mortality effects, will make treatments less effective.

The different life expectancies of men and women also have implications for the discounting effect. Both costs and benefits that occur in the future should be discounted. There is some disagreement regarding the appropriate discount rate. Standard practice is now to use a discount rate of 3%, with a sensitivity analysis that applies discount rates from 0% to 7% (2). If women, on net, have a longer life expectancy, then a higher discount rate will disproportionately reduce the overall effectiveness of the treatment in women relative to men. Conversely, a lower discount rate will favor women.

One key shortcoming of mortality as a measure of effectiveness is its bluntness as a measurement tool. Mortality distinguishes between those who live and those who die, but treats the outcome of care for all who survive as identical. Often, there is substantial variation among the survivors in recovery time and postrecovery health-related quality of life (HRQoL). Using measures of HRQoL can help to distinguish between treatments with similar mortality effects. However, the use of HRQoL when a treatment has a differential subgroup effect is problematic.

The most straightforward problem occurs when recovery times or nonfatal outcomes are subgroup-specific. For example, previous research has shown that some interventions are less effective in minority populations. There are many possible reasons for this disparity, including genetic differences, accessibility differences to other health care services, environmental differences (e.g., worse housing or the effect of income disparities). Regardless of the cause of the difference, the implication is that a treatment will be considered to have a lower benefit and will therefore be less cost-effective. Consider a surgical intervention that requires follow-up care. A minority person may have less access to transportation and therefore higher postsurgical morbidity rates. A narrow CEA would suggest redirecting resources away from minorities in order to maximize the output of dollars spent on health care.

A second complication with the use of measures of HRQoL in subgroup analysis is preference weights. Measures of HRQoL explicitly compare the quality of life in different health states. To create a measure of the relative quality of different health states, preference weights for different conditions are created. The preference weights vary depending on who is asked to rank the different health states. To calculate a gender-specific cost-effectiveness ratio, it would be reasonable to use gender-specific preference weights. Indeed, work in this area has already begun (5).

COST-EFFECTIVENESS OF CORONARY ARTERY STENTING IN WOMEN VS MEN

To illustrate the issues discussed in the previous section, this section examines the cost-effectiveness of stenting vs percutaneous transluminal coronary angioplasty

Table 1
Estimated Rates of Complications by Type and Gender for Coronary Stenting and PTCA

	Stents		PTCA	
	Men	Women	Men	Women
No complications	87.2%	83.3%	78.8%	68.1%
Repeat revascularization	9.0%	12.0%	14.0%	18.0%
CABG	2.9%	3.1%	6.0%	12.0%
Death	0.9%	1.6%	1.2%	1.9%

(PTCA) in women vs men. Stents have become an essential tool in the medical profession's treatments for CAD. Since 1996, stents have been implanted in the majority of percutaneous coronary revascularization procedures *(7)*. Men are more likely than women to receive a stent, although the rate of use in both genders has risen dramatically during the past 5 years *(8)*. Stenting increases the initial treatment cost (mostly owing to the device cost), but reduces the likelihood of high-cost complications, such as revascularization and coronary artery bypass surgery (CABG; *9*).

Although there have been numerous studies that examine the effectiveness and the cost-effectiveness of stents *(7)*, there is relatively little information regarding gender-specific cost-effectiveness. Women receiving either intervention tend to be older and have more complications (e.g, diabetes; *8,10–12*). Mehilli *(11)* reports that women have higher rates of poststent mortality (1.7% vs 0.8%), CAGB (0.9% vs 0.7%), and repeat angioplasty (2.3% vs 1.5%). Similarly, Peterson *(8)* reports higher in-hospital mortality for women (1.4% vs 0.9%) and higher rates of repeat revasculatization (4.8% vs 4.4%). Alfonso *(12)* also reports higher in-hospital mortality rates for women (6% vs 2%) and a higher overall complication rate (9% vs 4%).

This trend also holds true for PTCA: women tend to have higher mortality rates and higher complication rates. Robertson *(13)* reports that women had higher mortality rates (1.4% vs 1.1%) and higher CABG rates (3.3% vs 1.9%). Similarly, Malenka *(14)* reports higher mortality rates (1.6% vs 0.7%) and higher CABG rates (3.8% vs 3.1%), and Arnold *(15)* found women had an increased risk of death (1.1% vs 0.3%) and postangioplasty CABG (5.0% vs 4.5%). Women have also been found to have higher restenosis rates than men both with stenting (29% vs 26%) and without (52% vs 39%; *16*).

Published rates of mortality, restenosis, and CABG vary depending on the date of the study (because percutaneous coronary revascularization treatments both with and without stenting have been improving), sample characteristics, location, and study period (i.e., in-hospital, 1 year, etc.). Table 1 summarizes our estimate of the complication rates for a "typical" population for both stents and PTCA after 6 months. Women have been shown to have higher mortality rates for both treatments and higher rates of other complications.

Estimating differences in cost between gender is more tenuous given the paucity of available data. Cohen et al. *(17)* reports that stents are more expensive during the baseline hospitalization ($9738 vs $7506). More recently, Peterson *(9)* had a similar result with stents ($14,802) costing more than PTCA ($11,534) for a baseline hospitalization.

Gender will affect the treatment cost in several ways. First, the relative cost of the treatments may be different. For example, women are less likely to undergo multivessel

Table 2
Author's Calculation of the Cost of Stents vs PTCA by Gender

	Stents		PTCA	
	Men	Women	Men	Women
No complications	$15,000	$13,750	$11,250	$11,250
Repeat revascularization	$30,000	$27,500	$26,250	$25,000
CAGB	$40,000	$38,750	$36,250	$36,250
Death	$22,500	$21,375	$16,875	$18,000

treatment *(15)*. Women also tend to have a smaller diameter stenosis of the infarct-related artery *(16)*. Consequently, women will use fewer stents on average than men. It is also likely that women have a different average length of stay because of the higher mean age of treatment.

Table 2 presents our estimates of gender-specific costs of stents vs PTCA. The cost of a PTCA without complications is the same for both genders: $11,250. We assume that the cost of a typical stent is $1250. For men, the cost of receiving stents is slightly higher because we assume that men receive, on average, three stents versus two for women. For both genders in both treatment modalities, we assume that if there is a repeat revascularization, it includes stenting. The cost of the CAGB complication is equal to the cost of the initial treatment plus the $25,000 reported by Weintraub et al. *(18)* Finally, estimates of the in-hospital mortality cost were calculated using Medicare data and include both the cost of the treatment and the mean additional length of stay associated with death.

The benefit of the treatment is increased life expectancy. For the purposes of this exercise, we estimate that the average age at the time of the intervention for women is 69 and for men is 63. A 69-year-old woman has a life expectancy of 81 or 12 additional years. For a 63-year-old male, life expectancy is 78 or 15 additional years. Given the lowered mortality risk for women associated with stents, the expected increase in marginal life expectancy is 0.036 years. For men, with a slightly longer life expectancy, the expected increase in marginal life expectancy is 0.042 years.

Combining the results in Tables 1 and 2, we estimate that the mean cost of stenting for men is $17,143, whereas the cost of stenting for women is $16,297. The higher cost for men reflects the higher device cost. For PTCA, we estimate the average cost for men to be $14,918 and for women $16,853. The higher costs for women reflect their higher complication rates. These costs reflect those reported in a recent review of the PTCA research by Lecomte et al. *(19)*.

Table 3 presents our estimate of the incremental cost of stents, incremental increases in life expectancy, and cost per life year saved. For women, stents are cost-saving because the cost-savings associated with the reduction in complication rates because of stents overwhelms the cost increase associated with the device cost. For women, stents are unambiguously supported by our analysis: they both save lives and reduce resource use. For men, stents are likely not cost-effective. Although there are no precise guide-lines to appropriate cut-offs, one rule of thumb is that interventions that cost more than $40,000 per life year (the cost of treating mild hypertension) are not cost-effective *(20)*.

Table 3
Cost-Effectiveness of PTCA vs Stents by Gender

	Overall	Men	Women
Change in cost	$1391	2225	−556
Change in life years	0.040	0.042	0.036
Cost-effectiveness ratio	$34,775	$52,976	−$15,444

The overall result is borderline cost-effective. The majority of coronary interventions are in men; hence, the overall cost-effectiveness ratio is heavily weighted toward the male cost-effectiveness ratio.

CONCLUSION

Proponents of CEA suggest that all health care interventions should be evaluated and that health care resources should be targeted based on these analyses to maximize total population health given a set of resource constraints (21).

The role of gender as an independent predictor of mortality and morbidity is hotly debated, but differences in body size and baseline characteristics are widely accepted as independent predictors of mortality and morbidity in CAD (8). Specifically among CAD patients, women tend to be older and smaller than men with different lesion types and lengths, differences which lead to the cost ratios reported previously. As a result, stents are unambiguously cost-saving for women and, at best, are marginally cost-effective for men. A health system might very well approve this intervention for women, whereas reject it for men.

The notion that men will be prevented from receiving an intervention that would reduce their mortality risk when undergoing coronary revascularization will strike many as unfair. Indeed, although health professionals argue for CEA, surveys show that nonprofessionals reject CEA as a method to allocate health care resources even when the benefits of the system are clearly explained (22). Musgrove (23) argues that cost-effectiveness is only one of nine different criteria that could be used to allocate health resources. Among the alternatives are systems that focus on horizontal equity, which would argue for equal treatment based on gender, as well as the rule of rescue, which gives priority to life-saving interventions.

Yet, to not conduct subgroup analysis is equally troubling in its implications. In our example, men are not cost-effective and women are cost-saving. If we ignore gender and calculate a singe cost-effectiveness ratio, the overall ratio will be heavily tilted toward the male ratio because the majority of coronary interventions are performed on men. The overall cost per life year saved is marginally cost-effective. So, using an overall ratio in the name of equity might lead to the rejection of an intervention that, in women, not only saves lives, but also saves money. Increasing both costs and mortality rates seems an odd way to improve equity.

Subgroup analysis is relatively common in prevention programs because they are often targeted at particular populations. For example, AIDS prevention programs regularly focus on high-risk groups, such as homosexuals and drug addicts. Because these programs are only available to the subgroup, the CEA is conducted on the subgroup. But attitudes toward prevention may be different than attitudes toward curative treatments. If some groups have a higher risk of contracting an illness, it makes intuitive sense to make an extra effort to help those groups stay disease-free. But, once an illness has occurred, many reject the notion that care should be distributed based on associations between cost-effectiveness and gender or heart vessel size. Yet, only partially adopting the CEA framework may lead to illogical conclusions.

The long-standing assumption that health care interventions are equally effective in men and women has been pushed aside. It is now recognized that males and females with similar health problems will often report different symptoms and, once diagnosed, have different risk profiles. Researchers that investigate new health care interventions are now generally required to include men and women, as well as minorities. These studies will soon inundate the research community with data that allows calculation of subgroup-specific cost-effectiveness ratios. In theory, this will allow society to focus treatments on those who will receive the greatest benefit. But it is far from clear whether society is ready to have access to health care rationed based on gender or race.

REFERENCES

1. Gaziano J. Global burden of cardiovascular disease. In: Braunwald E, Zipes DP, Libby P (eds.). Heart Disease: A Textbook of Cardiovascular Medicine, 6th Edition. WB Saunders Publishing: 2001, pp. 1–17.
2. Weinstein M, Siegel J, Gold M, et al. for the Panel on Cost effectiveness in health and medicine. Recommendations of the Panel on Cost-Effectiveness in Health and Medicine. JAMA 1996;276:1253–1258.
3. Siegel J, Weinstein M, Russell L, Gold M for the Panel on Cost Effectiveness in Health and Medicine. Recommendations for reporting cost-effectiveness analyses. JAMA 1996;276:1339–1341.
4. Gafni G, Birch S. Equity considerations in utility-based measures of health outcomes in economic appraisals: an adjustment algorithm. J Health Econ 1991;10:329–342.
5. Schulpher M, Gafni A. Recognizing diversity in public preferences: the use of preference sub-groups in cost-effectiveness analysis. Health Econ 2001;10:317–324.
6. Gold M, Siegel J, Russell L, Weinstein M (eds.). Cost Effectiveness in Health and Medicine. Oxford Press, New York: 1996.
7. Suwaidi J, Berger P, Holmes D. Coronary artery stents. JAMA 2000;284:1828–1836.
8. Peterson ED, Lansky AJ, Kramer J, et al. National Cardiovascular Network Clinical Investigators. Effect of gender on the outcomes of contemporary percutaneous coronary intervention. Am J Cardiol 2001;88:359–364.
9. Peterson E, Cowper P, DeLong E, et al. Acute and long-term cost implications of coronary stenting. Interven Cardiol 1999;33:1610–1618.
10. Edwards F, Carey J, Grover F, et al. Impact of gender on coronary bypass operative mortality. Ann Thor Surg 1998;66:125–131.
11. Mehilli J, Kastrati A, Dirschinger J, et al. Differences in prognostic factors and outcomes between women and men undergoing coronary artery stenting. JAMA 2000;284:1799–1804.
12. Afonso F, Hernandez R, Banuelos C, et al. Initial results and long-term clinical and angiographic outcome of coronary stenting in women. Am J Cardiol 2000;86:1380–1383.
13. Robertson T, Kennard E, Mehta S, et al. Influence of gender on in-hospital clinical and angiographic outcomes and on one-year follow-up in the new approaches to coronary intervention (NACI) registry." Am J Cardiol 1997;80:26K–39K.
14. Malenka D, O'Connor G, Quinton H, et al. Differences in outcomes between women and men associated with percutaneous transluminal coronary angioplasty. Circulation 1996;94:II-99–II-103.
15. Arnold A, Mick M, Piedmonte M, Simpfendorfer C. Gender differences for coronary angioplasty. Am J Cardiol 1994;74:18–21.
16. Antoniucci D, Valenti R, Moschi G, et al. Sex-based differences in clinical and angiographic outcomes after primary angioplasty or stenting for acute myocardial infarction. Am J Cardiol 2001;87:289–293.
17. Cohen D, Krumholz H, Sukin C, et al. In-hospital and one-year economic outcomes after coronary stenting or balloon angioplasty: results from a randomized clinical trial." Circulation 1995;92:2480–2487.

18. Weintraub W, Becker E, Mauldin P, et al. "Costs of revascularization over eight years in the randomized and eligible patients in the emory angioplasty versus surgery trial (EAST)". Am J Cardiol 2000;86:747–752.

19. Lecomte P, McKenna M, Kennedy L, et al. International review of the utilisation and cost of percutaneious transluminal coronary angioplasty. Health Econ Preven Care 2001;2:118–127.

20. Cohen D. "Evaluation of the cost-effectiveness of coronary stenting: A societal prespective." Am Heart J 1999;137(5 Suppl):S133–S137.

21. Murray C, Evans D, Acharya A, Baltussen R. "Development of WHO guidelines on generalized cost-effectiveness analysis." Health Econ 2000;9:235–251.

22. Nord E, Richardson J, Street A, et al. "Who cares about cost? Does economic analysis impose or reflect social values?" Health Policy 1995;79–94.

23. Musgrove P. "Public spending on health care: how are different criteria related?" Health Policy 1999;47:207–223.

INDEX

425